Advances in Experimental Medicine and Biology

Volume 928

More information about this series at http://www.springer.com/series/5584

Subash Chandra Gupta · Sahdeo Prasad
Bharat B. Aggarwal
Editors

Anti-inflammatory Nutraceuticals and Chronic Diseases

Springer

Editors
Subash Chandra Gupta
Banaras Hindu University
Varanasi, Uttar Pradesh
India

Bharat B. Aggarwal
Inflammation Research Institute
San Diego, CA
USA

Sahdeo Prasad
University of Texas
MD Anderson Cancer Center
Houston, TX
USA

ISSN 0065-2598 ISSN 2214-8019 (electronic)
Advances in Experimental Medicine and Biology
ISBN 978-3-319-41332-7 ISBN 978-3-319-41334-1 (eBook)
DOI 10.1007/978-3-319-41334-1

Library of Congress Control Number: 2016947788

Printed on acid-free paper

This Springer imprint is published by Springer Nature
The registered company is Springer International Publishing AG Switzerland

Contents

About the Editors

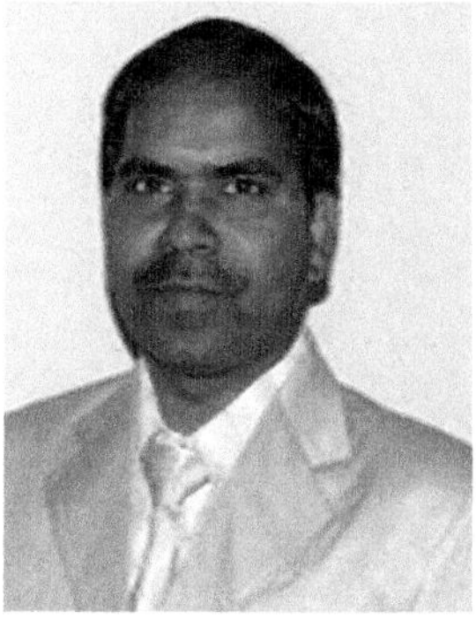

Dr. Subash Chandra Gupta is currently Assistant Professor at Department of Biochemistry, Institute of Science, Banaras Hindu University, India.

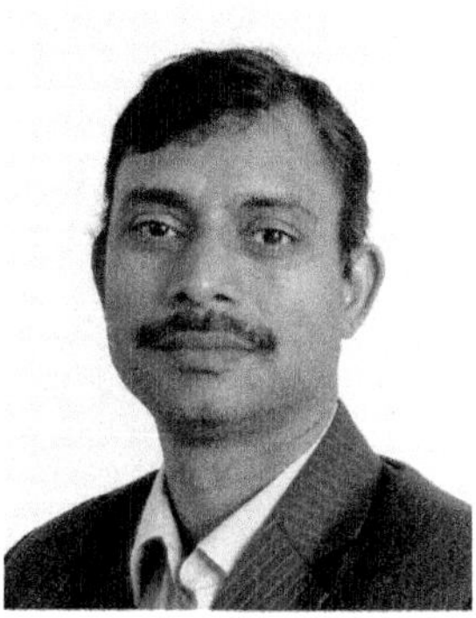

Dr. Sahdeo Prasad is currently at the Department of Experimental Therapeutics, The University of Texas MD Anderson Cancer Center, USA.

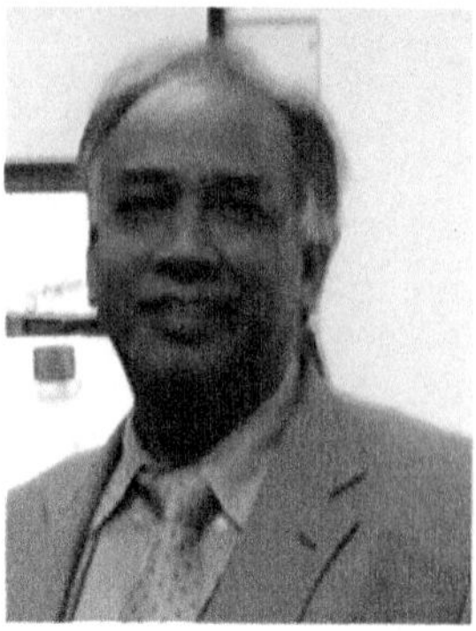

Dr. Bharat Aggarwal is currently Founding Director of Inflammation Research Institute, San Diego, CA, USA. He was a Ransom Horne, Jr., Distinguished Professor of Experimental Therapeutics, Cancer Medicine and Immunology, The University of Texas MD Anderson Cancer Center, USA.

Chapter 1
Curcumin and Its Role in Chronic Diseases

A. Kunwar and K.I. Priyadarsini

Abstract Curcumin, a yellow pigment from the spice turmeric, is used in Indian and Chinese medicine since ancient times for wide range of diseases. Extensive scientific research on this molecule performed over the last 3 to 4 decades has proved its potential as an important pharmacological agent. The antioxidant, anti-inflammatory, antimicrobial and chemopreventive activities of curcumin have been extended to explore this molecule against many chronic diseases with promising results. Further, its multitargeting ability and nontoxic nature to humans even up to 12 g/day have attracted scientists to explore this as an anticancer agent in the clinic, which is in different phases of trials. With much more scope to be investigated and understood, curcumin becomes one of the very few inexpensive botanical molecules with potent therapeutic abilities.

Keywords Curcumin · Antioxidant · Anti-inflammatory · Anticancer · Turmeric · Polyphenol

1.1 Introduction

Curcumin, a natural polyphenol, is one of the most investigated biomolecules from Mother Nature. Its natural source, *Curcuma longa* or turmeric is used in Indian Ayurvedic and Siddha medicines and also in Chinese medicines since thousands of years [3, 6, 22, 107]. Turmeric is a perennial plant of the ginger family, cultivated in tropical and subtropical regions of South Asia, and India is one of the largest producers of turmeric [35]. In Ayurveda, turmeric is used to treat ailments like arthritis, sprains, open wounds, acnes, stomach upset, flatulence, dysentery, ulcers,

A. Kunwar · K.I. Priyadarsini (✉)
Radiation and Photochemistry Division, Bhabha Atomic Research Centre,
Trombay, Mumbai 400085, India
e-mail: kindira@barc.gov.in

A. Kunwar
e-mail: kamit@barc.gov.in

S.C. Gupta et al. (eds.), *Anti-inflammatory Nutraceuticals and Chronic Diseases*,
Advances in Experimental Medicine and Biology 928,
DOI 10.1007/978-3-319-41334-1_1

jaundice, skin and eye infections. As a dietary agent, turmeric is regularly used as a spice and also as a coloring agent in Indian cuisine. Both turmeric and its active principle, curcumin, are permitted like other natural pigments and the food additive, E number for curcumin is E100. Depending on the origin and soil conditions, the percentage of curcuminoids in turmeric varies from 2 to 9 % of its dry weight. The word "curcuminoid" refers to a mixture of four polyphenols, such as curcumin, demethoxycurcumin and bis-demethoxy curcumin and cyclic curcumin. Out of these, curcumin is nearly 70 % of the total curcuminoids. In addition to these curcuminoids, turmeric also contains essential oils primarily composed of mono and sesquiterpenes, like turmerones, turmerol, etc. The strong yellow color of turmeric is mainly due to curcuminoids.

Historically, the first scientific report on isolation and chemical characteristics of curcumin was made in 1815 [115], and its molecular formula and chemical structure was published in 1910 [74]. Its first laboratory synthesis was demonstrated in 1913 [68], subsequently in 1964 a method for producing curcumin in high yields was published [80], and much later, its biosynthesis was understood [35]. Curcumin is extracted commercially from turmeric by solvent extraction with ethanol followed by column chromatography. Using high-performance liquid chromatography coupled with absorption, fluorescence and mass detectors, curcumin can be detected in nanomolar quantities in food samples and biological tissues [35, 90].

Apart from the ancient medicinal documents, early research report on therapeutic use of curcumin appears to date back to 1748; however, the first scientific document for treating human disease was reported in 1937 [79], wherein at least 67 patients were treated for chronic cholecystitis, using curcunat, which is equivalent of curcumin. In this study, oral administration for 3 weeks showed symptomatic improvement in all cases and radiologic improvement by cholecystogram in 18 patients. Interestingly, no ill effects were observed even when the treatment continued for several months. The efficacy of curcumin was attributed to its ability to cause the emptying of the gallbladder. Later in 1949, the antibacterial activity of curcumin [96] was established, since then and till 1970s there were very few reports on its biological activities [98, 106]. Initial research investigations were focused mostly on antioxidant and antibacterial activity and the first anticancer report in human participants was undertaken by Kuttan et al. [67]. However, after the report by Singh and Aggarwal [108], confirming the anti-inflammatory activity of curcumin by suppressing NF-κB activity, the pace of curcumin research has progressed systematically. With several encouraging results in rodent models, curcumin attracted researchers all over the world, to be developed as a potent anticancer drug. As per Pubmed website, (as of October 2015) there are 8247 articles reported with the word "curcumin" in the title, including 808 reviews and 141 clinical trials, out of these more than half have appeared in the last 5 years. It is well accepted by the scientific community that no other botanical molecule is as efficient and as scientifically celebrated as curcumin.

1.2 Physical, Chemical and Metabolic Reactions Influencing Curcumin Pharmacology

1.2.1 Physicochemical Properties

Curcumin is a diarylheptanoid, having three important functional moieties. It has two *o*-methoxyphenolic groups linked through a heptanoid linker consisting of an enone moiety and 1,3-diketone group in conjugation (Fig. 1.1). All these groups are involved in the biological activity of curcumin [35, 42, 88, 89]. Important physicochemical properties of curcumin are listed in Table 1.1. Like other β-diketones, curcumin exhibits keto-enol tautomerism, and in solution phase it mostly exists in the enol form [88]. Curcumin has three acidic protons two from the phenolic-OH groups (in the range 8.5–10.7) and one from the enolic OH (<8.5). Curcumin is yellow at neutral and acidic pH with absorption maximum ~420–430 nm and in alkaline solutions, it becomes red in color and the absorption maximum is shifted to 465 nm. It is practically insoluble in neutral and acidic

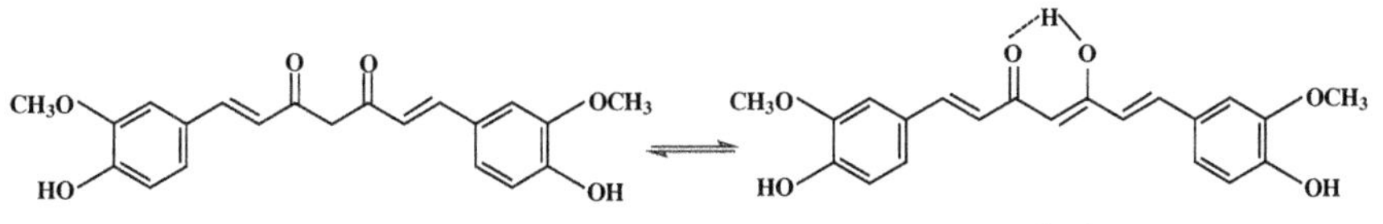

Fig. 1.1 Chemical structure of curcumin in keto and enol tautomeric forms

Table 1.1 Physico-chemical properties of curcumin

IUPAC name	(1E,6E)-1,7-bis (4-hydroxy-3-methoxy phenyl)-1,6-heptadiene 3,5-dione
Molecular formula	$C_{21}H_{20}O_6$
Molecular weight	368.39
Melting point	170–175 °C
Experimental dipole moment in dioxane	3.32 D
Absorption maximum and extinction coefficient fluorescence maximum in methanol	425 nm, 55,000 $dm^3\ mol^{-1}\ cm^{-1}$ 530 nm
Solubility	Insoluble in water Soluble in ethanol, methanol, chloroform, hexane, DMSO
Prototropic equilibrium constant (pKa) (three pKas)	pKa (1), Enolic proton: 7.7–8.5; pKa (2), Phenolic proton: 8.5–10.4; pKa (3), Phenolic proton: 9.5–10.7
log *P* value	~3.0
Color and odor	Yellow at neutral pH, red in alkaline pH; odorless

water, but is readily soluble in moderately polar solvents like methanol, acetonitrile, chloroform, dimethylsulfoxide (DMSO), etc. In aqueous solutions its solubility can be increased by the addition of surfactants, polymers, lipids and proteins. Because of the presence of serum albumin, clear curcumin solutions in micromolar concentration can be prepared in cell culture medium.

1.2.2 Chemical Structural Features Influencing the Biological Activity of Curcumin

Curcumin has three important functional groups, two *o*-methoxy phenolic groups, one enone moiety and an α,β-unsaturated diketone group. Each functional group has some specific role in crucial biological activity in curcumin. The *o*-methoxy phenolic-OH group of curcumin is primarily involved in direct scavenging of reactive oxygen species (ROS), where it donates an electron or hydrogen atom to the oxidizing radicals and the resultant curcumin phenoxyl radical acquires stability through the conjugation and resonating structures [87]. This phenoxyl radical is regenerated back to curcumin by water-soluble antioxidants like ascorbic acid making it an excellent chain-breaking antioxidant that has been reported to be at least ten times better than vitamin E. Curcumin binds to many biomolecules like proteins, lipids and DNA [42, 88]. The proteins that interact with curcumin include transcription factors, inflammatory molecules, kinases, tubulins, amyloid-β aggregates, adhesion molecules, growth factors, receptor proteins, protofilaments, prion proteins, etc. The experimentally reported dipole moment [84] and log P values (partition coefficient in octanol and water system) of curcumin (Table 1.1) indicate that the molecule has partial charge transfer character and is moderately polar to be soluble in lipid-like systems. Because of these properties and flexibility in its structure, curcumin binds to most of the biomolecules. The hydrophobic interactions and hydrogen-bonding interactions are mainly responsible for the efficient binding. It is still premature to clarify the role of any single moiety for these interactions but it appears that the orientation of the enolic group plays a crucial role.

The α,β-unsaturated β-diketo moiety of curcumin participates in nucleophilic addition reactions with molecules having functional groups like –SH, –SeH. This 1,4-addition reaction known as Michael addition reaction is of great significance in curcumin biology, like it reacts with glutathione (GSH) and depletes the GSH in cells [13]. Similarly through the reaction with the –SeH group, it inhibits thioredoxin reductase, an enzyme involved in cellular redox homeostasis [36].

Curcumin undergoes a fast chemical degradation in solution, where products like ferulic aldehyde, ferulic acid, vanillin, etc. are formed [102, 116]. The degradation occurs through the β-diketo moiety of curcumin and is increased in presence of light and decreased when solubilised in aqueous solutions along with lipids, proteins, surfactants, cyclodextrins, starch etc.

Metabolism of curcumin in mice produced varieties of products. Important products identified are curcumin glucuronide and curcumin sulfate along with reduction products like tetrahydrocurcumin, hexahydrocurcumin and octahydrocurcumin [11, 37, 56]. The orally administered curcumin undergoes conjugation whereas the systemically and/or intraperionial (i.p.) administered curcumin undergoes reduction. These processes occur by phase I and phase II enzymes like for example, phenol sulfur transferase enzyme is involved in sulfonation and alcohol dehydrogenase in reduction. Other minor products identified during curcumin metabolism are ferulic acid, dihydroferulic acid, etc. It is still not confirmed how enzymatic metabolism of curcumin competes with its chemical degradation, and there is a need to investigate the role of these metabolic and degradation products in the overall bioactivity of curcumin.

1.2.3 Curcumin–Metal Interactions: Role in Curcumin Biology

Curcumin binds to many metals and metalloproteins, and the binding is through covalent interactions, as the diketo group is an excellent metal chelator [89, 90, 117]. Binding of curcumin to metals ions has several biological consequences. Its binding to Al^{3+} ions is proposed to be one of the key factors involved in its role in preventing the pathogenesis of Alzheimer's disease (AD) [58]. Zn^{2+}-curcumin complex showed anticancer activity and Au^{3+} complexes exhibit anti-arthritic activity [99]. Curcumin–metal chelation can be used to reduce toxicity of heavy metals like Hg^{2+}, Cd^{2+}, Pb^{2+} [1, 81]. Several mixed ligand complexes of curcumin with metals like Cu^{2+}, Ni^{2+}, Mn^{3+}, Pd^{2+} are also finding applications as antioxidants, superoxide dismutase mimics and anticancer agents [15, 114]. Recently curcumin derived radiopharmaceuticals are being prepared and explored as new diagnostic and therapeutic agents. For example, $^{99m}Tc^{4+}$ and $^{68}Ga^{3+}$ complexes of curcumin reported to bind to amyloid-β (Aβ) fibrils and plaques, are being explored as novel radiodiagnostic agents for AD [12, 95].

1.2.4 Curcumin Bioavailability

The major issue concerning the development of curcumin based drugs is its extremely low bioavailability [9, 86]. Due to relatively low intestinal absorption and rapid metabolism in the liver, the oral bioavailability of curcumin is very low, while most of it is excreted through the feces within 3–6 h after administration. Even after oral administration in grams, no significant curcumin was detected in the plasma, and the highest curcumin levels were found in the intestines and detectable amounts were observed in the serum, but they fall below detection limit in other tissues. However, i.p. and intravenous (i.v.) administration has shown better

Table 1.2 Examples of important formulations used to enhance in vivo bioavailability of curcumin

Formulation	Piperine (20 mg/kg) + curcumin 2 g/kg)	Curcumin–phospholipid complex (100 mg/kg)	Cyclodextrin–curcumin	Pegylated-curcumin (2.5 mg/kg)	Curcumin–phosphatidylcholine (Mervia)
Increase in bioavailability	1.5-fold in serum	2.2-fold in plasma	1.8-fold in skin	2-fold in serum	5-fold increase in plasma

bioavailability than oral administration. The maximum tissue concentrations recorded after an i.p. injection of 100 mg/kg of curcumin was 73 ± 20, 200 ± 23, 9.1 ± 1.1, 16 ± 3, 8.4 ± 6.0, 78 ± 3 and 2.9 ± 0.4 nmol/g in liver, intestine mucosa, heart, lungs, muscle, kidneys, and brain respectively [85]. At 10 mg/kg i.v., maximum serum levels were 0.36 μg/ml, while in another study 2 mg/kg through tail vain showed plasma concentration of 6.6 μg/ml [9, 86]. Increasing the dose of curcumin did not result in higher bioabsorption. Being a lipophilic molecule, curcumin is expected to cross blood–brain barrier and reach brain tissue. However, dietary supplementation did not show significant accumulation in the brain tissue, but long-term supplementation of mice for nearly 4 months at a dose of 0.5–2 g/kg showed a maximum detectable concentration of 1.5 nmol/g in the brain tissue [9, 86].

The poor bioavailability of curcumin has thus emerged as one of the major limitations for its therapeutic applications. To increase the bioavailability of curcumin, researchers have developed several novel formulations. Important among these are liposomes, nanoemulsions, pegylation, polymers, hydrogels, cyclodextrins, piperine-combined, gold and mesoporous silica nanoconjugates and curcumin–iron oxide magnetic nanoparticles [9, 65, 71, 86, 89, 90, 105, 120]. Employing them a significant improvement, not only in the bioavailability of curcumin but also in its in vivo bioactivity was reported. Most of these formulations could be dispersed in aqueous buffer medium. There are several reports describing the preparation and characterization of these nano formulations. Important formulations that showed significant improvement in curcumin bioavailability are given in Table 1.2.

1.3 Modulation of Cell Signaling Pathways by Curcumin

All the biological activities/functions of a living cell are regulated by a dense network of signal transduction pathways. The components of signal transduction pathways are growth factors and their receptors, cytokines and their receptors, protein kinases, transcription factors and gene expression. Curcumin has been shown to affect many cellular or molecular pathways in executing its crucial biological activities. Figure 1.2 gives important signaling molecules involved in biological activities of curcumin. Some important results are discussed below.

Fig. 1.2 Important biological activities of curcumin and their associated major signaling molecules. The text in *green* and *red fonts* indicate upregulation and downregulation, respectively

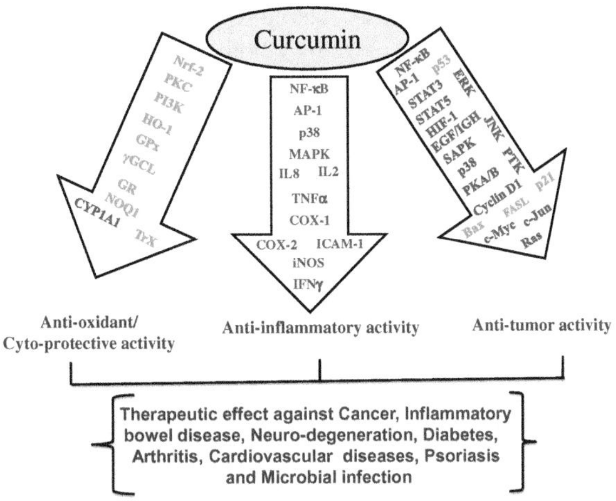

1.3.1 Growth Factors/Cytokines and Their Receptors

Growth factors/cytokines are proteins which upon binding to their specific receptors present on the plasma membrane of the cells stimulate multiple signal transduction pathways leading to the expression of genes controlling various cellular processes such as cell cycle, division, apoptosis, movement, inflammatory response to external stimuli, etc. One of the hallmarks of a cancer cell is the constitutive or increased expression of growth factors and their receptors inducing signals for the uncontrolled proliferation or the growth [46]. Recent studies provide evidence that curcumin targets such growth factors and their receptors to inhibit the growth and proliferation of cancer cells [4, 6, 49, 110]. For example, curcumin was reported to inhibit the effects of epidermal growth factor (EGF) and insulin growth factor (IGF) by downregulating the expression and tyrosine kinase activity of EGF and IGF receptors in colon cancer cells [93] and MCF-7 breast cancer cells [118]. Similarly curcumin has also been shown to downregulate the expression and activity of HER-2/erbB2/neu/p185, another member of the EGF receptor super family closely associated with breast, lung, kidney, and prostate cancers [52].

Further, the overexpression of other growth factors such as platelet-derived growth factor (PDGF), vascular endothelial growth factor (VEGF) and their receptors PDGFR and VEGFR, respectively have also been seen in many types of solid tumors [28, 39]. Park et al. [82] showed that curcumin inhibits PDGFR-induced proliferation of human hepatic myofibroblasts. In another study curcumin was shown to block the angiogenesis or the formation of new blood vessels in various cancer types by inhibiting both VEGF and VEGFR [28]. Some reports indicate that TNF acts as a growth factor for tumor cells. Similarly other cytokines such as IL6 and IL2 regulate the proliferation of T cells through the autocrine stimulation and play important roles in mounting the inflammatory response. Curcumin has been shown to negatively regulate the expression of these cytokines both at mRNA and protein levels by inhibiting the downstream signaling pathways [7, 19, 92]. These effects of curcumin have also been accounted for its ability to show the antitumor and the anti-inflammatory activities in various cellular and in vivo model systems.

1.3.2 Protein Kinases

Protein kinases are a class of enzymes, which activate the downstream signaling molecules through phosphorylation using ATP as a source of inorganic phosphate (Pi). They are the key transducers such as mitogen activated protein kinases (MAPKs)/extracellular signal regulated kinases (ERKs), protein kinase A (PKA), protein kinase B (PKB)/AKT, and protein kinase C (PKC), phosphatidyl inositol 3 phosphate kinase (PI3K), and mammalian target of rapamycin (mTOR) controlling cell growth, proliferation, cytoprotection, cytokines production and death [3, 4, 49, 110]. Interestingly, curcumin has been shown to modulate the expression and activity of MAPKs including ERKs, C-Jun, N terminal kinases (JNKs), p38 kinases, and the stress activated protein kinases (SAPK) in suppressing inflammation and cancer [49]. Although inhibitory effect of curcumin on MAPKs has been documented in several independent studies, there are also some reports, which indicate that curcumin activates JNKs leading to apoptosis or cell death in tumor cells [29]. Further, PI3K is the upstream regulator of PKB/AKT and the mTOR pathways playing a central role in the genesis of cancer. Recent studies have shown that curcumin inhibits proliferation/growth and induces apoptosis in tumor cells by inhibiting mTOR pathway and it is mediated through the suppression of PI3K and PKB/AKT. Additionally, the inhibitory effect of curcumin on mTOR signaling has also been attributed to its ability to activate adenosine monophosphate kinase (AMPK1), which senses cellular ATP levels and inhibits mTOR indirectly [122]. In a separate study, curcumin was shown to block the signals transmitted from EGFR by inhibiting the PI3K/AKT pathway in colon carcinoma cells [54]. On the contrary, curcumin activates the same PI3K and PKB/AKT signaling to induce the expression of antioxidant genes in pre-cancer cells and thus prevents both tumor initiation and promotion, a critical stage in carcinogenesis [61, 64]. Further, curcumin also modulates PKC differentially, depending on the cell type and nature of exogenous/endogenous stimuli. For example it has been shown to inhibit the tumor promoting action of 12-*o*-tetradecanoylphorbol-13-acetate (TPA) by inactivating PKC through oxidizing the vicinal thiols present within catalytic domain [72]. On the other hand, the chemopreventive activity of curcumin has been linked with its ability to activate PKC and the downstream p38 MAPK in human monocytes leading to induction of antioxidant genes [94].

1.3.3 Transcription Factors

Transcription factors are the cellular proteins, which upon activation through signaling cascades bind to the promoter/enhancer regions of their target genes and regulate their transcription/expression. Curcumin by modulating various signal transduction pathways affects the activation of a number of transcription factors such as nuclear factor-κB (NF-κB), activator protein-1 (AP-1), early growth response-1 (Egr-1), signal transducer and activator of transcription (STAT), peroxisome proliferator activated receptor-gamma (PPAR-γ), nuclear factor erythroid 2-related factor 2 (Nrf2), beta (β)-catenin and tumor suppressor p53 [19, 20, 24, 26, 57, 108, 110].

The NF-κB is reported to be constitutively activated in a variety of cancers and inflammatory disorders. Researchers working on the various aspects of biological activity have unanimously shown that curcumin is a strong suppressor of NF-κB activation [104, 108]. The inactivation of NF-κB by curcumin is mediated through the inhibition of IκBα kinase (IKK) directly and/or by modulating upstream signaling cascade [108]. AP-1 is another transcription factor associated with growth regulation, cell transformation, inflammation, and innate immune response. Curcumin suppresses the activation of AP-1 either by inhibiting the upstream kinases such as JNK, p38 and ERK or by directly interacting with AP-1 DNA binding motifs present in the promoter regions of the target genes [20]. The transcription factor Egr-1 is one of the immediate early induced gene products in response to growth factor or carcinogen mediated signaling. Curcumin suppresses the induction/de novo synthesis of Egr-1 protein in different cell types such as endothelial cells, fibroblast, and colon cancer cells [26]. The family of STAT proteins (STAT1-STAT7) performs the dual function of signal transducer as well as the transcription factor. Of the seven STAT proteins, the elevated activity of STAT3 and STAT5 has been mainly implicated in the angiogenic response and in growth of various cancer types. Curcumin has been found to inhibit the phosphorylation of STAT3 and STAT5 by upstream kinases (like janus kinase (JAK) and/or the growth factor/G-protein-coupled receptor kinases) and their subsequent translocation to nucleus there by suppressing the tumor cell proliferation and the pro-inflammatory immune responses [19, 25]. The protein PPAR-γ also plays the dual role of nuclear receptors of hormones and transcription factor. Curcumin has been shown to induce the expression of PPAR-γ in various cell types such as colon cancer cells [24] and hepatocytes leading to suppression of tumor cell proliferation, and the prevention of liver fibrosis and sepsis [119]. The transcription factor Nrf2 induces the expression of genes related to cytoprotection, antioxidant enzymes and phase II detoxification enzymes. Curcumin induces the antioxidant and cytoprotective responses in various cell types such as epithelial, monocytes, hepatocytes by activating Nrf2. The mechanism of activation is either through directly interacting with Keap-1 (inhibitor of Nrf2) or by positively regulating upstream kinases such as PI3K, PKC and MAPK [53, 94]. The β-catenin and p53 are some of other important transcription factors, which control the expression of genes involved in cell cycle progression and check points. Curcumin has been reported to induce as well as inhibit the transcriptional activity of β-catenin by differentially modulating the activity of glycogen synthase kinase-3 (GSK3) [57, 123]. The inhibition of β-catenin activation by curcumin has been liked with the suppression of tumor cell proliferation and the induction of apoptosis. Whereas curcumin mediated activation of β-catenin has been attributed toits anti-AD activity. The p53 protein is a tumor suppressor protein. Depending on cell type, curcumin regulates the level of p53 in different ways. For example, in normal thymocytes and myeloid leukemic cells, curcumin downregulates the expression of p53 and inhibits p53-induced apoptosis [45, 112]. In contrast to such studies, curcumin has been shown to upregulate p53 in colon, neuroblastoma, lymphoma, prostate, and human breast cancer cells to induce apoptosis [27, 110].

1.3.4 Gene Expression

Through modulating various signal transduction pathways, curcumin affects the expression of a number of genes [3, 4, 49, 110]. For example, the antioxidant and chemopreventive activities of curcumin have been attributed to the upregulated expression of hemeoxygenase-1 (HO-1), glutathione peroxidase (GPx), gamma-glutamyl-cysteine ligase (γGCL), and phase II detoxification enzymes like glutathione S transferase (GST), glutathione reductase (GR), NAD(P)H: quinonecidoreductase 1 (NOQ1), quinone reductase and epoxide hydrolase [53, 61, 62, 94, 103]. The anti-inflammatory activity of curcumin is associated with its ability to downregulate the expressions of genes like cyclooxygenase-1 (COX-1), cyclooxygenase-2 (COX-2), inducible nitrogen oxide synthase (iNOS), and cytokines such as interleukin-2 (IL-2), interferon-γ (IFNγ), tumor necrosis factor-α (TNFα), intracellular adhesion molecule-1 (ICAM-1), vascular adhesion molecule-1 (VCAM-1) and E-selectin [3, 51]. The anticancer effect of curcumin is mediated through downregulating the expressions of oncogenes (c-Met, c-Myc, c-Jun, Ras and Mdm2) and anti-apoptotic genes (Bcl_2, $BclX_L$, IAP, hTERT, Cyclin D1, survivin) and upregulating the expressions of tumor suppressor genes (p53, Rb, PTEN) and apoptotic genes (Bax, FASL and Bim) [49]. Additionally, curcumin has also been shown to affect the expression of genes like matrix metalloprotease-2,9 (MMP-2,9), macrophage inhibitor protein-1 (MIP-1), vascular endothelial growth factor (VEGF), endothelial growth factor (EGF), hypoxia-inducible factor-1 (HIF-1), p21, poly-ADP ribose polymerase (PRAP), growth arrest and DNA damage-inducible (GADD), cytochrome P450 (CYP1A1), and *p*-glycoprotein (pgp) associated with varied biological responses such as immunomodulation, angiogenesis, anti-tumor and drug metabolism [10, 14, 49, 78].

1.4 Biological Activities of Curcumin in Animal Models

Curcumin is one of the most extensively evaluated natural products in rodent models for therapeutic efficacy against various pathological conditions/diseases. Among the various activities, the effect of curcumin on carcinogenesis has been majorly studied in rodents [3, 63, 83, 110]. The transformation of a normal cell to cancerous cell is a complex process and occurs in three stages namely initiation, promotion and progression. Interestingly, oral administration of curcumin has been shown to affect all the three stages of carcinogenesis in chemical and/or genetic mice models of skin, stomach, duodenum, colon, liver, lung, and breast cancers [63, 83, 110]. Further, several reports are also available on the ability of topically applied curcumin to inhibit the tumor imitation and tumor promotion of skin carcinogenesis [30]. Similar effects of curcumin have been reported in Syrian golden hamsters, where it prevented chemical induced oral carcinogenesis [70]. In another interesting set of studies, oral curcumin was shown to inhibit the tumor progression in a xenograft model of human cancers of prostate, colon, pancreas, bladder and ovary [3, 110]. There are also reports indicating that curcumin inhibits metastasis of human breast cancer to the lungs in nude mice [5]. Taken together, curcumin has shown significant activity of inhibiting carcinogenesis in rodent models.

Curcumin has also been studied in rodent models for its effect on metabolic enzyme systems and antioxidant activity. For example in F344 mice, curcumin administered orally at a dosage of 270 mg/kg decreased the levels of metabolizing enzymes such as cytochrome p450 (CYP) isoforms CYP2B1 and CYP2E1 and prevented the *n*-nitrosomethylbenzamine (NMBA) induced oesophageal carcinogenesis [77]. Since the enzymes CYP2B1 and CYP2E1 are known to metabolize NMBA into an active carcinogen, the ability of curcumin to suppress their levels is in line with the hypothesis that curcumin inhibits carcinogenesis at initiation stage. Additionally, dietary curcumin is shown to play a role in preventing the early stage of carcinogenesis by inducing phase II enzymes such as GST and epoxy hydrolase in both mice and rat. Further, curcumin administration (75–300 mg/kg) in rodents is also associated with the increased expression of antioxidant enzymes like heme oxygenase (HO-1), glutathione peroxidase (GPx) and γ-glutamate cysteine ligase (γGCL) in liver, brain, small intestine and kidney tissues [8]. These effects of curcumin are associated with its ability to prevent nephrotoxicity in rats, reduce oxidative damage in the heart of diabetes-afflicted mice and brain of transgenic AD rats. It was also found to inhibit chemically induced hepatic injury and neurodegeneration in rats [8]. There are also studies indicating that curcumin lowered ROS production in vivo. For example, in mice the orally administered curcumin (100 mg/kg) prevented lipopolysaccharide induced inflammatory responses in liver by suppressing the expression of iNOS responsible for nitric oxide (NO) production [21]. Similarly, oral curcumin was also seen to prevent oxidative damage during indomethacin-induced gastric lesion by blocking inactivation of gastric peroxidase as well as directly scavenging peroxide (H_2O_2) and hydroxyl ($^{\cdot}OH$) radicals [23].

Oral curcumin is also effective against carrageenan-induced edema and enhanced wound-healing in diabetic rats and mice, documenting its anti-inflammatory activity. Some of the other potential biological effects of curcumin studied in rodent models through oral administration (50–300 mg/kg) include cardioprotective, neuroprotective, anti/pro-mutagenic, antifertility, antidiabetic, antifibrotic, anti-venom, anti-HIV, and anticoagulant activities [22].

1.5 Role of Curcumin in Chronic Diseases

It has been confirmed by several researchers that oxidative stress and oxidative damage are directly associated with chronic inflammation, which in turn leads to several chronic diseases, like cancer, metabolic, neurological, pulmonary, intestinal and cardiovascular diseases. Since curcumin has been identified as an important remedy against oxidative stress and inflammation, extensive research work has been undertaken to use curcumin against many chronic diseases. Important examples are mentioned briefly here [3, 51, 101].

Inflammatory bowel disease (IBD), symptomatic with severe diarrhea, pain, fatigue and weight loss, involves chronic inflammation of all or part of digestive tract. Both turmeric extract and polymer loaded curcumin formulations have been examined in animals and humans for treatment against IBD and many encouraging results were obtained without any side effects [18, 47, 48, 111]. In mice, oral administration of curcumin (100 mg/kg per day) for ten consecutive days prior to the induction of colitis by acetic acid and further continuation for 2 days showed decreased colon injury and ameliorated macroscopic and microscopic colitis sores. IBD patients treated with curcumin (550 mg twice daily for 1 month) showed decreased symptoms and inflammation indices, without any significant side effects.

Rheumatoid arthritis (RA), a long-lasting autoimmune disorder that primarily affects joints on both sides of the body, is a systemic chronic inflammatory disorder. To reduce arthritic reaction, it is essential to start early treatment and combination therapy. As a nonsteroid anti-inflammatory drug and antioxidant, curcumin has been examined as a potential therapy for RA, accordingly RA patients treated with curcumin showed significant symptomatic improvement [76, 90]. Similarly curcumin (500 mg) alone and in combination with diclofenac sodium (50 mg) administered in patients with RA showed best improvement in the overall disease scores. In a short term, a double-blind crossover study involving 18 young patients suffering from RA, oral curcumin at a daily dose of 12 g for 2 weeks exerted an anti-RA activity comparable to that of a standard drug phenylbutazone.

Diabetes mellitus (DM), commonly referred to as diabetes, is a metabolic disease in which there are high blood sugar levels over a prolonged period. Serious long-term complications include cardiovascular disease, stroke, chronic kidney failure, foot ulcers, and damage to the eyes. Effect of curcumin against diabetes was successfully demonstrated first in one patient in 1972 [109] and since then more than 200 papers have been published in this related subject [2, 73, 124]. Curcumin has been shown to reduce blood glucose and glycosylated hemoglobin levels and prevented weight loss in rodent models. Oral administration of curcumin (80 mg/kg) showed anti-hyperglycemic effect and improved insulin sensitivity. It was also effective in improving glucose intolerance. One or two contradicting effects were also reported, where intragastric administration of curcumin did not show any effect in blood glucose. Curcumin has been shown to reduce several other complications associated with diabetes like fatty liver, diabetic neuropathy, diabetic nephropathy, vascular diseases, musculoskeletal diseases and also islet viability.

Neurodegenerative diseases including Parkinson's and AD occur due to the progressive loss of structure or function of neurons, including death of neurons. Curcumin was considered as a potent drug mainly due to the fact that the epidemiological studies indicating reduced risk of AD amongst Indians consuming turmeric in their diet. In line with this, several experimental studies in mice models confirmed anti-AD effects of curcumin [44]. It significantly lowered the levels of oxidized proteins, IL-1β, insoluble and soluble plaque burden in AD transgenic Tg2576 mice brain. There are several ongoing clinical trials on the effect of curcumin for the prevention of AD. In one such study, daily intake of curcumin 1–4 g/day over 6 months found a trend towards increased serum Aβ levels which is considered as a possible clearance of Aβ plaques from the brain, but improvement in cognitive performance was not observed during the 6 months trial [16]. A few other studies indicate that curcumin also exhibits antidepressant and neuroprotective properties [32, 69, 75].

Psoriasis, a chronic skin disease, occurs when the immune system overreacts, causing inflammation and flaking of skin and is characterized by thick red and scaly lesions on any part of the body. Since ancient times turmeric has been used as a skin protectant in the Indian subcontinent. Further experimental evidences strongly indicate that curcumin is a potential natural product to suppress psoriasis by inhibiting the keratinocyte proliferation [59]. In a clinical trial, orally administered curcumin demonstrated therapeutic effects with no adverse reaction in patients with psoriasis and reduced psoriasis area and severity index [66]. Curcumin skin formulations are being marketed for skin diseases including psoriasis.

In addition to these important diseases, curcumin has been examined for treatment of other chronic diseases like cardiovascular diseases, allergy, asthma, bronchitis, kidney diseases, obesity, scleroderma, vitiligo, peptic ulcer, pylori infection and ophthalmic disorders and encouraging results are reported [3, 51]. The anticancer effects are discussed in detail in the next section.

1.6 Biological Activities of Curcumin in Humans

The remarkable success of curcumin as a therapeutic agent against various chronic diseases including cancer in preclinical studies has prompted clinicians to undertake many clinical trials in human subjects [4, 43, 97, 121]. As of October 2015, as many as 137 clinical trials with curcumin/turmeric extract are listed on a search engine (www.clinicaltrials.gov) of which 67 have been completed, 3 terminated, 9 withdrawn and rest are at recruitment (enrolment of human subjects) stage. Table 1. 3 gives the list of clinical trials from different countries and also the purpose. The maximum number of clinical trials has been reported from USA and the most common human disease evaluated is the cancer. The trials were primarily undertaken for safety and efficacy under different disease conditions. Important completed studies are discussed below.

The phase I clinical trials for safety evaluation of curcumin have indicated that its intake as high as 12 g/day orally for 3 months is safe. In order to determine the curcumin's maximum tolerated dose and safety, a dose-escalation trial has been recently completed. In this study, curcumin was administered to 24 healthy volunteers at a single oral dose ranging from 0.5 to 12 g and safety was assessed for 72 h after administration. Remarkably, only 7 out of 24 subjects showed minimal behavioral toxicities like diarrhea, headache, rash, and yellow stool. The pharmacokinetics studies in human (sample size ~1–30) involving healthy volunteers and the cancer/IBD/AD patients have revealed that the oral intake of curcumin (2–12 g/day) results in poor bioabsorption. However, in colorectal cancer (CRC) patients administered with 3.6 g of curcumin/day for 7 days, although indicated lower bioavailability in the tumor compared to normal tissue, the reduction in the levels of a DNA adduct, used as a biomarker, established that a daily dose of 3.6 g curcumin is pharmacologically efficacious against CRC [38]. Surprisingly, administration of oral curcumin at a similar daily dosage in patients suffering from hepatic metastases of CRC did not attain the pharmacologically effective concentration in the liver.

Due to multitargeting effects, curcumin has showed promising chemopreventive and therapeutic effects against a range of human malignancies such as colorectal cancer, aberrant crypt foci, familial adenomatous polyposis (FAP), pancreatic cancer, multiple myeloma, hepatocellular carcinoma, gastric cancer, and colon cancer in clinical trials. In the first study, topical curcumin applied, either as an ethanol extract or as an ointment, showed remarkable relief in 62 patients reported with external cancer lesions. Two phase I trials in CRC patients were conducted, one in 2001 with 15 patients with 36–180 mg daily for 4 months and another trial with 15 patients with escalated doses of 0.45–3.6 g daily for 4 months [100]. The drug was well tolerated by all except three patients with minor side effects along with improvement in the status of biological parameters indicating efficacy against CRC. In another study, CRC patients when treated with 0.36 g (in capsule form) curcumin daily for 10–30 days showed improvement in general health [50].

Curcumin was tested against pancreatic cancer with moderate results. In a single, blind, randomized, placebo-controlled study in 20 patients with 0.5 g curcumin with 5 mg piperine for 6 weeks showed reduction in oxidative stress with no significant effect in pain relief [33]. In another phase II clinical trial on 25 patients with advanced pancreatic cancer were treated orally with 8 g curcumin daily showed moderate results [31]. In another open-label phase II trial involving 17 patients with advance pancreatic cancer treated with 8 g of curcumin along with gemcitabine showed moderate results, while another recent study involving 21

Table 1.3 List of clinical trials with curcumin in patients with different diseases

Pathological conditions/diseases	Present status of clinical trials	No. of clinical trials	Study sites	Remarks/conclusions
Cancer (multiple myeloma, pancreatic cancer, FAP, colon cancer, colorectal cancer, leukemia, head and neck cell carcinoma, breast cancer, cancer lesions)	Completed	7	USA	Improvement in the histology of precancerous lesions Reduces markers (M1G DNA adducts) of colorectal cancer Decreases the number and size of polyps in FAP patients Despite low bioavailability curcumin shows biological activity against pancreatic, and multiple myeloma Reduces cancer lesions Safe in combination with other anticancer drugs
	Ongoing	22	USA, Puerto Rico, Canada, UK, Korea, India, Iran, Israel, Italy, France, Austria, Belgium	
	Withdrawn	4	USA	
Inflammatory bowel disease (IBD)/*H. pylori* infection/hepatic injury	Completed	5	USA, Israel, Korea	Reduces the levels of inflammatory cytokines and symptoms
	Ongoing	6	Israel, France, Itlay	
	Withdrawn			
Cardiovascular diseases and metabolic syndrome	Completed	7	France, Iran, Germany, Canada	Decreases serum levels of cholesterol and lipid peroxides, low density lipoprotein (LDL), ApoB Increases high density lipoprotein (HDL), ApoA
	Ongoing	5	Thailand, Canada, USA, Singapore	
	Withdrawn	1	USA	

(continued)

Table 1.3 (continued)

Pathological conditions/diseases	Present status of clinical trials	No. of clinical trials	Study sites	Remarks/conclusions
Neurodegenerative diseases, depression, optic neuropathy	Completed	7	Puerto Rico, India, China, Thailand, USA, Israel, Canada	Improves the cognitive functions and overall memory in patients with AD Improves inventory of depressive symptomatology self-rated version (IDS-SR30)
	Ongoing	9	USA, Israel, Iran, Canada	
	Withdrawn	2	Israel, USA	
Diabetes	Completed	4	Iran, USA, Sweden, India	Improves β cells function and decreases the level of serum fatty acids Decreases serum adipocyte-fatty acid binding protein (A-FABP) level Reduces atherogenic risk
	Ongoing	4	Thailand, Iran, USA	
	Withdrawn			
Radiotherapy/chemotherapy side effects	Completed	4	USA, Israel, India	Effective against radiotherapy/chemotherapy induced dermatitis, mucositis in cancer patients
	Ongoing	3	USA, Iran	
	Withdrawn			
Chronic kidney disease	Completed	1	USA	Improvement in the levels of inflammatory cytokines
	Ongoing	5	Canada, USA, Finland	
	Withdrawn			

(continued)

Table 1.3 (continued)

Pathological conditions/diseases	Present status of clinical trials	No. of clinical trials	Study sites	Remarks/conclusions
Allergy, asthma, bronchitis, oral disinfectant, cystic fibrosis	Completed	7	USA, Brazil, India	Decreases inflammation Effective anti-inflammatory mouthwash
	Ongoing			
	Withdrawn			
Rheumatoid arthritis (RA)	Completed	4	Belgium, France, USA, Thailand	Improvement in symptoms
	Ongoing	2	USA	
	Withdrawn			
Pancreatitis	Completed	1	USA	Improvement in symptoms and reduction in oxidative stress
	Ongoing			
	Withdrawn			
Psoriasis	Completed	2	USA	Decreases phosphorylase kinase activity a marker of psoriasis disease
	Ongoing	1	Italy	
	Withdrawn			
Bioavailability and pharmacokinetics	Completed	10	Germany, USA, Austria, Canada, Italy	Safe even at 12 g/day Poor bioavailability in serum and tissues
	Ongoing	2	USA, India	
	Withdrawn	2	Israel, USA	
General health benefits	Completed	8	USA, France, Korea	Dietary supplementation improves the levels of antioxidant enzymes and reduces oxidative stress Improves general health
	Ongoing	2	France, USA	
	Withdrawn			

gemcitabine resistant, patients were safe and seem to tolerate well [34, 60]. In a open-label phase I clinical trial, 14 patients with advanced and metastatic breast cancer were examined for feasibility and tolerability of curcumin in combination with docetaxel, based on which it has been recommended that 6 g curcumin/day for seven consecutive days for 3 weeks would be safe in combination with a standard dose of docataxel [17].

In a randomized double-blind study, curcumin (100 mg) in combination with isoflavin (40 mg) for 6 months in 85 patients showed synergism and suppressed prostrate specific antigen after treatment [55]. Curcumin was also examined against multiple myeloma and two clinical trials were completed. In one single blinded crossover pilot study in 26 patients with monoclonal gammopathy of undetermined significance (MGUS), curcumin showed therapeutic potential against MGUS [41]. In another study, involving 29 patients with asymptomatic, relapsed multiple myeloma, curcumin was found to be effective either alone or in combination with bioperine [113]. In a randomized open-label study involving 25 patients with chronic myeloid leukemia, curcumin (5 g) administered with imatinib (0.8 g) showed better efficacy in decreasing the nitric oxide levels. This suggested that curcumin can be used as an adjuvant to imatinib for the treatment of chronic myeloid leukemia patients [40]. Curcumin has also showed encouraging results in combination with other cancer drugs like paclitaxel, and cisplatin.

Oral curcumin has also been shown to prevent the *H. pylori* infection, a precursor of gastric cancer, prostatic intraepithelial neoplasia, a precursor of prostate cancer and to reduce the poly numbers and size in patients with FAP. The efficacy of curcumin against IBD has already been established in clinical trials. Similarly curcumin could effectively induce the gallbladder emptying and reduce gall stone formation, a potential risk factor for gallbladder cancer. In another study, oral curcumin (400 mg three times a day) compared to placebo showed much better anti-inflammatory response against spermatic cord edema in patients that underwent surgical repair of hernia and/or hydrocele.

Many other clinical trials against variety of other diseases have also been initiated and are being continued, interested readers may refer to some of the recent reviews on curcumin clinical trials [4, 43, 97, 121].

1.7 Conclusions

The natural product, "curcumin", a constituent of the golden spice, turmeric, a divine medicinal herb for the Indians, is now one of the highly researched molecules, very often referred by the modern scientists as "Cure-cumin". Extensive preclinical studies over the last three to four decades have established the therapeutic potential of curcumin against many diseases. Its multitargeting ability and direct interaction with signaling molecules have added advantage to exploit its use against several chronic diseases. In the clinic, curcumin has been found to be safe

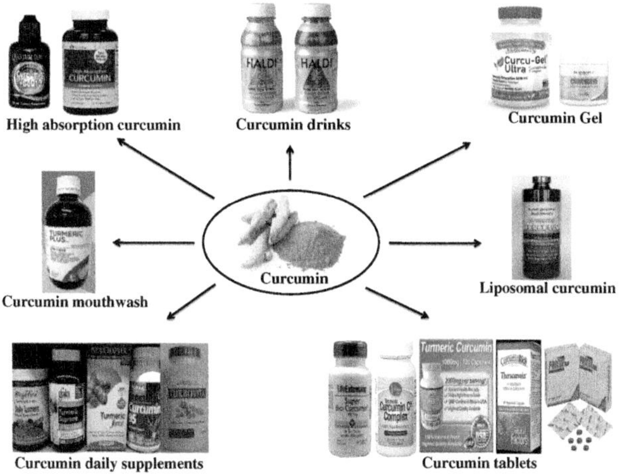

Fig. 1.3 Representative curcumin products in the market

and well tolerated by the patients under study. Its efficacy against diabetes, inflammatory bowel disease and arthritis are well proven in the clinic. Extensive clinical trials to develop curcumin as anticancer drug are still continuing, and the results are moderately encouraging, mainly due to complexity of the disease and low bioavailability of curcumin. To partly overcome this, new curcumin formulations with improved bioavailability are successfully designed and developed. More clinical trials with larger participants are warranted to translate the preclinical research to the clinical cancer medicine. Curcumin- and turmeric-based nutraceutical formulations are becoming very popular and more than hundred varieties of products in the form of drinks, capsules, creams, gels, food supplements are available in the market (Fig. 1.3 gives a few representative products). These products are recommended for both healthy people and also for patients undergoing treatment of chronic diseases. In view of all these gifted properties; it is not exaggerating to say that this inexpensive and innocuous dietary agent, a highly pleiotropic molecule, will be a "Panacea" in near future.

Acknowledgments The authors wish to express sincere thanks to Department of Atomic Energy, Government of India and acknowledge the contributions of many co-authors and students whose names appeared in the publications listed from our group.

References

1. Agarwal R, Goel SK, Behari JR (2010) Detoxification and antioxidant effects of curcumin in rats experimentally exposed to mercury. J Appl Toxicol 30:457–468
2. Aggarwal BB (2010) Targeting inflammation induced obesity and metabolic diseases by curcumin and other nutraceuticals. Annu Rev Nutr 30:173–199

3. Aggarwal BB, Sung B (2009) Pharmacological basis for the role of curcumin in chronic diseases: an age-old spice with modern targets. Trends Pharmacol Sci 30:85–94
4. Aggarwal BB, Kumar A, Bharti AC (2003) Anticancer potential of curcumin: preclinical and clinical studies. Anticancer Res 23:363–398
5. Aggarwal BB, Shishodia S, Takada Y et al (2005) Curcumin suppresses the paclitaxel induced nuclear factor-κB pathway in breast cancer cells and inhibits lung metastasis of human breast cancer in nude mice. Clin Cancer Res 11:7490–7498
6. Aggarwal BB, Sundaram C, Malini N et al (2007) Curcumin: the Indian solid gold. Adv Exp Med Biol 595:243–305
7. Aggarwal BB, Gupta SC, Sung B (2013) Curcumin: an orally bioavailable blocker of TNF and other pro-inflammatory biomarkers. Br J Pharmacol 169(8):1672–1692
8. Alrawaiq NS, Abdullah A (2014) A review of antioxidant polyphenol curcumin and its role in detoxification. Int J PharmTech Res 6:280–289
9. Anand P, Kunnumakkara AB, Newman RA, Aggarwal BB (2007) Bioavaialbility of curcumin: problems and promises. Mol Pharm 4:807–818
10. Arbiser JL, Klauber N, Rohan R, van LR, Huang MT, Fisher C, Flynn E, Byers HR (1998) Curcumin is an in vivo inhibitor of angiogenesis. Mol Med 4:376–383
11. Asai A, Miyazawa T (2000) Occurrence of orally administered curcuminoid as glucuronide and glucuronide/sulfate conjugates in rat plasma. Life Sci 67:2785–2793
12. Asti M, Ferrari E, Groci S et al (2014) ^{68}Ga-labelled curcuminoids complexes: characterisation of potential radiotracers for imaging of Alzheimer's disease. Inorg Chem 53:4922–4933
13. Awasthi A, Pandya U, Singhal SS et al (2000) Curcumin–glutathione interactions and the role of human glutathione *S*-transferase PI-1. Chem Biol Interact 128:19–38
14. Bae MK, Kim SH, Jeong JW et al (2006) Curcumin inhibits hypoxia-induced angiogenesis via down-regulation of HIF-1. Oncol Rep 15:1557–1562
15. Barik A, Mishra B, Shen L et al (2005) Evaluation of new copper–curcumin complex as superoxide dismutase mimic and its free radical reactions. Free Radic Biol Med 39:811–822
16. Baum L, Lam CW, Cheung SK et al (2008) Six month randomized placebo controlled double blind pilot clinical trial of curcumin in patients of Alzheimer disease. J Clin Psychopharmacol 28:110–113
17. Bayet-Robert M, Kwaitkowski F, Leheurteur M et al (2010) Phase I dose escalation trial of docataxel plus curcumin in patients with advanced metastatic breast cancer. Cancer Biol Ther 9:8–14
18. Beloqui A, Coco R, Memvanga PB et al (2014) pH sensitive nanoparticles for colonic delivery in inflammatory bowel disease. Int J Pharm 473:203–212
19. Bharti AC, Donato N, Aggarwal BB (2003) Curcumin (diferuloylmethane) inhibits constitutive and IL-6-inducible STAT3 phosphorylation in human multiple myeloma cells. J Immunol 171:3863–3871
20. Bierhaus A, Zhang Y, Quehenberger P et al (1997) The dietary pigment curcumin reduces endothelial tissue factor gene expression by inhibiting binding of AP-1 to the DNA and activation of NF-κB. Thromb Haemost 77:772–782
21. Chan MM, Huang HI, Fenton MR, Fong D (1998) In vivo inhibition of nitric oxide synthase gene expression by curcumin: a cancer preventive natural product with anti-inflammatory properties. Biochem Pharmacol 55:1955–1962
22. Chattopadhyay I, Biswas K, Bandyopadhyay U et al (2004) Turmeric and curcumin: biological actions and medicinal applications. Curr Sci 87:44–53
23. Chattopadhyay I, Bandyopadhyay U, Biswas K et al (2006) Indomethacin inactivates gastric peroxidase to induce reactive-oxygen-mediated gastric mucosal injury and curcumin protects it by preventing peroxidase inactivation and scavenging reactive oxygen. Free Radic Biol Med 40:1397–1408
24. Chen A, Xu J (2005) Activation of PPARγ by curcumin inhibits Moser cell growth and mediates suppression of gene expression of cyclin D1 and EGFR. Am J Physiol Gastrointest Liver Physiol 288:G447–G456

25. Chen WH, Chen Y, Cui GH et al (2004) Effect of curcumin on STAT5 signaling pathway in primary CML cells. Zhonghua Xue Ye Xue Za Zhi 12:572–576
26. Chen A, Xu J, Johnson AC (2006) Curcumin inhibits human colon cancer cell growth by suppressing gene expression of epidermal growth factor receptor through reducing the activity of the transcription factor Egr-1. Oncogene 25:278–287
27. Choudhuri T, Pal S, Das T, Sa G (2005) Curcumin selectively induces apoptosis in deregulated cyclin D1-expressed cells at G2 phase of cell cycle in a p53-dependent manner. J Biol Chem 280:20059–20068
28. Chua CC, Hamdy RC, Chua BH (2000) Mechanism of transforming growth factor-β1-induced expression of vascular endothelial growth factor in murine osteoblastic MC3T3-E1 cells. Biochim Biophys Acta 1497:69–76
29. Collett GP, Campbell FC (2004) Curcumin induces c-Jun N-terminal kinase-dependent apoptosis in HCT116 human colon cancer cells. Carcinogenesis 25:2183–2189
30. Conney AH (2003) Enzyme induction and dietary chemicals as approaches to cancer chemoprevention: the Seventh DeWitt S. Goodman lecture. Cancer Res 63:7005–7031
31. Dhillon N, Aggarwal BB, Newman RA et al (2008) Phase II trial of curcumin in patients with advanced pancreatic cancer. Clin Cancer Res 14:4491–4499
32. Kim DS, Kim JY, Han Y (2012) Curcuminoids in neurodegenerative diseases. CNS drug Discov 7:184–204
33. Durgaprasad S, Pai CG, Kumar V et al (2005) A pilot study of the antioxidant effect of curcumin in tropical pancreatic. Ind J Med Res 122:315–318
34. Epelbaum R, Schaffer M, Vizel B et al (2010) Curcumin and gemcitabine in patients with advanced pancreatic cancer. Nutr Cancer 62:1137–1141
35. Esatbeyoglu T, Huebbe P, Insa MA et al (2012) Curcumin—from molecule to biological function. Angew Chem Int Ed 51:5308–5332
36. Fang J, Jun L, Holmegren A (2005) Thioredoxin reductase is irreversibly modified by curcumin: a novel molecular mechanism for its anticancer activity. J Biol Chem 280:25284–25290
37. Garcea G, Jones DJ, Singh R et al (2004) Detection of curcumin and its metabolites in hepatic tissue and portal blood of patients following oral administration. Br J Cancer 90:1011–1015
38. Garcea G, Berry DP, Jones DJ et al (2005) Consumption of the putative chemopreventive agent curcumin by cancer patients: assessment of curcumin levels in the colorectum and their pharmacokinetic consequences. Cancer Epidemiol Biomarkers Prev 14:120–125
39. George D (2003) Targeting PDGF receptors in cancer–rationales and proof of concept clinical trials. Adv Exp Med Biol 532:141–151
40. Ghalaut VS, Sangwan L, Dahiya K et al (2012) Effect of imatinib therapy with and without turmeric powder on nitric oxide levels in chronic myeloid leukemia. J Oncol Pharm Pract 18:186–190
41. Golombick T, Diamond TH, Badmaev V et al (2009) The potential role of curcumin in patients with monoclonal gammopathy of undefined significance—its effect on paraproteinemia type I collagen bone turnover marker. Clin Cancer Res 15:5917–5922
42. Gupta S, Prasad S, Ji HK et al (2011) Multitargeting by curcumin as revealed by molecular interaction studies. Nat Prod Rep 28:1937–1955
43. Gupta SC, Patchva S, Aggarwal BB (2013) Therapeutic potential of curcumin: lessons learned from clinical trials. AAPS J 15:195–218
44. Hamaguchi T, Ono K, Yamada M (2010) Review: curcumin and Alzheimer's disease. CNS Neurosci Ther 16:285–297
45. Han SS, Chung ST, Robertson DA, Ranjan D, Bondada S (1999) Curcumin causes the growth arrest and apoptosis of B cell lymphoma by downregulation of egr-1, c-myc, bcl-XL, NF-κB, and p53. Clin Immunol 93:152–161
46. Hanahan D, Weinberg RA (2011) Hallmarks of cancer: the next generation. Cell 144: 646–674

47. Hanai H, Sugimoto K (2009) Curcumin has prospects for the treatment of inflammatory bowel disease. Curr Pharma Des 15:2087–2094
48. Hanai H, Iida T, Takeuchi K et al (2006) Curcumin maintenance therapy for ulcerative colitis randomized multicenter, double-blind placebo controlled trial. Clin Gastroentero Heatol 4:1502–1506
49. Hasima N, Aggarwal BB (2012) Cancer-linked targets modulated by curcumin. Int J Biochem Mol Biol 3:328–351
50. He ZY, Shi CB, Wen H et al (2011) Upregulation of p53 expression in cancer patients with colorectal cancer by administration of curcumin. Cancer Investig 29:208–213
51. He ZY, Yue Y, Zheng X, Zhang K, Chen S, Du Z et al (2015) Curcumin, inflammation, and chronic diseases: how are they linked? Molecules 20(5):9183–9213
52. Hong RL, Spohn WH, Hung MC (1999) Curcumin inhibits tyrosine kinase activity of p185neu and also depletes p185neu. Clin Cancer Res 5:1884–1891
53. Hoque M, Gong P, Killeen E, Green CJ, Foresti R, Alam J, Motterlini R (2003) Curcumin activates the haem oxygenase-1 gene via regulation of Nrf2 and the antioxidant-responsive element. Biochem J 371:887–895
54. Hussain AR, Al-Rasheed M, Manogaran PS et al (2006) Curcumin induces apoptosis via inhibition of PI3′-kinase/AKT pathway in acute T cell leukemias. Apoptosis 11:245–254
55. Ide H, Tokiwa S, Sakamaki K et al (2010) Combined inhibitory effects of soy isoflavons and curcumin on the production of prostate specific antigen. Prostate 70:1127–1133
56. Ireson RC, Jones DJL, Orr S et al (2002) Metabolism of the cancer chemopreventive agent curcumin in human and rat intestine. Cancer Epidemol Biomarkers Prev 11:105–111
57. Jaiswal AS, Marlow BP, Gupta N et al (2002) Beta-catenin-mediated transactivation and cell–cell adhesion pathways are important in curcumin (diferuylmethane)-induced growth arrest and apoptosis in colon cancer cells. Oncogene 21:8414–8427
58. Jiang T, Zhi X, Zhang Y, Pan L, Zhou P (2012) Inhibitory effect of curcumin on the Al(III)-induced A β(42) aggregation and neurotoxicity in vitro. Biochim Biophys Acta Mol Basis Dis 1822:1207–1215
59. Jun S, Yi Z, Jinhong H (2013) Curcumin inhibits imiquimod induced psoriasis like inflammation by inhibiting IL-1β and IL-6 production in mice. PLoS One 8:e67078
60. Kanai M, Yoshimura K, Asada M et al (2011) A phase I/II study of gemcitabine-based chemotherapy plus curcumin for patients with gemcitabine-resistant pancreatic cancer. Cancer Chemother Pharmacol 68:157–164
61. Kang ES, Woo IS, Kim HJ et al (2007) Up-regulation of aldose reductase expression mediated by phosphatidylinositol 3-kinase/Akt and Nrf2 is involved in the protective effect of curcumin against oxidative damage. Free Radic Biol Med 43:535–545
62. Kang ES, Kim GH, Kim HJ et al (2008) Nrf2 regulates curcumin-induced aldose reductase expression indirectly via nuclear factor-κB. Pharmacol Res 58:15–21
63. Kawamori T, Lubet R, Steele VE et al (1999) Chemopreventive effect of curcumin, a naturally occurring anti-inflammatory agent, during the promotion/progression stages of colon cancer. Cancer Res 59:597–601
64. Khan N, Afaq F, Mukhtar H (2008) Cancer chemoprevention through dietary antioxidants: progress and promise. Antioxid Redox Signal 10:475–510
65. Kunwar A, Barik A, Pandey R, Priyadarsini KI (2006) Transport of liposomal and albumin loaded curcumin to living cells: an absorption and fluorescence spectroscopic study. Biochim Biophys Acta (General) 1760:1513–1520
66. Kurd SK, Smith N, Van Voorhees A et al (2008) Oral curcumin in the treatment of moderate to severe psoriasis vulgaris, a prospective clinical trial. J Am Acd Dermatol 58:625–631
67. Kuttan R, Sreedharan PC, Joseph CD (1987) Turmeric and curcumin as topical agents in cancer therapy. Tumori 73:29–31
68. Lampe V, Milobedzka J (1913) Studien uber curucmin. Ber Dtsch Chem Ges 46:2235–2240
69. Lee WH, Loo CY, Bebawy M, Luk F, Mason RS, Rohanizadeh R (2013) Curcumin and its derivatives: their application in neuropharmacology and neuroscience in the 21st century. Curr Neuropharmacol 11(4):338–378

70. Li N, Chen X, Han C, Chen J (2002) Chemopreventive effect of tea and curcumin on DMBA-induced oral carcinogenesis in hamsters. Wei Sheng Yan Jiu 31:354–357
71. Li L, Braiteh FS, Kurzrock R (2005) Liposome-encapsulated curcumin: in vitro and in vivo effects on proliferation, apoptosis, signaling, and angiogenesis. Cancer 104:1322–1331
72. Liu JY, Lin SJ, Lin JK (1993) Inhibitory effects of curcumin on protein kinase C activity induced by 12-*O*-tetradecanoyl-phorbol-13-acetate in NIH 3T3 cells. Carcinogenesis 14:857–861
73. Meng BI, Li J, Cao H (2013) Antioixidant and anti-inflammatory activities of curcumin on diabetes mellitus and its complications. Curr Pharm Des 19:2101–2103
74. Milobedzka J, Kostanecki S, Lampe V (1910) Zur Kenntnis des Curcumins. Berichte der Deutschen Chemischen Gessellschaft 43:2163–2170
75. Monroy A, Lithgow GJ, Alavez S (2013) Curcumin and neurodegenerative diseases. BioFactors 39:122–132
76. Moon DO, Kim MO, Choi YH et al (2010) Curcumin attenuates inflammatory response in IL-1 bets induced human synovial fibroblasts and collagen induced arthritis in mouse model. Int Immunopharmacol 10:605–610
77. Mori Y, Tatematsu K, Koide A et al (2006) Modification by curcumin of mutagenic activation of carcinogenic *N*-nitrosamines by extrahepatic cytochromes P-450 2B1 and 2E1 in rats. Cancer Sci 97:896–904
78. Noorafshan A, Ashkani-Esfahani S (2013) A review of therapeutic effects of curcumin. Curr Pharm Des 19:2032–2046
79. Oppenheimer A (1937) Turmeric in biliary diseases. Lancet 229:619–621
80. Pabon HJ (1964) Synthesis of curcumin and related compounds. Rev Trav Chim 83:379–386
81. Pallikkavil R, Ummathur MS, Sreedharan S, Krishnankutty K (2013) Synthesis, characterization and antimicrobial studies of Cd(II), Hg(II), Pb(II), Sn(II) and Ca(II) complexes of curcumin. Main Group Met Chem 36:123–127
82. Park SD, Jung JH, Lee HW et al (2005) Zedoariae rhizome and curcumin inhibits platelet-derived growth factor-induced proliferation of human hepatic myofibroblasts. Int Immunopharmacol 5:555–569
83. Park W, Ruhul Amin ARM, Chen ZG, Shin DM (2013) New perspectives of curcumin in cancer prevention. Cancer Prev Res 6:387–400
84. Párkányi C, Stem-Beren MR, Martínez OR, Aaron JJ, MacNair MB, Arrieta AF (2004) Solvatochromic correlations and ground- and excited-state dipole moments of curcuminoid dyes. Spectrochim Acta A 60:1805–1810
85. Perkins S, Verschoyle RD, Hill K et al (2002) Chemopreventive efficacy and pharmacokinetics of curcumin in mouse, a model of familial adenomatous polyposis. Cancer Epidemiol Biomarkers Prev 11:535–540
86. Prasad S, Tyagi AK, Aggarwal BB (2014) Recent developments in delivery, bioavailability, absorption and metabolism of curcumin: the golden pigment from golden spice. Cancer Res Treat 46:2–18
87. Priyadarsini KI (1997) Free radical reactions of curcumin in model membranes. Free Radic Biol Med 23:838–884
88. Priyadarsini KI (2009) Photophysics, photochemistry and photobiology of curcumin: studies from organic solutions, bio-mimetics and living cells. J Photochem Photobiol C Chem Rev 10:81–96
89. Priyadarsini KI (2013) Chemical and structural features influencing the biological activity of curcumin. Curr Pharm Des 19:2093–2100
90. Priyadarsini KI (2014) The chemistry of curcumin: from extraction to therapeutic agent. Molecules 19:20091–20112
91. Ramadan G, El-Menshawy O (2013) Protective effects of ginger–turmeric rhizomes mixture on joint inflammation, atherogenesis, kidney disfunction and other complications in a rat model of human rheumatoid arthritis. Int J Rheum Dis 16:219–229

92. Ranjan D, Chen C, Johnston H, Jeon H, Nagabhushan M (2004) Curcumin inhibits mitogen stimulated lymphocyte proliferation, NFkappaB activation, and IL-2 signaling. J Surg Res 121:171–177
93. Reddy S, Rishi AK, Xu H et al (2006) Mechanisms of curcumin- and EGF-receptor related protein (ERRP)-dependent growth inhibition of colon cancer cells. Nutr Cancer 55:185–194
94. Rushworth SA, Ogborne RM, Charalambos CA, O'Connell MA (2006) Role of protein kinase C δ in curcumin-induced antioxidant response element-mediated gene expression in human monocytes. Biochem Biophys Res Commun 341(4):1007–1016
95. Sagnou M, Benaki D, Triantis C et al (2011) Curcumin as the OO bidentate ligand in "2 + 1" complexes with the [M(CO)(3)](+) (M = Re, ^{99m}Tc) tricarbonyl core for radiodiagnostic applications. Inorg Chem 50:1295–1303
96. Schraufstatter E, Bernt H (1949) Antibacterial action of curcumin and related compounds. Nature 164:456–457
97. Shanmugam MK, Rane G, Kanchi MM et al (2015) The multifaceted role of curcumin in cancer prevention and treatment. Molecules 20:2728–2769
98. Sharma OP (1976) Antioxidant activity of curcumin and related compounds. Biochem Pharmacol 25:1811–1812
99. Sharma KK, Chandra S, Basu DK (1987) Synthesis and antiarthritic study of a new orally active diferuloyl methane (curcumin) gold complex. Inorg Chim Acta 135:47–48
100. Sharma RA, Euden SA, Platton SL et al (2004) Phase I clinical trial of oral curcumin: biomarkers of systemic activity and compliance. Clin Cancer Res 10:6847–6854
101. Shehzad A, Rehman G, Lee YS (2013) Curcumin in inflammatory diseases. BioFactors 39:69–77
102. Shen L, Ji HF (2012) The pharmacology of curcumin: is it the degradation products? Trends Mol Med 18:138–143
103. Shen G, Xu C, Hu R et al (2006) Modulation of nuclear factor E2-related factor 2—mediated gene expression in mice liver and small intestine by cancer chemopreventive agent curcumin. Mol Cancer Ther 5:39–51
104. Shishodia S, Amin HM, Lai R, Aggarwal BB (2005) Curcumin (diferuloylmethane) inhibits constitutive NF-κB activation, induces G1/S arrest, suppresses proliferation, and induces apoptosis in mantle cell lymphoma. Biochem Pharmacol 70:700–713
105. Shoba G, Joy D, Joseph T, Majeed M, Rajendran R, Srinivas PSSR (1998) Influence of piperine on the pharmacokinetics of curcumin in animals and human volunteers. Planta Med 64:353–356
106. Shrimal RC, Dhawan BN (1973) Pharmacology of diferuloyl methane (curcumin), a non-steroidal anti-inflammatory agent. J Pharm Pharmacol 25:447–452
107. Singh S (2007) From exotic spice to modern drug? Cell 130:765–768
108. Singh S, Aggarwal B (1995) Activation of transcription factor NF-κB is suppressed by curcumin (Diferuloylmethane). J Biol Chem 270:24995–25000
109. Srinivasan M (1972) Effect of curcumin on blood sugar as seen in a diabetic subject. Ind J Med Sci 26:269–270
110. Strimpakos AS, Sharma RA (2008) Curcumin: preventive and therapeutic properties in laboratory studies and clinical trials. Antioxid Redox Signal 10:511–545
111. Taylor RA, Leonard MC (2011) Curcumin for inflammatory bowel disease, a review of human studies. Alt Med Rev 16:152–156
112. Tsvetkov P, Asher G, Reiss V, Shaul Y, Sachs L, Lotem J (2005) Inhibition of NAD(P)H: quinone oxidoreductase 1 activity and induction of p53 degradation by the natural phenolic compound curcumin. Proc Natl Acad Sci USA 102:5535–5540
113. Vadhan-Raj S, Weber D, Wang M et al (2007) Curcumin downregulates NF-κB and related genes in patients with multiple myeloma: results of phase 1/2 study. Blood 110:357a
114. Vajragupta O, Boonchoong P, Watanabe H et al (2003) Manganese complexes of curcumin and its derivatives: evaluation for the radical scavenging ability and neuroprotective activity. Free Radic Biol Med 35:1632–1644
115. Vogel HA, Pelletier J (1815) Curcumin-biological and medicinal properties. J Pharma 2:50

116. Wang YJ, Pan MH, Cheng AL et al (1997) Stability of curcumin in buffer solution and characterization of its degradation products. J Pharma Biomed Anal 15:1867–1876
117. Wanninger S, Lorenz V, Subhan A, Edelmann FT (2015) Metal complexes of curcumin—synthetic strategies, structures and medicinal applications. Chem Soc Rev 44:4986–5002
118. Xia Y, Jin L, Zhang B et al (2007) The potentiation of curcumin on insulin-like growth factor-1 action in MCF-7 human breast carcinoma cells. Life Sci 80:2161–2169
119. Xu J, Fu Y, Chen A (2003) Activation of peroxisome proliferator-activated receptor gamma contributes to the inhibitory effects of curcumin on rat hepatic stellate cell growth. Am J Physiol Gastrointest Liver Physiol 285:G20–G30
120. Yallapu MM, Ebeling MC, Khan S et al (2013) Novel curcumin-loaded magnetic nanoparticles for pancreatic cancer treatment. Mol Cancer Ther 12:1471–1480
121. Yang C, Su X, Liu A et al (2013) Advances in clinical study of curcumin. Curr Pharm Des 19:1966–1973
122. Yu S, Shen G, Kong TA (2006) Curcumin inhibits mTOR signaling by inhibiting protein kinase B/Akt and activating AMP-activated protein kinase (AMPK) in prostate cancer cell line PC-3. Proc Am Assoc Cancer Res 47:538
123. Zhang X, Yin WK, Shi XD, Li Y (2011) Curcumin activates Wnt/β-catenin signaling pathway through inhibiting the activity of GSK-3β in APPswe transfected SY5Y cells. Eur J Pharm Sci 42:540–546
124. Zhang D-W, Fu M, Gao S-H, Liu J-L (2013) Curcumin and diabetes: a systematic review. Evid Complement Altern Med 16:1–22

Chapter 2
Berberine and Its Role in Chronic Disease

Arrigo F.G. Cicero and Alessandra Baggioni

Abstract Berberine is a quaternary ammonium salt from the protoberberine group of isoquinoline alkaloids. It is found in such plants as *Berberis* [e.g. *Berberis aquifolium* (Oregon grape), *Berberis vulgaris* (barberry), *Berberis aristata* (tree turmeric)], *Hydrastis canadensis* (goldenseal), *Xanthorhiza simplicissima* (yellowroot), *Phellodendron amurense*[2] (Amur corktree), *Coptis chinensis* (Chinese goldthread), *Tinospora cordifolia*, *Argemone mexicana* (prickly poppy) and *Eschscholzia californica* (Californian poppy). In vitro it exerts significant anti-inflammatory and antioxidant activities. In animal models berberine has neuroprotective and cardiovascular protective effects. In humans, its lipid-lowering and insulin-resistance improving actions have clearly been demonstrated in numerous randomized clinical trials. Moreover, preliminary clinical evidence suggest the ability of berberine to reduce endothelial inflammation improving vascular health, even in patients already affected by cardiovascular diseases. Altogether the available evidences suggest a possible application of berberine use in the management of chronic cardiometabolic disorders.

Keywords Berberine · Antioxidant · Anti-inflammatory · Type 2 diabetes · Cardiovascular disease · Depression

2.1 Introduction

Cardiovascular diseases are yet the most common causes of death and one of the first causes of disability in industrialized countries and despite the efforts towards primary prevention of cardiovascular disease, many patients still remain at risk [1]. Lifestyle interventions such as diet and/or physical activity are the most

A.F.G. Cicero (✉) · A. Baggioni
Cardiovascular Disease Prevention Research Unit, Department of Medical and Surgical Sciences, S. Orsola-Malpighi University Hospital, Via Albertoni 15, 40138 Bologna, Italy
e-mail: arrigo.cicero@unibo.it

S.C. Gupta et al. (eds.), *Anti-inflammatory Nutraceuticals and Chronic Diseases*, Advances in Experimental Medicine and Biology 928,
DOI 10.1007/978-3-319-41334-1_2

cost-effective approach in delaying or preventing the onset of cardiovascular disease [2]. Moreover, people without a history of cardiovascular disease who lack common risk factors have a significantly greater risk of cardiovascular and all-cause mortality if they do not adhere to a healthy lifestyle [3]. However, lifestyle programs are often difficult to follow for long periods and some risk parameters, such as cholesterolemia, are relatively resistant to changes in dietary habits and physical activity [4]. On the other hand, a relatively large number of dietary supplements and nutraceuticals have been studied for their supposed or demonstrated ability to reduce cholesterolemia in humans [5]. The third National Cholesterol Educational Program suggested to integrate dietary supplements such as soluble fibres, omega-3 polyunsaturated fatty acids (PUFA), plant sterols and soy protein in the diet in order to achieve an optimal LDL-cholesterolemia [6]. These suggestions have been supported also by the recent new European guidelines of the management of dyslipidemias [7] that also cite some other nutraceuticals as potentially useful lipid-lowering substances. Since cardiovascular disease prevention needs a life course approach, both the tolerability and safety of dietary supplements/nutraceuticals used to control plasma cholesterol levels has to be adequately defined as well as the risk/benefit ratio of their assumption. A relatively large number of recent reviews already described the mechanism of action and the efficacy of the different nutraceuticals and botanicals with lipid-lowering effects [8–10]. In particular, Berberine (BBR) exhibits many different biological activities; among them, the best characterized are antioxidant, anti-inflammatory, cholesterol-lowering and anti-hyperglycemic effects.

2.1.1 Physico-Chemical and Pharmacological Properties of Berberine

Berberine is a quaternary ammonium salt from the group of isoquinoline alkaloids (2,3–methylenedioxy-9,10-dimethoxyprotoberberine chloride; $C_{20}H_{18}NO_4^+$) with a molar mass of 336.36122 g/mol [11]. It is highly concentrated in the roots, rhizomes and stem bark of various plants including *Coptis chinensis*, *Rhizoma coptidis*, *Hydrastis canadensis*, *Berberis aquifolium*, *Berberis vulgaris*, *Berberis aristata*, *Tinospora cordifolia*, *Arcangelisia flava* and *Cortex rhellodendri* [12]. Berberine is strongly yellow coloured, which explains the fact that in the past berberis species were used to dye wool, leather and wood. Under ultraviolet light, berberine shows a strong yellow fluorescence with a Colour Index of 75,160 [13].

Berberis vulgaris as well as other berberine-containing plants [14] are used medicinally in virtually all-traditional medical systems, and have a history of usage in Ayurvedic, Iranian and Chinese medicine dating back at least 3000 years [16]. Ancient Egyptians used barberry fruit with fennel seeds to ward off pestilent fevers [15]. Indian Ayurvedic physicians used barberry in the treatment of dysentery and traditional Iranian medicine uses its fruit as a sedative [15, 17]. In northern Europe, barberry was used to treat gall bladder and liver problems, while it was used in the treatment of abnormal uterine bleeds and rheumatism in Russia and Bulgaria [18, 19]. In North America, the Eclectics used barberry for treatment of malaria and as a general tonic [20]. Also, the American Indians found it effective in improving appetite and used its dried fruit as a gargle [21, 22].

Medicinal properties for all parts of the plant have been reported, including tonic, antimicrobial, antiemetic, antipyretic, antipruritic, antioxidant, anti-inflammatory, hypotensive, antiarrhythmic, sedative, antinociceptive, anticholinergic and cholagogue actions, and it has been used in some cases like cholecystitis, cholelithiasis, jaundice, dysentery, leishmaniasis, malaria and gall stones [23]. Furthermore, berberine has been used for treating diarrhoea and gastrointestinal disorders for a long time [24, 25]. It has multiple pharmacological effects including; antimicrobial activity against 54 microorganisms [26], inhibition of intestinal ion secretion and smooth muscle contraction, inhibition of ventricular tachyarrhythmia, reduction of inflammation, stimulation of bile secretion and bilirubin discharge [27].

Berberine has low bioavailability and poor absorption through the gut wall (<5 %) and bowel P-glycoprotein contributes to that, actively expelling the alkaloid from the lumen mucosal cells [28].

In a rat noncompartmental model [29], unbound berberine is transported to bile through active transportation and it is metabolized by P450 enzyme system in liver, with phase I demethylation and phase II glucuronidation. Berberine has four main metabolites identified in rats: berberrubine, thalifendine, demethyleneberberine and jatrorrhizine, and all of them have glucuronide conjugates [30]. Intestinal bacterial flora takes role in enterohepatic circulation of berberine and its conjugated metabolites [28]. On the other hand, very small amount of unchanged berberine is eliminated in urines [31].

As other alkaloids are present in *H. canadensis* extracts (i.e. hydrastine and canadine), berberine may inhibit cytochrome P450 2E1 (CYP2E1) [32] and 1A2 (CYP1A2) [33]. This inhibition is not related to a significant increase in pharmacological interactions since the largest part of the available drugs is not metabolized by these enzymatic systems.

2.1.2 Berberine Modulation of Cell Signalling Pathways

Berberine is a potent antioxidant and anti-inflammatory agent: these properties could be particularly relevant in the management of type 2 diabetes and cardiovascular diseases.

In metabolic disorders, as obesity and type 2 diabetes, increased oxidative stress is a common feature [34, 35]. It could induce or deteriorate insulin resistance and diabetes through multiple mechanisms. In the process of oxidative stress, excessive reactive oxygen species (ROS) are produced, mainly by mitochondria [36, 37]. They could cause damage and apoptosis of pancreatic islet β-cells and reduction of insulin secretion [38]. ROS also activate c-Jun N-terminal kinase (JNK), protein kinase C (PKC) and nuclear factor-κB (NF-κB), interfering with the insulin signalling pathway and causing insulin resistance [39–41]. In addition, oxidative stress also contributes to the development of chronic complications of diabetes, such as diabetic nephropathy, retinopathy and neuropathy [37].

Molecular mechanisms of berberine in reducing oxidative stress seem to be related with multiple cellular pathways (Fig. 2.1).

The NOX family of ROS-generating NADPH oxidases, a family of membrane-associated enzymatic complexes, is one of the major sources of ROS production in cells [42]; its activation is often associated to high levels of fatty acids, cholesterol, glucose or advanced glycation end products (AGEs) [43–45]. Among various NOX isoforms, berberine was reported to suppress the overexpression of NOX 2,4 and to decrease ROS production in macrophages and endothelial cells upon stimulation with inflammatory stimuli [46, 47]. In endothelial cells, berberine attenuated LDL oxidation induced by ROS and reduces the collapse of mitochondrial membrane potential, the chromosome condensation, the cytochrome C release and the caspase-3 activation [48]. Circulating endothelial

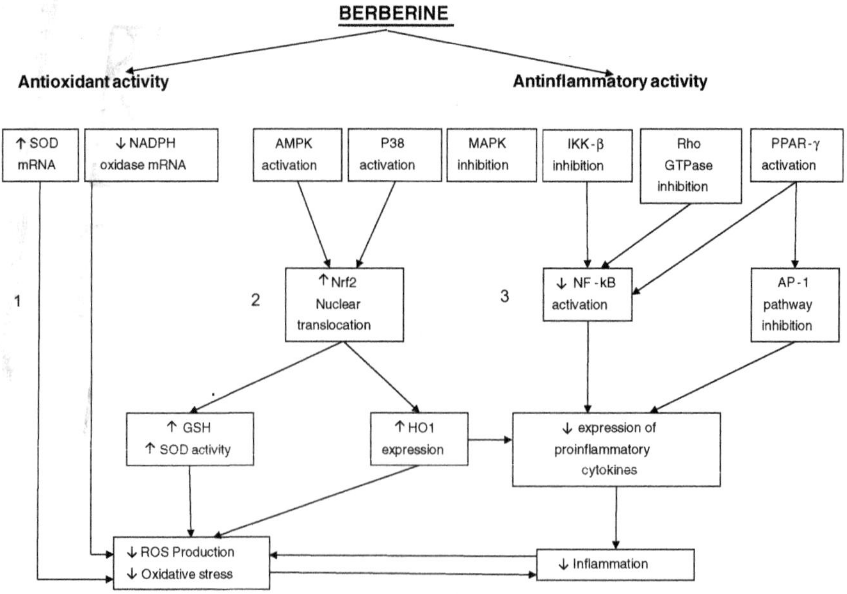

Fig. 2.1 Schematic illustration of the molecular mechanisms and pathways of Berberine in reducing oxidative stress and inflammation. *1* Berberine could inhibit oxidative stress by upregulation of SOD, and downregulation of NADPH oxidase expression. *2* Berberine administration induces the activation of the Nrf2 transcription. The effect of berberine on Nrf2 relies on the activation of AMPK, and P38 pathways. *3* Berberine could suppress inflammation by blocking the MAPK pathways in an AMPK-dependent manner, inhibiting the classic NF-κB transcription; inhibiting the Rho GTPase pathway, which plays a role in NF-κB regulation, and attenuating the transcription activity of AP-1, which was possible to be mediated by PPARγ activation

microparticles, vesicular structures found in plasma from patients with vascular diseases so utilized as a surrogate marker of endothelial dysfunction, are oxidative stress inducers; they promote upregulation of NOX4 expression and ROS production. It has been reported that berberine reversed NOX4-derived ROS production in human umbilical vein endothelial cells (HUVECs) [46].

NOX could be negatively regulated by adenosine monophosphate-activated protein kinase (AMPK) activation [49, 50]; in fact AMPK activators, such as metformin, may exert their cardiovascular protective function through NOX inhibition [51]. AMPK pathway is activated by berberine [52] and it seems to play a pivotal role in mediating its antioxidant activity [53, 54].

The AMPK is a ubiquitously expressed cellular energy sensor and an essential component of the adaptive response to cardiomyocyte stress that occurs during ischemia. AMPK plays also an important role in regulating function of NO synthesis in endothelial cells. In fact, AMPK is an upstream kinase of endothelial nitric oxide synthase (eNOS) which promotes the phosphorylation of eNOS at Ser1177 site as well as the formation of eNOS and HSP90 complex and NO production [55]. Zhang et al. [56] observed that in HUVECs berberine ameliorated palmitate-induced endothelial dysfunction by upregulating eNOS and downregulating of NOX4 through the activation of AMPK. In both cultured endothelial cells and blood vessels isolated from rat aorta berberine enhanced eNOS phosphorylation and attenuated high glucose-induced generation of ROS, cellular apoptosis, NF-κB activation and expression of adhesion molecules through AMPK signalling cascade activation, a key event in preventing oxidative and inflammatory signalling [57].

Besides NADPH oxidase downregulation and NO production, AMPK activation has been linked to upregulation of the antioxidant enzyme superoxide dismutase (SOD) [58, 59], which is dismutated to hydrogen peroxide. It was observed an increased SOD expression in berberine treated diabetic mice [60, 61]. Glutathione (GSH) is another antioxidant molecule which helps to maintain the balance of redox state in organisms and acting asco-substrate of glutathione peroxidase (GSH-Px) in the clearance of peroxides [62]. Berberine treatment promoted a GSH-Px and SOD hyperactivation in the liver of mice [63], attenuated ROS production and increased detoxifying enzymes GSH-Px and SOD in NSC34 motor neuron-like cells [64].

Recent studies revealed that berberine suppressed oxidative stress through induction of the nuclear factor erythroid-2-related factor-2 (Nrf2) pathway [65–67]. Nrf2 is a transcription factor which binds to antioxidative response elements (ARE) in DNA, leading to transcription of phase II enzymes and cytoprotective proteins genes such as NAD(P)H quinone oxidoreductase-1 (NQO-1) and heme oxygenase-1 (HO-1) with a wide range of activities in regulating redox state and energy metabolism in cells [68]. Now, Nrf2 is recognized as an important mediator of berberine in reducing oxidative stress, as blocking Nrf2 abolishes the antioxidant activity of berberine in macrophages and nerve cells [65–67]. The activation of AMPK, phosphatidylinositol 3-kinase (PI3K)/Akt and p38 kinase cellular pathways is involved in the effect of berberine on Nrf2, since the block of these pathways diminishes the stimulating effect of berberine on Nrf2 [65–67].

The anti-inflammatory activity of berberine was observed both in vitro and in vivo and was noted by the reduction of proinflammatory cytokines as well as acute phase proteins [69–78].

In cultured metabolically active cells (adipocytes and liver cells), immunocytes (macrophages and splenocytes) or pancreatic β-cells, berberine treatment reduced the production of TNF-α, IL-6, IL-1β, matrix metalloprotease 9 (MMP9), cyclooxygenase-2 (COX2), inducible NOS (iNOS), monocyte chemoattractant protein 1 (MCP-1) and C-reactive protein (CRP) and haptoglobin (HP) [70–100]. In insulin-resistant HepG2 cells, the anti-inflammatory activity of berberine was associated with its insulin-sensitizing effect. Berberine administration significantly decreased cytokine production, and reduced serine phosphorylation but increased insulin-mediated tyrosine phosphorylation of IRS in HepG2 cells treated with palmitate [71].

Berberine could reduce proinflammatory cytokines, acute phase protein and infiltration of inflammatory cells in animals with diabetes mellitus or insulin resistance, either induced by streptozocin injection/high-fat diet (HFD) feeding or spontaneously happened [69, 72, 74–76]. In these animal models, the anti-inflammatory activity of berberine was observed in different tissues like serum, liver, adipose tissue, and kidney and was associated with its effect against insulin resistance or diabetes mellitus [69, 72, 74–76]. Besides evidences from cultured cells and diabetic animal models, the anti-inflammatory effect of berberine was also observed in humans: the berberine dose of 1 g/day for 3 months significantly reduced the serum hsCRP and IL-6 level in patients with acute coronary syndrome following percutaneous coronary intervention [80].

Berberine suppresses inflammation through complex mechanisms. In addition to antioxidant activity, the AMPK pathway was also crucial for the anti-inflammatory efficacy of berberine [72]. Blocking AMPK could abolish the inhibitory effect of berberine on the production of proinflammatory cytokines, like inducible nitric oxide synthase (iNOS) and COX2 in macrophages [72]. Excessive iNOS in cells could cause overproduction of NO and had close relationship with the development of insulin resistance [82]. COX2 is a key enzyme for the synthesis of prostaglandins [81], which are important mediators for the pathogenesis of diabetes mellitus and diabetic nephropathy [82].

The anti-inflammatory activity of berberine was also associated with its inhibitory effect on the mitogen-activated protein kinase (MAPK) signalling pathways, which were activated by inflammatory stimuli [72, 83, 84]. The inhibitory effect of berberine on MAPKs was dependent on AMPK activation in macrophages [72]. It seems that conflicting results exist concerning the regulatory effect of berberine on MAPK signalling. Although some results suggested that berberine suppressed the inflammation through inhibiting MAPKs [72, 83, 84], others indicated that p38 kinase was activated by berberine which was considered important for berberine's efficacy against oxidative stress and inflammation [65–67].

The NF-κB pathway plays a key role in controlling inflammation [85]. In NF-κB signalling pathway, IκB kinase-β (IKK-β) could be activated by inflammatory stimuli like TNF-α, as well as nutritional factors like glucose and FFA [86]. The activation of IKK-β required phosphorylation of the serine residue at position 181

[87, 88]. In insulin-resistant 3T3-L1 adipocytes [89] and liver/adipose tissues from obese mice feed with HFD [74], berberine administration greatly reduced phosphorylation of ser^{181} and activation of IKK-β. In addition, the inhibitory effect of berberine on IKK-β required a cysteine residue at position 179 of IKK-β [89].

Recent studies proved that berberine could reduce renal inflammation in diabetic rats through inhibiting the Rho GTPase signalling pathway [69]. Rho GTPase is a member of the superfamily of small GTP binding proteins with multiple biological functions [90]; it was proven to positively regulate the NF-κB signalling pathway in diabetic rats [91]. Therefore, in addition to regulation of the classic NF-κB signalling pathway, berberine could inhibit NF-κB by suppressing Rho GTPase [69, 92]. Furthermore, the inhibitory effect of berberine on Rho GTPase relied on its antioxidant activity [69].

In addition to NF-κB, transcription factor activator protein 1 (AP-1) also played a role in the anti-inflammatory activity of berberine [93, 94]. Administration of berberine to macrophages or epithelial cells greatly attenuated the DNA binding activity of AP-1 and reduced the production of cytokines like MCP-1 and COX2 [93]. There were reports that the transcription stimulating activity of AP-1 and NF-κB could be inhibited by activation of peroxisome proliferator-activated receptor γ (PPARγ) [95–99].

2.1.2.1 Berberine Effects on Glucose Metabolism

In general, there are two distinct pathways to activate glucose uptake in peripheral tissues; one stimulated by insulin through the IRS-1/PI 3-kinase and the other by exercise or hypoxia via activation of AMP activated protein kinase (AMPK). In muscle, which is the major tissue responsible for whole body glucose disposal after liver, both pathways stimulate the translocation of glucose transporter-4 (GLUT4) to the cell membrane which accounts for the enhanced glucose uptake [100].

Current data suggest that the berberine effects are complex and may activate portions of both the insulin and the exercise-induced glucose uptake pathways [101]. In addition, berberine inhibits intestinal absorption of glucose, which also contributes to berberine glucose-lowering effect [102].

There is increasing evidence that the most widely expressed GLUT1, initially thought to be responsible only for basal glucose uptake, can be acutely activated by cell stressors such as azide [103, 104], osmotic stress [105, 106], methylene blue [107] and glucose deprivation [108, 109]. In particular, the acute activation of GLUT1 by hypoxia or azide has been attributed to activation of AMPK [110, 111]. In addition, it has been recently shown that peptide C activates GLUT1 transport activity in erythrocytes, establishing a potential link between GLUT1 activity and diabetes [112].

In cultured human liver cells and rat skeletal muscle, berberine increases insulin receptor mRNA expression through Protein kinase C-dependent activation of its promoter [113].

Since berberine was observed to act as an insulin-sensitizing agent in cultured cells [114], its activity has been compared with that of metformin in different animal models. In rat models of type 2 diabetes (T2DM), berberine shows to have equal or better fasting plasma glucose (FPG), insulin-resistance and low-density lipoprotein cholesterol (LDL-C) lowering activity than metformin by a mechanism involving retinol binding protein-4 (RBP-4) and (GLUT-4) [115, 116].

Berberine exhibited a high hypoglycemic potential; it has been shown that berberine activates AMPK with subsequent induction of glycolysis [117]. AMPK, as an intracellular energy receptor, has attracted more attention and become a new target for the treatment of diabetes and its cardiovascular complications due to its regulatory effect on endothelial cell function and energy homeostasis. In H9c2 myoblast cell line treated with insulin to induce insulin resistance, berberine attenuated the reduction in glucose consumption and glucose uptake at least in part via stimulation of AMPK activity [118]. berberine enhanced acute insulin-mediated GLUT4 translocation and glucose transport in insulin-resistant myotubes through activation of AMPK and PI3K pathway [119] (Fig. 2.2).

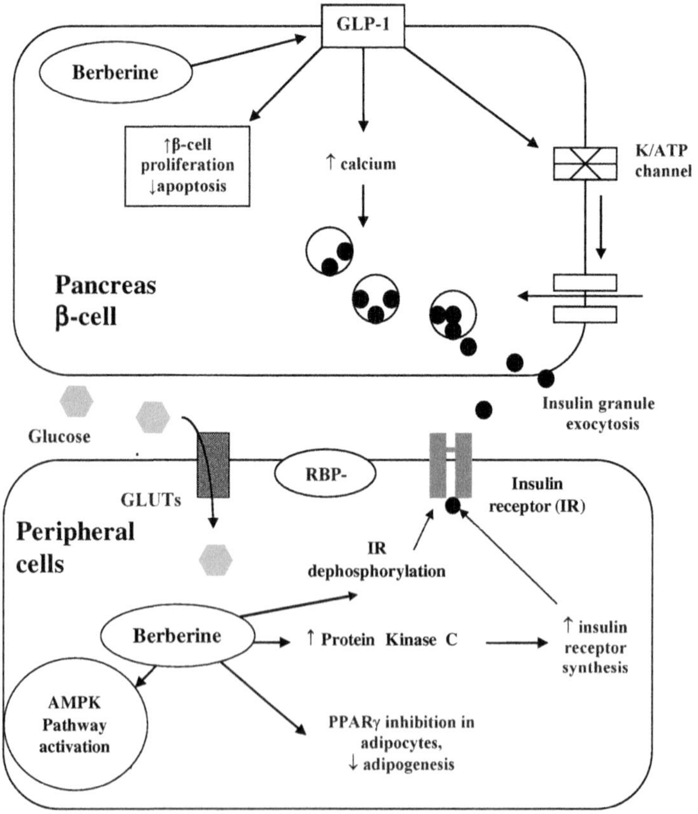

Fig. 2.2 Main glucose-lowering effects of berberine in the human cells. Berberine administration could decrease glycemia through the GLP-1 receptor activation in pancreas beta cells, the increase of Insulin Receptor expression and the AMPK-modulated Glut-4 translocation in peripheral cells

In a clinical study, the same group observed that berberine significantly lowered FPG, hemoglobin A1c, triglycerides and insulin levels in patients with T2DM as well as metformin and rosiglitazone (a combination commonly used for the T2DM therapy); the percentages of peripheral blood lymphocytes expressing InsR were significantly elevated after therapy [120].

In a recent meta-analysis of randomized clinical trials, berberine resulted to be safe and effective in the treatment of patients with T2DM [121].

2.1.2.2 Berberine Effects on Lipid Metabolism and Vascular Health

The cholesterol and triglycerides lowering effect of berberine has been clearly demonstrated by a recent meta-analysis of randomized clinical trials [122]. The lipid-lowering activity of berberine, in association with other nutraceuticals, has been also clearly confirmed in a relatively large number of randomized clinical trials [123, 124].

The supposed mechanism of action is the increased expression of the liver receptor for LDL mediated by the inhibition of the Pro-protein-convertase-subtilisin-kexin-9 (PCSK9) activity [125]. Besides its upregulation effect on the LDL receptor, berberine could also reduce triglycerides by AMP kinase activation and MAPK/ERK pathway blocking [126] (Fig. 2.3).

High levels of LDL and their oxidized counterpart, oxidized LDL (oxLDL), in the blood vessels represent a major risk factor for endothelial dysfunction and atherosclerosis [127]. Inactivity of LDL receptor (LDLR) or its low-level expression initiates accumulation of LDL in blood vessels [128]. On the other hand, the receptor of oxLDL, lectin-like oxidized low-density lipoprotein receptor-1 (LOX-1) identified as the main endothelial receptor for oxLDL also present in macrophages and smooth muscle cells (SMC), activates a proatherogenic cascade by inducing endothelial dysfunction, SMC proliferation, apoptosis and the transformation of macrophages into foam cells and platelet activation via NF-κB activation [129]. LOX-1 contains a lectin-like extracellular C-terminal domain which interacts with oxLDL, proteolytically cleaved and released as a soluble circulating form (sLOX-1) that reflects the increased expression of membrane-bound receptors and disease activities [130].

In human macrophage-derived foam cells treated with oxLDL, berberine inhibits the expression of LOX-1 [131] as well as the oxLDL uptake of macrophages and reduces foam cell formation in a dose-dependent manner [132] by activating the AMPK-SIRT1-PPARγ pathway [133]. Chi and colleagues demonstrated that berberine combined with atorvastatin is more effective in diminishing LOX 1 expression than atorvastatin alone in monocyte-derived macrophages both in vitro and in rats through modulation of endothelin-1 receptor [134].

Berberine improves also the survival of TNFα-treated endothelial progenitor cells (EPCs) via the activation of PI3K/AKT/eNOS transcription factor [135] possibly through AMPK activation. Wu and colleagues showed, both in vitro and in vivo that berberine reduces the leukocyte-endothelium adhesion and vascular cell

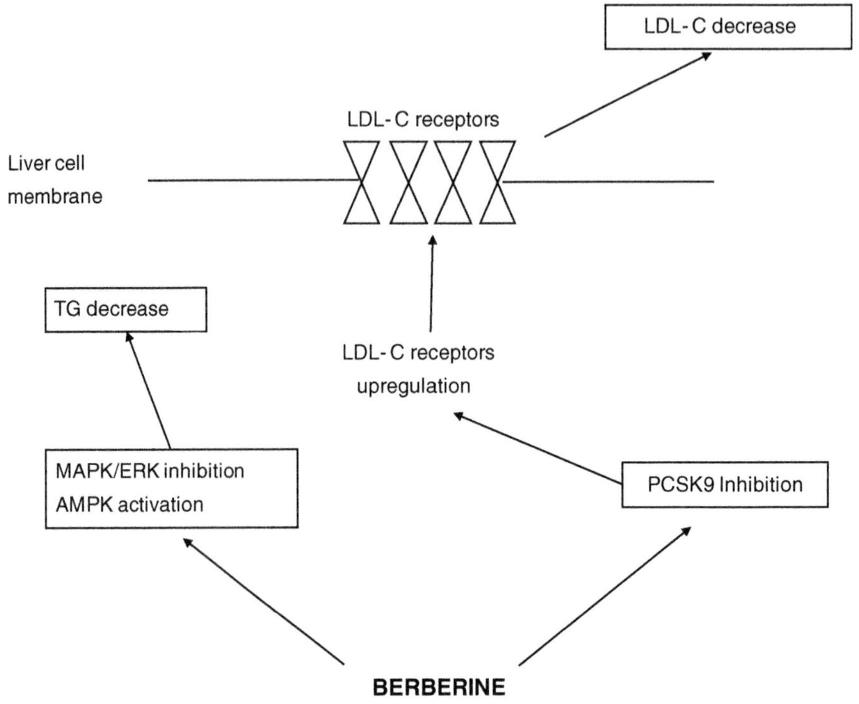

Fig. 2.3 Main lipid-lowering effects of berberine in the human liver cells. Berberine mainly decreases circulating LDLs by inducing LDLR expression in hepatic cells mediated by inhibition of PCSK9

adhesion molecule-1 (VCAM-1) expression induced by LPS. Berberine was further confirmed to inhibit the nuclear translocation and DNA binding activity of LPS-activated NF-κB signalling pathway [136].

2.1.2.3 Berberine and Central Nervous System Disorders

A large number of preclinical evidence support a possible role of berberine in the management of Alzheimer's disease, cerebral ischemia, mental depression, schizophrenia and anxiety, however the most part of these data have been obtained in purely experimental models [137]. Of particular interest is the potential antidepressant effect of berberine.

Berberine inhibited the immobility period in mice in both forced swim and tail-suspension test, two animal models of depression, in a dose independent manner [138, 139]. Among the reported bioactivities of berberine, there is the inhibition of monoamino oxidase (MAO)-A activity, [140] an enzyme catalyzing the oxidative deamination of catecholamines, and thus inhibiting degradation of these neurotransmitters. In fact acute and chronic administration of berberine in mice resulted in increased levels of norepinephrine, serotonin and dopamine, neurotransmitters induced by MAO-A enzyme [140]. In accordance with Kulkarni and colleagues data, Arora and Chopra [138] showed the protective antidepressant-like effect of berberine against the reserpine-induced biogenic amine depletion (a monoamine depletor commonly used to induce depression in animals. However, at the best of our knowledge, there are no available data on the evaluation of the potential antidepressant effects of berberine in humans [141].

2.1.2.4 Tolerability and Safety

Highly purified and concentrated berberine is safe, in fact, its Lethal Dose 50 (LD50) in mice is 25 mg/kg in mice [131].

Standard doses of berberine are usually well tolerated and adverse events are rare and mild. The most studied side effects are those on the gastrointestinal system. In fact, berberine and its derivatives can produce gastric lesions in animal models [142]. As shown by the determination of small intestinal transit time measurements by sorbitol and breath hydrogen test, berberine delays small intestinal transit time, and this may account for a part of its gastrointestinal side effects (but also of its antidiarrhoeal one) [143].

The main safety issue of berberine involves the risk of pharmacological interactions. In fact, berberine displaces bilirubin from albumin about tenfold more than phenylbutazone, thus any herb containing large amounts of berberine should be avoided in jaundiced infants and pregnant women [144]. Berberine also displaces warfarin, thiopental and tolbutamide from their protein binding sites, increasing their plasma levels [145].

Then, berberine can markedly increase blood levels of cyclosporine A because of CYP3A4 and P-glycoprotein inhibition in liver and gut wall, respectively, and because of the increase in gastric emptying time, thus causing increased cyclosporine A bioavailability and reduced metabolism [146]. In renal transplant recipients who take cyclosporine 3 mg/kg twice daily, the coadministration of berberine (0.2 g/day for three times a day for 3 months) increased the mean cyclosporine A AUC of 34.5 % and its mean half-life of 2.7 h [147].

Even if the main mechanism of berberine pharmacological interaction involves CYP3A4 and intestinal P-glycoprotein, it also inhibits CYP1A1, potentially interacting with drugs metabolized by this cytochrome isophorm as well. The impact of this observation in clinical practise has yet to be evaluated since the CYP1A1 metabolized drugs are relatively rare [148].

Overall, the assumption of berberine in dosages of 500–1000 mg/day has to be considered safe for the most part of subjects and the risk of clinically relevant pharmacological interaction is limited to cyclosporine and warfarin.

2.2 Conclusion

Berberine is a natural alkaloid with proven antioxidant, anti-inflammatory, glucose-lowering and lipid-lowering actions, both in animal models and in humans. Altogether, these effects support the need to study the effects of the long-term exposition to berberine for the management and prevention of numerous chronic diseases such as type 2 diabetes and atherosclerosis.

References

1. Banegas JR, López-García E, Dallongeville J et al (2011) Achievement of treatment goals for primary prevention of cardiovascular disease in clinical practice across Europe: the EURIKA study. Eur Heart J 32:2143–2152
2. Saha S, Gerdtham UG, Johansson P (2010) Economic evaluation of lifestyle interventions for preventing diabetes and cardiovascular diseases. Int J Environ Res Public Health 7:3150–3195
3. King DE, Mainous AG, Matheson EM, Everett CJ (2013) Impact of healthy lifestyle on mortality in people with normal blood pressure, LDL cholesterol, and C-reactive protein. Eur J Cardiovasc Prev Rehabil 20(1):73–79
4. Cicero AF, Derosa G, D'angelo A et al (2009) Gender-specific haemodynamic and metabolic effects of a sequential training programme on overweight-obese hypertensives. Blood Press 18:111–116
5. Cicero AF, Ertek S (2008) Natural sources of antidyslipidaemic agents: is there an evidence-based approach for their prescription? Med J Nutr Metab 2:85–93
6. NCEP Expert Panel (2001) Expert Panel on detection, evaluation and treatment of high blood cholesterol in adults. Executive summary of the third report of the National Cholesterol Education Program (NCEP) (Adult Treatment Panel III). J Am Med Assoc 285:2486–2497
7. Catapano AL, Reiner Z, De Backer G et al (2011) European Society of Cardiology (ESC); European Atherosclerosis Society (EAS). ESC/EAS Guidelines for the management of dyslipidaemias The Task Force for the management of dyslipidaemias of the European Society of Cardiology (ESC) and the European Atherosclerosis Society (EAS). Atherosclerosis 217:3–46
8. Hasani-Ranjbar S, Nayebi N, Moradi L et al (2010) The efficacy and safety of herbal medicines used in the treatment of hyperlipidemia: a systematic review. Curr Pharm Res 16:2935–2947
9. McGowan MP, Proulx S (2009) Nutritional supplements and serum lipids: does anything work? Curr Atheroscler Rep 11:470–476
10. Kim JY, Kwon O (2011) Culinary plants and their potential impact on metabolic overload. Ann NY Acad Sci 1229:133–139
11. Xia X, Weng J (2010) Targeting metabolic syndrome: candidate natural agents. J Diabetes 2:243–249
12. Birdsall TC, Kelly GS (1997) Berberine: therapeutic potential of an alkaloid found in several medicinal plants. Altern Med Rev 2:94–103
13. Vuddanda PR, Chakraborty S, Singh S (2010) Berberine: a potential phytochemical with multispectrum therapeutic activities. Expert Opin Investig Drugs 19:1297–1307
14. Souri E, Dehmobed-Sharifabadi A, Nazifia A, Farsam H (2004) Antioxidant activity of sixty plants from Iran. Iran J Pharm Res 13:55–59
15. Chevallier A (2001) The encyclopedia of medicinal plants. Dorling Kindersley, St Leonards, pp 234–237

16. Timothy CBN, Gregory S, Kelly ND (1997) Berberine: therapeutic potential of an alkaloid found in several medicinal plants. Altern Med Rev 13:94–103
17. Kunwar RM, Nepal BK, Kshhetri HB et al (2006) Ethnomedicine in Himalaya: a case study from Dolpa, Humla, Jumla and Mustang districts of Nepal. J Ethnobiol Ethnomed 13:27
18. Fatehi-Hassanabad Z, Jafarzadeh M, Tarhini A, Fatehi M (2005) The antihypertensive and vasodilator effects of aqueous extract from *Berberis vulgaris* fruit on hypertensive rats. Phytother Res 13(3):222–225
19. Ivanovska N, Philipov S (1996) Study on the anti-inflammatory action of *Berberis vulgaris* root extract, alkaloid fractions and pure alkaloids. Int J Immunopharmacol 13(10):553–561
20. Imanshahidi M, Hosseinzadeh H (2008) Pharmacological and therapeutic effects of Berberis vulgaris and its active constituent, Berberine. Phytother Res 13:999–1012
21. Mills S, Bone K (2000) Principals and practice of phytotherapy. Churchill Livingstone, Edinburgh, pp 338–341
22. Bone K (2003) A clinical guide to blending liquid herbs: herbal formulations for the individual patient. Churchill Livingstone, St Louis, pp 422–429
23. Khosrokhavar R, Ahmadiani AS (2010) Antihistaminic and anticholinergic activity of methanolic extract of barberry fruit (*Berberis vulgaris*) in the Guinea-Pig Ileum. J Med Plants 13:99–105
24. Akhter MH, Sabir M, Bhide NK (1979) Possible mechanism of antidiarrheal effect of berberine. Indian J Med Res 13:233–241
25. Rabbani GHBT, Knight J, Sanyal SC, Alam K (1987) Randomized controlled trial of berberine sulfate therapy for diarrhea due to enterotoxigenic *Escherichia coli* and *Vibrio cholera*. J Infect Dis 13:979–984
26. Amin AH, Subbaiah TV, Abbasi KM (1969) Berberine sulfate: antimidrobial activity, bioassay, and mode of action. Can J Microbiol 13:1067–1076
27. Sabir M (1971) Study of some pharmacological actions of berberine. Indian J Physiol Pharmacol 13:111–132
28. Pan GY, Wang GJ, Liu XD, Fawcett JP, Xie YY (2002) The involvement of P-glycoprotein in berberine absorption. Pharmacol Toxicol 91:193–197
29. Tsai PL, Tsai TH (2003) Hepatobiliary excretion of berberine. Drug Metab Dispos 32:405–412
30. Zuo F, Nakamura N, Akao T, Hattori M (2006) Pharmacokinetics of berberine and its main metabolites in conventional and pseudo germ-free rats determined by liquid chromatography/ion trap mass spectrometry. Drug Metab Dispos 34:2064–2072
31. Chen CM, Chang HC (1995) Determination of berberine in plasma, urine and bile by high performance liquid chromatograpy. J Chromatogr 665:117–123
32. Raner GM, Cornelious S, Moulick K et al (2007) Effects of herbal products on human cytochrome P450(2E1) activity. Food Chem Tox 45:2359–2365
33. Zhao X, Zhang JJ, Wang X et al (2008) Effect of berberine on hepatocyte proliferation inducible nitric oxide synthase expression, cytochrome 450 2E1 and 1A2 activities in diethylnitrosamine- and Phenobarbital-treated rats. Biomed Pharmacother 62:567–572
34. Furukawa S, Fujita T, Shimabukuro M et al (2004) Increased oxidative stress in obesity and its impact on metabolic syndrome. J Clin Investig 114(12):1752–1761
35. Bonnefont-Rousselot D (2002) Glucose and reactive oxygen species. Curr Opin Clin Nutr Metab Care 5(5):561–568
36. Alberici LC, Vercesi AE, Oliveira HC (2011) Mitochondrial energy metabolism and redox responses to hypertriglyceridemia. J Bioenerg Biomembr 43(1):19–23
37. Rösen P, Nawroth PP, King G et al (2001) The role of oxidative stress in the onset and progression of diabetes and its complications: a summary of a congress series sponsored by UNESCO-MCBN, the American diabetes association and the German diabetes society. Diab Metab Res Rev 17(3):189–212
38. Evans JL, Goldfine ID, Maddux BA, Grodsky GM (2003) Are oxidative stress—activated signaling pathways mediators of insulin resistance and β-cell dysfunction? Diabetes 52(1):1–8

39. Kaneto H, Xu G, Fujii N, Bonner-Weir S, Weir GC (2002) Involvement of c-Jun N-terminal kinase in oxidative stress-mediated suppression of insulin gene expression. J Biol Chem 277 (33):30010–30018
40. Scivittaro V, Ganz MB, Weiss MF (2000) AGEs induce oxidative stress and activate protein kinase C-β(II) in neonatal mesangial cells. Am J Physiol 278(4):F676–F683
41. Goldin A, Beckman JA, Schmidt AM, Creager MA (2006) Advanced glycation end products: sparking the development of diabetic vascular injury. Circulation 114(6):597–605
42. Frey RS, Ushio-Fukai M, Malik AB (2009) NADPH oxidase-dependent signaling in endothelial cells role in physiology and pathophysiology. Antioxid Redox Signal 11:791–810
43. Furukawa S, Fujita T, Shimabukuro M et al (2004) Increased oxidative stress in obesity and its impact on metabolic syndrome. J Clin Investig 114:1752–1761
44. Maiese K (2015) New insights for oxidative stress and diabetes mellitus. Oxid Med Cell Longev 2015:875961
45. Wu XD, Liu WL, Zeng K et al (2014) Advanced glycation end products activate the miRNA/RhoA/ROCK2 pathway in endothelial cells. Microcirculation 21(2):178–186
46. Cheng F, Wang Y, Li J et al (2013) Berberine improves endothelial function by reducing endothelial microparticles-mediated oxidative stress in humans. Int J Cardiol 167:936–942
47. Sarna LK, Wu N, Hwang SY, Siow YL, O K (2010) Berberine inhibits NADPH oxidase mediated superoxide anion production in macrophages. Can J Physiol Pharmacol 88:369–378
48. Hsieh S, Kuo WH, Lin TW et al (2007) Protective effects of berberine against low-density lipoprotein (LDL) oxidation and oxidized LDL-induced cytotoxicity on endothelial cells. J Agric Food Chem 55:10437–10445
49. Kim JE, Kim YW, Lee IK et al (2008) AMP-activated protein kinase activation by 5-aminoimidazole-4-carboxamide-1-β-D-ribofuranoside (AICAR) inhibits palmitate-induced endothelial cell apoptosis through reactive oxygen species suppression. J Pharmacol Sci 106:394–403
50. Wang S, Zhang M, Liang B et al (2010) AMPKα2 deletion causes aberrant expression and activation of NAD(P)H oxidase and consequent endothelial dysfunction in vivo: role of 26S proteasomes. Circ Res 106:1117–1128
51. Ceolotto G, Gallo A, Papparella I et al (2007) Rosiglitazone reduces glucose-induced oxidative stress mediated by NAD(P)H oxidase via AMPK-dependent mechanism. Arterioscler Thromb Vasc Biol 27:2627–2633
52. Lee KH, Lo HL, Tang WC et al (2014) A gene expression signature-based approach reveals the mechanisms of action of the Chinese herbal medicine berberine. Sci Rep 4:6394
53. Turner N, Li JY, Gosby A, To SW, Cheng Z, Miyoshi H et al (2008) Berberine and its more biologically available derivative, dihydroberberine, inhibit mitochondrial respiratory complex I: a mechanism for the action of berberine to activate AMP-activated protein kinase and improve insulin action. Diabetes 57(5):1414–1418
54. Li Z, Geng YN, Jiang JD, Kong WJ (2014) Antioxidant and anti-inflammatory activities of berberine in the treatment of diabetes mellitus. Evid Based Complement Alternat Med 2014:289264
55. Morrow VA, Foufelle F, Connell JM et al (2003) Direct activation of AMP-activated protein kinase stimulates nitric-oxide synthesis in human aortic endothelial cells. J Biol Chem 278:31629–31639
56. Zhang ZM, Jiang B, Zheng XX (2005) Effect of l-tetrahydropalmatine on expression of adhesion molecules induced by lipopolysaccharides in human umbilical vein endothelium cell. Zhongguo Zhong Yao Za Zhi 30(11):861–864
57. Wang Y, Huang Y, Lam KS et al (2009) Berberine prevents hyperglycemia-induced endothelial injury and enhances vasodilatation via adenosine monophosphate-activated protein kinase and endothelial nitric oxide synthase. Cardiovasc Res 82(3):484–492
58. Kukidome D, Nishikawa T, Sonoda K et al (2006) Activation of AMP-activated protein kinase reduces hyperglycemia-induced mitochondrial reactive oxygen species production and

promotes mitochondrial biogenesis in human umbilical vein endothelial cells. Diabetes 55:120–127
59. Xie Z, Zhang J, Wu J, Viollet B, Zou MH (2008) Upregulation of mitochondrial uncoupling protein-2 by the AMP-activated protein kinase in endothelial cells attenuates oxidative stress in diabetes. Diabetes 57(12):3222–3230
60. Chatuphonprasert W, Lao-ong T, Jarukamjorn K (2013) Improvement of superoxide dismutase and catalase in streptozotocin-nicotinamide-induced type 2-diabetes in mice by berberine and glibenclamide. Pharm Biol (Epub ahead of print). doi:10.3109/13880209.2013.839714
61. Lao-ong T, Chatuphonprasert W, Nemoto N, Jarukamjorn K (2012) Alteration of hepatic glutathione peroxidase and superoxide dismutase expression in streptozotocin-induced diabetic mice by berberine. Pharm Biol 50(8):1007–1012
62. Ceballos-Picot I, Witko-Sarsat V, Merad-Boudia M et al (1996) Glutathione antioxidant system as a marker of oxidative stress in chronic renal failure. Free Radic Biol Med 21:845–853
63. Abd El-Wahab AE, Ghareeb DA, Sarhan EE et al (2013) In vitro biological assessment of *Berberis vulgaris* and its active constituent, berberine: antioxidants, anti-acetylcholinesterase, anti-diabetic and anticancer effects. BMC Complement Altern Med 13:218
64. Hsu YY, Chen CS, Wu SN, Jong YJ, Lo YC (2012) Berberine activates Nrf2 nuclear translocation and protects against oxidative damage via a phosphatidylinositol 3-kinase/Akt-dependent mechanism in NSC34 motor neuron-like cells. Eur J Pharm Sci 46:415–425
65. Mo C, Wang L, Zhang J et al (2014) The crosstalk between Nrf2 and AMPK signal pathways is important for the anti-inflammatory effect of berberine in LPS-stimulated macrophages and endotoxin-shocked mice. Antioxid Redox Signal 20(4):574–588
66. Hsu YY, Tseng YT, Lo YC (2013) Berberine, a natural antidiabetes drug, attenuates glucose neurotoxicity and promotes Nrf2-related neurite outgrowth. Toxicol Appl Pharmacol 272(3):787–796
67. Bae J, Lee D, Kim YK et al (2013) Berberine protects 6-hydroxydopamine-induced human dopaminergic neuronal cell death through the induction of heme oxygenase-1. Mol Cells 35(2):151–157
68. Vomhof-Dekrey EE, PickloSr MJ (2012) The Nrf2-antioxidant response element pathway: a target for regulating energy metabolism. J Nutr Biochem 23(10):1201–1206
69. Xie X, Chang X, Chen L et al (2013) Berberine ameliorates experimental diabetes-induced renal inflammation and fibronectin by inhibiting the activation of RhoA/ROCK signaling. Mol Cell Endocrinol 381(1–2):56–65
70. Choi B-H, Ahn I-S, Kim Y-H et al (2006) Berberine reduces the expression of adipogenic enzymes and inflammatory molecules of 3T3-L1 adipocyte. ExpMol Med 38(6):599–605
71. Lou T, Zhang Z, Xi Z et al (2011) Berberine inhibits inflammatory response and ameliorates insulin resistance in hepatocytes. Inflammation 34(6):659–667
72. Jeong HW, Hsu KC, Lee JW et al (2009) Berberine suppresses proinflammatory responses through AMPK activation in macrophages. Am J Physiol Endocrinol Metab 296(4):E955–E964
73. Lin W-C, Lin JY (2011) Five bitter compounds display different anti-inflammatory effects through modulating cytokine secretion using mouse primary splenocytes in vitro. J Agric Food Chem 59(1):184–192
74. Shang W, Liu J, Yu X, Zhao J (2010) Effects of berberine on serum levels of inflammatory factors and inflammatory signaling pathway in obese mice induced by high fat diet. Zhongguo Zhong Yao Za Zhi 35(11):1474–1477
75. Chen Y, Wang Y, Zhang J, Sun C, Lopez A (2011) Berberine improves glucose homeostasis in streptozotocin-induced diabetic rats in association with multiple factors of insulin resistance. ISRN Endocrinol 2011:519371

76. Xing L-J, Zhang L, Liu T (2011) Berberine reducing insulin resistance by up-regulating IRS-2 mRNA expression in nonalcoholic fatty liver disease (NAFLD) rat liver. Eur J Pharmacol 668(3):467–471
77. Cui G, Qin X, Zhang Y et al (2009) Berberine differentially modulates the activities of ERK, p 38 MAPK, and JNK to suppress Th17 and Th1 T cell differentiation in type 1 diabetic mice. J Biol Chem 284(41):28420–28429
78. Chueh WH, Lin JY (2012) Protective effect of isoquinoline alkaloid berberine on spontaneous inflammation in the spleen, liver and kidney of non-obese diabetic mice through downregulating gene expression ratios of pro-/anti-inflammatory and Th1/Th2 cytokines. Food Chem 131(4):1263–1271
79. Zhang Y, Li X, Zou D et al (2008) Treatment of type 2 diabetes and dyslipidemia with the natural plant alkaloid berberine. J Clin Endocrinol Metab 93(7):2559–2565
80. Meng S, Wang LS, Huang ZQ et al (2012) Berberine ameliorates inflammation in patients with acute coronary syndrome following percutaneous coronary intervention. Clin Exp Pharmacol Physiol 39(5):406–411
81. Dubois RN, Abramson SB, Crofford L (1998) Cyclooxygenase in biology and disease. FASEB J 12(12):1063–1073
82. Mima A (2013) Inflammation and oxidative stress in diabetic nephropathy: new insights on its inhibition as new therapeutic targets. J Diab Res 2013:248563
83. Lee D, Bae J, Kim YK et al (2013) Inhibitory effects of berberine on lipopolysaccharide-induced inducible nitric oxide synthase and the high-mobility group box 1 release in macrophages. Biochem Biophys Res Commun 431(3):506–511
84. Zhou Y, Liu SQ, Yu L et al (2015) Berberine prevents nitric oxide-induced rat chondrocyte apoptosis and cartilage degeneration in a rat osteoarthritis model via AMPK and p38 MAPK signaling. Apoptosis 20(9):1187–1199
85. Gratas-Delamarche A, Derbré F, Vincent S, Cillard J (2014) Physical inactivity, insulin resistance, and the oxidative-inflammatory loop. Free Rad Res 48(1):93–108
86. Solinas G, Karin M (2010) JNK1 and IKKbeta: molecular links between obesity and metabolic dysfunction. FASEB J 24(8):2596–2611
87. Karin M (1999) Positive and negative regulation of IκB kinase activity through IKKβ subunit phosphorylation. Science 284(5412):309–313
88. Yi P, Lu FE, Xu LJ et al (2008) Berberine reverses free-fatty-acid-induced insulin resistance in 3T3-L1 adipocytes through targeting IKKβ. World J Gastroenterol 14(6):876–883
89. Pandey MK, Sung B, Kunnumakkara AB et al (2008) Berberine modifies cysteine 179 of IκBα kinase, suppresses nuclear factor-κB-regulated antiapoptotic gene products, and potentiates apoptosis. Cancer Res 68(13):5370–5379
90. Shi J, Wei L (2013) Rho kinases in cardiovascular physiology and pathophysiology: the effect of fasudil. J Cardiovasc Pharmacol 62(4):341–354
91. Xie X, Peng J, Chang X et al (2013) Activation of RhoA/ROCK regulates NF-κB signaling pathway in experimental diabetic nephropathy. Mol Cell Endocrinol 369(1–2):86–97
92. Remppis A, Bea F, Greten HJ et al (2010) Rhizoma Coptidis inhibits LPS-induced MCP-1/CCL2 production in murine macrophages via an AP-1 and NFκB-dependent pathway. Mediat Inflamm 2010:194896
93. Kuo CL, Chi CW, Liu TY (2004) The anti-inflammatory potential of berberine in vitro and in vivo. Cancer Lett 203(2):127–137
94. Schonthaler HB, Guinea-Viniegra J, Wagner EF (2011) Targeting inflammation by modulating the Jun/AP-1 pathway. Ann Rheum Dis 70(1):i109–i112
95. Ricote M, Li AC, Willson TM et al (1998) The peroxisome proliferator-activated receptor-γ is a negative regulator of macrophage activation. Nature 391(6662):79–82
96. Delerive P, Martin-Nizard F, Chinetti G et al (1999) Peroxisome proliferator-activated receptor activators inhibit thrombin-induced endothelin-1 production in human vascular endothelial cells by inhibiting the activator protein-1 signaling pathway. Circ Res 85(5):394–402

97. Pasceri V, Wu HD, Willerson JT, Yeh ETH (2000) Modulation of vascular inflammation in vitro and in vivo by peroxisome proliferator-activated receptor-γ activators. Circulation 101(3):235–238
98. Chen FL, Yang ZH, Liu Y et al (2008) Berberine inhibits the expression of TNFα, MCP-1, and IL-6 in AcLDL-stimulated macrophages through PPARγ pathway. Endocrine 33(3):331–337
99. Feng AW, Gao W, Zhou GR et al (2012) Berberine ameliorates COX-2 expression in rat small intestinal mucosa partially through PPARγ pathway during acute endotoxemia. Int Immunopharmacol 12(1):182–188
100. Krook A, Wallberg-Henriksson H, Zierath JR (2004) Sending the signal: molecular mechanisms regulating glucose uptake. Med Sci Sports Exerc 36:1212–1217
101. Kim SH, Shin EJ, Kim ED (2007) Berberine activates GLUT1-mediated glucose uptake in 3T3-L1 adipocytes. Biol Pharm Bull 30:2120–2125
102. Pan GY, Huang ZJ, Wang GJ et al (2003) The antihyperglycaemic activity of berberine arises from a decrease of glucose absorption. Planta Med 69:632–636
103. Shetty M, Loeb JN, Vikstrom K, Ismail-Beigi F (1993) Rapid activation of GLUT-1 glucose transporter following inhibition of oxidative phosphorylation in clone 9 cells. J Biol Chem 268:17225–17232
104. Rubin D, Ismail-Beigi F (2003) Distribution of Glutl in detergent-resistant membranes (DRMs) and non-DRM domains: effect of treatment with azide. Am J Physiol Cell Physiol 285:C377–C383
105. Barnes K, Ingram JC, Porras OH et al (2002) Activation of GLUT1 by metabolic and osmotic stress: potential involvement of AMP-activated protein kinase (AMPK). J Cell Sci 115:2433–2442
106. Barros LF, Barnes K, Ingram JC et al (2001) Hyperosmotic shock induces both activation and translocation of glucose transporters in mammalian cells. Pflugers Arch 442:614–621
107. Louters LL, Dyste SG, Frieswyk D et al (2006) Methylene blue stimulates 2-deoxyglucose uptake in L929 fibroblast cells. Life Sci 78:586–591
108. Kumar A, Xiao YP, Laipis PJ (2004) Glucose deprivation enhances targeting of GLUT1 to lipid rafts in 3T3-L1 adipocytes. Am J Physiol Endocrinol Metab 286:E568–E576
109. Roelofs B, Tidball A, Lindborg AE et al (2006) Acute activation of glucose uptake by glucose deprivation in L929 fibroblast cells. Biochimie 88:1941–1946
110. Jing M, Ismail-Beigi F (2007) Critical role of 5′-AMP-activated protein kinase in the stimulation of glucose transport in response to inhibition of oxidative phosphorylation. Am J Physiol Cell Physiol 292:C477–C487
111. Jing M, Cheruvu VK, Ismail-Beigi F (2008) Stimulation of glucose transport in response to activation of distinct AMPK signaling pathways. Am J Physiol Cell Physiol 295:C1071–C1082
112. Meyer JA, Froelich JM, Reid GE, Karunarathne WK, Spence DM (2008) Metal-activated C-peptide facilitates glucose clearance and the release of a nitric oxide stimulus via the GLUT1 transporter. Diabetologia 51:175–182
113. Kong WJ, Zhang H, Song DQ et al (2009) Berberine reduces insulin resistance through protein kinase C-dependent up-regulation of insulin receptor expression. Metabolism 58:109–119
114. Ko BS, Choi SB, Park SK et al (2005) Insulin sensitizing and insulin otropic action of berberine from *Cortidis rhizoma*. Biol Pharm Bull 28:1431–1437
115. Zhang W, Xu YC, Guo FJ, Meng Y, Li ML (2008) Antidiabetic effects of cinnamaldehyde and berberine and their impacts on retinol binding protein 4 expression in rats with type 2 diabetes mellitus. Chin Med J121:2124–2128
116. Ni WJ, Ding HH, Tang LQ (2015) Berberine as a promising anti-diabetic nephropathy drug: An analysis of its effects and mechanisms. Eur J Pharmacol 760:103–112
117. Yin J, Gao Z, Liu D, Liu Z, Ye J (2008) Berberine improves glucose metabolism through induction of glycolysis. Am J Physiol Endocrinol Metab 294:E148–E156

118. Chang W, Zhang M, Li J et al (2013) Berberine improves insulin resistance in cardiomyocytes via activation of 5′-adenosine monophosphate-activated protein kinase. Metabolism 62(8):1159–1167
119. Liu LZ, Cheung SC, Lan LL et al (2010) Berberine modulates insulin signaling transduction in insulin-resistant cells. Mol Cell Endocrinol 317(1–2):148–153
120. Zhang H, Wei J, Xue R et al (2010) Berberine lowers blood glucose in type 2 diabetes mellitus patients through increasing insulin receptor expression. Metabolism 59(2):285–292
121. Dong H, Wang N, Zhao L, Lu F (2012) Berberine in the treatment of type 2 diabetes mellitus: a systemic review and meta-analysis. Evidence-Based Complement Altern Med 2012:591654
122. Dong H, Zhao Y, Zhao L, Lu F (2013) The effects of berberine on blood lipids: a systemic review and meta-analysis of randomized controlled trials. Planta Med 79(6):437–446
123. Cicero AF, Tartagni E, Ertek S (2014) Nutraceuticals for metabolic syndrome management: from laboratory to benchside. Curr Vasc Pharmacol 12:565–571
124. Cianci A, Cicero AF, Colacurci N, Matarazzo MG, De Leo V (2012) Activity of isoflavones and berberine on vasomotor symptoms and lipid profile in menopausal women. Gynecol Endocrinol 28:699–702
125. Dong B, Li H, Singh AB, Cao A, Liu J (2015) Inhibition of PCSK9 transcription by berberine involves down-regulation of hepatic HNF1α protein expression through the ubiquitin-proteasome degradation pathway. J Biol Chem 290(7):4047–4058
126. Kong W, Wei J, Abidi P et al (2004) Berberine is a novel cholesterol-lowering drug working through a unique mechanism distinct from statins. Nat Med 10:1344–1351
127. Lubrano V, Balzan S (2014) LOX-1 and ROS, inseparable factors in the process of endothelial damage. Free Radic Res 48:841–848
128. Kong WJ, Liu J, Jiang JD (2006) Human low-density lipoprotein receptor gene and its regulation 4. J Mol Med 84:29–36
129. Cominacini L, Anselmi M, Garbin U et al (2005) Enhanced plasma levels of oxidized low-density lipoprotein increase circulating nuclear factor-kappa B activation in patients with unstable angina. J Am Coll Cardiol 46:799–806
130. Pirillo A, Catapano AL (2013) Soluble lectin-like oxidized low density lipoprotein receptor-1 as a biochemical marker for atherosclerosis-related diseases. Dis Markers 35:413–418
131. Guan S, Wang B, Li W, Guan J, Fang X (2010) Effects of berberine on expression of LOX-1 and SR-BI in human macrophage-derived foam cells induced by ox-LDL. Am J Chin Med 38:1161–1169
132. Huang Z, Dong F, Li S et al (2012) Berberine-induced inhibition of adipocyte enhancer-binding protein 1 attenuates oxidized low-density lipoprotein accumulation and foam cell formation in phorbol 12-myristate 13-acetate-induced macrophages. Eur J Pharmacol 690(1–3):164–169
133. Chi L, Peng L, Pan N, Hu X, Zhang Y (2014) The anti-atherogenic effects of berberine on foam cell formation are mediated through the upregulation of sirtuin 1. Int J Mol Med 34 (4):1087–1093
134. Chi L, Peng L, Hu X, Pan N, Zhang Y (2014) Berberine combined with atorvastatin downregulates LOX-1 expression through the ET-1 receptor in monocyte/macrophages. Int J Mol Med 34(1):283–290
135. Xiao M, Men LN, Xu MG et al (2014) Berberine protects endothelial progenitor cell from damage of TNF-α via the PI3K/AKT/eNOS signaling pathway. Eur J Pharmacol 743:11–16
136. Wu YH, Chuang SY, Hong WC et al (2012) Berberine reduces leukocyte adhesion to LPS-stimulated endothelial cells and VCAM-1 expression both in vivo and in vitro. Int J Immunopathol Pharmacol 25:741–750
137. Kulkarni SK, Dhir A (2010) Berberine: a plant alkaloid with therapeutic potential for central nervous system disorders. Phytother Res 24(3):317–324
138. Kulkarni SK, Dhir A (2008) On the mechanism of antidepressant-like action of berberine chloride. Eur J Pharmacol 589:163–172

139. Peng WH, Lo KL, Lee YH, Hung TH, Lin YC (2007) Berberine produces antidepressant-like effects in the forced swim test and in the tail suspension test in mice. Life Sci 81:933–938
140. Kong LD, Cheng CH, Tan RX (2001) Monoamine oxidase inhibitors from rhizoma of *Coptis chinensis*. Planta Med 67:74–76
141. Kumar A, Ekavali Chopra K et al (2015) Current knowledge and pharmacological profile of berberine: an update. Eur J Pharmacol 761:288–297
142. Kupeli E, Kosar M, Yesilada E, Hüsnü K, Başer C (2002) A comparative study on the anti-inflammatory, antinociceptive and antipyretic effects of isoquinoline alkaloids from the roots of Turkish berberis species. Life Sci 72:645–657
143. Chen C, Yu Z, Li Y, Fichna J, Storr M (2014) Effects of berberine in the gastrointestinal tract—a review of actions and therapeutic implications. Am J Chin Med 42(5):1053–1070
144. Chan E (1993) Displacement of bilirubin from albumin by berberine. Biol Neonat 63:201–208
145. Tan YZ, Wu AC, Tan BY et al (2002) Study on the interactions of berberine displace other drug from their plasma proteins binding sites. Chin Pharmacol Bull 18:576–578
146. Xin HW, Wu XC, Li Q et al (2006) The effects of berberine on the pharmacokinetics of cyclosporine A in healthy volunteers. Methods Find Exp Clin Pharmacol 28:25–29
147. Wu X, Lu Q, Xin H, Zhong M (2005) Effects of berberine on the blood concentration of cyclosporine A in renal transplanted recipients: clinical and pharmacokinetic study. Eur J Clin Pharmacol 61:567–572
148. Cicero AF, Tartagni E, Ertek S (2014) Safety and tolerability of injectable lipid-lowering drugs: a review of available clinical data. Expert Opin Drug Saf 13(8):1023–1030

Chapter 3
Emodin and Its Role in Chronic Diseases

B. Anu Monisha, Niraj Kumar and Ashu Bhan Tiku

Abstract Diseases, such as heart disease, stroke, cancer, respiratory diseases, and diabetes, are by far the leading cause of mortality in the world, representing 60 % of all deaths. Although substantial medical advances have been made and many therapeutic approaches proposed yet traditional medicine and medicinal plants find an important place in therapy. They have been providing invaluable solutions to the various health problems. Emodin (1,3,8-trihydroxy-6-methylanthraquinone) is a natural anthraquinone derivative found in various Chinese medicinal herbs. Traditionally, it has been used as an active constituent of many herbal laxatives. However, in the last few years, significant progress has been made in studying the biological effects of emodin at cellular and molecular levels and it is emerging as an important therapeutic agent. This review provides an overview of the modulatory effects of emodin in various diseases and cell signaling pathways, which may have important implications in its future clinical use.

Keywords Emodin · Bioavailability · Cancer · Anthraquinone · Radiosensitizer · Chemosesitizer

3.1 Introduction

Emodin is a member of natural compounds known as anthraquinones. Natural anthraquinones are found in diverse plant groups from higher plants to fungi and in some insects. More than half of the natural anthraquinones are found in lower fungi, mainly *Penicillium* and *Aspergillus* species and in lichens. Rest of them are found

B.A. Monisha
Department of Biomedical Science, Bharathidasan University,
Tiruchirappalli, Tamil Nadu 620024, India

N. Kumar · A.B. Tiku (✉)
Radiation and Cancer Therapeutics Lab, School of Life Sciences,
Jawaharlal Nehru University, New Delhi 110067, India
e-mail: abtiku@mail.jnu.ac.in

S.C. Gupta et al. (eds.), *Anti-inflammatory Nutraceuticals and Chronic Diseases*,
Advances in Experimental Medicine and Biology 928,
DOI 10.1007/978-3-319-41334-1_3

in higher plants and in isolated instances in insects [24, 131]. Among higher plants, plants belonging to families Rubiaceae, Rhamnaceae, Fabaceae, Polygonaceae, Bignoniaceae, Verbenaceae, Scrophulariaceae, and Liliaceae are rich sources of anthraquinones [134]. Emodin, rhein, chrysophanol, aloe-emodin, and physcion are the most common naturally occurring anthraquinonesin higher plants [24, 33].

The anthraquinone emodin is identified in 17 plant families distributed worldwide but is primarily reported in three plant species Fabaceae (*Cassia* spp.), Polygonaceae (*Rheum*, *Rumex,* and *Polygonum* spp.), and Rhamnaceae (*Rhamnus* and *Ventilago* spp.) [43]. Emodin (1,3,8-trihydroxy-6-methylanthraquinone) is present in bark, root, vegetative organ (stem, foliage), reproductive organ (flower, fruit, seeds, pods), and is produced as secondary metabolite by molds and lichens [120].

Although emodin was first described more than 75 years ago (reported as 'frangula-emodin,' [56], many of its diverse biological properties have been discovered in the last decade (see reviews by Srinivas et al. [120] and Shrimali et al. [117]). Emodin has also been reported to play a significant ecological role in the life of many plant species by mediating their interactions with their biotic and abiotic environment [43].

Emodin is a bioactive anthraquinone and has been an active constituent of many laxatives and Chinese herbal medicines [71, 73]. It has antitumour, antibacterial, diuretic, and vasorelaxant effects [39, 57, 175]. It induces growth inhibition in cancer cells but not in normal cells [98, 122, 162] and modulates cellular redox status in a dose- and time-dependent manner [58, 120, 163]. The photo-protective function of emodin against ultraviolet (UV) region of the solar radiation (290–400 nm) has also been reported [8]. Protective role of emodin against radiation-induced oxidative and DNA damage in murine splenocytes and in the concanavalin A (ConA)-induced hyperproliferation was also reported [109, 110]. It possesses immunosuppressive activities also [85, 142, 145]. Various pharmacological properties of emodin in both animal and human model systems have been tabulated (Tables 3.1, 3.2).

Emodin is highly effective in case of pancreatitis, asthma, myocarditis, arthritis, atherosclerosis, glomerulonephritis, Alzheimer's, hepatitis, and chronic obstructive lung disease [117, 156, 157]. It modulates various signaling pathways and produces many therapeutic effects (Table 3.3).

Besides the beneficial effects, emodin has been reported to cause some toxic side effects, such as genotoxicity, developmental toxicity, nausea, diarrhea, and renal failure. Recently, Sevcovicova et al. [108] showed emodin exhibited dual activities; on one side it was genotoxic inducing primary DNA lesions as well as gene mutations and on the other it exhibited DNA-protective activity via free radicals scavenging and reducing activities. Therefore, safety and effectiveness of emodin in naturopathic treatment is yet to be approved by the U.S. Food and Drug Administration (FDA). The present review is the compilation of the literature on effects of emodin in various disease conditions and the underlying molecular mechanisms.

Table 3.1 Therapeutic effects of emodin in animal model systems

Bioactivity	Model	Mechanism	References
Antibacterial, antiviral activity	*E.coli*, Mice, RAW 264.7 cell line	Anti-MRSA (Methicillin-resistant *Staphylococcus aureus*) effect via damaging cell membrane, affecting phospholipid membrane, and reducing the entry of CVB4 in a time-dependent manner	Alves et al. [2], Liu et al. [85], Liu et al. [86]
Anticancer effects	Mice xenografts bearing LS1034 (in vivo), SW1990 cells, Mice leukemia WEHI-3 cells, 4T1 and EO771 breast cancer cells, synthetic androgen receptor R1881cells, mice, rat, chick embryo, zebra fish, Mice bearing gall bladder carcinoma SGC-996, GBC-SD cells.	Promotes cell cycle arrest, induces apoptosis, inhibits cell proliferation, migration, differentiation, and downregulates androgen receptor Regulates the expression of NF-κB and NF-κB-regulated angiogenesis-associated factors, blocks the phosphorylation of KDR/Flk-1 and downstream effector molecules including FAK, ERK1/2, p38, Akt, endothelial nitric oxide synthase and stimulates phagocytosis and macrophage recruitment in vivo	Ljubimov et al. [87], Wang et al. [143], Kaneshiro et al. [51], Kwak et al. [60], He et al. [35], Li et al. [71, 73], Wang et al. [140, 141], Chang et al. [9], Lin et al. [78, 79], Ma et al. [91], Li et al. [68, 74, 76], Jia et al. [45]
Anti-inflammatory activity	Mouse mammary epithelial cells, rat epithelial cells, rats, mice	Inhibiting receptor expression and common inflammatory pathways, such as inhibiting NF-κB activation and TNF-α production, reducing neutrophil infiltration, and cytokine production	Li et al. [76], Zhu et al. [177], Ni et al. [100, 101], Sharma and Tiku [109], Yang et al. [161], Chen et al. [11], Han et al. [32], Li et al. [69, 70, 75, 77], Pang et al. [104]

(continued)

Table 3.1 (continued)

Bioactivity	Model	Mechanism	References
Antiallergic activity	Mice	Acts primarily on Syk to suppress downstream signaling events and mast cell activation and prevents cardiac inflammation, oxidative stress, and thrombotic complications	Lu et al. [88], Nemmar et al. [99]
Anti-hyperlipidaemic activity	C57BL/6 J male mice, rat, STZ-induced diabetic mice.	Enhances CPT-1 expression along with increased AMPK and ACC protein expression, protects against diabetic cardiomyopathy by phosphorylation and regulation of AKT/GSK-3β signaling pathway	Zhao et al. [173], Feng et al. [26], Tzeng et al. [133], Wu et al. [148, 150]
Therapy for hepatic failure	D-galactosamine-sensitized mice, Liquid fructose feeding rats	Deactivates MAPKs and NF-κB signaling pathways, and inhibits TNF-α production	Yin et al. [165], Li et al. [75]
Therapy for bone remodeling and arthritis	Mice	Suppresses osteoclast differentiation and the bone-resorbing activity of mature osteoclasts by inhibiting RANKL-induced NF-κB, c-Fos, and NFATc1 expression	Hwang et al. [41], Zhu et al. [177], Kang et al. [52], Kim et al. [54]
Treats schizophrenia	Rodent	Attenuates phosphorylation of ErbB1 and ErbB2 and EGF receptor signaling	Mizuno et al. [96]
Cure for gall bladder disorder	Guinea pig gall bladder smooth muscle, In vivo and in vitro in SGC996 gall bladder carcinoma cell lines	Inhibits voltage dependent potassium current in gall bladder smooth muscle cell model	Wu et al. [151], Li et al. [74]

Table 3.2 Therapeutic effects of emodin in human model systems

Bioactivity	Models	Mechanism	References
Antitumor agent	Human HCC cells, MCF-7 cells and MDA-MB-231 cells, PC3 prostate cancer cells, Human Umbilical Vein Endothelial Cells (HUVECs) Human skin squamous cell carcinoma, HSC5 cells, Prostrate and Lung cancer cells, Parental human ovarian adenocarcinoma cell line COC1 and its cDDP-resistant derivative COC1/DDP, human hepatoma cell line SMMC-7721, HL-60 cells, MCF-7cells, Human NSCLC cell lines, PC9, H1299, H1650, and H1975, Human breast (MDA-MB-435s, and MDA-MB-468) cancer cells, HepG2, BGC, AGS, HELF Retina capillary endothelial cells, HUVECs, LS1034 human colon cancer cells, LS1034 tumor xenografts model, Her2 over expressed cancer cell lines, Human Gastric cancer cell lines (SGC996, SGC7901, MKN 45,) gall bladder carcinoma GBC-SD cells, MCF-7/ADR	Downregulates VEGF, inhibits Integrin Linked Kinase expression through AMPKα-mediated reduction of Sp1 and c-Jun proteins Downregulates TGF-β signaling pathway, Blocks Her2/neu binding to Hsp90, resulting in proteasomal degradation of Her2/neu Effects ERCCI expression, inhibits the expression of ABCG2, decreases the level of PRL-3 expression, downregulates MRP1, and generates ROS	Huang et al. [40], Kaneshiro et al. [51], Wang et al. [138, 140, 141], Yan et al. [158], Ma et al. [91] He et al. [34], Ok et al. [102], Fu et al. [27], Sun and Bu [127], Li et al. [74], Jelassi et al. [44], Ma et al. [90], Sui et al. [123], Thacker and Karunagaran [129], Masaldan and Iyer [93], Deng et al. [19], Hwang et al. [42], Zhang et al. [169, 172], Tang et al. [128], Chihara et al. [16], Jun et al. [49]

(continued)

Table 3.2 (continued)

Bioactivity	Models	Mechanism	References
Apoptotic agent	Human breast cancer cells Bcap-37 and ZR-75-30, SW1990, Panc-1, HPNE cells and ECs, Human Hepatoma cell lines HepG2/C3A (ATCC CRL-1074), PLC/PRF/5 (ATCC CRL - 8024), and SK-HEP-1 (ATCC HTB-52), SW1990 cells, HeLa cells	Induces apoptosis by intrinsic mitochondrial and extrinsic death receptor pathways, activates caspase and PARP, increases levels of p53 and Bax, and decreases levels of Bcl-2 Regulates the expression of NF-κB and NF-κB-regulated angiogenesis-associated factors Inhibits the expression of cyclin B1 and Cdc2 to mediate the G2/M arrest in cell cycle	Shieh et al. [115], Wei et al. [147], Lin et al. [78, 79], Yaoxian et al. [162], Zu et al. [178]
Cytotoxic agent	HeLa cells, Human Multiple Myeloma cell lines, U266, and IM-9	Generates intracellular ROS and inhibits interleukin-6-induced JAK2/STAT3 pathway selectively	Wang et al. [144], Muto et al. [98]
Anti-antherosclerosis agent	Vascular smooth muscle cell (VSMC)	Inhibits proliferation of VSMC via caspase dependent apoptosis	Heo et al. [36]
Barrier protective effects	Intestinal epithelial cells	Attenuates intestinal epithelial barrier dysfunction by inhibiting the HIF-1α and NF-κB signaling pathways	Lei et al. [67]

Table 3.3 Therapeutic effects of emodin in chronic diseases and mechanisms of action

Diseases	Mechanism	References
Allergy	Inhibits TNF-α secretion through the inhibition of PKC or PKC-IKK2 pathways	Lu et al. [88], Kim et al. [53], Nemmar et al. [99]
Cancer	Targets PI3K/Akt pathway Downregulates TGF-β signaling pathway and Inhibits β-catenin/Akt Downregulates cytoprotective ERK and Akt cascade Elevates the levels of Bax, reduces Bcl-2 and activates caspase-2, -3, and -9, Suppresses the activation of $P210^{BCR-ABL}$ downstream signaling pathways including CrkL, Akt/mTOR and MEK/ERK Inhibits TOR signaling pathway and blocks autophagy Inhibits ILK expression through AMPKα-mediated reduction of Sp1 and c-Jun proteins and suppresses the activation of MAPK signaling pathways Inhibits Wnt signaling pathway like (i) regulating the regulators-p300 and HBP1 (ii) increasing reactive oxygen species	Su et al. [121], Olsen et al. [103], Hsu et al. [37], Yan et al. [158], Way et al. (2014), Thacker and Karunagaran [129, 130], Li et al. [77], Deng et al. [19], Hu et al. [38], Tang et al. [128], Sun et al. [124]
Cardiovascular diseases	Enhances mitochondrial antioxidant components and inducesTNF-α upregulation and cardiomyocyte apoptosis Suppresses pro-inflammatory cytokines TNF-α and IL-1β due to inhibition of NF-κB activation Inhibits IL-23/IL-17 inflammatory axis, Th17cell proliferation and viral replication mRNA/protein	Du et al. [23], Wu et al. [149], Song et al. [119], Chen et al. [10, 12, 14], Jiang et al. [46]
Diabetes	Regulates PPAR-γ and AKT/GSK-3β signaling pathway	Xue et al. [155], Wang et al. [142, 145], Wu et al. [148, 150], Arvindekar et al. [3]
Kidney diseases	Activates autophagy by modulating AMPK/mTOR signaling pathways	Gao et al. [27], Liu et al. [81]
Liver diseases	Increases the mRNA levels of PPAR-γ Inhibits p38 MAPK-NF-κB pathway leading to suppression of hepatic IFN-γ, TNF-α, IL-1β, IL-12, IL-6, iNOS, ITGAM, CCL2, and MIP-2, MIP-2 receptor, and CXCR2	Zhan et al. [167], Dong et al. [20], Meng et al. [94], Dong et al. [22], Lin et al. [81], Dang et al. [18], Dong et al. [22], Lee et al. [61], Tzeng et al. [133], Liu et al. [84], Xue et al. [156]

(continued)

Table 3.3 (continued)

Diseases	Mechanism	References
	Enhances CPT-1 expression along with increase in AMPK and ACC protein expression and phosphorylation	
Lung diseases	Inactivates NF-κB and p38 MAPK pathway	Xiao et al. [153], Xue et al. [157], Sun et al. [125], Yin et al. [164]
Neurological disorders	Downregulates PI3K/Akt/GSK-3β signaling pathway, promotes PI3K/Akt-dependent CREB phosphorylation and activates class III PI3K/Beclin-1/B-cell lymphoma 2 pathway	Gao et al. [28], Li et al. [72], Yang et al. [160], Park et al. [105], Sun and Liu [126]
Other diseases	Inhibits NF-κB and MAPKs signal pathways, Blocks HIF-1α/NF-κB-COX-2 signaling pathways, Interferes with ROS-ERK1/2/p38 signal pathway Upregulates PPAR-γ expression Inhibits AP-1 signaling pathway	Lee et al. [63], Ha et al. [31], Chu et al. [17], Li et al. [68, 74, 76], Lee et al. [66], Lei et al. [67], Chen et al. [12], Pang et al. [104]

3.2 Chemical Structure, Biophysical Properties, and Bioavailability

The basic chemical structure of anthraquinone is an anthracene ring (tricyclic aromatic) with two ketone groups in position C9 and C10. The chemical structure of emodin is depicted in Fig. 3.1 Zhang et al. [171] examined the relationship between the chemical structure and the activity of emodin and proposed that one methyl, one hydroxy, and one-carbonyl functional groups are critical for the biological activities of emodin. The keto forms of emodin are less stable than the enol form, because the latter is stabilized by *p*-conjugation in the B ring. These differences in stability between the enol and keto forms indicate that the contribution of

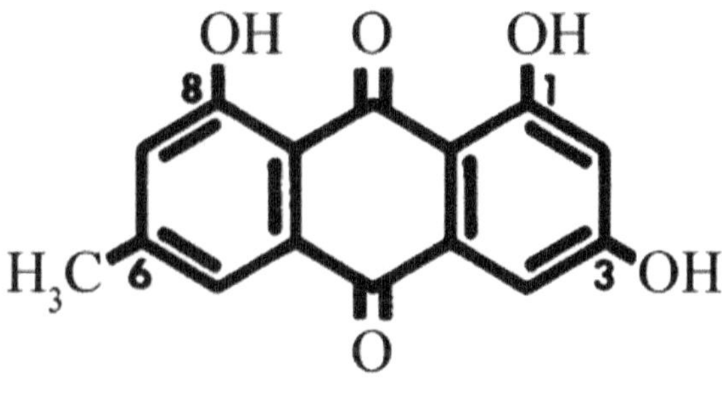

Fig. 3.1 Structure of emodin, 1,3,8-trihydroxy-6-methyl-anthraquinone

the keto forms can be considered negligible for emodin as a free molecule. It is clear that emodin appears to be a planar molecule and the most stable radical in the gas phase is the 3-OH species. Despite planarity of radical structures, there is no significant electronic delocalisation between adjacent rings [92].

Emodin–DNA interaction mainly involves intercalation of emodin between bases and with PO_2 backbone. Interaction occurs mainly through Ade and Thy bases and PO_2 backbone of double helix. Binding constant for emodin–DNA is 5.59×10^{-3} M^{-1} [107]. Emodin has low DNA-binding affinity and has low cytotoxicity against various cancer cells. Addition of pyrazole ring and certain chemical groups like polymethyleneamine, sugar with anthraquinone chromophore result in increased binding affinity and cytotoxicity against various cancers. Chain of varying length, polarity, charge, rigidity, and steric bulk may impart different DNA binding affinity. Emodin with mono-cationic amino side chain has stronger cytotoxic potential against cancer cells than di-cationic amino side chain, as indicated by cytotoxicity potency index (IC_{50}) value [154].

Absorption, excretion, tissue distribution, and metabolism of emodin were studied after a single oral administration of C^{14}-labeled emodin (50 mg/kg) in rat model [4]. Emodin was quickly absorbed from the gastrointestinal tract. Radioactivity in the peripheral blood reached a peak 2 h after administration, and within 24 h subsequently decreased to 30 % of the peak value. In two cannulated rats, biliary excretion reached a maximum at approximately 6 h and amounted to 49 % dose within 15 h; 70 % of biliary activity was in the form of conjugated emodin. Urinary excretion amounted to 18 and 22 % dose, in 24 and 72 h, respectively and most metabolites in pooled urine found were free emodin and emodic acid. Emodin glycosides are carried unabsorbed to the large intestine (because of its chemical structure) where metabolism to the active aglycone takes place by intestinal bacterial flora. The aglycone damages epithelial cells, which leads directly and indirectly to changes in absorption, secretion, motility and exerts its laxative effect [97, 135].

In Male Sprague-Dawley rats orally administered PC *Polygonum cuspidatum* a widely used Chinese medicine which contains resveratrol and emodin, it was found that the sulfates/glucuronides of resveratrol and emodin were the major forms in circulation and in most assayed organs after oral intake [78, 79]. With regard to tissue distribution emodin was detected as sulfates/glucuronides in lung and kidney, as free form in liver, but was not detectable in brain and heart [113, 114]. In rats poor oral bioavailability of emodin is thought to be the result of intestinal and hepatic glucuronidation [83]. The activity and positional preference of glucuronidation of anthraquinones varies with organs, species, substrate concentrations, UGT isoforms, and the substitution at b-positions [148, 150]. Generally, the conjugated metabolites are recognized as the inactive product of drugs, however, now there are increasing evidences showing that the conjugated metabolites of polyphenols demonstrate various bioactivities [25, 111, 112, 116, 159, 166]. Emodin which mainly exists as conjugated metabolite in the circulation and in most organs, needs to be extensively investigated in future.

3.3 Role of Emodin in Various Chronic Disorders

3.3.1 Allergy

Emodin plays an important role in allergic diseases like asthma, rhinitis, and atopic dermatitis [47, 88]. Asthma is a respiratory disease associated with symptoms like airway hyper responsiveness, mucus hypersecretion, and bronchial inflammation [139]. Emodin can be a therapeutic agent in treating allergic airway inflammation. It inhibited ovalbumin-induced increase in eosinophil counts and hypersecretion of mucus from goblet cells in air way passage [17]. Emodin also exhibited antiallergic activities via increasing the stability of the cell membrane and inhibiting extracellular Ca^{2+} influx [142, 145].

Mast cells play a major role in allergic diseases. Emodin lowered mast cell-dependent passive anaphylactic reaction in Ig-E sensitized mice and inhibited degranulation, generation of eicosanoid, and secretion of cytokines in dose-dependent manner in mast cell [53, 88, 117]. Mast cell degranulation inhibition occurred via attenuation of protein kinase C and IκB kinase 2 signaling pathway [53].

3.3.2 Arthritis

Rheumatoid arthritis is a chronic inflammatory disease that causes damage to the joints and is characterized by inflammation and infiltration of inflammatory cells into synovial tissue and joint destruction. One of the major transcriptional pathways involved in joint inflammation is the nuclear factor-κB (NF-κB) pathway. Emodin exerted anti-inflammatory effects in collagen-induced arthritic mice through inhibition of the NF-κB pathway and has shown therapeutic value for the treatment of rheumatoid arthritis [41, 177]. Synovial angiogenesis is the main characteristic feature of rheumatoid arthritis. Emodin decreased expression of various angiogenesis-related genes like vascular endothelial growth factor (VEGF), HIF-1α, and cyclooxygenase 2 [31]. Emodin considerably inhibited IL-1β and lipopolysaccharide (LPS)-stimulated proliferation of RA synoviocytes under hypoxic condition and reduced the production of pro-inflammatory cytokines (TNF-α, IL-6 and IL-8), prostaglandin E2, and matrix metalloproteinase (MMP-1, MMP-13) [31, 117].

Emodin treatment was also helpful in treatment of osteoporosis as it stimulated osteoblast formation and inhibited osteoclastogenesis. Mice treated with emodin showed decrease of LPS-induced bone loss and increased bone formation [54]. Emodin is emerging as a potential therapeutic agent to treat arthritis, fractures, muscle injury, and pain [41, 152, 177].

3.3.3 Cancer

Recent studies on emodin are mostly focused on its antitumor properties. These efforts led to unraveling both the effect of emodin against cancer development and the underlying molecular mechanisms involved. A number of studies have demonstrated that emodin inhibited the growth and proliferation of various cancer cells derived from different tumors, such as cervical, breast, lung, colorectal, and prostate cancers (Tables 3.1, 3.2). After evaluation with other anthraquinone derivatives, including emodin 1-O-β-D-glucoside, physcion 1-O-β-D-glucoside, and physcion, C1 and C3 position of emodin was supposed to be important for its antitumor function [59]. Meanwhile, emodin displayed over 25-fold differential cytotoxicity against ras-transformed bronchial epithelial cells to the normal human bronchial epithelial cells [6]. Emodin also evoked a less or no cytotoxic effect in several normal cells, together with human fibroblast-like lung WI-38 cells, HBL-100 cells derived from normal human breast tissue and three primary cultured rat normal cells [115, 170]. Recently, Sharma and Tiku [109] reported noncytotoxic effects on murine splenocytes up to 100 μM of emodin. These observations suggested that normal cells might be more resistant to emodin-induced cytotoxicity than cancer cells. Cells contain various pathways designed to protect them from the genomic instability or toxicity that can result when their DNA is damaged. A pivotal role in this response is played by checkpoint proteins that control the normal passage of cells through the cell cycle. The effect of emodin on cell cycle has been demonstrated on various cancer cells. In Her2/neu-over expressing MDA-MB-453 breast cancer cells emodin azide methyl derivative (AMAD) triggered mitochondrial-dependent cell apoptosis involving caspase-8-mediated Bid cleavage. This derivative-induced G0/G1 arrest by blocking Her2/neu binding to Hsp90. This was associated with decreasing protein expression of c-Myc, Cyclin D1, CDK4, and p-Rb [123, 158, 169]. Emodin-induced G2/M phase arrest in v-ras-transformed cells [6] and the human hepatoma cell line HepG2/C3A cells [115]. Elevation of p53 and p21 expression might be involved in this G2/M arrest [115]. In addition to G2/M phase arrest, emodin was reported to block the G1 to S phase of the cell cycle in human colon carcinoma HCT-15 cells [50] and breast cancer MDA-MB-453 cells [170]. It downregulated Wnt signaling pathway in human colorectal cancer cells SW480 and SW620 [129]. Emodin attenuated radioresistance in the HepG2 cells via upregulation of the apoptotic signals and downregulation of the proliferative signals [42]. Emodin also inhibited the lung metastasis of human breast cancer in a mouse xenograft model, and inhibited the invasion of MDA-MB-231 cells associated with the downregulation of MMP-2, MMP-9, uPAR, and uPA expression as well as decreased activity of p38 and ERK [124]. Combination of emodin with curcumin synergistically inhibited survival, proliferation, and invasion of breast cancer cells and cervical cancer [130].

Apoptosis could be a potential general mechanism of the anti-proliferative and antineoplastic effects of emodin. A number of studies have demonstrated that emodin is capable of inducing apoptotic cell death in various cancer cells [120].

Several studies revealed that emodin-induced apoptosis was mediated by reactive oxygen species (ROS) generated from the semiquinone [48, 121], however there was a report that emodin-induced apoptosis, ROS-independently [13]. It is believed that the quinoid structure of emodin could be activated to the semiquinone radical intermediate, which in turn could react with oxygen to generate ROS and induce oxidative stress [121]. The generation of ROS may contribute to mitochondrial injury, reduction of mitochondrial transmembrane potential, cytochrome c and Smac release, and subsequent caspase activation resulting in apoptosis [5].

Several groups examined the role of Bcl-2 family members to further explore the mitochondria-related pathway involved in emodin-induced apoptosis. Emodin treatment significantly increased expression level of Bax and Bak, pro-apoptotic protein, and caused Bax mitochondrial translocation preceding apoptosis [48]. Besides, anti-apoptotic protein Bcl-2 was also involved in emodin-induced apoptosis: first, emodin caused a significant decrease in Bcl-2 expression; second, ectopic expression of Bcl-2 markedly blocked emodin-induced apoptosis [68, 178]. Additionally, PKC-δ and ε may also be involved in emodin-induced apoptosis. It appeared that PKC was downstream of caspase-3 in the emodin-induced apoptosis [62]. The inhibitory effects of emodin on tumor-induced metastasis and angiogenesis in human breast cancer were caused by inhibition of MMPs and VEGFR-2, which may be associated with the downregulation of Runx2 transcriptional activity [44, 89, 124].

Emodin also potentiates the anticancer effects of cisplatin on gallbladder and ovarian cancer cells through ROS-dependent pathway [90, 140]. Emodin co-treatment was found to downregulate multidrug-resistance-associated protein-1 (MRP-1) and increase the sensitivity of SGC996 cells to cisplatin, carboplatin, or oxaliplatin [74, 140, 141]. Emodin was also found to be a potential agent for radio-sensitization of hepatocellular carcinoma (HCC) HepG-2 cells [42, 169].

Alternatively emodin protects cultured human kidney (HEK 293) cells and murine splenocytes against cisplatin-induced and gamma radiation-induced oxidative stress, respectively [109, 136]. Theses reported studies showed that emodin can have differential effects on normal cells and cancerous cells.

3.3.4 Cardiovascular Diseases

Myocarditis is an inflammatory disease of heart that leads to heart failure. Inflammation and autoimmunity is the major cause of myocarditis. Emodin is a promising candidate for treatment of myocarditis. The severity of myocarditis was reduced by treatment with emodin. In a murine acute myocardial infarction model, emodin reduced the myocardial infarct size [149]. In rat model of experimental autoimmune myocarditis, it inhibited NF-κB activity there by reducing the level of pro-inflammatory cytokines TNF-α, IL-1β [119]. Besides it protected against viral myocarditis by inhibiting IL-23/IL-17 inflammatory axis, Th17 cell proliferation, and viral replication in mice [46]. Emodin was found to inhibit CVB3 replication (causal agent of viral myocarditis) by inhibiting CVB3 VP1 protein translation. The fundamental signaling pathways involved in inhibition of CVB3 VP1 protein translation include Akt-mTORC1-4EBP1, mTORC1-p70S6K, ERK1/2-p90RSK, and Ca^{2+}-calmodulin (Ca^{2+}-CaM) cascades. Therefore, these pathways might be the targets for emodin [168].

Atherosclerosis a chronic inflammatory disease characterized by the presence of atherosclerotic plaque in the arterial intima can lead to hardening and narrowing of the major arteries. Emodin inhibited NF-κB activation and TNF-α-induced migration, proliferation and MMP-2, MMP-9 expression in rat aortic smooth muscle cells (RASMCs) [95]. It also had beneficial effects on stability of atherosclerotic plaque in Apo-E deficient mice (apo-E has anti-atherosclerosis property) and was found to inhibit the expression of M-CSF and MMP-9, whereas it enhanced the PPAR-γ expression [174]. Cardiovascular protective actions of emodin have been attributed to activation of cardiac natriuretic hormone secretion.

In isolated rabbit atria, emodin heighted atrial natriuretic peptide (ANP) secretion via inhibition of L-type calcium channels and activation of potassium ATP channels [176]. C-reactive protein (CRP) an inflammatory molecule plays a direct role in atherogenesis. Emodin was also found to inhibit Hcy-induced CRP generation in vascular smooth muscles cells via ROS-ERK1/2/p38 signaling pathway and upregulated PPARγ expression [104]. The above-mentioned results provide a rationale for the use of emodin in the treatment of cardiovascular homeostasis and other heart diseases.

3.3.5 Diabetes

Diabetes mellitus is a disease characterized by chronic hyperglycemia, disorders of lipid, carbohydrates, and microvascular pathology of retina, renal glomerulus, and peripheral nerves. Emodin injected intraperitoneally for 3 weeks to diabetic mice (high fat fed diet) and low dose of streptozotocin (STZ) showed significantly reduced blood glucose, triglycerides, and cholesterol in serum. qRT-PCR results further confirmed that emodin significantly elevated the mRNA expression level of PPAR-γ (regulates the mRNA expressions of LPL, FAT/CD36, resistin, and FABPs (ap2) in liver and adipocyte tissues) [155]. Emodin at a concentration of 3 and 30 μm/L suppressed 11-dehydrocorticosterone-induced lipolysis and adipogenesis, respectively without affecting corticosterone-induced lipolysis and adipogenesis [142, 145]. Emodin also reduced the activation of glucocorticoid, which is insulin antagonizing hormone by inhibiting 11β-hydroxysteroid dehydrogenase type 1 (11β-HSD1) in 3T3-L1 adipocyte cells in a concentration-and time-dependent manner. Adiponectin is an important insulin-sensitizing adipokine, emodin lead to assembly of high-molecular weight adiponectin and increased the ratio of high-molecular adiponectin (possesses insulin-sensitizing activity) to total adiponectin in 3T1-L1 adipocytes [10, 14]. SREBP-1 and SREBP-2 (transcription factor involved in biosynthesis of cholesterol, fatty acid, and triglyceride) mRNA level was also significantly reduced in the liver and adipose tissue after emodin treatment [69].

Emodin may also be a potential medication in treating the glucose dependent structural and functional abnormalities in peritoneal membrane. Emodin regulated the undesirable effects of concentrated glucose on human peritoneal mesothelial cells by suppression of protein kinase C (PKC) activation and cyclic AMP response element binding protein (CREB) phosphorylation [7]. Emodin was found to protect against diabetic cardiomyopathy by regulating AKT/GSK-3β signaling pathway [148, 150]. In the presence of high-glucose concentration human umbilical vein endothelial cells (HUVECs) cultured with 3 μm of emodin showed protection from endothelial cytotoxicity by suppressing MAPK pathway and inhibiting chemokine ligand 5 (CCL5) expression [30].

Autoimmune diabetes (AID) is a metabolic disease that progresses through an intricate relationship of environmental, genetic, and immune factor. Emodin was able to suppress the chemotactic activity of leukocytes at the insulitis stage (inflammation of the islets of Langerhans) of AID development [15].

3.3.6 Kidney Diseases

Emodin was also found to have beneficial effects in renal dysfunction. In diabetic nephropathy it inhibited activation of p38 MAPK pathway and downregulated the expression of fibronectin. This effect was independent of the blood glucose level [137]. Emodin was able to protect mice from drug-induced kidney injury. In cyclosporine-induced kidney nephropathy emodin prevented the overexpression of Protein Kinase Casein Kinase II (PKCK2) which has a role in apoptosis [118]. In LPS treated NRK-52E cells (Rat kidney epithelial cells) it inhibited TLR2-mediated NF-κB signaling pathway [70]. Emodin was found to ameliorate cisplatin-induced apoptosis of rat renal tubular cells in vitro through modulating the AMPK/mTOR signaling pathways and activating autophagy. Emodin may have therapeutic potential for the prevention of drug-induced nephrotoxicity [81].

3.3.7 Liver Ailments

Emodin has been found to be beneficial in various liver ailments like fructose-induced nonalcoholic fatty liver in rat, Con A-induced liver injury, and LPS-induced fulminant hepatic failure. High carbohydrate/high fat diet fed mice treated with emodin were protected from hepatosteatosis and metabolic derangement. The mechanism involved were modulation of glutathione homeostasis and TNF-α inhibition [1]. Con A-induced hepatic injury is a well-characterized murine model with a pathophysiology similar to that of human viral and autoimmune hepatitis. Emodin pretreatment protected against Con A-induced liver injury in mice, partially through inhibition of both the infiltration of CD4(+) and F4/80(+) cells and the activation of the p38 MAPK-NF-κB pathway in CD4(+) T cells and macrophages [156, 165]. Emodin was capable of improving the lipid accumulation through the ERS-SREBP1c pathway in fructose-induced nonalcoholic fatty liver disease [75]. Thus emodin might be applied as a potential candidate for the prevention and intervention of liver diseases. However, in a recent study toxic effects of emodin were reported in idiosyncratic liver injury model by Tu et al. [132]. Emodin-potentiated liver injury induced by noninjurious dose of LPS. The mechanisms underlying this effect are yet to be fully understood.

3.3.8 Lung Diseases

Emodin is considered as a potential pulmonary protective agent against lung toxicity induced by particulate air pollution. Particulate air pollution is related with inflammation, impairment of lung function, and oxidative stress. In lung diseases emodin reduced oxidative stress and increased the expression and activity of HO-1, Nrf-2 [99, 157]. Besides acute lung injury is a very well-known fatal disease. Emodin has been reported to repress LPS-induced pulmonary inflammation, pulmonary oedema, and can be used to treat acute lung injury (ALI) and acute respiratory distress syndrome (ARDS) [153].

3.3.9 Neurological Disorders

Abnormality in cytokine signaling is implicated in the neuropathology and emodin has been reported to be an effective neuroprotective drug. Subchronic oral administration of emodin (50 mg/kg) to an epidermal growth factor (EGF)-induced schizophrenia rat model, resulted in suppressed acoustic startle responses and abolished prepulse inhibition deficits. Emodin was found to both attenuate EGF receptor signaling and ameliorate behavioral deficits [96]. Accumulation of β-amyloid is an important step in pathogenesis of Alzheimer's disease. Emodin treatment protected cultured cortical neurons from $A\beta_{25-35}$-induced toxicity and inhibited abnormal aggregation of tau protein into paired helical filaments. The mechanism mediating this neuroprotective effect involve the upregulation of Bcl-2, the activation ER/PI3K/Akt pathway as well as the inhibition of JNK1/2 phosphorylation induced by $A\beta_{25-35}$ [82, 126].

Chronic emodin (20, 40 and 80 mg/kg) treatments remarkably improved depression-like behavior in chronic unpredictable mild stress (CUMS) mice. Abnormal activation of hypothalamic–pituitary–adrenal (HPA) axis is an important marker of depression. Antidepressant activity of emodin was mediated, at least in part, by the upregulating Glucocorticoid Respotor (GR) and Brain Derived Neurotrophic Factor (BDNF) levels in hippocampus [72]. Epilepsy is another chronic brain dysfunction syndrome. COX-2, N-Methyl-D-Aspartate (NMDA) receptor, and P-glycoprotein have a synergic relationship in the pathogenesis of epilepsy. Epileptic seizures are tightly associated with upregulated MDR1 gene, and emodin showed good antagonistic effects on epileptic rats, possibly through inhibition of NMDA-mediated overexpression of MDR1 and its associated genes [160]. Neurite outgrowth is an important marker of neuronal differentiation. Emodin-induced neurite outgrowth in Neuro2a cell by P13K/Akt/GSK3β signaling pathway [105]. Future studies aiming at precisely understanding the cellular mechanisms involved in the neuroprotective effects of emodin could open new avenues for the treatment of various neurodegenerative diseases, and other neuronal disorders.

3.3.10 Other Diseases

Emodin has been reported to have anti-inflammatory effects in both in vitro and in vivo system (Tables 3.1, 3.2). Emodin when administered intraperitoneally reduced LPS-induced mammary gland injury in mastitis [76]. Emodin has also proved to be a potential candidate in treating serious vascular inflammatory diseases, such as sepsis and septic shock and had anti-inflammatory effects in sepsis mouse model in vivo [64, 65]. Emodin inhibited inflammation in intestinal epithelial cells by blocking HIF-1α/NF-κB-COX-2 signaling pathways [67]. Emodin also lessened ocular tissue inflammation and fibrosis by inhibition of NF-κB pathway after eye injury [11, 55]. Lee et al. [66] reported anti-inflammatory effects of emodin derivative [6-O-β-D-glucoside emodin (EG)] in vitro in human umbilical vein endothelial cells (HUVECs) as well as in mice. Recently, Han et al. [32] reported that emodin attenuated NLRP3 inflammasome activation, leading to decreased secretion of cleaved IL-1β, and blocking of the inflammasome-induced pyroptosis. Ocular neovascularization is the origin of blindness related with ischemic retinal ataxia in conjunction with proliferative diabetic retinopathy (PDR), retinopathy of prematurity (ROP) and age-related macular degeneration. The induction of angiogenesis in retina is due to VEGF. Emodin-$MgSiO_3$ nanoparticles could inhibit the expression of both VEGF gene and protein effectively and can be an effective therapy for eye-related disorders [106].

3.3.11 Conclusions and Future Perspective

A detailed survey of the literature evaluating the efficacy of emodin in various disorders, suggests that it can modulate multiple signaling pathways. The primary signaling pathways affected by emodin are involved in cell proliferation, apoptosis, differentiation, and have role in inflammation (Fig. 3.2). On one hand it inhibits antiapoptotic pathways and prosurvival signals, and on the other can reduce

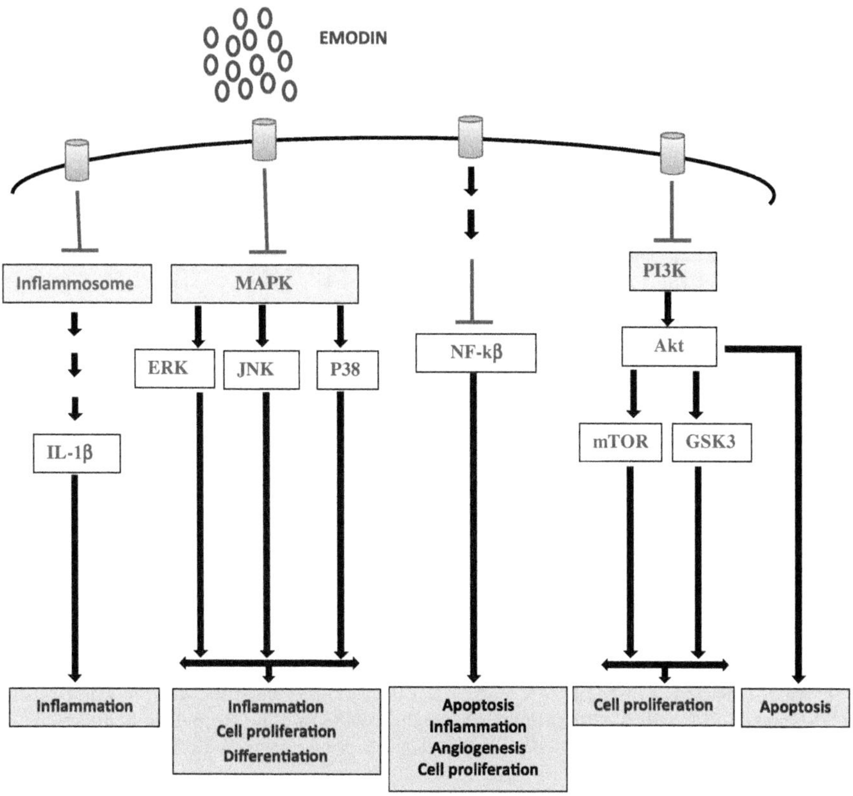

Fig. 3.2 Common signaling pathways downregulated by emodin

cytotoxic effects through upregulation of autophagy. It can be an effective adjuvant in cancer therapy by acting as a radiosensitizer making cancer cells more susceptible to radiation, and at the same time protecting the normal cells. In combination with various chemo therapeutic drugs it increases their efficacy and over comes drug resistance in various cancers. The primary transcription factor downregulated by emodin in different disorders is NF-κB that further regulates production/transcription of cytokines (TNF-α, IL-6), cell adhesion molecules and MMPs that have important role in various chronic disorders (Fig. 3.3). Recently, emodin has been found to regulate energy metabolism. It upregulates transcription factor PPAR-γ that is involved in regulation of adipogenesis and thus can be helpful in treating metabolic disorders. Thus emodin has potential to be an important drug molecule. However, the therapeutic potential of emodin is limited by its low bioavailability. Literature survey on methods to improve the bioavailability of emodin shows work in this direction has just started and emodin loaded nanoparticles and chemical modification of emodin could be a way forward.

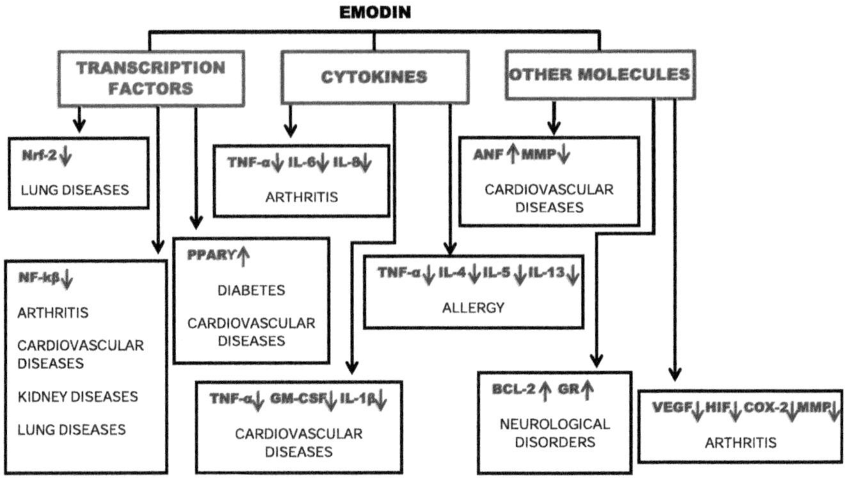

Fig. 3.3 Molecules modulated (upregulated ↑/downregulated ↓) by emodin in different chronic disorders

References

1. Alisi A, Pastore A, Ceccarelli S, Panera N, Gnani D, Bruscalupi G, Massimi M, Tozzi G, Piemonte F, Nobili V (2012) Emodin prevents intrahepatic fat accumulation, inflammation and redox status imbalance during diet-induced hepatosteatosis in rats. Int J Mol Sci 13:2276–2289
2. Alves DS, Perez-Fons L, Estepa A, Micol V (2004) Membrane-related effects underlying the biological activity of the anthraquinones emodin and barbaloin. Biochem Pharmacol 68: 549–561
3. Arvindekar A, More T, Payghan PV, Laddha K, Ghoshal N, Arvindekar A (2015) Evaluation of anti-diabetic and alpha glucosidase inhibitory action of anthraquinones from Rheum emodi. Food Funct 6(8):2693–2700
4. Bachmann M,. Schlatter C (1981) Metabolism of [^{14}C] emodin in the rat. Xenobiotica 11(3):217–225
5. Bras M, Queenan B, Susin SA (2005) Programmed cell death via mitochondria: different modes of dying. Biochemistry (Mosc) 70:231–239
6. Chan TC, Chang CJ, Koonchanok NM, Geahlen RL (1993) Selective inhibition of the growth of ras-transformed human bronchial epithelial cells by emodin, a protein-tyrosine kinase inhibitor. Biochem Biophys Res Commun 193:1152–1158
7. Chan TM, Leung JK, Tsang RC, Liu ZH, Li LS, Yung S (2003) Emodin ameliorates glucose-induced matrix synthesis in human peritoneal mesothelial cells. Kidney Int 64(2):519–533
8. Chang LC, Sheu HM, Huang YS, Tsai TR, Kuo KW (1999) A novel functions of emodin. enhancement of the nucleotide excision repair of UV- and cisplatin-induced DNA damage in human cells. Biochem Pharmacol 58:49–57
9. Chang YC, Lai TY, Yu CS, Chen HY, Yang JS, Chueh FS, Lu CC, Chiang JH, Huang WW, Ma CY, and Chung JG (2011) Emodin induces apoptotic death in murine myelomonocytic leukemia WEHI-3 cells in vitro and enhances phagocytosis in leukemia mice in vivo. Evid Based Complem Altern Med. Article ID 523596

10. Chen C, Liang Z, Chen Q, Li ZG (2012) Irbesartan and emodin on myocardial remodelling in Gold Blatt hypertensive rats. J Cardiovasc Pharmacol 60(4):375–380
11. Chen G, Zhang J, Zhang H, Xiao Y, Kao X, Liu Y, Liu Z (2015) Anti-Inflammatory effect of emodin on lipopolysaccharide-induced keratitis in wistar rats. Int J ClinExp Med 8(8):12382–12389
12. Chen Q, Pang L, Huang S, Lei W, Huang D (2014) Affects of emodin and irbesartan on ventricular fibrosis in Gold Blatt hypertensive rats. Pharmacies 69(5):374–378
13. Chen YC, Shen SC, Lee WR, Hsu FL, Lin HY, Ko CH, Tseng SW (2002) Emodin induces apoptosis in human promyeloleukemic HL-60 cells accompanied by activation of caspase 3 cascades but independent of reactive oxygen species production. Biochem Pharmacol 64:1713–1721
14. Chen Z, Zhang L, Yi J, Li Z (2012) Promotion of adiponectin multimerization by emodin: A novel AMPK activator with PPARγ-agonist activity. J Cell Biochem 113(11):3547–3558
15. Chien SC, Wu YC, Chen ZW, Yang WC (2015) Naturally occurring anthraquinones: chemistry and therapeutic potential in autoimmune diabetes. Evid Based Complem Altern Med, Article ID 357357
16. Chihara T, Shimpo K, Beppu H, Yamamoto N, Kaneko T, Wakamatsu K, Sonoda S (2015) Effects of aloe-emodin and emodin on proliferation of the MKN45 human gastric cancer cell line. Asian Pac J Cancer Prev 16(9):3887–3891
17. Chu X, Wei M, Yang X, Cao Q, Xie X, Guan M, Wang D, Deng X (2012) Effects of an anthraquinone derivative from Rheum Officinale Baill, Emodin, on airway responses in a murine model of asthma. Food Chem Toxicol 50(7):2368–2375
18. Dang SS, Zhang X, Jia XL, Cheng YA, Song P, Liu EQ, He Q, Li ZF (2008) Protective effects of emodin and astragalus polysaccharides on chronic hepatic injury in rats. Chin Med J (Engl) 121(11):1010–1014
19. Deng G, Ju X, Meng Q, Yu ZJ, Ma LB (2015) Emodin inhibits the proliferation of PC3 prostate cancer cells in vitro via the notch signalling pathway. Mol Med Rep 12(3): 4427–4433
20. Dong H, Lu FE, Gao ZQ, Xu LJ, Wang KF, Zou X (2005) Effects of emodin on treating murine nonalcoholic fatty liver induced by high caloric laboratory chaw. World J Gastroenterol 11(9):1339–1344
21. Dong H, Lu FE, Gao ZQ (2006) Experimental Study on effects of emodin on nonalcohoalic fatty liver induced by high fat diet in rats. Zhongguo Zhong Xi Yi Jie He Za Zhi 26 suppl: 64–67
22. Dong MX, Jia Y, Zhang YB, Li CC, Geng YT, Zhou L, Li XY, Liu JC, Niu YC (2009) Emodin protects rat liver from CCl(4)-induced fibrogenesis via inhibition of hepatic stellate cells activation. World J Gastroenterol 15(38):4753–4762
23. Du Y, Ko KM (2006) Effects of pharmacological preconditioning by emodin/oleanolic acid treatment and/or ischemic preconditioning on mitochondrial antioxidant components as well as the susceptibility to ischemia-reperfusion injury in rat hearts. Mol Cell Biochem 288(1–2): 135–142
24. Evans WC (1996) Treas and evanspharmacognosy, 4th edn. W.B. Saunders Company, London
25. Fang SH, Hou YC, Chang WC, Hsiu SL, Chao PD, Chiang BL (2003) Morin sulphates/ glucuronides exert anti-inflammatory activity on activated macrophages and decreased the incidence of septic shock. Life Sci 743–756
26. Feng Y, Huang SL, Dou W, Zhang S, Chen JH, Shen Y, Shen JH, Leng Y (2010) Emodin, a natural product, selectively inhibits 11b-hydroxysteroid dehydrogenase type 1 and ameliorates metabolic disorder in diet-induced obese mice. Br J Pharmacol 161:113–126
27. Fu JM, Zhou J, Shi J, Xie JS, Huang L, Yip AY, Loo WT, Chow LW, Ng EL (2012) Emodin affects ERCC1 expression in breast cancer cells. J Transl Med 19(10 Suppl 1):S7
28. Gao J, Wang F, Wang W, Su Z, Guo C, Cao S (2014) Emodin suppresses hyperglycaemia-induced proliferation and fibronectin expression in mesangial cells via inhibiting cflip. PLoS ONE 9(4):e93588

29. Gao Y, Liu H, Deng L, Zhu G, Xu C, Li G, Liu S, Xie J, Liu J, Kong F, Wu R, Li G, Liang S (2011) Effect Of emodin on neuropathic pain transmission mediated by P2X2/3 receptor of primary sensory neurons. Brain Res Bull 84(6):406–413
30. Gao Y, Zhang J, Li G, Xu H, Yi Y, Wu Q, Song M, Bee YM, Huang L, Tan M, Liang S, Li G (2015) Protection of vascular endothelial cells from high glucose-induced cytotoxicity by emodin. Biochem Pharmacol 94(1):39–45
31. Ha MK, Song YH, Jeong SJ, Lee HJ, Jung JH, Kim B, Song HS, Huh JE, Kim SH (2011) Emodin inhibits proinflammatory responses and inactivates histone deacetylase 1 in hypoxic rheumatoid synoviocytes. Biol Pharm Bull 34(9):1432–1437
32. Han JW, Shim DW, Shin WY, Heo KH, Kwak SB, Sim EJ, Jeong JH, Kang TB, Lee KH (2015) Anti-inflammatory effect of emodin via attenuation of NLRP3 inflammasome activation. Int J Mol Sci 16:8102–8109
33. Harborne JB, Baxter H, Moss GP (1999) Phytochemical dictionary. A handbook of bioactive compounds from plants, 2nd edn. Taylor & Francis, London
34. He L, Bi JJ, Guo Q, Yu Y, Ye XF (2012) Effects of emodin extracted from chinese herbs on proliferation of non-small cell lung cancer and underlying mechanisms. Asian Pac J Cancer Prev 13(4):1505–1510
35. He Z, He MF, Ma SC, But PP (2009) Anti-angiogenic effects of rhubarb and its anthroquinone derivatives. J Ethnopharmacol 121313–121317
36. Heo SK, Yun HJ, Park WH, Park SD (2008) Emodin inhibits TNF-A-induced human aortic smooth-muscle cell proliferation via caspase and mitochondrial-dependent apoptosis. J Cell Biochem 105(1):70–80
37. Hsu CM, Hsu YA, Tsai Y (2010) Emodin inhibits the growth of hepatoma cells: finding the common anti-cancer pathway using Huh7, Hep3B, Andhepg2 cells. Biochem Biophys Res Commun 392(4):473–478
38. Hu H, Sun W, Gu LB, Tu Y, Liu H (2015) Molecular mechanism of emodin on inhibiting autophagy induced by HBSS in renal tubular cells. Zhongguo Zhong Yao ZaZhi 40(10): 1965–1970
39. Huang HC, Chu SH, Chao-Lee PD (1991) Vasorelaxants from Chinese herbs, emodin and scoparone, possess immunosuppressive properties. Eur J Pharmacol 198:211–213
40. Huang LY, Hu JD, Chen XJ, Zhu LF, Hu HL (2005) Effects of emodin on the proliferation inhibition and apoptosis induction in HL-60 cells and the involvement of c-myc gene. Zhonghua Xue Ye XueZaZhi 26(6):348–351
41. Hwang JK, Noh EM, Moon SJ, Kim JM, Kwon KB, Park BH (2013) Emodin suppresses inflammatory responses and joint destruction in collagen-induced arthritic mice. Rheumatology (Oxf Engl) 52(9):1583–1591
42. Hwang SY, Heo K, Kim JS, Im JW, Lee SM, Cho M, Kang DH, Heo J, Lee JW, Choi CW, Yang K (2015) Emodin attenuates radio-resistance induced by hypoxia in HepG2 cells via the enhancement of PARP1 cleavage and inhibition of JMJD2B. Oncol Rep 33(4): 1691–1698
43. Izhaki I (2002) Emodin—a secondary metabolite with multiple ecological functions in higher plants. New Phytol 155:205–217
44. Jelassi B, Anchelin M, Chamouton J, Cayuela ML, Clarysse L, Li J, Gore J, Jiang LH, Roger S (2013) Anthraquinone emodin inhibits human cancer cell invasiveness by antagonizing P2X7 receptors. Carcinogenesis 34(7):1487–1496
45. Jia X, Fang Yu, Wang J, Iwanowycz S, Saaoud F, Wang Y, Hu J, Wang Q, Fan D (2014) Emodin suppresses pulmonary metastasis of breast cancer cells accompanied with decreased macrophage recruitment and M2 polarization in the lungs. Breast Cancer Res Treat 148 (2):291–302
46. Jiang N, Liao W, Kuang X (2014) Effects of emodin on IL-23/IL-17 inflammatory axis, Th17 cells and viral replication in mice with viral myocarditis. J South Med Univ 34(3):373–378
47. Jin JH, Ngoc TM, Bae KH, Kim YS, Kim HP (2011) Inhibition of experimental atopic dermatitis by rhubarb (rhizomes of rheum tanguticum) and 5-lipoxygenase inhibition of its major constituent. Emodin Phytother Res 25(5):755–775

48. Jing X, Ueki N, Cheng J, Imanishi H, Hada T (2002) Induction of apoptosis in hepatocellular carcinoma cell lines by Emodin. Jpn J Cancer Res 93:874–882
49. Jun C, Niu X, Chen Y, Hu Q, Shi G, Wu H, Wang J, Yi J (2008) Emodin-induced generation of reactive oxygen species inhibits RhoA activation to sensitize gastric carcinoma cells to anoikis. Neoplasia 10:41–51
50. Kamei H, Koide T, Kojima T, Hashimoto Y, Hasegawa M (1998) Inhibition of cell growth in culture by quinones. Cancer Biother Radiopharm 13(3):185–188
51. Kaneshiro T, Morioka T, Inamine M, Kinjo T, Arakaki J, Chiba I, Sunagawa N, Suzui M, Yoshimi N (2006) Anthraquinone derivative emodin inhibits tumor-associated angiogenesis through inhibition of extracellular signal-regulated kinase 1/2 phosphorylation. Eur J Pharmacol 553:46–53
52. Kang DM, Yoon KH, Kim JY, Oh JM, Lee M, Jung ST, Juhng SK, Lee YH (2014) CT imaging bio-marker for evaluation of emodin as a potential drug on LPS-mediated osteoporosis mice. Acad Radiol 21(4):457–462
53. Kim DY, Kang TB, Shim DW, Sun X, Han JW, Ji YE, Kim TJ, Koppula S, Lee KH (2014) Emodin attenuates A23187-induced mast cell degranulation and tumor necrosis factor-A secretion through protein kinase C and Iκb kinase 2 signaling. Eur J Pharmacol 723:501–506
54. Kim JY, Cheon YH, Kwak SC, Baek JM, Yoon KH, Su M, Oh LJ (2014) Emodin regulates bone remodelling by inhibiting osteoclastogenesis and stimulating osteoblast formation. J Bone Miner Res 29(7):1541–1553
55. Kitano AI, Saika S, Yamanaka O, Ikeda K, Okada Y, Shirai K, Reinach PS (2007) Emodin suppression of ocular surface inflammatory reaction. Invest Ophthalmol Vis Sci 489 (11):5013–5022
56. Kogl F, Postowsky JJ (1925) Untersuchungen üuber Pilzfarbstoffe. II. Uber die Farbstaffe des blutroten Hautkorpfes (Dermocybe sanquinea Wulf.). Justus LiebigsAnnalen der Chemie 444:1–7
57. Koyama M, Kelly TR, Watanabe KA (1988) Novel type of potential anticancer agents derived from chrysophanol and emodin. J Med Chem 31:283–284
58. Kuo TC, Yang JS, Lin MW, Hsu SC, Lin JJ, Lin HJ (2009) Emodin has cytotoxic and protective effects in rat C6 glioma cells: roles of Mdr1a and nuclear factor B in cell survival. J Pharmacol Exp Ther 330(3):736–744
59. Kuo YC, Sun CM, Ou JC, Tsai WJ (1997) A tumor cell growth inhibitor from polygonum hypoleucum ohwi. Life Sci 61(23):2335–2344
60. Kwak HJ, Park MJ, Park CM, Moon SI, Yoo DH, Lee HC, Lee SH, Kim MS, Lee HW, Shin WS, Park IC, Rhee CH, Si Hong (2006) Emodin inhibits vascular endothelial growth factor-A-induced angiogenesis by blocking receptor-2 (KDR/Flk-1) phosphorylation. Int J Cancer 118:2711–2720
61. Lee BH, Huang YY, Duh PD, Wu SC (2012) Hepatoprotection of emodin and polygonum multiflorum against Ccl(4)-induced liver injury. Pharm Biol 50(3):351–359
62. Lee HZ (2001) Protein kinase C involvement in aloe-emodin- and emodin-induced apoptosis in lung carcinoma cell. Br J Pharmacol 134:1093–1102
63. Lee J, Jung E, Lee J, Huh S, Hwang CH, Lee HY, Kim EJ, Cheon JM, Hyun CG, Kim YS, Park D (2006) Emodin inhibits TNF alpha-induced MMP-1 expression through suppression of activator protein-1 (AP-1). Life Sci 79:2480–2485
64. Lee W, Ku SK, Kim TH, Bae JS (2013) Emodin-6-O-B-D-glucoside inhibits HMGB1-induced inflammatory responses in vitro and in vivo. Food Chem Toxicol 52:97–104
65. Lee W, Ku SK, Bae JS (2013) Emodin-6-O-B-D-glucoside down-regulates endothelial protein C receptor shedding. Arch Pharm Res 36(9):1160–1165
66. Lee W, Ku SK, Lee D, Lee T, Bae JS (2014) Emodin-6-O-B-D-glucoside inhibits high-glucose-induced vascular inflammation. Inflammation 37(2):306–313
67. Lei Q, Qiang F, Chao D, Di W, Guoqian Z, Bo Y, Lina Y (2014) Amelioration of hypoxia and LPS-induced intestinal epithelial barrier dysfunction by emodin through the suppression of the NF-Kb and HIF-1α signaling pathways. Int J Mol Med 34(6):1629–1639

68. Li D, Zhang N, Cao Y, Zhang W, Su G, Sun Y, Liu Z, Li F, Liang D, Liu B, Guo M, Fu Y, Zhang X, Yang Z (2013) Emodin ameliorates lipopolysaccharide-induced mastitis in mice by inhibiting activation Of NF-Kb and mapks signal pathways. Eur J Pharmacol 705(1–3): 79–85
69. Li J, Chen Y, Chen B, Chen C, Qiu B, Zheng Z, Zheng J, Liu T, Wang W, Hu J (2015) Inhibition of 32Dp210 cells harboring T315I mutation by a novel derivative of emodin correlates with down-regulation of BCR-ABL and its downstream signalling pathways. J Cancer Res Clin Oncol 141(2):283–293
70. Li J, Ding L, Song B, Xiao X, Qi M, Yang Q, Yang Q, Tang X, Wang Z, Yang L (2015) Emodin improves lipid and glucose metabolism in high fat diet-induced obese mice through regulating Srebp pathway. Eur J Pharmacol S0014–2999(15):30383–30386
71. Li J, Liu P, Mao H, Wanga A, Zhang X (2009) Emodin sensitizes paclitaxel-resistant human ovarian cancer cells to paclitaxel-induced apooptosis in vitro. Oncol Rep 21(6):1605–1610
72. Li M, Fu Q, Li Y, Li S, Xue J, Ma S (2014) Emodin opposes chronic unpredictable mild stress induced depressive-like behaviour in mice by upregulating the levels of hippocampal glucocorticoid receptor and brain-derived neurotrophic factor. Fitoterapia 98:1–10
73. Li WY, Chan SW, Guo DJ, Chung MK, Leung TY, Yu PH (2009) Water extract of rheum officinale baill. Induces apoptosis in human lung adenocarcinoma A549 and human breast cancer MCF-7 cell lines. J Ethnopharmacol 124:251–256
74. Li WY, Chan RY, Yu PH, Chan SW (2013) Emodin induces cytotoxic effect in human breast carcinoma MCF-7 cell. Pharm Biol 51(9):1175–1181
75. Li X, Xu Z, Wang S, Guo H, Dong S, Wang T, Zhang L, Jiang Z (2015) Emodin ameliorates hepatic steatosis through endoplasmic reticulum-stress sterol regulatory element-binding protein 1c pathway in liquid fructose-feeding rats. Hepatol Res. doi:10.1111/hepr.12538
76. Li XX, Dong Y, Wang W, Wang HL, Chen YY, Shi GY, Yi J, Wang J (2013) Emodin as an effective agent in targeting cancer stem-like side population cells of gallbladder carcinoma. Stem Cells Dev 22(4):554–566
77. Li Y, Xiong W, Yang J, Zhong J, Zhang L, Zheng J, Liu H, Zhang Q, Ouyang X, Lei L, Yu X (2015) Attenuation of inflammation by emodin in lipopolysaccharide-induced acute kidney injury via inhibition of toll-like receptor 2 signal pathway. IJKD 9:202–208
78. Lin SP, Chu PM, Tsai SY, Wu MH, Hou YC (2012) Pharmacokinetics and tissue distribution of resveratrol, emodin and their metabolites after intake of polygonum cuspidatum in rats. J Ethnopharmacol 144(3):671–676
79. Lin SZ, Wei WT, Chen H, Chen KJ, Tong HF, Wang ZH, Ni ZL, Liu HB, Guo HC, Liu DL (2012) Antitumor activity of emodin against pancreatic cancer depends on its dual role: promotion of apoptosis and suppression of angiogenesis. PLoS ONE 7(8):e42146
80. Lin YL, Wu CF, Huang YT (2008) Phenols from the roots of rheum palmatumattenuate chemotaxis in rat hepatic stellate cells. Planta Med 74(10):1246–1252
81. Liu H, Gu LB, Tu Y, Hu H, Huang YR, Sun W (2016) Emodin ameliorates cisplatin-induced apoptosis of rat renal tubular cells in vitro by activating autophagy. Acta Pharmacol Sin 37:235–245
82. Liu T, Jin H, Sun QR, Hu HT (2010) Neuroprotective effects of emodin in rat cortical neurons against β-amyloid-induced neurotoxicity. Brain Res 1347(C):149–156
83. Liu W, Feng Q, Li Y, Ye L, Hu M, Liu Z (2012) Coupling of UDP-glucuronosyltransferases and multidrug resistance-associated proteins is responsible for the intestinal disposition and poor bioavailability of emodin. Toxicol Appl Pharmacol 265(3):316–324
84. Liu Y, Chen X, Qiu M, Chen W, Zeng Z, Chen Y (2014) Emodin ameliorates ethanol-induced fatty liver injury in mice. Pharmacology 94(1–2):71–77
85. Liu Z, Wei F, Chen LJ, Xiong HR, Liu YY, Luo F, Hou W, Xiao H, Yang ZQ (2013) Invitro and invivo studies of the inhibitory effects of emodin isolated from polygonum cuspidatum on coxsakievirus b_4. Molecules 18(10):11842–11858
86. Liu Z, Ma N, Zhong Y, Yang Zhan-qin Y (2015) Antiviral effect of emodin from Rheum palmatus against coxaskievirus $B_5$and human respiratory syncytial virus in vitro. J Huazhong University Sci Technol (Medical Sciences) 35:916–922

87. Ljubimov AV, Caballero S, Agoki AM, Pinna LA, Grant MB (2004) Involvement of protein kinase CK2 in angiogenesis and retinal neovascularization. Invest Ophthalmol Vis Sci 45:4583–4591
88. Lu Y, Yang JH, Li X, Hwangbo K, Hwang SL, Taketomi Y, Murakami M, Chang YC, Kim CH, Son JK, Chang HW (2011) Emodin, a naturally occurring anthroquinone derivative, suppresses IGE-mediated anaphylactic reaction and mast cell activation. Biochem Pharmacol 82(11):1700–1708
89. Ma J, Lu H, Wang S, Chen B, Liu Z, Ke X, Liu T, Fu J (2015) the anthraquinone derivative emodin inhibits angiogenesis and metastasis through downregulating Runx2 activity in breast cancer. Int J Oncol 46(4):1619–1628
90. Ma J, Yang J, Wang C, Zhang N, Dong Y, Wang C, Wang Y, Lin X (2014) Emodin augments cisplatin cytotoxicity in platinum-resistant ovarian cancer cells via ros-dependent MRP1 downregulation. Biomed Res Int: Article ID 107671, 8 p
91. Ma Y-S, Weng SW, Lin MW, Lu CC, Chiang JH, Yang JS, Lai KC, Lin JP, Tang NY, Lin JG, Chung JG (2012) Antitumor effects of emodin on LS1034 human colon cancer cells in vitro and in vivo: roles of apoptotic cell death and LS1034 tumor xenografts model. Food Chem Toxicol 50:1271–1278
92. Markovic ZS, Manojlovic NT (2009) DFT study on the reactivity of OH groups in emodin. Monatsh Chem 140:1311–1318
93. Masaldan S, Iyer VV (2014) Exploration of effects of emodin in selected cancer cell lines: enhanced growth inhibition by ascorbic acid and regulation of LRP1 and AR under hypoxia-like conditions. J Appl Toxicol 34(1):95–104
94. Meng KW, Lv Y, Yu L, Wu SL, Pan CE (2005) Effects of emodin and double blood supplies on liver regeneration of reduced size graft liver in rat model. World J Gastroenterol 11 (19):2941–2944
95. Meng L, Yan D, Xu W, Ma J, Chen B, Feng H (2012) Emodin inhibits tumor necrosis factor-α-induced migration and inflammatory responses in rat aortic smooth muscle cells. Int J Mol Med 29(6):999–1006
96. Mizuno M, Kawamura H, Takei N, Nawa H (2008) The anthraquinone derivative emodin ameliorates neurobehavioral deficits of a rodent model for schizophrenia. J Neural Transm (Vienna) 115(3):521–530
97. Mueller SO, Schmitt M, Dekant W, Stopper H, Schlatter J, Schreier P, Lutz WK (1999) Occurrence of emodin, chrysophanol and physcion in vegetables, herbs and liquors. Genotoxicity and anti-genotoxicity of the anthraquinones and of the whole plants. Food Chem Toxicol 37:481–491
98. Muto A, Hori M, Sasaki Y, Saitoh A, Yasuda I, Maekawa T, Uchida T, Asakura K, Nakazato T, Kaneda T, Kizaki M, Ikeda Y, Yoshida T (2007) Emodin has a cytotoxic activity against human multiple myeloma as a janus-activated kinase 2 inhibitor. Mol Cancer Ther 6(3):987–994
99. Nemmar A, Al-Salam S, Yuvaraju S, Beegam S, Ali BH (2015) Emodin mitigates diesel exhaust particles-induced increase in airway resistance, inflammation and oxidative stress in mice. Respir Physiol Neurobiol 15(215):51–57
100. Ni Q, Sun K, Chen G, Shang D (2014) In vitro effects of emodin on peritoneal macrophages that express membrane-bound CD14 protein in a rat model of severe acute pancreatitis/systemic inflammatory response syndrome. Mol Med Rep 9:355–359
101. Ni Q, Zhang W, Sun K, Yin C, An J, Shang D (2014) In vitro effects of emodin on peritoneal macrophage intercellular adhesion molecule-3 in a rat model of severe acute pancreatitis/systemic inflammatory response syndrome. Biomed Rep 2(1):63–68
102. Ok S, Kim SM, Kim C, Nam D, Shim BS, Kim SH, Ahn KS, Choi SH, Ahn KS (2012) Emodin inhibits invasion and migration of prostate and lung cancer cells by downregulating the expression of chemokine receptor CXCR4. Immunopharmacol Immunotoxicol 34(5): 768–778

103. Olsen B, Bjørling-Poulsen M, Guerra B (2007) Emodin negatively affects the phosphoinositide 3-kinase/AKT signalling pathway: a study on its mechanism of action. Int J Biochem Cell Biol 39:227–237
104. Pang X, Liu J, Li Y, Zhao J, Zhang X (2015) Emodin Inhibits homocysteine-induced CReactive protein generation in vascular smooth muscle cells by regulating PPARγ expression and ROS-ERK1/2/p38 signal pathway. PLoS ONE 10(7):e0131295
105. Park SJ, Jin ML, An HK, Kim KS, Ko MJ, Kim CM, Choi YW, Lee YC (2015) Emodin induces neurite outgrowth through PI3K/Akt/GSK-3β-mediated signaling pathways in Neuro2a cells. Neurosci Lett 19(588):101–107
106. Ren H, Zhu C, Li Z, Yang W, Song E (2014) Emodin-loaded magnesium silicate hollow nanocarriers for anti-angiogenesis treatment through inhibiting VEGF. Int J Mol Sci 15 (9):16936–16948
107. Saito ST, Silva G, Pungartnik C, Brendel M (2012) Study of DNA-emodin interaction by FTIR and UV–Vis spectroscopy. J Photochem Photobiol B 4(111):59–63
108. Sevcovicova A, Bodnarova K, Loderer D, Imreova P, Galova E, Miadokova E (2014) Dual activities of emodin—DNA protectivity vs mutagenicity. Neuro Endocrinol Lett 35(Suppl 2): 149–154
109. Sharma R, Tiku AB (2014) Emodin, an anthraquinone derivative, protects against gamma radiation-induced toxicity by inhibiting DNA damage and oxidative stress. Int J Radiat Biol 90(4):275–283
110. Sharma R, Tiku AB (2015) Emodin inhibits splenocyte proliferation and inflammation by modulating cytokine responses in a mouse modelsystem. J Immunotoxicol 13(1):20–26
111. Shia CS, Juang SH, Tsai SY, Chang PH, Kuo SC, Hou YC, Chao PD (2009) Metabolism and pharmacokinetics of anthraquinones in Rheum palmatum in rats and ex vivo antioxidant activity. Planta Med 75:1386–1392
112. Shia CS, Hou YC, Tsai SY, Huieh PH, Leu YL, Chao PD (2010) Differences in pharmacokinetics and ex vivo antioxidant activity following intravenous and oral administrations of emodin to rats. J Pharm Sci 99(4):2185–2195
113. Shia CS, Tsai SY, Lin JC, Li ML, Ko MH, Chao PD, Huang YC, Hou YC (2011) Steady-state pharmacokinetics and tissue distribution of anthraquinones of rhei rhizoma in rats. J Ethnopharmacol 137(3):1388–1394
114. Shia CS, Hou YC, Juang SH, Tsai SY, Hsieh PH, Ho LC, Chao PD (2011) Metabolism And Pharmacokinetics Of San-Huang-Xie-Xin-Tang, a polyphenol-rich Chinese medicine formula, in rats and ex-vivo antioxidant activity. Evid Based Complement Altern Med. Article ID 721293
115. Shieh DE, Chen YY, Yen MH, Chiang LC, Lin CC (2004) Emodin-induced apoptosis through P53-dependent pathway in human hepatoma cells. Life Sci 74(18):2279–2290
116. Shirai M, Kawai Y, Yamanishi R, Kinoshita T, Chuman H, Terao J (2006) Effect of a conjugated quercetin metabolite, quercetin 3-glucuronide, on lipid hydroperoxide-dependent formation of reactive oxygen species in differentiated PC-12 cells. Free Radic Res 40(10): 1047–1053
117. Shrimali D, Shanmugam MK, Kumar AP, Zhang J, Tan BK, Ahn KS, Sethi G (2013) Targeted abrogation of diverse signal transduction cascades by emodin for the treatment of inflammatory disorders and cancer. Cancer Lett 341(2):139–149
118. Son YK, Lee SM, An WS, Kim KH, Rha SH, Rho JH, Kim SE (2013) The role of protein kinase CK2 in cyclosporine-induced nephropathy in rats. Transplant Proc 45(2):756–762
119. Song ZC, Wang ZS, Bai JH, Li Z, Hu J (2012) Emodin, a naturally occurring anthraquinone, ameliorates experimental autoimmune myocarditis in rats. Tohoku J Exp Med 227(3):225–230
120. Srinivas G, Babykutty S, Prasanna Sathiadevan PP, Srinivas P (2007) Molecular mechanism of emodin action: transition from laxative ingredient to an antitumor agent. Inc. Med Res Rev 27(5):591–608
121. Su YT, Chang HL, Shyue SK, Hsu SL (2005) Emodin induces apoptosis in human lung adenocarcinoma cells through a reactive oxygen species-dependent mitochondrial signaling pathway. Biochem Pharmacol 70(2):229–241

122. Subramaniam A, Shanmugam MK, Ong TH, Li F, Perumal E, Chen L, Vali S, Abbasi T, Kapoor S, Ahn KS, Kumar AP, Hui KM, Sethi G (2013) Emodin inhibits growth and induces apoptosis in an orthotopic hepatocellular carcinoma model by blocking activation of STAT3. Br J Pharmacol 170(4):807–821
123. Sui JQ, Xie KP, Zou W, Xie MJ (2014) Emodin inhibits breast cancer cell proliferation through the Erα-MAPK/Akt-Cyclin D1/Bcl-2 signaling pathway. Asian Pac J Cancer Prev 15 (15):6247–6251
124. Sun Y, Wang X, Zhou Q, Lu Y, Zhang H, Chen Q, Zhao M, Su S (2015) Inhibitory effect of emodin on migration, invasion and metastasis of human breast cancer MDA-MB-231 cells in vitro and in vivo. Oncol Rep 33(1):338–346
125. Sun Y, Sun L, Liu S, Song J, Cheng J, Liu J (2015) Effect of emodin on aquaporin 5 expression in rats with sepsis-induced acute lung injury. J Tradit Chin Med 35(6):679–684
126. Sun YP, Liu JP (2015) Blockade of emodin on amyloid-B 25-35-induced neurotoxicity in Aβpp/PS1 mice and PC12 cells through activation of the class III phosphatidylinositol 3-Kinase/Beclin-1/B-cell lymphoma 2 pathway. Planta Med 81(2):108–115
127. Sun ZH, Bu P (2012) Downregulation of phosphatase of regenerating liver-3 is involved in the inhibition of proliferation and apoptosis induced by emodin in the SGC-7901 human gastric carcinoma cell line. Exp Ther Med 3(6):1077–1081
128. Tang Q, Zhao S, Wu J, Zheng F, Yang L, Hu J, Hann SS (2015) Inhibition of integrin-linked kinase expression by emodin through crosstalk of Ampkα and ERK1/2 signaling and reciprocal interplay of Sp1 and C-Jun. Cell Signal 27:1469–1477
129. Thacker PC, Karunagaran D (2014) Emodin suppresses Wnt signaling in human colorectal cancer cells SW480 and SW620. Eur J Pharmacol 5(742):55–64
130. Thacker PC, Karunagaran D (2015) Curcumin and emodin down-regulate TGF-β signaling pathway in human cervical cancer cells. PLoS ONE 10(3):e0120045
131. Thomson RH (1987) Naturally occurring quinines. III. Recent advances. London
132. Tu C, Gao D, Li XF, Li CY, Li RS, Zhao YL, Li N, Jia GL, Pang JY, Cui HR, Ma ZJ, Xiao XH, Wang JB (2015) Inflammatory stress potentiates emodin-induced liver injury in rats. Front Pharmacol 23(6):233
133. Tzeng TF, Lu HJ, Liou SS, Chang CJ, Liu IM (2012) Emodin, a naturally occurring anthraquinone derivative, ameliorates dyslipidemia by activating AMP-activated protein kinase in high-fat-diet-fed rats. Evid Based Complement Altern Med 2012:781812
134. Van den Berg AJJ, Labadie RP (1989) Quinones. In: Deypm H (ed) Methods in plant biochemistry, vol 1. Plant phenolics. Academic Press, London, pp 451–491
135. van Gorkom BA, De Vries EG, Karrenbeld A, Kleibeuker JH (1999) Anthranoid laxatives and their potential carcinogenic effects. Aliment Pharmacol Ther 13(4):443–452
136. Waly MI, Ali BH, Al-Lawati I, Nemmar A (2013) Protective effects of emodin against cisplatin-induced oxidative stress in cultured human kidney (HEK 293) cells. J Appl Toxicol 33:626–630
137. Wang J, Huang H, Liu P, Tang F, Qin J, Huang W, Chen F, Guo F, Liu W, Yang B (2006) Inhibition of phosphorylation of P38 MAPK involved in the protection of nephropathy by emodin in diabetic rats. Eur J Pharmacol 553(1–3):297–303
138. Wang RT, Yin H, Dong SB, Yuan W, Liu YP, Liu C (2014) Research progress of emodin anti-gallbladder carcinoma. Zhongguo Zhong Yao Za Zhi Zhongguo Zhong Yao Za Zhi 39 (11):1976–1978
139. Wang T, Zhong XG, Li YH, Jia X, Zhang SJ, Gao YS, Liu M, Wu RH (2015) Protective effect of emodin against airway inflammation in the ovalbumin-induced mouse model. Chin J Integr Med. 21(6):431–437
140. Wang W, Sun Y, Li X, Li H, Chen Y, Tian Y, Yi J, Wang J (2011) Emodin potentiates the anticancer effect of cisplatin on gallbladder cancer cells through the generation of reactive oxygen species and the inhibition of survivin expression. Oncol Rep 26(5):1143–1148
141. Wang W, Sun YP, Huang XZ, He M, Chen YY, Shi GY, Li H, Yi J, Wang J (2010) Emodin enhances sensitivity of gallbladder cancer cells to platinum drugs via glutathion depletion and MRP1 downregulation. Biochem Pharmacol 79(8):1134–1140

142. Wang W, Zhou Q, Liu L, Zou K (2012) Anti-allergic activity of emodin on IgE-mediated activation in RBL-2H3 cells. Pharmacol Rep 64(5):1216–1222
143. Wang XH, Wu SY, Zhen YS (2004) Inhibitory effects of emodin on angiogenesis. Yao Xue Xue Bao 39(4):254–258
144. Wang XJ, Yang J, Cang H, Zou YQ, Yi J (2005) Gene expression alteration during redox dependent enhancement of arsenic cytotoxicity by emodin in hela cells. Cell Res 15(7): 511–522
145. Wang YJ, Huang SL, Feng Y, Ning MM, Leng Y (2012) Emodin, an 11β-hydroxysteroid dehydrogenase type 1 inhibitor, regulates adipocyte function in vitro and exerts anti-diabetic effect in Ob/Ob mice. Acta Pharmacol Sin 33(9):1195–1203
146. Way TD, Husang JT, Chou CH, Huang CH, Yang MH, Ho CT (2014) Emodin represses tWIST 1-induced epithelial-mesenchymal transitions in head and neck squamous cell carcinoma cells by inhibiting the β-catenin and Akt pathways. Eur J Cancer 50:366–378
147. Wei WT, Chen H, Ni ZL, Liu HB, Tong HF, Fan L, Liu A, Qiu MX, Liu DL, Guo HC, Wang ZH, Lin SZ (2011) Antitumor and apoptosis-promoting properties of emodin, an anthraquinone derivative from rheum officinale baill, against pancreatic cancer in mice via inhibition of Akt activation. Int J Oncol 39(6):1381–1390
148. Wu W, Hu N, Zhang Q, Li Y, Li P, Yan R (2014) In vitro glucuronidation of five rhubarb anthraquinones by intestinal and liver microsomes from humans and rats. Chem Biol Interact 5(219):18–27
149. Wu Y, Tu X, Lin G, Xia H, Huang H, Wan J, Cheng Z, Liu M, Chen G, Zhang H, Fu J, Liu Q, Liu DX (2007) Emodin-mediated protection from acute myocardial infarction via inhibition of inflammation and apoptosis in local ischemic myocardium. Life Sci 81(17–18): 1332–1338
150. Wu Z, Chen Q, Ke D, Li G, Deng W (2014) Emodin protects against diabetic cardiomyopathy by regulating the AKT/GSK-3β signaling pathway in the rat model. Molecules 19(9):14782–14793
151. Wu ZX, Yu BP, Xu L (2009) Emodin inhibits voltage-dependent potassium current in guinea pig gallbladder smooth muscle. Basic Clin Pharmacol Toxicol 105(3):167–172
152. Xiang MX, Xu Z, Su HW, Hu J, Yan YJ (2011) Emodin-8-O-B-D-glucoside from polygonum amplexicaule D. Don Var. Sinense Forb promotes proliferation and differentiation of osteoblastic MC3T3-E1 cells. Molecules 16(1):728–737
153. Xiao M, Zhu T, Zhang W, Wang T, Shen YC, Wan QF, Wen FQ (2014) Emodin ameliorates LPS-induced acute lung injury, involving the inactivation of NF-κB in mice. Int J Mol Sci 15 (11):19355–19368
154. Xing JY, Song GP, Deng JP, Jiang LZ, Xiong P, Yang BJ, Liu SS (2015) Antitumor effects and mechanism of novel emodin rhamnoside derivatives against human cancer cells in vitro. PLoS One 10(12):e0144781
155. Xue J, Ding W, Liu Y (2010) Anti-diabetic effects of emodin involved in the activation of PPARγ on high-fat diet-fed and low dose of streptozotocin-induced diabetic mice. Fitoterapia 81(3):173–177
156. Xue J, Chen F, Wang J, Wu S, Zheng M, Zhu H, Liu Y, He J, Chen Z (2015) Emodin protects against concanavalin a-induced hepatitis in mice through inhibiting activation of the p38 MAPK-NF- κB signaling pathway. Cell Physiol Biochem 35(4):1557–1570
157. Xue WH, Shi XQ, Liang SH, Zhou L, Liu KF, Zhao J (2015) Emodin attenuates cigarette smoke induced lung injury in a mouse model via suppression of reactive oxygen species production. J Biochem Mol Toxicol 29(11):526–532
158. Yan YY, Zheng LS, Zhang X, Chen LK, Singh S, Wang F, Zhang JY, Liang YJ, Dai CL, Gu LQ, Zeng MS, Talele TT, Chen ZS, Fu LW (2011) Blockade of Her2/neu binding to Hsp90 by emodin azide methyl anthraquinone derivative induces proteasomal degradation of Her2/neu. Mol Pharm 8(5):1687–1697
159. Yang JH, Hsia TC, Kuo HM, Chao PD, Chou CC, Wei YH, Chung JG (2006) Inhibition of lung cancer cell growth by quercetin glucuronides via G2/M arrest and induction of apoptosis. Drug Metab Dispos 34(2):296–304

160. Yang T, Kong B, Kuang Y, Cheng L, Gu J, Zhang J, Shu H, Yu S, Yang X, Cheng J, Huang H (2015) Emodin plays an interventional role in epileptic rats via multidrug resistance gene 1 (MDR1). Int J Clin Exp Pathol 8(3):3418–3425
161. Yang Z, Zhou E, Wei D, Li D, Wei Z, Zhang W, Zhang X (2014) Emodin inhibits LPS-induced inflammatory response by activating PPAR-γ in mouse mammary epithelial cells. Int Immunopharmacol 21(2):354–360
162. Yaoxian W, Hui Y, Yunyan Z, Yanqin L, Xin G, Xiaoke W (2013) Emodin induces apoptosis of human cervical cancer hela cells via intrinsic mitochondrial and extrinsic death receptor pathway. Cancer Cell Int 13(1):71
163. Yen G-C, Duh P-D, Chuang D-Y (2000) Antioxidant activity of anthraquinones and anthrone. Food Chem 70(4):437–441
164. Yin JT, Wan B, Liu DD, Wan SX, Fu HY, Wan Y, Zhang H, Chen Y (2016) Emodin alleviates lung injury in rats with sepsis. J Surg Res. doi:10.1016/j.jss.2015.12.049
165. Yin X, Gong X, Jiang R, Kuang G, Wang B, Zhang L, Xu G, Wan J (2014) Emodin ameliorated lipopolysaccharide-induced fulminant hepatic failure by blockade of TLR4/MD2 complex expression in D-galactosamine-sensitized mice. Int Immunopharmacol 23(1):66–72
166. Yoshino S, Hara A, Sakakibara H, Kawabata K, Tokumura A, Ishisaka A, Kawai Y, Terao J (2011) Effect of quercetin and glucuronide metabolites on the monoamine oxidase-A reaction in mouse brain mitochondria. Nutrition 27(7–8):847–852
167. Zhan Y, Wei H, Wang Z, Huang X, Xu Q, Li D, Lu H (2001) Effects of emodin on hepatic fibrosis in rats. Zhonghua Gan Zang Bing Za Zhi 9(4):235–236
168. Zhang HM, Wang F, Qiu Y, Ye X, Hanson P, Shen H, Yang D (2016) Emodin inhibits coxsackievirus B3 replication via multiple signalling cascades leading to suppression of translation. Biochem J 473(4):473–485. doi:10.1042/BJ20150419
169. Zhang K, Jiao K, Zhu Y, Wu F, Li J, Yu Z (2015) Effect of emodin on proliferation and cell cycle of human oral squamous carcinoma Tca8113 cells in vitro. Nan Fang Yi Ke Da Xue Xue Bao 35(5):665–670
170. Zhang L, Chang CJ, Bacus SS, Hung MC (1995) Suppressed transformation and induced differentiation of HER-2/neu-overexpressing breast cancer cells by emodin. Cancer Res 55 (17):3890–3898
171. Zhang L, Lau YK, Xi L, Hong RL, Kim DS, Chen CF, Hortobagyi GN, Chang C, Hung MC (1998) Tyrosine kinase inhibitors, emodin and its derivative repress HER-2/neu-induced cellular transformation and metastasis-associated properties. Oncogene 16(22):2855–2863
172. Zhang X, Chen Y, Zhang T, Zhang Y (2015) Inhibitory effect of emodin on human hepatoma cell line Smmc-7721 and its mechanism. Afr Health Sci 15(1):97–100
173. Zhao XY, Qiao GF, Li BX et al (2009) Hypoglycaemic and hypolipidaemic effects of emodin and its effect on L-type calcium channels in dyslipidaemic-diabetic rats. Clin Exp Pharmacol Physiol 36(1):29–34
174. Zhou M, Xu H, Pan L, Wen J, Guo Y, Chen K (2008) Emodin promotes atherosclerotic plaque stability in Fat fed Apolipoprotein –E deficient mice. Tohoku J Exp Med 215(1):61–69
175. Zhou XM, Chen QH (1988) Biochemical study of chinese rhubarb XXII. Inhibitory effect of anthraquinone derivatives on sodium-potassium-atpase of a rabbit renal medulla and their diuretic action. Acta Pharmacol Sin 23:17–20
176. Zhou GH, Zhang F, Wang XN, Kwon OJ, Kang DG, Lee HS, Jin SN, Cho KW, Wen JF (2014) Emodin accentuates atrial natriuretic peptide secretion in cardiac atria. Eur J Pharmacol 15(735):44–51
177. Zhu X, Zeng K, Qiu Y, Yan F, Lin C (2013) Therapeutic effect of emodin on collagen-induced arthritis in mice. Inflammation 36(6):1253–1259
178. Zu C, Zhang M, Xue H, Cai X, Zhao L, He A, Qin G, Yang C, Zheng X (2015) Emodin induces apoptosis of human breast cancer cells by modulating the expression of apoptosis-related genes. Oncol Lett 10(5):2919–2924

Chapter 4
Ursolic Acid and Chronic Disease: An Overview of UA's Effects On Prevention and Treatment of Obesity and Cancer

Anna M. Mancha-Ramirez and Thomas J. Slaga

Abstract Chronic diseases pose a worldwide problem and are only continuing to increase in incidence. Two major factors contributing to the increased incidence in chronic disease are a lack of physical activity and poor diet. As the link between diet and lifestyle and the increased incidence of chronic disease has been well established in the literature, novel preventive, and therapeutic methods should be aimed at naturally derived compounds such as ursolic acid (UA), the focus of this chapter. As chronic diseases, obesity and cancer share the common thread of inflammation and dysregulation of many related pathways, the focus here will be on these two chronic diseases. Significant evidence in the literature supports an important role for natural compounds such as UA in the prevention and treatment of chronic diseases like obesity and cancer, and here we have highlighted many of the ways UA has been shown to be a beneficial and versatile phytochemical.

Keywords Cancer · Obesity · Inflammation · Ursolic acid · Triterpenoids · Phytonutrients

4.1 Introduction

Over the past 50 years, trends in lifestyle and diet have drastically affected the way human beings experience disease and aging. Tragically, the modern western diet is poorly balanced and composed of many nutrient-deficient foods. With this in mind,

A.M. Mancha-Ramirez
Department of Cellular and Structural Biology, The University of Texas Health Science Center San Antonio, 7703 Floyd Curl Drive, San Antonio, TX 78229, USA
e-mail: manchaa@livemail.uthscsa.edu

T.J. Slaga (✉)
Department of Pharmacology, The University of Texas Health Science Center San Antonio, 7703 Floyd Curl Drive, San Antonio, TX 78229, USA
e-mail: slagat@uthscsa.edu

S.C. Gupta et al. (eds.), *Anti-inflammatory Nutraceuticals and Chronic Diseases*,
Advances in Experimental Medicine and Biology 928,
DOI 10.1007/978-3-319-41334-1_4

it is not surprising that chronic disease poses a serious worldwide problem, and one that has undoubtedly risen from a stark dissonance between today's modern diet and that which our ancestors once thrived upon.

The modern western diet is characterized by an excess of salt and refined sugar, and the readily available low cost, high calorie, nutrient foods that are part of a typical western diet are believed to be a key component in the increasing obesity epidemic [77, 116]. Specifically, based on data obtained from the National Health and Nutrition Examination Survey, some of the most concerning issues with the typical modern western diet include an increased uptake of refined grains, added sugars, and saturated fats [81]. Moreover, it has been suggested that some of the modern agricultural practices and over-processed nature of the typical western diet has contributed to the nutrient deficiency seen in many components of regularly consumed food products [116].

As the link between diet and lifestyle and the increased incidence of chronic disease has been well established in the literature, it makes sense to direct our attention to phytonutrients as meaningful therapeutic agents for the prevention and treatment of chronic illnesses such as those discussed in this chapter. Natural remedies derived from plants play an important role both in the prevention of chronic disease development and in the treatment of chronic inflammation-driven diseases. Moreover, plant-derived compounds have been the primary source of medication for centuries in the Asian subcontinent [3, 7].

Significant evidence in the literature suggests that persistent inflammation is the primary initiating factor that causes major chronic disease. Unfortunately, novel approaches towards prevention or treatment of chronic diseases is still moving quite slowly [1]. It is well known that phytonutrients derived from plants and their extracts have been widely used in Eastern medicine for thousands of years for a variety of illnesses included but not limited to hypertension, inflammation, and of course cancer [58, 74]. Modern epidemiological studies have shown that consumption of nutrient-rich fruit and vegetable-based diets can decrease the risk of many diseases including metabolic syndrome and cancer [10, 43, 70, 128]. One such powerful and versatile phytonutrient is ursolic acid (UA), a pentacyclic triterpene that can be found in apples and rosemary, among other sources [40]. In this chapter, we will discuss this phytonutrient in great detail including the multitude of ways UA has shown great efficacy in both metabolic disorder maladies as well as against several types of cancer (Fig. 4.1).

When considering the importance of chronic illness, for perspectives sake, let us picture a crowded football stadium where every seat is filled; now, imagine that the people in this stadium represent the population of the United States. According to a 2012 CDC report, approximately half of the fans in our imaginary stadium had one or more chronic health condition(s), and one in four had two or more chronic health conditions. Stepping away from our stadium analogy, this translates to approximately 117 million Americans, half of the adult population, who were living with chronic illnesses in 2012. Of the ten most common chronic diseases, this chapter will focus on cancer, obesity, and other illnesses that result from the latter, such as those associated with metabolic syndrome. Perhaps after using our imagination for the

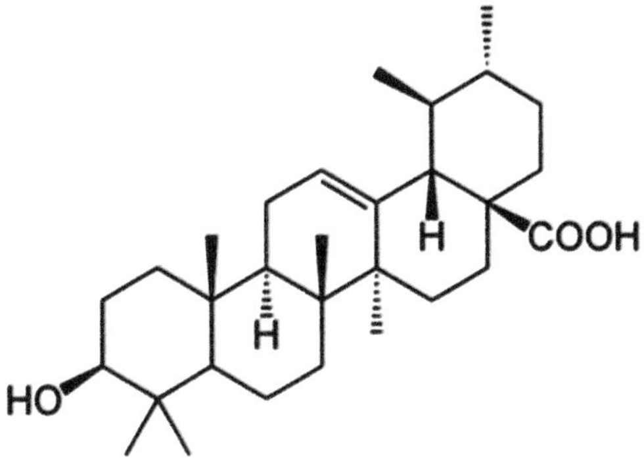

Fig. 4.1 Chemical structure of ursolic acid (UA) [123]

football stadium exercise, it is not difficult to see why chronic diseases and conditions are among the costliest of all health problems. However, what *is* difficult to discern is why we have not managed to diminish this increasing trend of chronic illness when much of it can be prevented. The unfortunate trend in poor diet choices coupled with incredibly busy lifestyles, which do not leave any room for regular exercise, has led to a startling incidence in obesity and subsequently, the rise of metabolic syndrome in the western world. Metabolic syndrome is a generalized term for maladies such as hypertension, heart disease, and type II diabetes, all of which are typically developed as a consequence of an individual having low physical activity, resulting in obesity. Interestingly, there are several different types of cancer including colon and breast cancer where risk factor is greatly increased by being overweight or obese. Consequently, there is growing evidence supporting a strong link between metabolic syndrome and an increased risk of developing cancer, making it quite easy to see how these two chronic illnesses are tightly intertwined.

4.1.1 A Brief Overview of Obesity and Metabolic Syndrome

According to the World Health Organization, being overweight is one of the top 10 risk conditions in the world, and one which will affect upwards of one billion people by 2030 [37]. Perhaps the most devastating aspect of this chronic illness is the fact that obesity brings about so many different comorbidities that can significantly compromise a patient's quality of life; one highly relevant example of this is diabetes. Current predictions for the prevalence of diabetes suggest that this disease will globally increase from 285 million in 2010 to 439 million in 2030 [101]. Not only has diabetes quickly become an epidemic, but the other characteristic aspects of the disease such as damage to tissue in the liver, kidney, adipose tissue, pancreas, and vasculature as a result of pro-inflammation and oxidative stress, generate unique problems of their own [14]. It is vital to remember that the pathogenesis of obesity is extremely complex and can be caused by a variety of factors such as a genetic predisposition, metabolism, physiology, endocrine problems, and behavioral issues

[134]. While obesity is traditionally considered fundamental to the development of type II diabetes, it is now known that both insulin resistance and hyperinsulinemia are part of this process as well [134]. As current antidiabetic drugs have minimal efficacy and can often possess safety concerns, the need to identify novel therapies for this devastating disease is immense. If new antidiabetic agents, ideally derived from natural compounds, can be identified and utilized, these could hold great promise for the hundreds of millions of individuals currently seeking better management of diabetes.

4.1.2 A Brief Overview of Cancer

"Cancer" is considered a rather oversimplified term for upwards of 100 malignant neoplastic diseases [96]. As cancer is a multifactorial disease with many complicated and intertwined causal pathways, choosing effective targets, and developing novel therapies can be incredibly difficult. Despite significant time, money, and effort put forth over the past several decades, the American Cancer Society reported in 2013 that cancer still remains the second leading cause of death in the United States. The startling difficulties of developing novel effective treatments coupled with the fact that it is still one of the leading causes of death in the United States, has directed a significant portion of research towards cancer chemoprevention. Chemoprevention utilizes specific natural or synthetic chemical compounds to inhibit or reverse carcinogenesis and/or to suppress the development of cancer [95]. As many studies have shown that the incidence of cancer could potentially be decreased by chemoprevention, this strategy has become one that is heavily investigated. Importantly, the majority of the chemopreventive agents currently being evaluated are natural products or their derivatives. Many natural compounds, or *phytonutrients*, have already been found to exhibit cancer chemopreventive activities both in vitro and in vivo [49, 86]. Of course, one of the most beneficial aspects of utilizing phytonutrients for chemoprevention is their nontoxic nature, which is vastly different from traditional cancer therapies.

4.2 Mechanistic Links Between Obesity, Metabolic Syndrome Diseases, and Cancer

Although cancer and obesity are two entirely different diseases by definition, they share many cellular signaling pathways that play a part in their pathogenesis. Moreover, both cancer and obesity-related diseases share a very important aspect of pathogenesis, which is inflammation. Chronic inflammation has been linked with most chronic illnesses including cancer, cardiovascular disease, diabetes, obesity, and neurologic disease [3]. Significant epidemiological evidence shows an increased risk of acquiring several different types of cancer which is greatly increased by being overweight or obese [5]. Specifically, a wide variety of cancers, including high-grade prostate cancer, colorectal cancer, postmenopausal breast cancer, and melanoma have been shown to be linked to obesity in epidemiological studies [15, 25, 92, 105]. As you might expect, just as obesity and diabetes have been shown to be associated with increase cancer incidence, conversely, exercise, and decreased caloric intake have been shown to be associated with decreased cancer incidence. It is well known that calorie restriction and exercise aid in the prevention of obesity and diabetes, but both have also been correlated with decreased cancer incidences in many epidemiological studies and can directly inhibit tumor formation in certain cancer models [48, 75, 79]. For example, calorie restriction was able to prevent tumor formation in various mouse models of cancer including the breast, colon, brain, prostate, and chemically induced skin cancer [24, 69, 102].

When there is excess dietary intake in an individual, the result is excess fat storage and improper processing of glucose and lipids [32]. The peptide hormone insulin is secreted by the β cells of the pancreas and its job is to maintain normal blood glucose levels by facilitating cellular glucose uptake, regulating carbohydrate, lipid, and protein metabolism and promoting cell division and growth [122]. The goal of insulin in healthy humans is to increase glucose uptake and tell the liver to shut down the process of gluconeogenesis. Conversely, in overweight or obese humans, this process is derailed by chronic exposure to high levels of glucose and free fatty acids. Obesity-associated inflammation regulates insulin resistance in target cells, ultimately resulting in more insulin production in order to reduce blood glucose and fatty acid levels [51, 122]. The end result of the increased demand for insulin production is the breakdown of insulin-producing β-cells in the pancreas, and ultimately type II diabetes (Fig. 4.2).

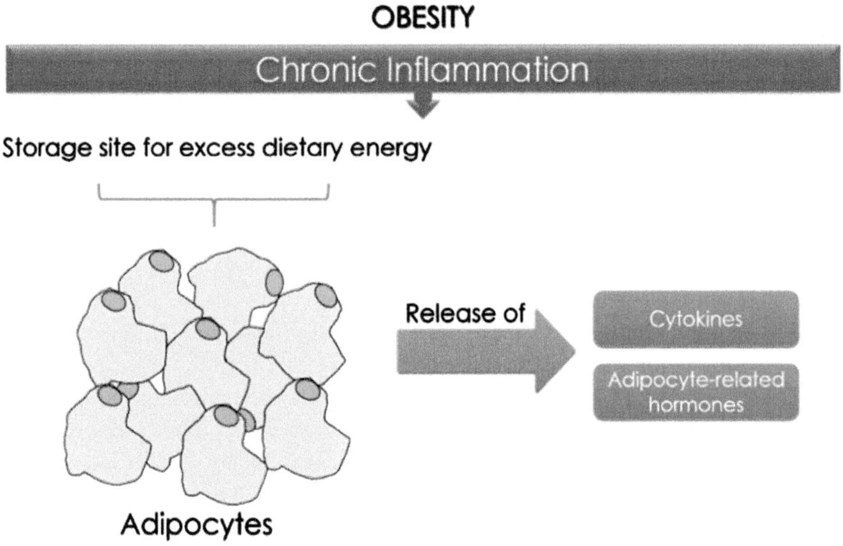

Fig. 4.2 The role of obesity and chronic inflammation in cytokine and hormone release

Excess dietary energy is stored in the adipocytes, and as this process occurs, cytokines are released along with adipocyte-related hormones which affect systemic vasculature [28, 106, 115]. Of the cytokines released via the process described above, some of the most notable are angiogenin, vascular endothelial growth factor, endostatin, tumor necrosis factor-α, and interleukin (IL)-6 [28, 106, 115].

This release of cytokines that takes place results in the activation of various signaling pathways including nuclear transcription factor κB (NFκB) [8, 112]. NFκB is a ubiquitous transcription factor that normally resides in the cytoplasm, but when activated, is translocated to the nucleus, where it induces transcription of many genes [2]. In terms of obesity and NFκB, the obese state in general is associated with increased systemic inflammatory cytokine production and chronic activation of NFκB [55, 71]. In addition to its role in metabolic disorders, NFκB is also upregulated in a multitude of human cancers and contributes to tumor promotion [19, 47, 62, 72, 109, 110]. The activated form of NFκB is capable of mediating cancer, atherosclerosis, diabetes, arthritis, and many other inflammatory diseases [2]. Specifically, the NFκB pathway is one of the most important signaling pathways involved in immunity, inflammation, proliferation, and anti-apoptotic defenses. In terms of cancer, inhibition of NFκB leads to downregulation of proteins involved in anti-apoptotic defense mechanisms utilized by cancer cells such as Bcl-2, Bcl-xL, and c-FLIP; this process thereby promotes apoptotic cell death in cancer cells [58]. The activation of IKKβ plays a major role in inflammation induced tumor promotion and progression [126]. Experimental studies have shown the NFκB activity is necessary for the formation of a number of tumor types [38]. Increased NFκB activation may provide a link between obesity, diabetes, and a range of tumor types [90, 91, 113].

It is well known that AMP-activated protein kinase (AMPK) is a fuel-sensing enzyme that is activated by changes in the AMP/ATP ratio. The role of this enzyme is to increase cellular ATP generation and diminish ATP use for less critical processes depending upon the situation [93]. In addition to glucose transport, lipid and protein synthesis, and fuel metabolism, AMPK is also responsible for regulating a myriad of other physiological processes including but not limited to cellular growth and proliferation, mitochondrial function, and factors linked to insulin resistance, including inflammation, oxidative and ER stress, and autophagy [93]. AMPK restores ATP levels by inhibiting anabolic processes like fatty acid synthesis and gluconeogenesis and activating catabolic processes like fat oxidation and glucose uptake [117]. Significant evidence in the literature supports a definite link between dysregulation of AMPK and insulin resistance in both rodents and humans. In addition, common antidiabetic drugs, as well as insulin-sensitizing hormones like adiponectin, function via AMPK [23, 76, 121, 124, 136]. It has also been shown that AMPK suppresses NFκB activities in different systems through a variety of mechanisms, and antidiabetic drugs have also shown NFκB-suppressing properties as a consequence of AMPK activation [9, 94, 133]. As many studies have shown that calorie restriction can prevent tumor formation in various mouse models of cancer, the link between obesity and cancer is one that is well represented in the literature. Calorie restriction models have prevented tumor formation in brain, colon, breast, prostate, and chemically mediated skin cancer [11, 12, 24, 69, 102]. It has been suggested that the anticancer effects of calorie restriction and exercise may be mediated by the energy sensor AMPK [67].

Additional mechanistic links between metabolic syndrome and cancer include as we would expect, many of the cell signaling pathways related to inflammation such as TNF-α. Additionally, interleukin-6 (IL-6) is also shown to be elevated in obesity and is positively correlated with BMI [50]. Increased IL-6 levels, as seen in obesity models, leads to induced JAK-STAT3 signal transduction and stimulates cell proliferation, differentiation, and metastasis [21, 125]. Data related to insulin resistance and mechanistic links to cancer suggest that insulin resistance may lead to a poorer response to cancer treatment and possibly a more aggressive phenotype in patients with preexisting diabetes [66].

4.3 An Overview of Ursolic Acid

Ursolic acid (UA), 3β-hydroxy-olea-12-en-28-oic acid, is a pentacyclic triterpenoid that is derived from various different sources such as berries, leaves, flowers, and fruits of medicinal plants such as *Eriobotrya japonica, Calluna vulgaris, Rosmarinus officinalis,* and *Eugenia jambolana* [64]. The pentacyclic triterpenoids contain six isoprene units, the basic molecular formula $C_{30}H_{48}O_x$, and they have five rings in their skeleton [40]. One of the benefits of UA is that it is widely distributed in the plant kingdom [84]. Significant evidence in the literature suggests that consumption of fruits and vegetables rich in triterpenoids have shown beneficial effects against a variety of inflammation-driven diseases including several different types of cancer such as breast, colon, and pancreas [3, 99] (Table 4.1).

Classified according to the number of isoprene units, the terpenoid compounds are a large class of natural agents that are synthesized in plants by cyclization of squalene [123]. Specifically, pentacyclic triterpenoids have been shown in the literature to have a myriad of functions, however the effective concentrations to produce different cellular effects varies depending upon the exact phytonutrient in question [126]. Some of the effects that pentacyclic triterpenoids have been cited as eliciting include the induction of the anti-inflammatory response, cytoprotective effects, and apoptotic effects [126]. Triterpenoids are capable of affecting multiple signaling pathways, and the pentacyclic triterpenoids are particularly studied in the literature having proven to have many useful clinical properties. The precise mechanism by which UA derives its various efficacious properties is still unknown, however it is believed that the presence of α,β-unsaturated carbonyl moieties significantly enhances the potency of this specific class of terpenoids [126]. Additionally, pentacyclic triterpenoids have the ability to inhibit multiple targets, a trait that is suggested to be mediated by the reversible Michael addition of these phytonutrients to exposed nucleophilic groups of various susceptible signaling proteins [126]. NF-κB, STAT3, Bcl-2, Bax, ICAM-1, p53, and PKC are all examples of molecular targets of UA for anticancer and anti-inflammatory activities

Table 4.1 Various medicinal plants containing ursolic acid (adapted from [6])

Botanical name	Common name
Ocimum sanctum L.	Holy Basil (Tulsi)
Eriobotrya japonica	Loquat
Vaccinium macrocarpon	Cranberry
Harpagophytum procumbens DC	Devil's Claw
Sambucus nigra L.	Elder flowers (European variety)
Mentha piperita L.	Peppermint leaves
Eugenia jambolana	Java plum
Perilla frutescens	Beefsteak plant
Apocynaceae *Lavandula augustifolia* Mill.	Lavender
Origanum vulgare L.	Oregano
Malus domestica	Different apples
Melissa officinalis	Lemon balm
Rosmarinus officinalis	Rosemary
Plantago major	Greater plantain
Thymus vulgaris L.	Thyme
Crataegus laevigata (Poir) DC	Hawthorn
Coffea arabica	Coffee
Calluna vulgaris	Heather
Eucalyptus spp.	Eucalyptus

[126]. Although the focus here is on chronic illnesses, cancer and obesity, UA has also been shown to be effective in treatment of chronic diseases related to cardiovascular conditions, atherosclerosis, and osteoporosis [126].

UA is a phytonutrient with great versatility and is capable of multiple biological functions; however one potential drawback to its potential use is that despite low toxicity, it has low water solubility [127]. To overcome this potential drawback and improve upon its activity and bioavailability, many studies have been carried out in order to identify structural modifications to achieve this goal. Specifically, UA derivatives with modifications at the 3-OH and/or 17-COOH positions demonstrate significant antitumor effects both in vitro and in vivo suggesting that these modifications can enhance the bioavailability of UA [13, 26, 80]. Additionally, structural studies have also shown that modification of UA with a piperazine group, specifically a piperazine moiety at the C-28 position, can elicit a better inhibitory effect on cancer cell growth [22, 100]. Overall, of the many reported UA analogs which have been developed to date, some of the most important modifications include those on the positions of C-3/C-28, C-11, C-17, and C-28, and modifications on C-2/C-3 positions and ring A [16].

Although there have not been any detailed studies on pure UA and its absorption and distribution, one study investigating the intestinal uptake of UA (from the ethanolic extract of *Sanbucus chinesis*) reported that a dose contributing 80 mg/kg body weight, UA had about 0.6 % oral bioavailability in rats [59]. Moreover, the half-life was found to be about 4.3 h, and UA was detected in kidney tissue (3.51 ± 0.57 nmol/mg) after oral administration of 0.2 % UA in the diet to rats over a period of 11 weeks [59]. There are not any published studies on acute and/or subacute toxicity of UA alone, but one study looked at a mixture of UA and oleanolic acid (OA), a similar compound, also a triterpenoid [39, 107]. They found that a single subcutaneous injection of OA (1.0 g/kg) to mice or rats during a 5-day period did not cause mortality. Moreover, during multiple administrations of OA (180 mg/kg, p.o.) for 10 days, no abnormalities were observed in brain, heart, lung, liver, kidney, thyroid, testes, spleen, or intestines [39, 107]. Several studies aimed at evaluating UA and/or OA found that these compounds also do not cause irritation or inflammation when given either topically to the skin or in the diet [31, 39, 53, 59, 64, 107]. UA does not lead to liver damage or elevated liver enzymes which relate to possible liver damage, and in fact, it is a very potent hepatoprotective component of several medicinal herbs [29, 60, 68, 104]. UA has a wide range of pharmaceutical properties and is a secondary plant metabolite usually present in the stem, bark, leaves, or fruit peel [123].

UA and its isomer oleanolic acid (OA) have been shown to have many valuable abilities including inhibition of tumorigenesis, inhibition of tumor promotion, and inhibition of angiogenesis. Moreover, UA and OA have been shown to possess antiatherosclerotic, anti-inflammatory, hepatoprotective, gastroprotective, and cardiovascular treatment abilities [83]. UA is considered to be nutritionally important in the prevention of several chronic diseases, including diabetes and cancer, but of course is not limited to only these two illnesses [56, 64]. Used because of its diverse healing properties in traditional Chinese medicine for centuries, UA has in recent years been studied in great detail in order to elucidate the exact mechanisms of action by which it exerts its health beneficial effects, however the precise nature of these mechanisms have yet to be determined [123]. Studies aimed at predicting the molecular targets of UA have been carried out which analyze the signaling pathways of the predicted targets of UA. Bioinformatic data from these studies demonstrated that there were 611 possible molecular proteins as targets for interaction with UA, and more than 49 functional clusters responding to it as well [36]. Notably, there were 76 pathways that were significantly enriched such as MAPK, p53, and mTOR pathways [36].

In addition to effects in cancer and obesity, which are the focus of this chapter, UA has also been shown to have an effect on the liver, on muscle and fat, exhibit anti-atherogenic and cardioprotective effects, and antimicrobial activity. A very potent hepatoprotective component of several medicinal herbs, UA is capable of protecting the liver from chloroform-induced injury and against D-galactosamine-induced liver injury in rats [29, 60, 68, 104]. Recent studies have also shown that UA alone or in combination with resveratrol were effective in preventing obesity and fatty liver disease in mice fed a high-fat diet (Digiovanni and Slaga, unpublished results). UA alone has been shown to elicit an antifibrotic effect in the liver, but the exact targets for this mechanism have not yet been discerned [36]. Many UA containing plants have anti-bacterial and antifungal activity; in fact, UA has been shown to have antimicrobial activity against several strains of staphylococci [4, 130]. Finally, UA is a potent inhibitor of components of metabolic syndrome such as hypertension, triglyceride levels, and accumulation of inflammatory monocytes and associated atherosclerosis [41, 42, 108, 114].

4.4 Ursolic Acid and Its Effects on Obesity and Metabolic Syndrome

Among other traditional Chinese medicinal agents such as anthraquinones, several terpenes including UA have proven to be effective antiobesity agents. It is proposed that these phytonutrients can aid against obesity by modulating body weight, blood glucose levels, triglycerides, and total cholesterol [134]. Recently, it has been demonstrated that UA along with several of its other triterpenoid family members, can improve insulin signaling by enhancing insulin receptor β subunit phosphorylation and Akt in vitro [46, 61, 132]. UA has also been shown to promote glucose uptake from the bloodstream into peripheral tissues through upregulation of GLUT4 [20, 33, 119]. One study investigating the ability of UA to promote glucose uptake found that UA achieved this by enhancing the translocation of GLUT4 to the plasma membrane in 3T3-L1 adipocytes [46]. A final mechanism by which UA is suggested to aid in lowering blood glucose levels is by lowering endogenous glucose production through gluconeogenesis inhibition [14].

Another important target when considering insulin resistance therapies is PTP1B, a molecule that negatively regulates insulin signaling. Targeting PTP1B is a very useful approach because it can inhibit the PI3K/Akt signaling pathway to induce insulin resistance by inhibition of the translocation of GLUT4 to the plasma membrane [111]. Many studies have evaluated several triterpenoids including UA for their ability to act as PTP1B inhibitors, and several in vitro findings suggest that UA can directly inhibit PTP1B and improve insulin sensitivity [61, 78, 88].

Studies utilizing rodents on a high-fat diet showed UA's ability to normalize blood glucose levels in animals characterized by diet-induced obesity or diabetes [73, 89]. One particular study utilized a hypertensive rat model, and showed that UA was able to lower resting glucose, LDL cholesterol, and triglycerides to near control levels; it also raised antioxidant enzymes and HDL cholesterol after 6 weeks of treatment [108]. UA also reversed high-fat diet-induced NFκB signaling and deficits in metabolic signaling in mice [54, 89]. One study produced findings which suggest UA may function via a similar mechanism as exercise, due to results showing that UA stimulates glucose uptake and activates AMPK in insulin resistant cells [34].

Among the many comorbidities associated with metabolic syndrome, in patients with type II diabetes, hyperglycemia promotes an increase in free radicals and a decrease in antioxidants leading to lipid peroxidation [14]. It is well established that free radicals such as reactive oxygen species can have negative effects as they can ultimately lead to cellular dysfunction [30]. Animal studies showed that treatment with UA was able to decrease liver damage caused by oxidative stress inducing chemicals such as carbon tetrachloride [65]. Moreover, UA, and other triterpenoids were also able to increase the activities of the antioxidant enzymes superoxide dismutase and glutathione peroxidase [68, 118]. Another significant complication of diabetes is diabetic nephropathy, and therefore UA was tested to determine what effect it would have on renal function in streptozotocin-induced diabetes. The study looking at diabetic nephropathy found that UA significantly prevented biochemical and histopathologic changes in the kidneys associated with diabetes, and lowered NF-κB activity and renal oxidative stress levels [63]. Finally, phase 2 clinical studies evaluating the effect of UA on insulin sensitivity and metabolic syndrome were carried out in 2015 but the results have not yet been published. Despite the fact that recent studies have demonstrated that UA does exert an antiobesity effect, the mechanisms of action are still under investigation. Currently, several of the proposed mechanisms and targets include inhibition of PTP1B, lipolysis stimulation via cAMP-dependent PKA pathway modulation, modulation of the LKB1/AMPK pathway, and regulation of adipogenic differentiation [42, 57, 82, 89, 120].

4.5 Ursolic Acid and Its Effects on Cancer

With regards to cancer, UA has been studied in great detail. However, the precise mechanisms of the many anticancer effects of UA and corresponding molecular targets for these capabilities are still under investigation. UA has been shown to have a variety of anticancer capabilities, including the ability to suppress proliferation of several different types of tumor cells, induce apoptosis, and inhibit tumor promotion, metastasis, and angiogenesis in cancer animal models [98]. Several mechanisms which have been elucidated for the above mentioned anticancer abilities of UA thus far and include the ability to suppress multiple cell signaling pathways such as growth factor receptor activation (EGFR), signaling through IKK/NF-κB, Akt/mTOR, Cox-2, STAT3, MMP9, and VEGF [97, 126, 131].

4.5.1 Ursolic Acid and Cancer: Notable in vitro Studies

UA has shown great efficacy as an anticancer therapy in many in vitro models, many of which are accomplished via inhibition of DNA replication, caspase activation, inactivation of protein tyrosine kinases, induction of Ca^{2+} release, and finally via NFκB mediated downregulation of the cellular inhibitor of apoptosis gene [98]. UA has been reported to induce apoptosis in diverse cell lines via its immunomodulatory and anti-inflammatory actions [123]. In B16F10 and A375 melanoma cells, the combination of UA with chloroquine was able to synergistically decreased cell viability [45]. Additionally, studies carried out in mouse skin papilloma and carcinoma cell lines have indicated that the cytotoxic effects of UA can be enhanced with *p*-glycoprotein inhibitors [44].

Cranberry-derived UA showed potent anti-proliferative activities against HepG2 liver cancer cells and MCF7 breast cancer cells [35]. UA-mediated apoptosis of human bladder cancer cells was strongly suppressed by AMPK knockdown [135]. Additionally, UA reduced the viability of human colon cancer cell lines [27]. UA has also shown great promise in breast cancer studies as well, with an ability to strongly decrease viability of a breast cancer cell line with an associated inhibition of NFκB, as well as, a decrease size of breast cancer xenografts in murine models [129].

Similar in vitro effects of UA have been seen in prostate cancer models as well [99]. Notably, it was found that UA was able to suppress NFκB activation induced by numerous carcinogens, such as TNFα, phorbol ester, okadaic acid, H_2O_2, and cigarette smoke [103]. Inhibition of NFκB activation was mediated via IKK kinase activation, IκBα phosphorylation and degradation, p65 phosphorylation, p65 nuclear translocation, and NFκB dependent reporter gene expression [98]. Results from multiple myeloma in vitro studies showed that UA was able to inhibit both constitutive and IL-6-inducible STAT3 activation, which was mediated through the inhibition of upstream kinases C-SRC, JAK1, JAK2, and ERK1/2 [85]. Moreover, they also showed that UA could induce expression of the SHP-1 protein, while knockdown of SHP-1 via RNA interference was able to suppress the induction of SHP-1 and reverse the inhibition of STAT3 activation. The results from the Pathak group suggest a critical role of SHP-1 in the mechanism of action of UA, and show that it can be effective in suppressing important inflammatory networks including NFκB, STAT3, and AKT [85].

4.5.2 Ursolic Acid and Cancer: Notable in vivo Studies

In addition to the extensive work that has been carried out investigating the efficacy of UA in in vitro cancer models, significant evidence supporting the versatility and usefulness of UA has also been amassed in in vivo studies as well. For example, the effect of UA was evaluated on early stages of skin tumorigenesis utilizing a two-stage carcinogenesis SENCAR mouse model, and found topical application of UA alone and/or in combination with calcium D-glutarate during the promotion stage was able to inhibit tumor multiplicity and tumor incidence [52]. Results from this study showed that UA is a potent inhibitor of skin tumor promotion and inflammatory signaling in skin cancer and potentially other epithelial cancers in humans as well [52]. UA isolated from *P. frutescens* was also evaluated in a two-stage skin carcinogenesis mouse model, and was found to significantly inhibit skin tumor promotion by the tumor promoting agent, TPA [17, 18]. Specifically, pretreatment with UA resulted in a 42 % inhibition of papilloma formation [17, 18]. Furthermore, when UA was used in combination with resveratrol, a phytochemical present in grapes, berries, peanuts, and red wine, the combination was found to have a greater inhibitory effect on skin tumor promotion by TPA in a mouse model than with either agent used independently [17, 18]. Mechanistic studies into the enhanced inhibitory effects observed in the UA + resveratrol combination showed an upregulation of tumor suppressor genes such as p21 and PDCD4 as well as a dramatic increase of *p*-AMPKα and its downstream target *p*-Ulk1-^{ser555} [17, 18].

In a prostate cancer DU145 xenograft nude mouse model, one group analyzed whether UA could inhibit the growth of prostate cancer and found that UA was able to significantly suppress the tumor growth in vivo following 6 weeks of treatment [99]. Also noteworthy in this xenograft prostate cancer study was that at the endpoint of the experiment, there was no significant change in body weight of UA-treated mice suggesting that UA is a nontoxic compound when administered to mice. Results from this in vivo prostate cancer mouse model showed a substantial decrease in VEGF expression and an increase in caspase-3 expression in UA-treated mice, suggesting that perhaps UA is functioning as an anti-angiogenic and pro-apoptotic agent against prostate cancer in this model [99]. Additionally, UA, when administered by gavage, also decreased incidence of chemically induced preneoplastic lesions in rat colon [27] (Fig. 4.3).

Finally, a phase I trial was carried out in 2015 to evaluate the multiple-dose safety and antitumor activity of UA liposomes (UAL) in patients with advanced solid tumors. UA liposome is a new antitumor drug that has significant potential therapeutic value as it utilizes liposomes to overcome the poor solubility of UA, increase the therapeutic efficiency, reduce the side effects, and enhance the bioavailability of the drug. Results from this clinical trial demonstrate that UAL treatment of patients with advanced solid tumors via multiple-dose and consecutive

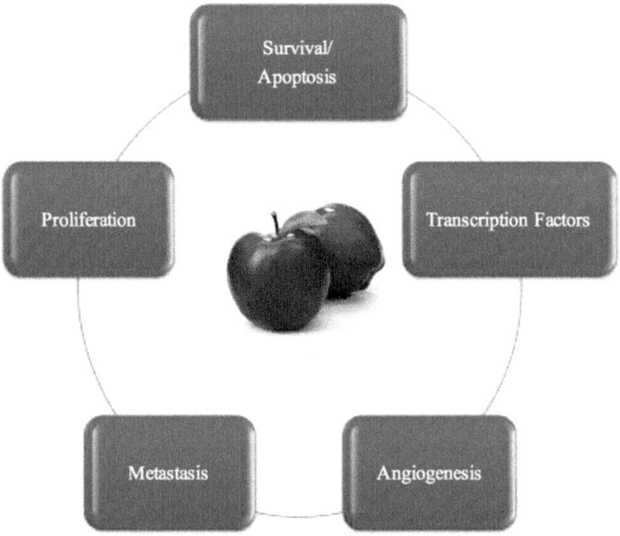

Fig. 4.3 An overview of the many oncogenic targets UA has been shown to modulate

14-day intravenous infusion every 21 days was safe. Additionally, the preliminary antitumor activity of UAL was evaluated for the first time in a clinical setting and their results indicate UAL may be able to potentially improve patient remission [87].

4.6 Conclusion

As obesity, metabolic syndrome, and cancer have been shown to have similar mechanistic links, this presents a useful avenue for novel preventive and therapeutic strategies aimed at fighting these chronic diseases. Dysregulation of important cell signaling pathways occurs during the constant state of inflammation during obesity, and this has been linked to an increased overall risk of certain cancers such as breast and colorectal cancer. Moreover, as discussed earlier, patients with preexisting conditions brought on by obesity, such as insulin resistance, tend to respond more poorly to traditional chemotherapeutic agents than otherwise healthy individuals. As cancer is a multifactorial disease, it is vital to investigate novel therapeutic compounds that exhibit efficacy against key pathways often dysregulated in cancer pathogenesis. Due to the unique nature of each individual cancer development, multi-targeting therapies from natural resources are vital for targeting cancer development and progression. Triterpenoids such as UA offer unique and novel drug platforms for development due to the fact that they have been shown to target critical inflammatory proteins for the prevention and treatment of cancer. As these phytonutrient have been shown to be nontoxic, it is their safety and ability to affect various key targets that makes compounds like UA very desirable as a starting point for future drug development. It is quite possible that triterpenes such as UA could be used in conjunction with commonly used chemotherapeutic agents to allow for perhaps a decrease in the chemotherapeutic dose, less adverse effects of the chemotherapeutic agent, or even synergistic effects between UA and the drug. While there is significant data in the literature to support an important role for UA in cancer prevention/therapy, future clinical investigations are needed to further validate these findings. Here, we have discussed in detail the various ways in which UA has shown great potential as an anticancer agent in many different types of cancer; many of these results have significant clinical implications as UA has been shown to target key cancer pathways.

UA is not only capable of acting as an anticancer compound, but it also has been shown to have versatile antiobesity properties which we have described in detail. These effects appear to be partially mediated by inhibition of NFκB and/or activation of AMPK, but due to the many various effects of UA seen in both cancer and obesity, the precise mechanisms of action for these effects are still unclear. Although diet and exercise plus a highly controlled blood glucose level is currently the recommended treatment for obesity and type II diabetes, one of the major drawbacks of this standard of care is of course compliance. Where patients may exhibit poor compliance with a recommended course of diet and exercise, pharmacological agents targeting key disease pathways such as those targeted by UA could significantly aid in the prevention/of obesity and obesity-related comorbidities in addition to diet and exercise regimens.

Significant evidence in the literature supports an important role for natural compounds such as UA in the prevention and treatment of chronic diseases like obesity and cancer, and here we have highlighted many of the ways UA has been shown to be a beneficial and versatile phytochemical in both of these diseases. Although there is extensive data in the literature to support the efficacious nature of UA in cancer and obesity, there is still significant work to be done in more mechanistic-oriented research in order to determine the mechanisms by which this versatile and effective compound exerts its action. Moreover, it is great importance to undergo further structural studies of UA in order to develop novel derivatives which may exhibit increased bioavailability while still maintaining the same efficacy and low toxicity seen in the parent compound. As the link between diet and lifestyle and the increased incidence of chronic disease has been well established in the literature, it is extremely vital to investigate the use of phytonutrients as meaningful therapeutic agents for the prevention and treatment of chronic illnesses such as those discussed in this chapter as well as to elucidate the mechanisms by which they elicit their action.

References

1. Aggarwal B, Van Kuiken ME, Iyer LH, Harijumar KB, Sung B (2009) Molecular targets of nutraceuticals derived from dietary spices: potential role in suppression of inflammation and tumorigenesis. Exp Biol Med 234:825–849
2. Aggarwal B, Shishodia S (2004) Suppression of the nuclear factor-κB activation pathway by spice-derived phytochemicals. Ann NY Acad Sci 1030:434–441
3. Aggarwal B, Shishodia S (2006) Molecular targets of dietary agents for prevention and therapy of cancer. Biochem Pharmacol 71:1397–1421
4. Anisimov MM, Shcheglov VV, Strigina LI et al (1979) Chemical structures and antifungal activity of a number of triterpenoids. Biol Bull Acad Sci USSR 6:464–468
5. Aridiacono B, Iiritano S, Nocera A, Possidente K, Nevolo M, Ventura V, Foti D, Chiefari E, Brunetti A (2012) Insulin resistance and cancer risk: an overview of the pathogenic mechanisms. Exp Diabetes Res 2012:1–12
6. Babalola I, Shode F (2013) Ubiquitous ursolic acid: a potential pentacyclic triterpene natural product. J Pharmacogn Phytochem 2:214–222
7. Balunas MJ, Kinghorn AD (2005) Drug discovery from medicinal plants. Life Sci 78: 431–441
8. Bastard JP, Maachi M, Lagathu C, Kim MJ, Caron M, Vidal H (2006) Recent advances in the relationship between obesity, inflammation, and insulin resistance. Eur Cytokine Netw 1:4–12
9. Bess E, Fisslthaler B, Fromel T, Fleming I (2011) Nitric oxide-induced activation of the AMP-activated protein kinase α2 subunit attenuates IκB kinase activity and inflammatory responses in endothelial cells. PLoS One 6:e20848
10. Bessaoud F, Daures J (2008) Dietary factors and breast cancer risk: a case control study among a population in southern France. Nutr Cancer 60:177–187

11. Birt DF, Pelling JC, White LT, Dimitroff K, Barnett T (1991) Influence of diet and calorie restriction on the initiation and promotion of skin carcinogenesis in SENCAR mouse model. Cancer Res 51:1851–1854
12. Blando J, Moore T, Hursting S, Jiang G, Saha A, Beltran L (2011) Dietary energy balance modulates prostate cancer progression in Hi-Myc mice. Cancer Prev Res 4:2002–2014
13. Brenner DA (2011) Molecular pathogenesis of liver fibrosis. Trans Am Clin Climatol Assoc 120:361–368
14. Camer D, Yu Y, Szabo A, Huang XF (2014) The molecular mechanisms underpinning the therapeutic properties of oleanolic acid, its isomer and derivatives for type 2 diabetes and associated complications. Mol Nutr Food Res 58:1750–1759
15. Campbell PT, Jacobs ET, Ulrich CM, Figueiredo JC, Poynter JN, McLaughlin JR et al (2010) Case–control study of overweight, obesity, and colorectal cancer risk, overall and by tumor microsatellite instability status. J Natl Cancer Inst 6:391–400
16. Chen H, Gai Y, Wang A, Zhou X, Zheng Y, Zhou J (2015) Evolution in medicinal chemistry of ursolic acid derivatives as anticancer agents. Eur J Med Chem 92:648–655
17. Cho J, Rho O, Junco J, Carbajal S, Siegel D, Slaga T, DiGiovanni J (2015) Effect of combined treatment with ursolic acid and resveratrol on skin tumor promotion by 12-*O*-tetradecanoylphorbol-13-acetate. Cancer Prev Res 8:817–825
18. Cho J, Tremmel L, Rho O, Camelio A, Siegel D, Slaga T, DiGiovanni J (2015) Evaluation of pentacyclic triterpenes found in *Perilla frutescens* for inhibition of skin tumor promotion by 12-*O*-tetradecanoylphorbol-13-acetate. Oncotarget 6:39292–39306
19. Cogswell PC, Guttridge DC, Funkhouse WK, Baldwin AS (2000) Selective activation of NF-κB subunits in human breast cancer: potential roles for NF-κB 2/p52 and for Bcl-3. Oncogene 19:1123–1131
20. Cong LN, Chen H, Li YH, Zhou LX et al (1997) Physiological role of Akt in insulin-stimulated translocation of GLUT4 in transfected rat adipose cells. Mol Endocrinol 11:1881–1890
21. Darnell JE Jr, Kerr IM, Stark GR (1994) Jak-STAT pathways and transcriptional activation in response to IFNs and other extracellular signaling proteins. Science 264:1415–1421
22. Dong HY, Yang X, Xie JJ, Xiang LP, Li YF, Ou MR, Chi T, Liu ZH, Yu SH, Gao Y, Chen JZ, Shao JW, Jia L (2015) UP12, a novel ursolic acid derivative with potential for targeting multiple signaling pathways in hepatocellular carcinoma. Biochem Pharmacol 93:151–162
23. Fediuc S, Pimenta AS, Gaidhu MP, Ceddia RB (2008) Activation of AMP-activated protein kinase, inhibition of pyruvate dehydrogenase activity, and redistribution of substrate partitioning mediate the acute insulin-sensitizing effects of troglitazone in skeletal muscle cells. J Cell Physiol 215:392–400
24. Fernandes G, Chandrasekar B, Troyer DA, Venkatraman JT, Good RA (1995) Dietary lipids and calorie restriction affect mammary tumor incidence and gene expression in mouse mammary tumor virus/v-Ha-ras transgenic mice. Proc Natl Acad Sci 92:6494–6498
25. Freedland SJ, Platz EA (2007) Obesity and prostate cancer: making sense out of apparently conflicting data. Epidemiol Rev 29:88–97
26. Friedman SL (2008) Mechanisms of hepatic fibrogenesis. Gastroenterology 134(6): 1655–1669
27. Furtado RA, Rodrigues EP, Araujo FR, Oliveira WL, Furtado MA et al (2008) Ursolic acid and oleanolic acid suppress preneoplastic lesions induced by 1,2-dimethylhydrazine in rat colon. Toxicol Pathol 36:576–580
28. Galic S, Oakhill JS, Steinberg GR (2009) Adipose tissue as an endocrine organ. Mol Cell Endocrinol 285:115–122
29. Gan KH, Lin CN (1988) Studies on the constituents of Formosan gentianaceous plants. XI. Constituents of Gentiana flavor-maculata and tripterospermum Taiwanese and the cento-hepatotoxic activities of ursolic acid derivatives. Chin Pharmaceut J 40:77–84
30. Gao D, Li Q, Li Y, Liu Z et al (2009) Antidiabetic and antioxidant effects of oleanolic acid from *Ligustrum lucidum* Ait in alloxan-induced diabetic rats. Phytother Res 23:1257–1262

31. Garrido JC, Cevallos GAC, Siciliano LG et al (2012) Acute and subacute toxicity (28 day) of a mixture of ursolic acid and oleanolic acid obtained from Bouvard interminfolia in mice. Bull Latinoam Caribe Plantas Medic Aromat 11(1):91–102
32. Guarente L (2006) Sirtuins as potential targets for metabolic syndrome. Nature 444:868–874
33. Hajduch E, Alessi DR, Hemmings BA, Hundal HS (1998) Constitutive activation of protein kinase B alpha by membrane targeting promotes glucose and system A amino acid transport, protein synthesis, and inactivation of glycogen synthase kinase 3 in L6 muscle cells. Diabetes 47:1006–1013
34. He Y, Li Y, Zhao T, Wang Y, Sun C (2013) Ursolic acid inhibits adipogenesis in 3T3-L1 adipocytes through LKB1/AMPK pathway. PLoS One 8:1–12
35. He X, Liu RH (2006) Cranberry phytochemicals: isolation, structure elucidation, and their antiproliferative and antioxidant activities. J Agric Food Chem 54:7069–7074
36. He W, Shi F, Zhou Z-W, Li B, Zhang K, Zhang X et al (2015) A bioinformatic and mechanistic study elicits the antifibrotic effect of ursolic acid through the attenuation of oxidative stress with the involvement of ERK, PI3K/Akt, and p38 MAPK signaling pathways in human hepatic stellate cells and rat liver. Drug Des Dev Ther 9:3989–4104
37. Hill JO, Wyatt HR, Reed GW, Peters JC (2003) Obesity and the environment: where do we go from here? Science 299:853–855
38. Huang S, Pettaway CA, Uehara H, Bucana CD, Fidler IJ (2001) Blockade of NF-κB activity in human prostate cancer cells is associated with suppression of angiogenesis, invasion, and metastasis. Oncogene 31:4188–4197
39. Hunan Med Inst (1975) Pharmacological studies of hepatoprotective compounds from *Swertia mileenses*. Trad Med (Zhang Chao Yao) 6:47–62
40. Jager S, Trojan H, Kopp T, Laszczyk MN, Scheffler A (2009) Pentacyclic triterpene distribution in various plants—rich sources for a new group of multi-potent plant extracts. Molecules 14:2016–2031
41. Jang SM, Yee ST, Choi J et al (2009) Ursolic acid enhances the cellular immune system and pancreatic β-cell function in streptozotocin-induced diabetic mice fed a high-fat diet. Int Immunopharmacol 9(1):113–119
42. Jayaprakasam B, Olson LK, Schutzki RE, Tai MH, Nair M (2006) Amelioration of obesity and glucose intolerance in high-fat-fed C57BL/6 mice by anthocyanins and ursolic acid in cornelian cherry (*Cornus mas*). J Agric Food Chem 54:243–248
43. Jedrychowski W, Maugeri U, Popiela T, Kulig J, Sochacka-Tatara E, Pac A, Sowa A, Musial A (2010) Case–control study on beneficial effect of regular consumption of apples on colorectal cancer risk in a population with relatively low intake of fruits and vegetables. Eur J Cancer Prev 19:42–47
44. Junco J, Mancha A, Malik G, Wei S, Kim DJ, Liang H, Slaga TJ (2013) Resveratrol and *p*-glycoprotein inhibitors enhance the anti-skin cancer effects of ursolic acid. Mol Cancer Res 11:1521–1529
45. Junco J, Mancha-Ramirez A, Malik G, Wei S, Kim DJ, Liang H, Slaga TJ (2015) Ursolic acid and resveratrol synergize with chloroquine to reduce melanoma cell viability. Melanoma Res 25:103–112
46. Jung SH, Ha YJ, Shim EK, Choi SY et al (2007) Insulin-mimetic and insulin-sensitizing activities of a pentacyclic triterpenoid insulin receptor activator. Biochem J 403:243–250
47. Karin M (2009) NF-κB as a critical link between inflammation and cancer. Cold Spring Harb Perspect Biol 1:a000141
48. Kelley DE, Wing R, Buonocore C, Sturis J, Polonsky K, Fitzsimmons M (1993) Relative effects of calorie restriction and weight loss in noninsulin-dependent diabetes mellitus. J Clin Endocrinol Metab 5:1287–1293
49. Kelloff GJ, Crowell JA, Steele VE, Lubet RA, Malone WA, Boone CW, Kopelovich L, Et Hawk, Lieberman R, Lawrence JA, Ali I, Viner JL, Sigman CC (2000) Progress in cancer chemoprevention: development of diet-derived chemopreventive agents. J Nutr 130: 467S–471S

50. Kern PA, Ranganathan S, Li C, Wood L, Ranganathan G (2001) Adipose tissue tumor necrosis factor and interleukin-6 expression in human obesity and insulin resistance. Am J Physiol 280:E745–E751
51. Kloppel E, Sinzato YK, Damasceno DC, Volpato GT, Campos KE (2015) Effect of maternal obesity on insulin action in male adult offspring rats. Diabetol Metab Syndr 7:A127
52. Kowalczyk MC, Junco J, Kowalczyk P, Tostykh O, Hanausek M, Slaga TJ, Walaszek Z (2013) Effects of combined phytochemicals on skin tumorigenesis in SENCAR mice. Int J Oncol 43:911–918
53. Kowalczyk MC, Walaszek Z, Kowalczyk P et al (2009) Differential effects of several phytochemicals and their derivatives on murine keratinocytes in vitro and in vivo: implications for skin cancer prevention. Carcinogenesis 30(6):1008–1015
54. Kunkel SD, Elmore CJ, Bongers KS, Ebert SM, Fox DK, Dyle MC, Bullard SA, Adams CM (2012) Ursolic acid increases skeletal muscle and brown fat and decreases diet-induced obesity, glucose intolerance and fatty liver disease. PLoS One 7:1–8
55. Lappas M, Yee K, Permezel M, Rice GE (2005) Sulfasalazine and BAY 11-7082 interfere with the nuclear factor-κB and kinase pathway to regulate the release of proinflammatory cytokines from human adipose tissue and skeletal muscle in vitro. Endocrinology 3: 1491–1497
56. Lee J, Yee ST, Kim JJ, Choi MS, Kwon EY, Seo KI, Lee MK (2010) Ursolic acid ameliorates thymic atrophy and hyperglycemia in streptozotocin-nicotinamide-induced diabetic mice. Chem Biol Interact 188:635–642
57. Li Y, Xing D, Chen Q, Chen W (2010) Enhancement of chemotherapeutic agent-induced apoptosis by inhibition of NF-κB using ursolic acid. Int J Cancer 127:462–473
58. Li-Weber M (2010) Targeting apoptosis pathways in cancer by Chinese medicine. Cancer Lett 332:304–312
59. Liao Q, Yang W, Jia Y et al (2005) LC-MS Determination and pharmacokinetic studies of ursolic acid in rat plasma after administration of the traditional Chinese medicinal preparation Lu–Ying extract. Yakugaku Zasshi 125(6):47–62
60. Lin CN, Chung MI, Gan KH (1988) Novel anti-hepatotoric principles of *Solanun incanum* L. Planta Med 54:222
61. Lin ZH, Zhang Y, Zhang YN, Shen H et al (2008) Oleanolic acid derivative NPLC441 potently stimulates glucose transport in 3T3-L1 adipocytes via a multi-target mechanism. Biochem Pharmacol 76:1251–1262
62. Lind DS, Hochwald SN, Malaty J, Rekkas S, Hebig P, Mishra G (2001) Nuclear factor-κB is upregulated in colorectal cancer. Surgery 130:363–369
63. Ling C, Jinping L, Xia L, Renyong Y (2013) Ursolic acid provides kidney protection in diabetic rats. Curr Ther Res 75:59–63
64. Liu J (1995) Pharmacology of oleanolic acid and ursolic acid. J Ethnopharmacol 49:57–68
65. Liu J, Liu Y, Mao Q, Klaassen CD (1994) The effects of 10 triterpenoid compounds on experimental liver injury in mice. Fundam Appl Toxicol 22:34–40
66. Louie SM, Roberts LS, Nomura DK (2013) Mechanisms linking obesity and cancer. Biochim Biophys Acta 1831:1499–1508
67. Lupertz R, Chovolou Y, Kampkotter A, Watjen W, Kahl R (2008) Catalase overexpression impairs TNF-α induced NF-κB activation and sensitizes MCF-7 cells against TNF-α. J Cell Biochem 103:1497–1511
68. Ma XH, Zhao YC, Yin L et al (1986) Studies on the preventive and therapeutic effects of ursolic acid on acute hepatic injury in rats. Acta Pharm Sin 21:332–335
69. Mai V, Colbert LH, Berrigan D, Perkins SN, Pfeiffer R, Lavigne JA (2003) Calorie restriction and diet composition modulate spontaneous intestinal tumorigenesis in Apc(Min) mice through different mechanisms. Cancer Res 63:1752–1755
70. Martin C, Zhang Y, Tonelli C, Petroni K (2013) Plants, diet, and health. Annu Rev Plant Biol 64:19–46

71. Maury E, Noel L, Detry R, Brichard SM (2009) In vitro hyperresponsiveness to tumor necrosis factor-α contributes to adipokyne dysregulation in omental adipocytes of obese subjects. J Clin Endocrinol Metab 4:1393–1400
72. McNulty SE, del Rosario R, Cen D, Meyskens FL Jr, Yang S (2004) Comparative expression of NFκB proteins in melanocytes of normal skin vs. benign intradermal naevus and human metastatic melanoma biopsies. Pigment Cell Res 17:173–180
73. de Melo CL, Queiroz MG, Fonseca SG, Bizerra AM et al (2010) Oleanolic acid, a natural triterpenoid improves blood glucose tolerance in normal mice and ameliorates visceral obesity in mice fed a high-fat diet. Chem Biol Interact 185:59–65
74. Meng Q, Niu Y, Niu X, Roubin RH, Hanrahan JR (2009) Ethnobotany, phytochemistry, and pharmacology of the genus *Caragana* use in traditional Chinese medicine. J Ethnopharmacol 124:350–368
75. Molfino A, Cascino A, Conte C, Ramaccini C, Rossi F, Laviano A (2010) Caloric restriction and L-carnitine administration improves insulin sensitivity in patients with impaired glucose metabolism. J Parent Enteral Nutr 34:295–299
76. Musi N, Hirshman MF, Nygren J, Svanfeldt M, Bavenholm P, Rooyackers O et al (2002) Role of AMP-activated protein kinase in mechanism of metformin action. J Clin Investig 108:1167–1174
77. Myles I (2014) Fast food fever: reviewing the impacts of the Western diet on immunity. Nutr J 13:1–17
78. Na M, Oh WK, Kim YH, Cai XF et al (2006) Inhibition of protein tyrosine phosphatase 1B by diterpenoids isolated from *Acanthopanax koreanum*. Bioorg Med Chem Lett 16: 3061–3064
79. Nakano Y, Oshima T, Sasaki S, Higashi Y, Ozono R, Takenaka S, Miura F et al (2001) Calorie restriction reduced blood pressure in obesity hypertensives by improvement of autonomic nerve activity and insulin sensitivity. J Cardiovasc Pharmacol 38:69–74
80. Novo E, Cannito S, Paternostro C, Bocca C, Miglietta A, Parola M (2014) Cellular and molecular mechanisms in liver fibrogenesis. Arch Biochem Biophys 548:20–37
81. Nowlin SY, Hammer MJ, D'Eramo Melkus G (2012) Diet, inflammation, and glycemic control in type 2 diabetes: an integrative review of the literature. J Nutr Metab 2012:1–28
82. Ntambi JM, Young-Cheul K (2000) Adipocyte differentiation and gene expression. J Nutr 130:3122S–3126S
83. Ovesna Z, Kozics K, Slamenova D (2006) Protective effects of ursolic acid and oleanolic acid in leukemic cells. Mutat Res 600:131–137
84. Padua TA, de Abreu P, Costa T, Nakamura MJ, Valente LM, Henriques M, Siani A, Rosas E (2013) Anti-inflammatory effects of methyl ursolate obtained from a chemically derived crude extract of apple peels: potential use in rheumatoid arthritis. Arch Pharmacol Res 37:1487–1495
85. Pathak AK, Bhutani M, Nair AS, Ahn KS, Chakraborty A, Kadara H, Guha S, Sethi G, Aggarwal BB (2007) Ursolic acid inhibits STAT3 activation pathway leading to suppression of proliferation and chemosensitization of human multiple myeloma cells. Mol Cancer Res 5:943–955
86. Pezzuto JM (1997) Plant-derived anticancer agents. Biochem Pharmacol 53:1121–1133
87. Qian Z, Wang X, Song Z, Zhang H, Zhou S, Zhao J, Wang H (2015) A phase i trial to evaluate the multiple-dose safety and antitumor activity of ursolic acid liposomes in subjects with advanced solid tumors. BioMed Res Int 2015:1–7
88. Ramirez-Espinosa JJ, Rios MY, Lopez-Martinez S, Lopez-Vallejo F et al (2011) Antidiabetic activity of some pentacyclic acid triterpenoids, role of PTP-1B: in vitro, in silico, and in vivo approaches. Eur J Med Chem 46:2243–2251
89. Rao VS, de Melo CL, Queiroz MGR, Lemos TLG et al (2011) Ursolic acid, a pentacyclic triterpene from *Sambucus australis*, prevents abdominal adiposity in mice fed a high-fat diet. J Med Food 14:1375–1382
90. Renehan AG, Roberts DL, Dive C (2008) Obesity and cancer: pathophysiological and biological mechanisms. Arch Physiol Biochem 114:71–83

91. Rial NS, Choi K, Nguyen T, Snyder B, Slepian MJ (2012) Nuclear factor κB: a novel cause for diabetes, coronary artery disease and cancer initiation and promotion? Med Hypotheses 78:29–32
92. Rodriguez C, Freedland SJ, Deka A, Jacobs EJ, McCullough ML, Patel AV et al (2007) Body mass index, weight change, and risk of prostate cancer in the Cancer Prevention Study II Nutrition Cohort. Cancer Epidemiol Biomarkers Prev 16:63–69
93. Ruderman NB, Carling D, Prentki M, Cacicedo JM (2013) AMPK, insulin resistance, and the metabolic syndrome. J Clin Investig 123:2764–2772
94. Salminen A, Lehtonen M, Suuronen T, Kaarniranta K, Huuskonen J (2008) Terpenoids: natural inhibitor sof NF-κB signaling with anti-inflammatory and anticancer potential. Cell Mol Life Sci 65:2979–2999
95. Sarkar FH, Li YW (2007) Targeting multiple signal pathways by chemopreventive agents for cancer prevention and therapy. Acta Pharmacol Sin 28:1305–1315
96. Senn HJ, Kerr D (2011) Chronic non-communicable diseases, the European Chronic Disease Alliance—and cancer. Ann Oncol 22:248–249
97. Shanmugam M, Dai X, Kumar AP, Tan B, Sethi G, Bishayee A (2013) Ursolic acid in cancer-prevention and treatment: molecular targets, pharmacokinetics and clinical studies. Biochem Pharmacol 85:1579–1587
98. Shanmugam M, Nguyen A, Kumar AP, Tan B, Sethi G (2012) Targeted inhibition of tumor proliferation, survival, and metastasis by pentacyclic triterpenoids: potential role in prevention and therapy of cancer. Cancer Lett 320:158–170
99. Shanmugam M, Rajendran P, Li F, Nema T, Vali S, Abbasi T, Kapoor S, Sharma A, Kumar A, Ho P, Hui K, Sethi G (2011) Ursolic acid inhibits multiple cell survival pathways leading to suppression of growth of prostate cancer xenograft in nude mice. J Mol Med 89:713–727
100. Shao JW, Dai YC, Xue JP, Wang JC, Lin FP, Guo YH (2011) In vitro and in vivo anticancer activity evaluation of ursolic acid derivatives. Eur J Med Chem 46:2652–2661
101. Shaw JE, Sicree RA, Zimmet PZ (2010) Global estimates of the prevalence of diabetes for 2010 and 2030. Diabetes Res Clin Pract 87:4–14
102. Shelton LM, Huysentruyt LC, Mukherjee P, Seyfreid TN (2010) Calorie restriction as an anti-invasive therapy for malignant brain cancer in the MV mouse. ASN Neurosci 2:e00038
103. Shishodia S, Majumdar S, Banerjee S, Aggarwal B (2003) Ursolic acid inhibits nuclear factor-κB activation induced by carcinogenic agents through suppression of IκBα kinase and p65 phosphorylation: correlation with down-regulation of cyclooxygenase 2, matrix metalloproteinase 9, and cyclin D1. Cancer Res 63:4375–4383
104. Shuckla B, Viser S, Patnaik GK et al (1992) Hepatoprotective activity in the rat of ursolic acid isolated from *Eucalyptus* hybrid. Phytother Res 6:74–79
105. Siddiqui AA (2011) Metabolic syndrome and its association with colorectal cancer: a review. Am J Med Sci 3:227–231
106. Silha JV, Krsek M, Suchurda P, Murphy LJ (2005) Angiogenic factors are elevated in overweight and obese individuals. Int J Obes 29:1308–1314
107. Singh GB, Singh S, Bani S et al (1992) Anti-inflammatory activity of oleanolic acid in rats and mice. J Pharm Pharmacol 44:456–458
108. Somova LO, Nadar A, Rammanan P et al (2003) Cardiovascular antihyperlipidemic and antioxidant effects of oleanolic and ursolic acids in experimental hypertension. Phytomedicine 10(2–3):115–121
109. Sovak MA, Bellas RE, Kim DW, Zanieski GJ, Rogers AE, Traish AM et al (1997) Aberrant nuclear factor-κB/Rel expression and the pathogenesis of breast cancer. J Clin Invest 100:2952–2960
110. Suh J, Rabson AB (2004) NF-κB activation in human prostate cancer: important mediator or epiphenomenon? J Cell Biochem 91:100–117
111. Sun T, Wang Q, Yu ZG, Zhang Y et al (2007) Hyrtiosal, a PTP1B inhibitor from the marine sponge *Hyrtios erectus*, shows extensive cellular effects on PI3K/AKT activation, glucose transport, and TGF β/Smad2 signaling. Chem Biol Chem 8:187–193

112. Tilg H, Moschen AR (2008) Inflammatory mechanisms in the regulation of insulin resistance. Mol Med 14:222–231
113. Tornatore L, Thotakura AK, Bennett J, Moretti M, Franzoso G (2012) The nuclear factor κB signaling pathway: integrating metabolism with inflammation. Trends Cell Biol 22:557–566
114. Ullevig SL, Zhao Q, Zamora D et al (2011) Ursolic acid protects diabetic mice against monocyte dysfunction and accelerated atherosclerosis. Atherosclerosis 219(2):409–416
115. Vaccharajani V, Granger DN (2009) Adipose tissue: a motor for the inflammation associated with obesity. Int Union Biochem Mol Biol 61:424–430
116. Via M (2012) The malnutrition of obesity: micronutrient deficiencies that promote diabetes. Endocrinology 2012:1–8
117. Violett B, Lantier L, Devin-Leclerc J, Hebrard S, Amouyal C, Mournier R et al (2009) Targeting the AMPK pathway for the treatment of type 2 diabetes. Front Biosci 14: 3380–3400
118. Wang X, Li YL, Wu H, Liu JZ et al (2011) Antidiabetic effect of oleanolic acid: a promising use of a traditional pharmacological agent. Phytother Res 25:1031–1040
119. Wang QH, Somwar R, Bilan PJ, Liu Z et al (1999) Protein kinase B Akt participates in GLUT4 translocation by insulin in L6 myoblasts. Mol Cell Biol 19:4008–4018
120. White UA, Stephens JM (2010) Transcriptional factors that promote formation of white adipose tissue. Mol Cell Endocrinol 318:10–14
121. Whitehead JP, Richards AA, Hickman IJ, Macdonald GA, Prins JB (2006) Adiponectin—a key adipokine in the metabolic syndrome. Diabetes Obes Metab 8:264–280
122. Wilcox G (2005) Insulin and insulin resistance. Clin Biochem Rev 26:19–28
123. Wozniak L, Skapska S, Marszalek K (2015) Ursolic acid—a pentacyclic triterpenoid with a wide spectrum of pharmacological activities. Molecules 20:20614–20641
124. Xiao X, Su G, Brown SN, Chen L, Ren J, Zhao P (2010) Peroxisome proliferator-activated receptors gamma and alpha agonists stimulate cardiac glucose uptake via activation of AMP-activated protein kinase. J Nutr Biochem 21:621–626
125. Yadav A, Kumar B, Datta J, Teknos TN, Kumar P (2011) IL-6 promotes head and neck tumor metastasis by inducing epithelial-mesenchymal transition via the JAK-STAT3-SNAIL signaling pathway. Mol Cancer Res 9:1658–1667
126. Yadav VR, Prasad S, Sung B, Kannappan R, Aggarwal B (2010) Targeting inflammatory pathways by triterpenoids for prevention and treatment of cancer. Toxins 2:2428–2466
127. Yang X, Li Y, Jiang W, Ou M, Chen Y, Xu Y, Wu Q, Zheng Q, Wu F, Wang L, Zou W, Zhang YJ, Shao J (2015) Synthesis and biological evaluation of novel ursolic acid derivatives as potential anticancer prodrugs. Chem Biol Drug Des 86:1397–1404
128. Yang G, Zheng W, Xiang Y, Gao J, Li H, Zhang X, Gao Y, Shu X (2011) Green tea consumption and colorectal cancer risk: a report from the Shanghai Men's Health Study. Carcinogenesis 32:1684–1688
129. Yeh CT, Wu CH, Yen GC (2010) Ursolic acid, a naturally occurring triterpenoid, suppresses migration and invasion of human breast cancer cells by modulating c-Jun N-terminal kinase, Akt and mammalian target of rapamycin signaling. Mol Nutr Food Res 54:1285–1295
130. Zaletova N, Shchavlinskii A, Tolkachev O, Vichkanova S, Fateeva T, Krutikova N, Yartseva I, Klyuev N (1987) Preparation of some derivatives of ursolic acid and their antimicrobial activity. Chem Abs 106:18867e
131. Zang LL, Wu BN, Lin Y, Wang J, Fu L, Tang ZY (2014) Research progress of ursolic acid's anti-tumor actions. Chin J Integr Med 20:72–79
132. Zhang W, Hong D, Zhou Y, Zhang Y et al (2006) Ursolic acid and its derivative inhibit protein tyrosine phosphatase 1B, enhancing insulin receptor phosphorylation and stimulating glucose uptake. Biochim Biophys Acta 1760:1505–1512
133. Zhang Y, Qiu J, Wang X, Xia M (2011) AMP-activated protein kinase suppresses endothelial cell inflammation through phosphorylation of transcriptional coactivator p300. Arterioscler Thromb Vasc Biol 31:2897–2908

134. Zhang WL, Zhu L, Jiang JG (2014) Active ingredients from natural botanicals in the treatment of obesity. Obes Rev 15:957–967
135. Zheng QY, Jin FS, Yao C, Zhang T, Zhang GH, Ai X (2012) Ursolic acid-induced AMP-activated protein kinase (AMPK) activation contributes to growth inhibition and apoptosis in human bladder cancer T24 cells. Biochem Biophys Res Commun 419:741–747
136. Zhou G, Myers R, Li Y, Chen Y, Shen X, Fenyk-Melody J et al (2001) Role of AMP-activated protein kinase in mechanism of metformin action. J Clin Investig 108: 1167–1174

Chapter 5
Tocotrienol and Its Role in Chronic Diseases

Kok-Yong Chin, Kok-Lun Pang and Ima-Nirwana Soelaiman

Abstract Tocotrienol is a member of vitamin E family and is well-known for its antioxidant and anti-inflammatory properties. It is also a suppressor of mevalonate pathway responsible for cholesterol and prenylated protein synthesis. This review aimed to discuss the health beneficial effects of tocotrienol, specifically in preventing or treating hyperlipidaemia, diabetes mellitus, osteoporosis and cancer with respect to these properties. Evidence from in vitro, in vivo and human studies has been examined. It is revealed that tocotrienol shows promising effects in preventing or treating the health conditions previously mentioned in in vivo and in vitro models. In some cases, alpha-tocopherol attenuates the biological activity of tocotrienol. Except for its cholesterol-lowering effects, data on the health-promoting effects of tocotrienol in human are limited. As a conclusion, the encouraging results on the health beneficial effects of tocotrienol should motivate researchers to explore its potential use in human.

Keywords Bone · Cancer · Cholesterol · Diabetes · Glucose · Osteoporosis · Tocopherol · Tocotrienol · Vitamin E

K.-Y. Chin · I.-N. Soelaiman (✉)
Department of Pharmacology, Universiti Kebangsaan Malaysia Medical Centre, Universiti Kebangsaan Malaysia, Jalan Yaacob Latif, Bandar Tun Razak, Cheras, 56000 Kuala Lumpur, Malaysia
e-mail: imasoel@ppukm.ukm.edu.my

K.-L. Pang
Biomedical Science Programme, School of Diagnostic and Applied Health Sciences, Faculty of Health Sciences, Universiti Kebangsaan Malaysia, Jalan Raja Abdul Aziz, 50300 Kuala Lumpur, Malaysia

S.C. Gupta et al. (eds.), *Anti-inflammatory Nutraceuticals and Chronic Diseases*, Advances in Experimental Medicine and Biology 928,
DOI 10.1007/978-3-319-41334-1_5

5.1 Tocotrienol

Tocotrienol and tocopherol are collectively known as tocochromanols, or commonly as vitamin E. They share a similar chemical structure, consisting of a chromanol ring and a long carbon tail. The difference between tocotrienol and tocopherol is that the carbon tail of tocotrienol contains three double bonds (an unsaturated farnesyl tail), whereas the carbon tail of tocopherol contains only single bonds (a saturated phytyl tail). The difference in the long carbon tail dictates the difference in biological activity between these two compounds. Similar to tocopherol, tocotrienol can be further divided into 4 isomers (alpha, beta, gamma and delta) based on the position of the methyl side chain on the chromanol ring. Beta- and gamma-tocotrienols are structural isomers and possess the same number of methyl group on the chromanol ring. Alpha-tocotrienol has an additional methyl group whereas delta-tocotrienol has one less methyl group on the chromanol ring compared to beta- and gamma-tocotrienol [6, 14] (Fig. 5.1).

Tocotrienol and tocopherol isomers are found together in a wide variety of plants. Tocotrienol is more commonly found in the fruit and seed. Some of the natural sources that yield the highest amount of tocotrienol include seeds of *Bixa orellana* (achiote, annatto) (1.53 mg/g dry weight), *Zea mays* (maize) (1.42 mg/g dry weight), *Garcinia mangostana* (purple mangosteen) (1.33 mg/g dry weight) and oil of *Elaeis guineensis* (oil palm) (1.08 mg/g dry weight). Latex of *Hevea brasiliensis* (rubber tree) (2.59 mg/g dry weight) also contains high amount of tocotrienol, but this is not found in other latex-producing plants (summarized by Müller et al. [98]). Usually alpha-tocopherol is found together with tocotrienol isomers in varying proportions in natural sources. In palm oil, the proportion of alpha-tocopherol is around 30 % of the total vitamin E content [111]. In rice bran, the average percentage of tocotrienol with respect to total vitamin E content is 61 %

Fig. 5.1 Chemical structure of vitamin E isomers

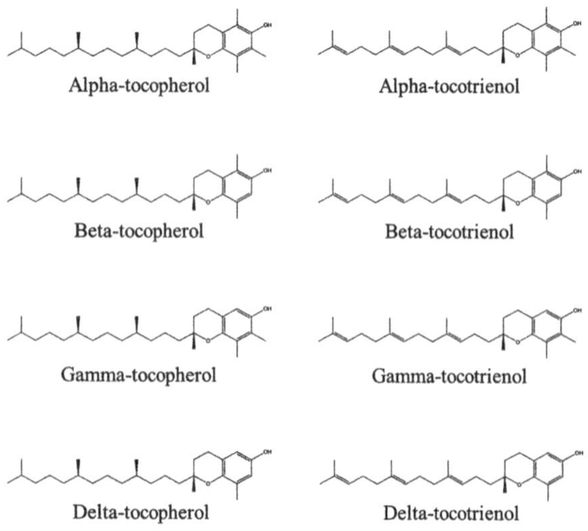

[156]. Vitamin E derived from the seed of *Bixa orellana* contains 10 % gamma-tocotrienol and 90 % delta-tocotrienol with no traceable amount of alpha-tocopherol [42]. Several studies on the tocotrienol content of common food have been performed [31, 157]. The tocotrienol intake has been found to be very low (1.9–2.1 mg/person/day) compared to alpha-tocopherol (8–10 mg/day/person) in a Japanese study. This amount is insufficient compared to the doses used in experimental studies to achieve the health-promoting benefits of tocotrienol. Currently, the recommended dietary allowance (RDA) for vitamin E is 15 mg (22.4 IU) for male and female aged 14 years and above [61]. This estimation is based on alpha-tocopherol because it is the only fraction retained in the blood. The RDA for tocotrienol has not been established.

The absorption of tocotrienol is increased with fat-rich food because it is a lipophilic compound [185]. Tocotrienol and tocopherol are absorbed in the lumen of the small intestine, whereby they enter the enterocytes via passive diffusion, and secreted into the lymphatics [43]. They are transported in the form of chylomicron. The release of vitamin E isomers from the liver to the blood stream is regulated by alpha-tocopherol transporter protein. The transfer protein has the highest affinity towards alpha-tocopherol (100 % binding affinity towards RRR-alpha-tocopherol) and lower binding affinity towards other vitamin E isomers (12 % towards alpha-tocotrienol, 38 % towards beta-tocopherol, 9 % towards gamma-tocopherol and 2 % towards delta-tocopherol) [53]. Tocotrienol is distributed by the bloodstream to various tissues. Significant accumulation of tocotrienol can be found in the adipose and skin tissue, as demonstrated by rodent experiments [72, 147]. Similar to tocopherols, tocotrienols are also metabolised and excreted in the form of carboxyethyl-hydroxychromans [81].

Tocotrienol features a variety of biological activities, which enable it to be used as a candidate agent to prevent chronic diseases. The prominent antioxidant and anti-inflammatory properties of tocotrienol will be discussed in the following sections. Tocotrienol is also a known suppressor of the mevalonate pathway involved in cholesterol synthesis, bone metabolism and carcinogenesis. This will be discussed in the respective sections.

5.2 Antioxidant Effects of Tocotrienol

Oxidants such as reactive oxygen species (ROS) and reactive nitrogen species (NOS) are essential for defence against infectious agents, for cell signalling and for redox homeostasis [170]. They are balanced by endogenous and exogenous antioxidants in our body, such as antioxidant enzymes, vitamins, thiols and glutathione. Oxidative stress occurs when the production of oxidants overwhelms the production of antioxidants in our body [152, 153]. Free radical species are capable of damaging macromolecules such as carbohydrate, protein and DNA in the body and generate more free radicals, thereby forming a vicious cycle [48]. Many adverse health conditions, such as neurodegeneration [12], diabetes mellitus [9], cardiovascular disease [82] and osteoporosis [20], have been linked to oxidative stress. This highlights a possible role of tocotrienol, a strong antioxidant, in preventing these oxidative stress-related diseases.

Both tocotrienol and tocopherol exert their free radical scavenging activity by donating phenolic hydrogen at the sixth position of the chromanol ring [113]. Tocotrienol has been shown to be a superior membrane antioxidant compared to its tocopherol counterpart [161]. This is due to the uniform distribution of tocotrienol in the membrane and its stronger ability to disorder membrane lipids, thus enhancing its recycling efficiency [145]. In studies using lipid peroxidation in microsomes extracted from rat liver, Serbinova et al. showed that the antioxidant effect of alpha-tocotrienol was 40–60 times stronger than alpha-tocopherol [145]. They attributed the superior antioxidant effect of tocotrienol to its higher recycling efficacy from chromanoxyl radicals, uniform distribution in the membrane bilayers and stronger disordering of membrane lipids structure, resulting in a higher efficacy in its interaction with free radicals [145]. Palozza et al. showed that tocotrienol isomers inhibited lipid peroxidation, ROS production and heat shock protein expression in rat liver microsomal membrane and in RAT-1 immortalized fibroblasts challenged with free radicals [121]. The effectiveness of delta-tocotrienol was found to be greater than gamma-tocotrienol, and similar between gamma- and alpha-tocotrienol [121]. It was proposed that decreased methylation of the chromanol ring, as in delta-tocotrienol, allowed the molecule to be better incorporated into cell membranes [121]. Kamat et al. showed that palm tocotrienol significantly reduced the lipid and protein peroxidation products in the microsomal extracts of the brain and liver from rats [66, 67]. Among the individual isomers, they identified that gamma-tocotrienol had the highest antioxidant efficacy compared to delta- and alpha-tocotrienol [66, 67].

The antioxidant properties of tocotrienol were also demonstrated in cell culture studies. Tan et al. showed that alpha-tocotrienol prevented the decrease of glutathione and mitochondrial depolarization induced by hydrogen peroxide in hepatocytes [166]. The increase of cellular ROS and malondialdehyde, a lipid peroxidation product, induced by hydrogen peroxide and paracetamol in hepatocytes were also suppressed by alpha-tocotrienol. Nizar et al. showed that gamma-tocotrienol prevented the apoptosis of primary osteoblast induced by hydrogen peroxide [115]. In a subsequent experiment, they showed that this was achieved by the preservation of cellular antioxidant defence system, such as superoxide dismutase, catalase and glutathione peroxidase, and the reduction of lipid peroxidation product in the treated cells [1].

Tocotrienol also exhibited its antioxidant effect in animal models. Nesaretnam et al. demonstrated that long-term feeding of rats with diet containing palm oil rich in tocotrienol significantly reduced the peroxidation potential of hepatic mitochondria and microsomes compared to corn oil control [106]. The initial rate of lipid peroxidation was also found to be slower in the palm oil supplemented group compared to the corn oil control [106]. Lee et al. showed that rats supplemented with tocotrienol-rich fraction at 25 or 50 mg/kg body weight for 28 days and forced to undergo a swimming endurance test showed higher liver superoxide dismutase, catalase and glutathione peroxidase activity but lower liver lipid peroxidation and reduced liver and muscle protein carbonyl levels compared to the vehicle and alpha-tocopherol (25 mg/kg body weight) groups [79]. Supplementation of alpha-tocotrienol (0.04 % weight diet) for one month in rats fed with vitamin E-deficient diet reduced the level of hydroxyoctadecadienoic acid and isoprostane, both markers of lipid peroxidation, in plasma and various organs of the rats [186].

The limited examples presented above showcased the antioxidant potential of tocotrienol ex vivo and in vivo. The role of tocotrienol in suppressing oxidative stress in relation to specific diseases will be discussed separately in the later sections.

5.3 Anti-inflammatory Effects of Tocotrienol

Inflammation has been implicated in the pathogenesis of various diseases, such as cardiovascular disease [80], diabetes mellitus [35], rheumatoid arthritis [30] and osteoporosis [99]. Prostaglandin and leukotriene generated from arachidonic acid are important mediators of the inflammatory process. Prostaglandin E2 (PGE2) synthesized by cyclooxygenase (COX) 1 and 2 are important in activating cytokine formation, apart from eliciting pain and fever. Leukotriene B4 is another important chemotactic agent synthesized by 5-lipoxygenase (5-LOX). Nuclear factor kappa-B, JAK–STAT6/3 (signal transducer and activator of transcription 6/3) and CCAAT-enhancer binding protein β (C/EBPβ) are transcription factors vital in inducing the expression of proinflammatory cytokines (reviewed by Jiang [63]).

Wu et al. showed that palm tocotrienol-rich fraction inhibited the release of nitric oxide and PGE2 in lipopolysaccharide (LPS)-treated human monocytic cells [181]. This was achieved by the suppression of inducible nitric oxide synthase and COX-2 (but not COX-1) expression by tocotrienol-rich fraction [181]. Concurrently, the production of interleukin-4, interleukin-8 and tumor necrosis factor-alpha was suppressed by tocotrienol treatment [181]. Using LPS-treated murine peritoneal macrophages, Ng and Ko demonstrated that tocotrienol-rich fraction inhibited the production of nitric oxide, PGE2 and proinflammatory cytokines, such as tumor necrosis factor-alpha, interferon-gamma, interleukin-1 beta and interleukin-6 in these cells [110]. This contributed to the suppressed protein expression of inducible nitric oxide synthase, COX (but not COX-1) and nuclear factor kappa-B [110]. They further showed that the anti-inflammatory effects of tocotrienol-rich fraction were better than alpha-tocopherol and alpha-tocopheryl acetate [110]. Yam et al. compared the anti-inflammatory effects between alpha-tocopherol, tocotrienol-rich fraction and individual tocotrienol isomers (alpha-, gamma- and delta-tocotrienol) in LPS-treated RAW 264.7 murine macrophages [183]. Yam et al. found that tocotrienol-rich fraction and all three tocotrienol isomers inhibited interleukin-6 and nitric oxide production [183]. Only alpha-tocotrienol could suppress the production of tumor necrosis factor-alpha. Tocotrienol-rich fraction, alpha- and delta-tocotrienol lowered the production of PGE2 [183]. The gene expression of COX-2 was downregulated by tocotrienol-rich fraction and individual isomers but not by alpha-tocopherol [183]. Wang and Jiang showed that gamma-tocotrienol inhibited LPS-induced interleukin-6 production in murine RAW267.4 macrophages by blocking the activation of nuclear factor kappa-B [177]. It also suppressed the LPS induced upregulation of C/EBPβ needed for IL-6 production and the expression of its target gene, granulocyte-colony stimulating factor [177]. These effects could be replicated in bone marrow derived macrophages [177]. Wang et al. further showed that gamma-tocotrienol blocked the activation of nuclear factor kappa-B by upregulating its inhibitor, A20, via modulating the synthesis of sphingolipids involved in inflammatory response [178].

In an vivo study, Qureshi et al. showed that 4-week consumption of diet containing tocotrienol derived from annatto seeds (100 ppm) in aged and young mice inhibited the inflammation induced by LPS alone or in combination with interferon-gamma or interferon-beta [133]. This was evidenced by a reduced nitric oxide and tumour necrosis factor-alpha level in the treated group [133]. This was achieved by suppression of genes related to proinflammatory cytokines, such as interleukin-1 beta, interleukin-1 alpha, interleukin-1 RA, interleukin-6, interleukin-12, COX-2, tumor necrosis factor-alpha etc. [133]. In another experiment, Qureshi et al. compared the anti-inflammatory effects of alpha-, gamma- and delta-tocotrienol in LPS-treated BALB/c mice [129]. A dose-dependent decrease of tumor necrosis factor-alpha synthesis was observed in all tocotrienol-treated groups [129]. The inhibition was strongest in the delta-tocotrienol group [129]. Using peritoneal macrophages derived from these mice, it was shown that delta-tocotrienol could suppress the LPS-induced gene expression of tumor necrosis factor-alpha, interleukin-1 beta, interleukin-6 and inducible nitric oxide synthase [129]. Heng et al. demonstrated that supplementation of tocotrienol mixture 400 mg daily for 16 weeks caused a significant reduction of interleukin-1 and tumor necrosis factor-alpha in a group of subjects (aged 20–60 years) with metabolic syndrome [50]. Supplementation of tocotrienol 15 mg daily for 4 weeks significantly decreased the high-sensitivity C-reactive protein in a group of patients with type-2 diabetes [47].

The role of tocotrienol in suppressing inflammation in individual diseases will be discussed in detail in later sections.

5.4 Tocotrienol as a Hypocholesterolemic Agent

The mevalonate pathway is responsible for the synthesis of cholesterol and other isoprenoids. The determining step in this multi-cascade pathway is the synthesis of 3-hydroxy-3-methyglutaryl-CoA (HMG-CoA) from acetyl-CoA via the enzyme HMG-CoA reductase (HMGR). The expression of HMGR is in turn regulated by sterol regulatory element-binding proteins (SREBPs), whereby the absence of sterol isoprenoids in the cells upregulates its expression (reviewed by Buhaescu and Izzedine [17]). Cholesterol is carried in lipoproteins with specific apolipoproteins which direct the load to specific tissues. Excretion of cholesterol occurs in the form of bile acid. The rate-determining enzyme in this process is cholesterol-7-alpha-hydroxylase [65]. Hypercholesterolemia is an important contributing factor to cardiovascular disease and coronary heart disease [159].

Tocotrienol is known as an inhibitor of the mevalonate pathway. The structure of tocotrienol with its three double bonds is similar to farnesyl, the compound preceding the formation of squalene in cholesterol synthesis [122]. Tocotrienol promotes the formation of farnesol from farnesyl, thus reducing the formation of squalene [122]. Gamma- and delta-tocotrienol have been shown to regulate HMGR in different ways [155]. Delta-tocotrienol stimulates ubiquitination and degradation of HMGR and blocks processing of SREBPs, while gamma-tocotrienol is more selective in enhancing HMGR degradation than blocking SREBP processing [155]. In other studies, gamma-tocotrienol has been shown to stimulate apolipoprotein B degradation by decreasing its translocation into the endoplasmic reticulum lumen [168]. This also causes a reduction in the number of apolipoprotein B in lipoprotein particles [168]. Gamma- and delta-tocotrienol have also been demonstrated to downregulate the expression of genes involved in lipid homeostasis, such as DGAT2. APOB100, SREBP1/2 and HMGR [190]. These tocotrienols also enhance efflux of low density lipoprotein (LDL) cholesterol through increasing LDL receptor expression [190]. Gamma-tocotrienol has been shown to decrease triglyceride (TG) level in liver cells by decreasing the expression of fatty acid synthase, SERBP1 and increasing the expression of carnitine palmitoyl transferase 1A [19] (Fig. 5.2).

The effects of tocotrienol on lipid profile have been tested in several animal models of dyslipidaemia. Different species of animals have been used, including chicken, swine and rodents (rats, hamsters, guinea pigs). Qureshi et al. found that chicken supplemented with delta-tocotrienol (50 ppm for 4 weeks) showed reduced level of total and LDL cholesterol [130]. It also suppressed the lipid elevating effects of dexamethasone and potentiated the TG-lowering effects of riboflavin [130]. Using chickens fed with different dosage (50–2000 ppm) of vitamin E isomers and mixtures, Yu et al. showed that gamma- and delta-tocotrienol reduced the level of total and LDL cholesterol most significantly, followed by tocotrienol-rich fraction and alpha-tocotrienol [188]. Alpha-tocopherol did not exhibit lipid-lowering effects in their experiment [188]. In another experiment, Qureshi and Peterson demonstrated that a combination of tocotrienol-rich fraction (50 ppm) and lovastatin (50 ppm) for 4 weeks suppressed HMGR activity more effectively than lovastatin alone in chickens [125]. The combination was also more effective in reducing serum total and LDL cholesterol, apolipoprotein B, TG, thromboxane B2 and platelet factor 4 than individual treatments [125]. Qureshi et al. also showed that alpha-tocopherol attenuated the inhibition of HMGR by gamma-tocotrienol in chickens [124]. They concluded that the effective preparation of tocotrienol mixture to maximize its hypocholesterolemic effects should contain 15–20 % alpha-tocopherol and 60 % gamma- or delta-tocotrienol [124]. In an experiment using genetically hypercholesterolemic swines, Qureshi et al. showed that 6 weeks treatment of 50 mg tocotrienol-rich fraction derived from rice bran, gamma-tocotrienol, desmethyl (d-P21-T3) or didesmethyl (d-P25-T3) tocotrienol individually could cause

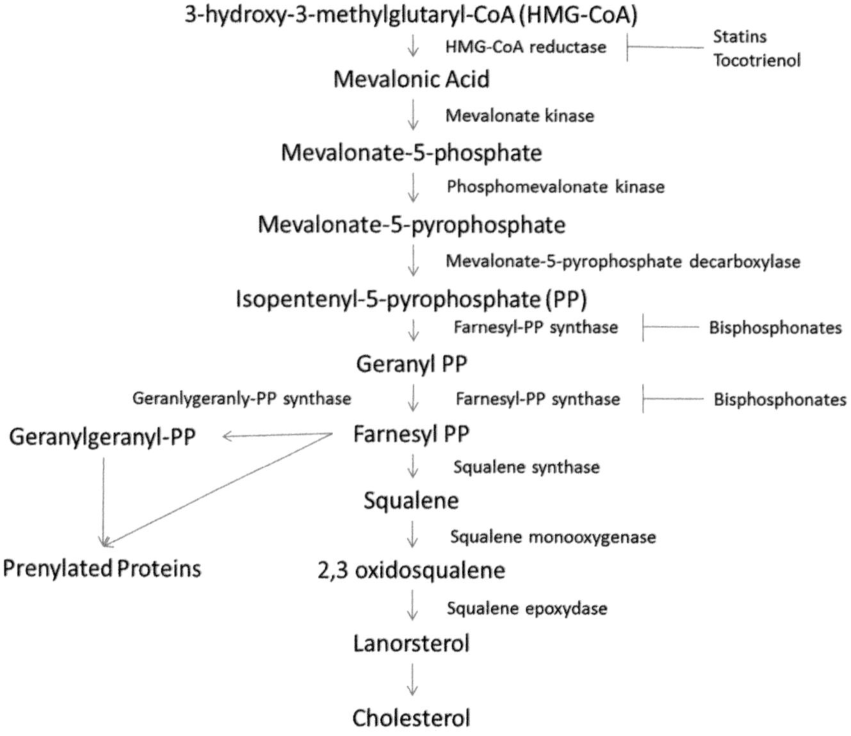

Fig. 5.2 The role of tocotrienol in suppressing cholesterol synthesis

significant reduction in serum total and LDL cholesterol, TG, apolipoprotein B, platelet factor 4, thromboxane B2, glucose and glucagon [126]. These tocotrienols also lowered HMGR activity but did not affect cholesterol-7-alpha-hydroxylase activity [126]. After termination of the treatment, the cholesterol-lowering effects of tocotrienols persisted for 10 weeks [126]. In another study using palm tocotrienol-rich fraction (50 mg/g diet for 42 days), genetically hypercholesterolemic swine responded to the treatment by showing a significant decrease in serum total and LDL cholesterol, apolipoprotein B, thromboxane B2 and platelet factor 4 [127]. However, the effects on normal swine were limited to reduction of total cholesterol and apolipoprotein B [127]. The activity of HMGR in adipose tissue was reduced with treatment in both normal and hypercholesterolemic swine [127].

In experiment using rats, hamsters or genuine pigs, tocotrienol was shown to prevent diet or chemical-induced hyperlipidaemia. Burdeos et al. demonstrated that F344 rats on high fat diet receiving 5 or 10 mg rice bran tocotrienol per day for 3 weeks showed a reduction in TG and phospholipid hydroperoxides (oxidative stress marker) in the liver and plasma [18]. This reduction could be due to suppressed production and accumulation of TG by the hepatocytes [18]. However, the cholesterol level did not change in these rats [18]. In a similar experiment by

Watkins et al., rats were fed with an atherogenic diet for 6 weeks and the treatment groups received 50 mg gamma-tocotrienol and 500 mg alpha-tocopherol per kg diet [179]. The treatment group showed lower plasma cholesterol, LDL, very-low-density lipoprotein (VLDL), TG, malondialdehyde and fatty acid hydroperoxides [179]. Minhajuddin et al. demonstrated that rats on a 3-week atherogenic diet showed significant reduction in TG, total and LDL cholesterol, malondialdehyde and conjugated dienes after supplementation with tocotrienol-rich fraction (8–48 mg/kg) for 1 week [91]. The activity of HMGR was suppressed with atherogenic diet, probably due to physiological feedback mechanism [91]. Supplementation of tocotrienol-rich fraction led to further reduction in the activity of HMGR [91].

Using a chemically induced hypercholesterolemic model, Iqbal et al. showed that supplementation of rice bran tocotrienol-rich fraction (10 mg/kg/day) significantly suppressed the increase in plasma total and LDL cholesterol in rats administered with 7,12-dimethylbenz[alpha]anthracene [62]. It also suppressed the activity and protein mass of hepatic HMGR [62]. Salman Khan et al. demonstrated that Tocomin, a palm tocotrienol mixture, reduced the level of plasma lipoproteins, cholesterol, apolipoprotein B, small dense LDL and LDL in inflammation-induced hypercholesterolemia in Syrian hamsters [142]. In the same experiment using computational modelling, they showed that the inhibition of HMGR was greater with delta-tocotrienol, followed by gamma-, beta- and alpha-tocotrienol [142]. Raederstorff et al. compared the hypocholesterolemic effects of pure gamma-tocotrienol and tocotrienol mixture in hamsters [134]. They found that both gamma-tocotrienol (at 58 and 263 mg/kg) and tocotrienol mixture (at 263 mg/kg) reduced plasma total and LDL cholesterol but TG and high density lipoprotein (HDL) cholesterol were not affected [134]. Thus, the hypocholesterolemic effect of pure gamma-tocotrienol was greater than the tocotrienol mixture [134]. Khor and Ng showed that presence of alpha-tocopherol might attenuate the hypocholesterolemic effect of tocotrienol [74]. In male hamsters fed with diet containing low-dose alpha-tocopherol (30 ppm), the activity of HMGR was inhibited [74]. However, diet containing high-dose alpha-tocopherol (81 ppm) significantly stimulated the activity of HMGR [74]. On the other hand, in guinea pigs treated with 10 mg tocotrienol (i.p.), showed significant inhibition of HMGR activity but mixture of 5 mg alpha-tocopherol and 10 mg tocotrienol caused less inhibition [74]. This observation in turn validated the experiment of Qureshi et al. using chickens [124]. In a further experiment using guinea pigs injected with palm olein triglycerides containing either tocotrienol or alpha-tocopherol, Khor et al. indicated that tocotrienol (1–5 mg) significantly reduced the activity of liver microsomal HMGR and cholesterol-7-alpha-hydroxylase [73]. The inhibition by alpha-tocopherol was less effective [73]. Furthermore, the inhibitory effect of alpha-tocopherol was lost at 5 mg [73]. At a higher dose (50 mg), alpha-tocopherol significantly elevated the activity of HMGR and reduced the inhibitory effects of tocotrienol [73].

Effects of tocotrienol supplementation on lipid profile in humans were heterogeneous. This could be due to the differences in the composition of the tocotrienol mixture used, population studied, diet of the subjects, etc. In an earlier study using palm vitamin E (containing 18 mg tocopherols and 42 mg tocotrienols), Tan et al. showed that supplementation for 30 days lowered serum total and LDL cholesterol but the TG and HDL cholesterol were not affected [167]. However, this is not a randomized controlled trial and the number of subjects was small. Qureshi et al. showed that palm vitamin E at 200 mg caused a reduction in serum total and LDL cholesterol, apolipoprotein B, thromboxane, platelet factor 4 and glucose in subjects during the four week-treatment [128]. A separate hypocholesterolemic group given 200 mg gamma-tocotrienol showed greater reduction in total cholesterol compared to palm vitamin E group [128]. Daud et al. demonstrated that supplementation of tocotrienol for 16 weeks (180 mg tocotrienols with 40 mg tocopherols) decreased the normalized plasma TG and increased HDL in patients undergoing chronic hemodialysis [36]. These changes might be associated with higher plasma apolipoprotein and lower cholesteryl-ester transfer protein activity [36]. It should be noted that the results of this study was not adjusted for medication used by the subjects. Chin et al. showed that when elderly (>50 years) and young (<50 years) subjects were supplemented with tocotrienol-rich fraction (160 mg/day, containing 74 % tocotrienols and 26 % tocopherols) for 6 months, the elderly subjects responded better by showing an increase in HDL cholesterol compared to placebo group [29]. The products of oxidation, such as protein carbonyl and advance-glycation end products, were also reduced only in the elderly subjects [29]. Baliarsingh et al. supplemented 19 type 2 diabetic subjects with hyperlipidemia with tocotrienol-rich fraction (3 mg/kg body weight) for 60 days and total lipids, total and LDL cholesterol were reduced with treatment [11]. In the study by Qureshi et al., hypercholesterolemic subjects on American Heart Association step 1 diet were supplemented with rice bran tocotrienol-rich fraction at different doses (25–200 mg/kg) [132]. They observed that 100 mg/kg tocotrienol-rich fraction produced maximum decrease in total and LDL cholesterol, apolipoprotein B and TG compared to baseline [132]. In another study, Qureshi demonstrated that hypercholesterolemic subjects on American Heart Society step 1 diet supplemented with rice bran tocotrienol-rich fraction and lovastatin in combination for 25 weeks showed more significant reduction than individual treatments [131]. The combination of alpha-tocopherol and lovastatin did not produce similar changes [131].

Tomeo et al. supplemented subjects presented with hyperlipidemia, cerebrovascular disease and carotid stenosis with 300 mg palm vitamin E (16 mg alpha-tocopherol and 40 mg tocotrienols in 240 mg palm olein) for 18 months [169]. Apparent carotid atherosclerotic regression was found in supplemented subjects while some controls showed progression [169]. Malondialdehyde was decreased in the treatment group but was increased in the placebo group [169]. However, no changes in total and LDL cholesterol, TG and HDL were found in both groups [169]. In men with mildly elevated serum lipid level, supplementation of tocotrienol (4 capsules daily for 6 weeks, each containing 35 mg tocotrienols and 20 mg alpha-tocopherol) produced no significant effects on serum LDL and HDL cholesterol, TG, lipoprotein a, lipid peroxide, platelet aggregation velocity and maximum aggregation, and thromboxane B2 formation compared to men receiving 20 mg alpha-tocopherol only [90]. In the study of O'Byrne et al., subjects followed a low-fat diet for 4 weeks, then were randomized into treatment groups receiving placebo, alpha-, gamma-, delta-tocotrienol acetate supplements (250 mg/d) for 8 weeks while were still maintained on the low-fat diet [120]. It was found that alpha-tocotrienol increased the in vitro LDL oxidation resistance and decreased its rate of oxidation [120]. However, tocotrienol treatments did not affect total and LDL cholesterol, and apolipoprotein B level [120]. In another study, hypercholesterolemic men and women were randomized to receive three different brands of tocotrienol from palm or rice bran, or the placebo. The subjects were put on the American Heart Association Step 1 diet, 21 days before and throughout the trial period [101]. There were no significant changes in lipid profile between placebo and treatment after 28 days [101]. Rasool et al. observed that in healthy male subjects taking placebo or tocotrienol-rich vitamin E at 80, 160 and 320 mg/day for 2 months, arterial compliance, plasma total antioxidant status, serum total and LDL cholesterol were not different among the groups [136].

5.5 Tocotrienol as Antidiabetic Agent

Diabetes mellitus represents a group of chronic metabolic conditions characterized by increased blood glucose. Type 1 diabetes results from the destruction of beta-cell in the pancreas due to autoimmunity, thus causing cessation in insulin production. Type 2 diabetes is caused by abnormal resistance of the body to the action of insulin, and the insufficiency of insulin production to overcome this resistance. It is estimated that 5–10 % of the total diabetes cases belong to type 1 and 90–95 % belong to type 2. Diabetes can affect many organ systems and lead to serious complications such as damage to the nervous, renal, cardiovascular system and the eyes [38]. Oxidative stress and inflammation are involved in the development and exacerbation of diabetic complications [39].

The antidiabetic effects of tocotrienol have been explored mainly in animal studies. Diabetes is mostly induced by streptozotocin (STZ), a chemical that can cause cellular ATP reduction, inhibition of insulin production, DNA alkylation and death of pancreatic beta cells [75]. Tocotrienol has been shown to improve the glycemic status and diabetic complications in many instances. Wan Nazaimoon et al. showed that a diet enriched with tocotrienol-rich fraction (1 g/kg diet) significantly reduced the blood glucose level and glycated haemoglobin of STZ-induced diabetic male rats [176]. However, serum-advanced glycation end product and malondialdehyde were not affected [176]. Matough et al. showed that supplementation of tocotrienol-rich fraction at 200 mg/kg body weight for 4 weeks in STZ-induced diabetic rats reduced the plasma glucose level [85]. The supplementation also increased the erythrocytic superoxide dismutase and glutathione levels but decreased the level of reduced glutathione and malondialdehyde [85]. Comet assays revealed reduced DNA damage in the supplemented group [85].

Tocotrienol was shown to prevent diabetic nephropathy in several animal models. Kuhad and Chopra showed that tocotrienol mixture at 25, 50 and 100 mg/kg for 8 weeks dose-dependently reduced diabetic proteinuria, polyuria and increased serum creatinine and blood urea nitrogen levels and their clearance [77]. The improvement in renal profile was accompanied by a dose-dependent decrease in lipid peroxidation product and an increase in non-protein thiol, superoxide dismutase and catalase activity in the kidney [77]. Nitrosative stress in the kidney was also decreased with tocotrienol supplementation as evidenced by a lower nitric oxide level [77]. Tocotrienol was shown to reduce the level of tumor necrosis factor-alpha associated with renal hypertrophy and hyperfunction, transforming growth factor-beta associated with renal fibrosis and the expression of nuclear factor kappa-b p65 subunit indicative of inflammation in the nuclear fraction and apoptosis in the kidney [77]. Siddiqui et al. compared the hypoglycemic effects of tocotrienol-rich fraction derived from palm oil and rice bran oil in two separate experiments [151]. Diabetic male rats were treated with either 200 mg/kg body weight palm oil tocotrienol or rice bran tocotrienol [151]. Both treatments were found to reduce the fasting blood glucose and percentage of glycosylated haemoglobin [151]. Improvements in renal profile, indicated by reductions in serum creatinine and urine protein level, were also seen in both treatment groups [151]. Histopathological examination revealed that both tocotrienol-rich mixtures prevented glomerular hypertrophy, mesangial expansion, tubular atrophy, tubular basement membrane thickening and proteinaceous cast formation in the lumen [151]. The improvement could be attributed to the antioxidative properties of tocotrienol, as evidenced by the decrease in lipid peroxidation products and the increase in superoxide dismutase and catalase activity in the kidney with tocotrienol treatment [151]. Overall, efficacy of tocotrienol from palm was higher compared to rice bran [151]. In the second experiment, Siddiqui et al. fed male Wistar rats with high fat diet for 5 weeks, then switched them to standard diet and induced diabetes in them with STZ at the same time [150]. The hypoglycemic effects between 16-week supplementation with palm tocotrienol at 200 mg/kg body weight and rice bran tocotrienol 400 mg/kg body weight were compared [150]. In agreement with their previous findings, palm and rice bran tocotrienol prevented the rise of blood glucose level as early as week 6 [150]. Percentage of glycosylated hemoglobin was also reduced by both treatments [150]. They also suppressed the increase in TG, total, LDL and VLDL cholesterol and elevated the HDL cholesterol level [150]. Improvement in renal profile, indicated by decreased urinary creatinine and blood urea nitrogen and increased creatinine clearance, was seen with both treatments [150]. These positive changes might be related to improved oxidative status in the kidney (reduced malondialdehyde level, increased superoxide dismutase, catalase, glutathione peroxidase and reductase activities) [150]. In addition, the protein expression of collagen type IV, transforming growth factor-beta and fibronectin related to renal fibrosis were reduced significantly by palm tocotrienol [150]. This was accompanied by an improvement in renal histopathology in both treatment groups [150]. Palm tocotrienol, even though at a lower dosage, exhibited higher efficacy in preventing diabetic nephropathy than rice bran tocotrienol [150].

The presence of cardiovascular risk factors, such as hypertension and hypercholesterolemia, in diabetic patients lead to poorer outcomes compared to those without [38]. In fact, the risk for cardiovascular death is nearly doubled in diabetic patients compared with the non-diabetic [21]. As described in the earlier section, tocotrienol is an effective hypocholesterolemic agent and its effectiveness has been proven in chemical and diet-induced hypercholesterolemic models. Several animal studies also demonstrated that the hypocholesterolemic effect of tocotrienol persisted in diabetic model, accompanied by other cardio and vascular protective effects. Budin et al. fed STZ-induced diabetic rats with palm tocotrienol-rich fraction 200 mg/kg body weight for 8 weeks and observed positive changes in risk factors for cardiovascular disease [16]. Adverse changes in fasting blood glucose, HbA1c and lipid profile were attenuated in the tocotrienol-treated group [16]. Besides, malondialdehyde-4-hydroxynonenal in aorta and plasma, and DNA damage in lymphocytes were reduced and plasma superoxide dismutase activity was increased with tocotrienol treatment [16]. Tocotrienol also reduced the degenerative changes in aortic wall by reducing the proliferation and degeneration of vascular smooth muscle cells and defects in the aortic walls [16]. Using a diet-induced diabetic rat model, Patel et al. showed that co-supplementation of alpha-lipoic acid (1.6 g/kg diet) and palm tocotrienol-rich fraction (0.84 g/kg diet) for 8 weeks could prevent and reverse the increase in plasma glucose, systolic blood pressure, interstitial collagen deposition in the left ventricle, diastolic stiffness and plasma malondialdehyde [123].

Tocotrienol was able to prevent diabetic-associated neuropathy. Kuhad and Chopra et al. showed that tocotrienol mixture at 25, 50 and 100 mg/kg for 10 weeks could prevent the increase in plasma glucose in STZ-induced diabetic rats [76]. Transfer latency and percentage of time spend in the target quadrant in a water maze were decreased in all tocotrienol treated groups compared to the control, indicating better memory and learning performance [76]. This was attributed to decreased oxidative stress, indicated by a reduction in lipid peroxide level and an increase in non-protein thiols, superoxide dismutase and catalase activity, and decreased nitrosative stress indicated by reduced nitric oxide level in the cerebral cortex and hippocampus [76]. Inflammation was also prevented by tocotrienol supplementation, as evidenced by decreased protein expression of interleukin-1b and p65 subunit of nuclear factor kappa-B in the brain [76]. The reduction in both oxidative stress and inflammation led to reduced apoptosis of the neurons [76]. In the subsequent experiment, Kuhad and Chopra supplemented STZ-induced diabetic rats with 25, 50 and 100 mg/kg tocotrienol mixture and assessed the effects on hyperalgesia [78]. Tocotrienol mixture prevented the reduction in nociceptive threshold in the diabetic rats, indicated by increased tolerance for thermal and mechanical stimuli, and tactile allodynia [78]. They also found that lipid peroxide and total nitric oxide levels were reduced; while non-protein thiol levels and activities of superoxide dismutase and catalase were increased in the sciatic nerve with tocotrienol treatment [78]. Inflammation was also reduced with tocotrienol treatment, indicated by a reduction in tumor necrosis factor-alpha, transforming growth factor-1 beta and interleukin-1 beta in the sciatic nerve [78]. Apoptosis indicated by caspase 3 expression was also decreased in the sciatic nerve [78].

There are limited studies attempted to validate the hypoglycemic effects of tocotrienol in humans and the results are heterogenous. In a longitudinal study (median follow-up period 10.2 years) assessing the intake of antioxidants and the risk of type 2 diabetes in 29,133 Finnish male smokers aged 50–69 years, Kataja-Tuomola et al. found that all tocotrienol isomers were not associated with the risk of the disease after multiple adjustment. This could be contributed to the low levels of tocotrienols in the subjects [71]. In the study of Baliarsingh et al., type 2 diabetic subjects supplemented with tocotrienol-rich fraction (3 mg/kg body weight) for 60 days showed no changes in fasting and postprandial plasma sugar, HbA1c and serum creatinine [11]. This could be due to the limited number of subjects in this study ($n = 19$) and the low dose of tocotrienol. In a study by Haghighat et al., type 2 diabetic subjects taking non-insulin medication were randomized to take 15 mg/day tocotrienol mixture or blank canola oil with meals for 4 weeks [47]. It was observed that urinary microalbumin and serum high-sensitivity C-reactive protein were significantly lowered in the tocotrienol group compared to the placebo, indicating a better renal profile and a reduced risk for cardiovascular disease [47].

5.6 Tocotrienol as Antiosteporotic Agent

Osteoporosis is a metabolic bone disease characterized by low bone mass and deterioration of bone microarchitecture, which subsequently leads to fragility fracture [68]. Despite the high prevalence in women, osteoporosis affects men as well, with female to male ratio of 6:1 [64]. Osteoporosis is a result of the imbalanced bone remodelling process consisting of bone resorption regulated by osteoclast and bone formation regulation by osteoblast. Sex hormone deficiency is the predominant condition underlying the imbalance in bone remodelling, although recent studies have switched the focus to the role of oxidative stress and inflammation [2, 84]. Oxidative stress and inflammation inhibit differentiation of osteoblast (osteoblastogenesis), but promote differentiation of osteoclast (osteoclastogenesis) [2, 10, 171]. Hence, an antioxidant and anti-inflammatory agent like tocotrienol putatively has beneficial effects in preventing bone loss.

The effects of tocotrienol in promoting differentiation of osteoblast and suppressing the differentiation of osteoclast have been demonstrated in cell culture studies. Ha et al. demonstrated that alpha-tocotrienol but not alpha-tocopherol could suppress osteoclastogenesis in an osteoblast-bone marrow co-culture [46]. This was brought about by an inhibition of receptor activator of nuclear factor kappa-b (RANKL) expression in osteoblasts [46]. In osteoclasts, alpha-tocotrienol suppressed the RANKL-mediated differentiation process by inhibiting c-Fos expression via suppression of extracellular signal-regulated kinases and nuclear factor kappa-b activation [46]. Alpha-tocotrienol also prevented the bone resorption activity of mature osteoclasts [46]. Brook et al. compared the suppressive effects of different tocotrienol isomers (alpha, gamma and delta) on human-derived CD14+ cells [15]. It was found that gamma and delta-tocotrienol were effective in suppressing the formation of osteoclast-like cells and the resorbing activity of these cells was significantly inhibited. Gamma-tocotrienol was found to be with less toxic to CD14+ cells, indicating that it is safer compared to delta-tocotrienol [15].

The effectiveness of tocotrienol in preventing bone loss has been demonstrated in several animal models of osteoporosis. The methods of assessing bone health in the animals included densitometry which measures bone mineral density; histomorphometry which measures bone structure, cells and mineralization activity; biomechanical test which measures the stiffness and strength of the bone; bone mineral concentration and serum bone remodelling markers which measure the bone formation and resorption activity (reviewed in [24, 27]).

Norazlina supplemented ovariectomized rats with palm vitamin E, which was rich in tocotrienol at either 30 or 60 mg/kg body weight for 8 months and measured the femoral and vertebral bone mineral density [118]. It was found palm vitamin E prevented the decline of bone mineral density in both supplemented groups [118]. Muhammad et al. observed that palm tocotrienol at 60 mg/kg body weight for 8 weeks could improve bone structural indices (increased bone volume and trabecular number, and decreased trabecular separation) in an oestrogen-deficient model of osteoporosis induced by ovariectomy [96]. A decrease in osteoclast number was found in the tocotrienol supplemented group [96]. The effects of alpha-tocopherol at 60 mg/kg body weight were found to be comparable with palm tocotrienol [96]. In a subsequent experiment, Muhammed et al. supplemented the ovariectomized rats with tocotrienol-rich fraction (60 mg/kg for 8 weeks) and found that it improved bone structural indices (increased bone volume and trabecular thickness, and decreased trabecular separation) [97]. Its effects were comparable to calcium (15 mg/kg) and oestrogen treatment (64.5 μg/kg) [97]. Aktifanus et al. demonstrated that tocotrienol-rich fraction at 60 mg/kg body weight for 8 weeks improved bone dynamic indices (decreased single-labelled surface, increased double-labelled surface, mineral apposition rate and bone formation rate) in ovariectomized rats [8]. The effects of tocotrienol were better than oestrogen replacement (64.5 μg/kg body weight) [8]. Using palm tocotrienol at 60 mg/kg body weight for 8 weeks, Soelaiman et al. demonstrated similar findings and its effects were superior to calcium supplementation (1 % calcium in drinking water ad libitum) [154]. Abdul-Majeed et al. supplemented ovariectomized rats with annatto tocotrienol (60 mg/kg body weight for 8 weeks) or in combination with lovastatin (11 mg/kg body weight for 8 weeks) [3, 4]. Annatto tocotrienol alone was found to improve bone structural (increased bone volume, trabecular number and trabecular thickness, decreased trabecular separation) and cellular indices (increased osteoblast number, osteoid surface and osteoid volume, and decreased osteoclast number and eroded surface), bone biomechanical strength (increased load, strain, stress and Young's modulus) and bone remodelling markers (increased osteocalcin, a bone formation marker and decreased type-1 C-terminal telopeptide crosslink, a bone resorption marker) [3, 4]. The combination of annatto tocotrienol and lovastatin further improved these variables, suggesting an additive or synergistic effect between the two compounds [3, 4]. Deng et al. supplemented ovariectomized mice with 100 mg/kg emulsified gamma-tocotrienol subcutaneously. The supplemented mice showed significant improvements in femoral bone mineral density, bone structural (increased bone volume, trabecular number, trabecular thickness and decreased trabecular separation), dynamic (increased mineral apposition rate and bone formation rate) and cellular indices (increased osteoblast number and decreased osteoclast number) [37]. Elevated gene expression of transcription factors runt-2 and osterix in the bone of supplemented groups suggested increased osteoblast differentiation [37]. This was coupled with increased gene expression of osteoprotegerin and decreased gene expression of RANKL, indicating an inhibition of osteoclast formation [37]. Feeding mevalonate (25 mg/kg body weight) to the supplemented group abolished all the beneficial effects of tocotrienol treatment, suggesting the involvement of mevalonate pathway in the protective action of tocotrienol on bone [37].

Using an orchidectomy-induced testosterone deficient model of osteoporosis, Ima-Nirwana et al. showed that supplementation of palm vitamin E at 30 mg/kg for 8 months prevented the deterioration of femoral and vertebral bone mineral density and calcium level [58]. Other studies also showed that annatto tocotrienol at 60 mg/kg could prevent deterioration of bone cancellous microarchitecture assessed with X-ray microtomography (decreased trabecular separation), bone structural (increased bone volume and trabecular number, decreased trabecular separation), dynamic (decreased single-labelled surface, increased double-labelled surface) and cellular (increased osteoblast number, osteoid surface and osteoid volume, decreased osteoclast number and eroded surface) indices [25, 28]. This was brought about by increased gene expression of alkaline phosphatase, beta-catenin, collagen type 1 alpha 1 and osteopontin, indicating increased osteoblast activity [28]. However, no significant changes in bone resorption genes were observed [28]. Annatto tocotrienol was less efficacious compared to supraphysiological testosterone enanthate injection (7 mg/kg weekly) in the same experiment [28].

Smoking is a non-modifiable risk factor for osteoporosis. In a model of osteoporosis induced by nicotine, Hermizi et al. showed that supplementation of either tocotrienol-rich fraction or gamma-tocotrienol at 60 mg/kg body weight improved bone structural (increased bone volume and trabecular thickness), dynamic (reduced single-labelled surface and increased mineral apposition rate and bone formation rate) and cellular indices (reduced osteoclast and eroded surface) [51]. Abukhadir et al. indicated that these positive changes were brought about by the ability of tocotrienol to reverse nicotine-induced suppression of runt-2, osterix and bone morphogenetic protein-2 [5]. Tocotrienol also inhibited nicotine-induced elevation of interleukin-1 and interleukin-6 [117, 119]. Nazrun et al. demonstrated that palm tocotrienol at 100 mg/kg was able to increase trabecular thickness, bone formation rate, osteoblast number and decrease eroded surface in the osteoporotic animal [7, 105]. This effect was also brought about by the suppression of interleukin-1 and interleukin-6 by tootrienol [7]. The effects of tocotrienol in preventing bone loss due to glucocorticoid treatment were also studied. Ima-Nirwana and Fakhrurazi supplemented palm vitamin E in dexamethasone-treated adrenalectomized male rats and observed no significant changes on bone mineral density and bone calcium level [56]. In a subsequent attempt, supplementation of gamma-tocotrienol at 60 mg/kg body weight for 8 weeks increased the fourth lumbar vertebra bone calcium content in dexamethasone-treated adrenalectomized male rats [59]. Alpha-tocopherol at the same dose did not exert a similar effect [59].

The beneficial effects of tocotrienol were also shown in healthy male rats supplemented with alpha-tocopherol, delta-tocotrienol or gamma-tocotrienol at 60 mg/kg for 8 weeks [89, 149]. Gamma-tocotrienol supplementation improved all bone structural, dynamic and cellular indices and biomechanical strength while alpha-tocopherol and delta-tocotrienol only improved some of the indices, indicating a superior bone-anabolic effect of gamma-tocotrienol over the other vitamin E isomers [89, 149]. Maniam et al. showed that palm tocotrienol at 100 mg/kg for 4 months reduced malondialdehyde and increased glutathione peroxidase activity in the bone of healthy male rats. Alpha-tocopherol at the same dose did not exert similar effects on bone [83].

Despite there are many observational studies on the association between vitamin E and bone health, most studies measured the intake and blood level of alpha-tocopherol. Vitamin E (alpha-tocopherol) was associated with increased bone mineral density or a reduced fracture risk in most studies [26]. However, there has been no report on the effects of tocotrienol on bone health in humans to date. The suggested mechanism of tocotrienol in preventing bone loss is summarized in Fig. 5.3.

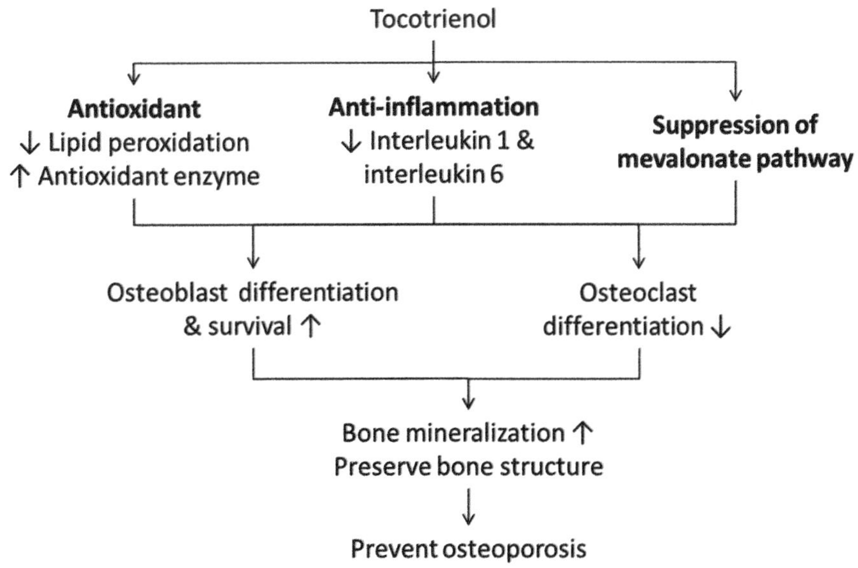

Fig. 5.3 The antiosteoporotic mechanism of tocotrienol

5.7 Anticancer Activity

Anticancer activity of vitamin E was discovered and studied extensively since the first experimental evidence of inhibition of tumorigenesis by vitamin E rich palm oil [164]. Anticancer property of tocotrienol was found to be independent of its antioxidant property [32, 162]. Tocotrienol isomer with lower antioxidant properties like delta- and gamma-tocotrienol usually showed greater potency in killing cancerous cells. Based on quantitative structure–activity relationship studies, chromanol structure and phytyl carbon tail were shown to be essential in apoptosis induction [13]. Decreasing methyl groups on the chromanol head increased anti-proliferative potency of tocotrienol (delta-tocotrienol > gamma-tocotrienol > beta-tocotrienol > alpha-tocotrienol) [162]. Shortening the unsaturated phytyl tail of gamma-tocotrienol by one isoprenyl unit also resulted in greater apoptotic activity [13]. In silico analysis suggested that esterification of lysine with gamma-tocotrienol could enhanced its anticancer activity [114]. Tocotrienol metabolites such as carboxyethyl-hydroxychromans were found to be a less effective anti-proliferative agent [34].

Besides that, tumor cell uptake and intracellular accumulation of tocotrienol also determine its anticancer activity. Due to the lipophilic nature of tocotrienols, they are readily transferred between the membranes and accumulated in cells in a time and concentration-dependent manner [187]. Studies have shown that serum physiological tocotrienol level was usually low or absent due to slow absorption, rapid metabolism and lack of a specific carrier protein [164]. Besides that, tocotrienol is highly tissue-dependent and it is only found in a few tissues/organs like the liver and pancreas [52, 55]. Interestingly, in animal models, gamma-tocotrienol and delta-tocotrienol were found to accumulate in tumors [52, 55]. Different tocotrienol isomers possess different cellular accumulation tendency, i.e. delta > gamma > alpha-tocotrienol [52, 87, 88, 116, 141, 144]. This might explain the poor anticancer activity of alpha-tocotrienol.

Tocotrienol and tocotrienol-rich fraction were demonstrated to induce anti-proliferation and apoptosis selectively in several cancerous cell lines originating from the mammary gland [32, 41, 44, 87, 109, 146, 173–175, 189], lung [70, 86, 184], liver [49, 52, 140, 141, 172], prostate [33, 86, 158], melanoma [22, 86], colon [40, 182] and leukemic cells [100]. The inhibitory potency of tocotrienol-rich fraction, tocotrienol isoforms or their succinate synthetic derivatives in different cancerous cells generally follows the order of delta- >gamma- and beta- >alpha-tocotrienol [22, 33, 40, 52, 140, 172]. Studies also demonstrated that tocotrienol possessed little or no adverse effect on normal cell viability or growth in in vitro [49, 70, 87, 88, 141, 158, 184] or animal models [112, 135, 137]. In animal studies, tocotrienols and tocotrienol-rich fraction were also demonstrated to reduce tumor load. Oral administration of 0.05 % tocotrienol-rich vitamin E mixture significantly reduced liver and lung carcinogenesis in C3H/He mice and 4NQO-treated ddY mice model [172]. Gamma-tocotrienol or delta-tocotrienol diet (0.1 %) significantly delayed tumor growth in C3H/HeN mice inoculated subcutaneously with murine hepatoma MH134 cells [52]. There was no apparent adverse effect and insignificant body and tissue weight changes in animals fed with 0.1 % of gamma-tocotrienol or delta-tocotrienol diet [52].

Studies also demonstrated that tocotrienol as a farnesol-mimetic molecule and HMGR inhibitor possessed great potential to produce synergistic anticancer activity with other chemotherapeutic agents [86]. Combination of low concentration of gamma-tocotrienol with several individual statins synergistically inhibited HMGR activity and Rap1A & Rab6 prenylation [174]. Besides that, combination of tocotrienol with flavonoids such as genistein, naringenin, hesperetin, tangeretin, nobiletin, quercetin, apigenin, epigallocatechin gallate or resveratrol demonstrated synergistic activity in inhibiting human breast cancer MCF7 or/and MDA-MB-435 cells proliferation, which was enhanced further with the addition of tamoxifen [45, 54]. The combination of tocotrienol with docetaxel also resulted in higher proportion of apoptotic cells [22]. Combination of tocotrienols with tamoxifen increased the arrest of DNA synthesis and triggered an endoplasmic reticulum (ER)-independent anti-proliferation event in the breast cancer cells [44, 189]. Combination of tocotrienol isomers (delta-tocotrienol and gamma-tocotrienol) was also found to induce cell death synergistically in DU145 and PC3 [33]. In animal studies, gamma-tocotrienol also acted synergistically with lovastatin to reduce tumor load in C57BL/6 mice inoculated with B16 cells [86].

There are limited clinical trials on tocotrienol and cancer conducted to date. Malaysian Palm Oil Board had conducted two clinical trials on the efficacy of tocotrienol in breast cancer patients [107]. The first study was conducted to identify tocopherol and tocotrienol concentrations in malignant and benign adipose tissues of breast cancer patients after a palm oil diet. The results revealed a higher concentration of tocotrienols (alpha-, delta- and gamma-isomers), in the adipose tissues of patients with benign breast lumps compared with that of patients with malignant tumors [107]. The second study was a 5-year double-blind, placebo-controlled pilot trial conducted to compare tamoxifen with or without tocotrienol-rich fraction on early breast cancer [108]. The risk of dying due to breast cancer decreased by 70 % and risk of recurrence decreased by 20 % in patients taking the adjuvant tocotrienol and tamoxifen compared with the patients receiving only tamoxifen [107]. However, there was no significant association between adjuvant tocotrienol therapy with breast cancer survival rate [108].

5.7.1 Tocotrienol-Induced Caspase Activation and Mode of Cell Death

Caspases are constitutively present in cells in an inactive precursor form, the procaspases [164]. In receptor-mediated apoptosis, there is early activation of death receptors (Fas, TNF or TRAIL) which lead to caspase-8 activation. In mitochondria-mediated apoptosis, there are apoptotic signals from damaged DNA or loss of mitochondrial membrane potential, which will lead to activation of caspase-9. Initiator caspases (caspase-8 and -9) activate effector caspases (caspase-3, -6, and -7) which will then execute the cells by cleaving DNA, PARP and other structural proteins [164]. Both death receptor- [33, 140, 141] and mitochondria-mediated [22, 33, 103, 139, 160, 165, 182, 184] pathway of apoptosis induced by tocotrienol-rich fraction, tocotrienol isomers, ether or succinate synthetic derivatives were reported. Tocotrienol-rich fraction and tocotrienol isomer-induced apoptosis are selective and greatly dependent on cell types and treatment conditions. It might involve the upregulation of Bax and tBid protein with the increased of Bax/Bcl-2 ratio [140].

Besides that, gamma-tocotrienol was also found to induce caspase-12 activation in +SA cellular apoptosis [173]. Caspase-12 activation is closely associated with endoplasmic reticulum ER stress-mediated cell death. Further experiments identified an early involvement of PERK/eIF2a/ATF4 phosphorylation and CHOP-dependent TRB3-mediated ER stress response pathway in gamma-tocotrienol-induced +SA cellular apoptosis [173]. Furthermore, gamma-tocotrienol, delta-tocotrienol, gamma-tocotrienol succinate and delta-tocotrienol succinate were also found to trigger caspase-independent cell death in DU145, PC3 and LNCap cells whereby the event of apoptosis could not be abrogated by general caspase inhibitors [33].

5.7.2 Tocotrienol-Induced Upstream Apoptotic Pathway Modulation

The inhibition of HMGR by tocotrienol not only suppresses cholesterol synthesis but also inhibits cell proliferation via prenylation of Ras, RhoA or Rap1A signalling molecules through generation of prenyl intermediates [184]. Farnesyl side chain of tocotrienol is essential for the post-transcriptional suppression of HMGR. Gamma-tocotrienol was shown to downregulate HMGR levels in +SA cells via post-translational protein degradation [173]. However, the gamma-tocotrienol-induced downregulation of HMGR was not able to block Rap1A & Rab6 prenylation and trigger +SA cell death [174]. Delta-tocotrienol-induced growth arrest might be due to HMGR inhibition, causing marked decrease of cyclin D1/cyclin-dependent kinase CDK4 complex but not cyclin E/CDK2 complex, which subsequently reduced the phosphorylation of retinoblastoma RB protein and E2F1 expression [41, 103].

6-*O*-carboxypropyl-alpha-tocotrienol (alpha-T3E) was more potent compared to alpha-tocotrienol in inducing apoptosis in A549 cells and H28 cells [70, 184]. 6-*O*-carboxypropyl-alpha-tocotrienol also harbours the similar farnesyl side chain and might possess HMG-CoA reductase inhibitory activity. 6-*O*-carboxypropyl-alpha-tocotrienol can inhibit RhoA geranyl-geranylation and Ras molecules farnesylation, subsequently blocking MEK, ERK and p38 phosphorylation and lead to cyclin D and Bcl-xL downregulation during G1 arrest and apoptosis [160, 174, 184].

Besides that, 6-*O*-carboxypropyl-alpha-tocotrienol also inactivated Src kinase via phosphorylation at Tyr527 site and dephosphorylation at Tyr416 site, which decreased the phosphorylated form of EGFR and its activity [70]. Another study revealed that gamma-tocotrienol inhibited PI3k/PDK-1/Akt pathway via suppression of EGFR (ErbB3)-receptor tyrosine phosphorylation [143]. 6-*O*-carboxypropyl-alpha-tocotrienol also inhibited Stat-3 activation which might be due to Src kinase inactivation [70]. 6-*O*-carboxypropyl-alpha-tocotrienol was shown to partially inhibit Src kinase. However, this was inadequate to trigger cell death on A549 cells under hypoxia [69]. Survival and invasion capacity of A549 cells under hypoxia were suppressed by 6-*O*-carboxypropyl-alpha-tocotrienol via inhibition of the Src/HIF-2alpha/PAI-1 and PI3k/PDK-1/Akt signalling pathways [69]. Gamma-tocotrienol was also demonstrated to inhibit PI3k/PDK-1/Akt pathway and subsequently suppressed the FLIP level [163]. Gamma-tocotrienol also induced +SA cells apoptosis via TRB3-mediated ER stress [173]. TRB3 inhibited Akt signalling pathway and this also contributed to the decrease of Akt activity [173].

Combination of gamma-tocotrienol with several individual statins also synergistically induced +SA cells growth arrest and apoptosis which was associated with inactivation of ERK, p38, JNK MAP kinases and Akt kinases [174, 175]. Downstream Stat-3 inactivation leads to similar downregulation of cyclin D1 and Bcl-xL [69]. Therefore, HMG-CoA reductase might be involved in upstream regulation of RhoA/Ras, Src/HIF-2alpha/PAI-1 and PI3k/Akt pathway.

Previous studies demonstrated that tocotrienol-rich fraction, alpha-, gamma- and delta-tocotrienol inhibited proliferation and induced apoptosis in human breast cancer MCF-7, MDA-MB-435 and MDA-MB-231 cells, regardless of their oestrogen receptor status [32, 41, 44, 109, 189]. Delta-tocotrienol was showed to downregulate cyclin B1 and CDK1 expression in MDA-MB-231 cellular growth arrest [41]. Combination of gamma-tocotrienol with either epigallocatechin gallate or resveratrol suppressed MCF-7 cell proliferation via downregulation of cell cycle regulatory proteins E2F, CDK4 and cyclin D1 [54]. In vitro and in silico studies revealed that gamma- and delta-tocotrienol specifically bound and activated estrogen receptor β signalling molecule [32]. Activated estrogen receptor β served as an upstream signal of apoptosis and suppressed ER alpha-mediated cell survival and proliferation [32]. Estrogen receptor β upregulated MIC-1, cathepsin D and EGR-1 mRNAs expression which triggered subsequent caspase-regulated cell death [32].

Epidermal growth factor (EGF)-dependent mitogenesis is associated with the activation of phospholipid-dependent protein kinase C (PKC) and cyclic AMP (cAMP)-dependent proteins [88]. Tocotrienol-rich fraction, alpha-, gamma-, and delta-tocotrienol induced apoptosis and inhibit the proliferation of EGF-induced preneoplastic mammary epithelial CL-S1 cells, neoplastic mammary epithelial-SA cells and +SA cells [87, 146, 174, 175]. Tocotrienol-rich fraction also reduced EGFR-independent and cAMP-dependent EGF-induced G-protein mitogenic signalling in CL-S1 cells [162]. Combination of tocotrienol-rich fraction with G-protein stimulants (cholera and pertussis toxin) or cAMP agonists (forskolin and 8-Br-cAMP) completely reversed anti-proliferative effects of tocotrienol-rich fraction on CL-S1 cells [162]. Besides that, tocotrienol was shown to inhibit PKC, adenylate cyclase and cyclic AMP-dependent protein activation which might be related to its anti-proliferative effects [23, 88, 94]. Delta- and beta-tocotrienol could inhibit PKC activity leading to transcriptional inhibition of c-myc and hTERT, thus reducing telomerase activity [40]. In addition, gamma-tocotrienol also induced downregulation of Id family proteins and EGFR protein with concomitant activation of JNK MAP kinase pathway [22]. Alpha-tocotrienol but not its acetate analogue was able to inhibit intrinsic cellular 20S proteasome activity which might contribute to THP-1 anti-proliferation activity [100]. Tocotrienol-rich fraction, alpha-, gamma- and delta-tocotrienol might serve as potent DNA synthesis inhibitors with the rank order of gamma-tocotrienol > delta-tocotrienol > alpha-tocotrienol [189].

5.7.3 Tocotrienol-Induced Anti-angiogenesis and Anti-invasion

Anti-angiogenic therapy has recently emerged as a strategy for cancer therapy. As oxidative stress is an important factor in angiogenesis, it is possible that established antioxidants such as tocotrienol may minimize the formation of new blood vessels [60]. An in vitro study revealed that tocotrienol significantly inhibited the proliferation and tube formation of BAEC as well as FGF- or VEGF-induced HUVEC cells in the order of delta- >beta- >gamma- >alpha-tocotrienol [60, 93–95, 103, 180]. Tocotrienol also suppressed VEGF secretion in colon carcinoma cells DLD-1 and HepG2 cells under normoxic and hypoxic conditions in the order of delta- >beta- >gamma- >alpha-tocotrienol [148]. In vivo studies revealed that tocotrienol-rich oil was able to inhibit DLD-1 cells-induced angiogenesis via mouse dorsal air sac (DAS) assay [93, 103]. Tocotrienol-rich fraction and delta-tocotrienol were also demonstrated in vivo to possess anti-angiogenic effects as assessed by chick embryo chorioallantoic membrane (CAM) assay [94, 103, 180]. Tocotrienol-rich fraction supplementation also suppressed serum VEGF level in BALB/c mice inoculated with mouse mammary cancer 4T1 cells which indicated its potential anti-angiogenic activity [180].

Western blotting analysis identified that anti-angiogenic activity of delta-tocotrienol was mediated via apoptosis induction and inactivation of PI3K/PDK/Akt pathway [93]. The inactivation of PI3K/PDK/Akt pathway then suppressed the phosphorylation of ERK1/2, eNOS, and GSK3 alpha/beta and increased the phosphorylated ASK-1 and p38 and p21 which were associated with apoptosis [103]. Besides that, DNA microarray analysis revealed that delta-tocotrienol also downregulated VEGF receptor expression and subsequently blocked intracellular VEGF signalling (phospholipase C-gamma and PKC) in HUVEC cells [94]. Delta-tocotrienol also managed to suppress IL-8 and angiogenic factor secretion and downregulate HIF-1 alpha and IL-8 mRNA in hypoxic conditions [148]. The downregulation of hypoxia-induced HIF-1 alpha expression then inhibited VGEF transcriptional activation [148]. Furthermore, tocotrienol was demonstrated to inhibit human and mice DNA polymerase λ activity in the order of delta- >beta- >gamma- >alpha-tocotrienol [95]. Tocotrienol-induced DNA polymerase λ inhibition required direct binding of tocotrienol to N-terminal region of polymerase [95]. Inhibition of DNA polymerase λ might be closely related to anti-angiogenic activity of tocotrienol.

Tocotrienol-rich fraction and tocotrienols also possessed anti-migration and anti-invasion properties. Delta-tocotrienol inhibited HUVEC and BAEC cells migration as shown in scratch assay test [92, 180]. Delta-tocotrienol also demonstrated profound inhibitory effect on human monocyte U937 cells adhesion to HAECs via blockage of HAECs surface VCAM-1 mRNA and expression [102]. Both alpha-tocotrienol and gamma-tocotrienol suppressed VCAM-1 expression, which inhibited human monocyte THP-1 cells adhesion to endothelial HUVEC cells with the order of alpha-tocotrienol > gamma-tocotrienol [116]. Gamma-tocotrienol also inhibited melanoma cells invasion via restoration of E-cadherin and gamma-catenin expression, together with downregulation of Snail, alpha-SMA, vimentin and twist expression [22].

The anticancer mechanism of tocotrienol is summarized in Fig. 5.4.

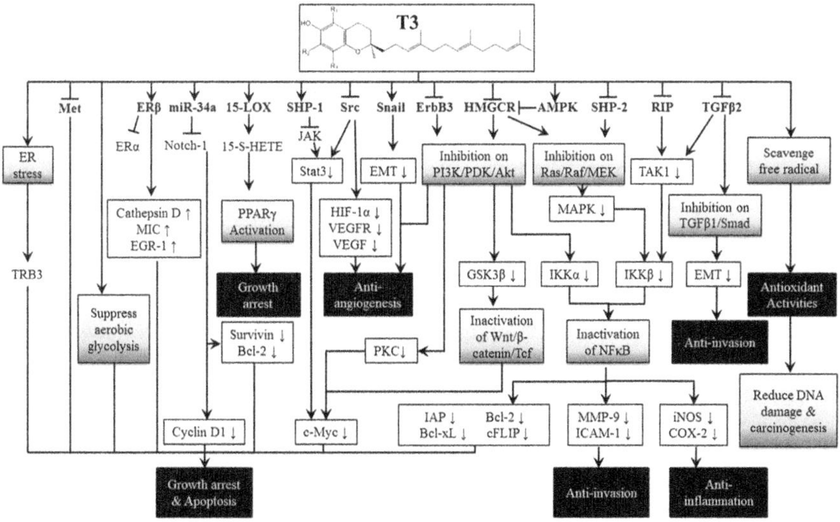

Fig. 5.4 The anticancer mechanism of tocotrienol

5.8 Safety of Tocotrienol

A toxicity study conducted by Ima-Nirwana et al. in the mice revealed that palm tocotrienol at the doses of 500 and 1000 mg/kg body weight (oral) for 14 days (subacute) and 42 days (subchronic) increased the bleeding the clotting time [57]. After conversion based on body surface area [138], this is equivalent to 40.54 and 81.08 mg/kg in humans. Nakamura et al. observed changes in haematology, blood serum enzyme levels and organ histology in rats fed with palm tocotrienol (0.75–3 % weight of diet) for 13 weeks [104]. The no-observed-adverse-effect level derived from this study was 120 mg/kg body weight for male rats and 130 mg/kg body weight for female rats [104]. This is equivalent to 19.46 mg/kg in men and 21.08 mg/kg in women. In view of these studies, it is recommended that patients who are taking anticoagulants such as warfarin, heparin and aspirin to refrain from using tocotrienol because it may increase haemorrhagic risk. Prolonged use of tocotrienol at high dose should also be avoided because it may exert adverse effects on the liver. Taking these into consideration, the use of tocotrienol is relatively safe. The highest dose used in human recorded in this review is 400 mg [47], equivalent to 5.71 mg/kg for a 70 kg adults, which is far below the toxic doses.

5.9 Conclusion

The two groups of vitamin E, the tocotrienols and the tocopherols possess distinct similarities and differences. These differences may be seen even between isomers within the same group. Extensive in vivo and in vitro studies on vitamin E mixtures from various natural sources, as well as the pure isomers, have been done. Most of these studies have shown beneficial effects of the tocotrienol and tocopherol isomers in varying degrees. The source of the naturally occurring vitamin E mixtures are from palm oil, rice bran or annatto oil. However, in the reported literature, the vitamin E mixtures differ in composition, some consisting of mixtures of tocopherols and tocotrienols, while some are mixtures of tocotrienol isomers only. The doses used also differ between studies. Even experiments using individual tocotrienol or tocopherol isomers differ in their effective doses. Thus, it is not easy to summarize the results, but in general the preclinical literature shows that tocotrienols are beneficial in metabolic disease conditions associated with elevated free radicals and inflammatory cytokines, such as dyslipidaemia, diabetes mellitus and osteoporosis. Some clinical trials on tocotrienols and dyslipidaemia have been reported, while none on diabetes mellitus or osteoporosis are available so far. Data from the available clinical trials are inconclusive, and generally the beneficial effects are slight and not as significantly obvious as the effects seen in the in vivo and in vitro studies. This begs the question as to whether dose of the tocotrienols used in the human studies were too low, or the duration of treatment insufficient, or even whether the sampling methods were adequate. Another cause for the discrepancy could be that the distribution and metabolism of the tocotrienols differ between humans and the rodent models used. It will be interesting to see whether the same sort of observations will be seen in clinical trials on the effects of tocotrienols in diabetics or in osteoporotic patients.

Many well-reported studies on the anticancer effects of tocotrienol were found in the literature. Most of these studies are in vitro studies using cancer cell lines. Most of the studies are on breast cancer cells, while some studies are on liver, colon, lung and leukaemic cell lines. The mechanisms have been elucidated as being apoptotic and anti-angiogenetic. The anticancer effects of tocotrienol are thought to be separate from the antioxidant and anti-inflammatory effects. Limited animal studies have been done using genetically modified mice, and only two reported clinical trials on the effects of tocotrienols on breast cancer are found in literature. Again the data from the human studies are scant and inconclusive.

From the above review, tocotrienol presents an exciting possibility as an alternative or adjuvant therapy for diseases associated with increased oxidative stress and inflammation, such as dyslipidaemia and diabetes. Its application in preventing osteoporosis in humans still awaits results from clinical trial. More coordinated, well-designed clinical trials are needed to determine the effects on humans, however, the consistently beneficial effects in in vivo studies indicate that the potential for human therapeutic use is real. As for the anticancer properties, the potential for use presents a real challenge to researchers. The apoptotic and anti-angiogenetic properties seen in the cell culture studies appears very promising and can be the alternative to the stressful chemotherapy, or at least as an adjuvant to reduce the side-effects of chemotherapy.

Acknowledgements This work is supported by Universiti Kebangsaan Malaysia via grants GGPM-2015-036.

References

1. Abd Manan N, Mohamed N, Shuid AN (2012) Effects of low-dose versus high-dose gamma-tocotrienol on the bone cells exposed to the hydrogen peroxide-induced oxidative stress and apoptosis. Evid Based Complement Altern Med 2012:680834
2. Abdelmagid SM, Barbe MF, Safadi FF (2015) Role of inflammation in the aging bones. Life Sci 123:25–34
3. Abdul-Majeed S, Mohamed N, Soelaiman I-N (2012) Effects of tocotrienol and lovastatin combination on osteoblast and osteoclast activity in estrogen-deficient osteoporosis. Evid Based Complement Altern Med 2012:960742
4. Abdul-Majeed S, Mohamed N, Soelaiman IN (2015) The use of delta-tocotrienol and lovastatin for anti-osteoporotic therapy. Life Sci 125:42–48
5. Abukhadir SSA, Mohamed N, Makpol S, Muhammad N (2012) Effects of palm vitamin e on bone-formation-related gene expression in nicotine-treated rats. Evid Based Complement Altern Med 2012:656025
6. Aggarwal BB, Sundaram C, Prasad S, Kannappan R (2010) Tocotrienols, the vitamin E of the 21(St) Century: it's potential against cancer and other chronic diseases. Biochem Pharmacol 80(11):1613–1631

7. Ahmad NS, Khalid BAK, Luke DA, Ima Nirwana S (2005) Tocotrienol offers better protection than tocopherol from free radical-induced damage of rat bone. Clin Exp Pharmacol Physiol 32(9):761–770
8. Aktifanus AT, Shuid AN, Rashid NH et al (2012) Comparison of the effects of tocotrienol and estrogen on the bone markers and dynamic changes in postmenopausal osteoporosis rat model. Asian J Anim Vet Adv 7(3):225–234
9. Atli T, Keven K, Avci A et al (2004) oxidative stress and antioxidant status in elderly diabetes mellitus and glucose intolerance patients. Arch Gerontol Geriatr 39(3):269–275
10. Baek KH, Oh KW, Lee WY et al (2010) Association of oxidative stress with postmenopausal osteoporosis and the effects of hydrogen peroxide on osteoclast formation in human bone marrow cell cultures. Calcif Tissue Int 87(3):226–235
11. Baliarsingh S, Beg ZH, Ahmad J (2005) The therapeutic impacts of tocotrienols in type 2 diabetic patients with hyperlipidemia. Atherosclerosis 182(2):367–374
12. Barnham KJ, Masters CL, Bush AI (2004) Neurodegenerative diseases and oxidative stress. Nat Rev Drug Discov 3(3):205–214
13. Birringer M, EyTina JH, Salvatore BA, Neuzil J (2003) Vitamin E analogues as inducers of apoptosis: structure-function relation. Br J Cancer 88(12):1948–1955
14. Brigelius-Flohe R, Kelly FJ, Salonen JT, Neuzil J, Zingg JM, Azzi A (2002) The European perspective on vitamin E: current knowledge and future research. Am J Clin Nutr 76(4):703–716
15. Brooks R, Kalia P, Ireland DC, Beeton C, Rushton N (2011) Direct inhibition of osteoclast formation and activity by the vitamin E isomer gamma-tocotrienol. Int J Vitam Nutr Res 81 (6):358–367
16. Budin SB, Othman F, Louis SR, Bakar MA, Das S, Mohamed J (2009) The effects of palm oil tocotrienol-rich fraction supplementation on biochemical parameters, oxidative stress and the vascular wall of streptozotocin-induced diabetic rats. Clinics (Sao Paulo) 64(3):235–244
17. Buhaescu I, Izzedine H (2007) Mevalonate pathway: a review of clinical and therapeutical implications. Clin Biochem 40(9–10):575–584
18. Burdeos GC, Nakagawa K, Kimura F, Miyazawa T (2012) Tocotrienol attenuates triglyceride accumulation in Hepg2 cells and F344 rats. Lipids 47(5):471–481
19. Burdeos GC, Nakagawa K, Watanabe A, Kimura F, Miyazawa T (2013) Gamma-tocotrienol attenuates triglyceride through effect on lipogenic gene expressions in mouse hepatocellular carcinoma hepa 1-6. J Nutr Sci Vitaminol (Tokyo) 59(2):148–151
20. Callaway DA, Jiang JX (2015) Reactive oxygen species and oxidative stress in osteoclastogenesis, skeletal aging and bone diseases. J Bone Miner Metab 33(4):359–370
21. Campbell PT, Newton CC, Patel AV, Jacobs EJ, Gapstur SM (2012) Diabetes and cause-specific mortality in a prospective cohort of one million U.S. adults. Diabetes Care 35 (9):1835–1844
22. Chang PN, Yap WN, Lee DT, Ling MT, Wong YC, Yap YL (2009) Evidence of Γ-tocotrienol as an apoptosis-inducing, invasion-suppressing, and chemotherapy drug-sensitizing agent in human melanoma cells. Nutr Cancer 61(3):357–366
23. Chatelain E, Boscoboinik DO, Bartoli G-M et al (1993) Inhibition of smooth muscle cell proliferation and protein kinase C activity by tocopherols and tocotrienols. Biochim Biophys Acta (BBA) Mol Cell Res 1176(1–2):83–89
24. Chin K-Y, Ima-Nirwana S (2012) Vitamin E as an antiosteoporotic agent via receptor activator of nuclear factor kappa-B ligand signaling disruption: current evidence and other potential research areas. Evid Based Complement Altern Med 2012:747020
25. Chin KY, Abdul-Majeed S, Fozi NF, Ima-Nirwana S (2014) Annatto tocotrienol improves indices of bone static histomorphometry in osteoporosis due to testosterone deficiency in rats. Nutrients 6(11):4974–4983
26. Chin KY, Ima-Nirwana S (2014) The effects of alpha-tocopherol on bone: a double-edged sword? Nutrients 6(4):1424–1441
27. Chin KY, Ima-Nirwana S (2015) the biological effects of tocotrienol on bone: a review on evidence from rodent models. Drug Des Devel Ther 9:2049–2061

28. Chin KY, Ima Nirwana S (2014) The effects of annatto-derived tocotrienol supplementation in osteoporosis induced by testosterone deficiency in rats. Clin Interv Aging 9:1247–1259
29. Chin SF, Ibahim J, Makpol S et al (2011) Tocotrienol rich fraction supplementation improved lipid profile and oxidative status in healthy older adults: a randomized controlled study. Nutr Metab (Lond) 8(1):42
30. Choy EHS, Panayi GS (2001) Cytokine pathways and joint inflammation in rheumatoid arthritis. N Engl J Med 344(12):907–916
31. Chun J, Lee J, Ye L, Exler J, Eitenmiller RR (2006) Tocopherol and tocotrienol contents of raw and processed fruits and vegetables in the United States Diet. J Food Compos Anal 19 (2–3):196–204
32. Comitato R, Nesaretnam K, Leoni G et al (2009) A novel mechanism of natural vitamin E tocotrienol activity: involvement of Erβ signal transduction. Am J Physiol Endocrinol Metab 297:E427–E437
33. Constantinou C, Hyatt JA, Vraka PS et al (2009) Induction of caspase-independent programmed cell death by vitamin E natural homologs and synthetic derivatives. Nutr Cancer 61(6):864–874
34. Conte C, Floridi A, Aisa C, Piroddi M, Floridi A, Galli F (2004) Γ-tocotrienol metabolism and antiproliferative effect in prostate cancer cells. Ann N Y Acad Sci 1031:391–394
35. Dandona P, Aljada A, Bandyopadhyay A (2004) Inflammation: the link between insulin resistance, obesity and diabetes. Trends Immunol 25(1):4–7
36. Daud ZA, Tubie B, Sheyman M et al (2013) Vitamin E tocotrienol supplementation improves lipid profiles in chronic hemodialysis patients. Vasc Health Risk Manag 9:747–761
37. Deng L, Ding Y, Peng Y et al (2014) Γ-tocotrienol protects against ovariectomy-induced bone loss via mevalonate pathway as Hmg-Coa reductase inhibitor. Bone 67:200–207
38. Deshpande AD, Harris-Hayes M, Schootman M (2008) Epidemiology of diabetes and diabetes-related complications. Phys Ther 88(11):1254–1264
39. Di Marco E, Jha JC, Sharma A, Wilkinson-Berka JL, Jandeleit-Dahm KA, de Haan JB (2015) Are reactive oxygen species still the basis for diabetic complications? Clin Sci (Lond) 129(2):199–216
40. Eitsuka T, Nakagawa K, Miyazawa T (2006) Down-regulation of telomerase activity in Dld-1 human colorectal adenocarcinoma cells by tocotrienol. Biochem Biophys Res Commun 348(1):170–175
41. Elangovan S, Hsieh TC, Wu JM (2008) Growth inhibition of human Mda-Mb-231 breast cancer cells by Δ-tocotrienol is associated with loss of cyclin D1/Cdk4 expression and accompanying changes in the state of phosphorylation of the retinoblastoma tumor suppressor gene product. Anticancer Res 28:2641–2648
42. Frega N, Mozzon M, Bocci F (1998) Identification and estimation of tocotrienols in the annatto lipid fraction by gas chromatography-mass spectrometry. J Am Oil Chem Soc 75 (12):1723–1727
43. Gee PT (2011) Unleashing the untold and misunderstood observations on vitamin E. Genes Nutr 6(1):5–16
44. Guthrie N, Gapor A, Chambers AF, Carroll KK (1997) Inhibition of proliferation of estrogen receptor-negative Mda-Mb-435 and -Positive Mcf-7 human breast cancer cells by palm oil tocotrienols and tamoxifen, alone and in combination. J Nutr 127:544S–548S
45. Guthrie N, Gapor A, Chambers AF, Carroll KK (1997) Palm oil tocotrienols and plant flavonoids act synergistically with each other and with tamoxifen in inhibiting proliferation and growth of estrogen receptor-negative Mda-Mb-435 and -positive Mcf-7 human breast cancer cells in culture. Asia Pac J Clin Nutrition 6(1):41–45
46. Ha H, Lee JH, Kim HN, Lee ZH (2011) Alpha-tocotrienol inhibits osteoclastic bone resorption by suppressing rankl expression and signaling and bone resorbing activity. Biochem Biophys Res Commun 406(4):546–551
47. Haghighat N, Vafa M, Eghtesadi S, Heidari I, Hosseini A, Rostami A (2014) The effects of tocotrienols added to canola oil on microalbuminuria, inflammation, and nitrosative stress in

patients with type 2 diabetes: a randomized, double-blind, placebo-controlled trial. Int J Prev Med 5(5):617–623
48. Halliwell B (1994) Free radicals, antioxidants, and human disease: curiosity, cause, or consequence? Lancet 344(8924):721–724
49. Har CH, Keong CK (2005) Effects of tocotrienols on cell viability and apoptosis in normal murine liver cells (Bnl Cl.2) and liver cancer cells (Bnl 1me A.7r.1), in Vitro. Asia Pac J Clin Nutr 14(4):374–380
50. Heng KS, Hejar AR, Johnson Stanslas J, Ooi CF, Loh SF (2015) Potential of mixed tocotrienol supplementation to reduce cholesterol and cytokines level in adults with metabolic syndrome. Malays J Nutr 21(2):231–243
51. Hermizi H, Faizah O, Ima-Nirwana S, Ahmad Nazrun S, Norazlina M (2009) Beneficial effects of tocotrienol and tocopherol on bone histomorphometric parameters in Sprague-Dawley male rats after nicotine cessation. Calcif Tissue Int 84(1):65–74
52. Hiura Y, Tachibana H, Arakawa R et al (2009) Specific accumulation of Γ- and Δ-tocotrienols in tumor and their antitumor effect in vivo. J Nutr Biochem 20(8):607–613
53. Hosomi A, Arita M, Sato Y et al (1997) Affinity for alpha-tocopherol transfer protein as a determinant of the biological activities of vitamin E analogs. FEBS Lett 409(1):105–108
54. Hsieh TC, Wu JM (1992) Suppression of cell proliferation and gene expression by combinatorial synergy of Egcg, resveratrol and Γ-tocotrienol in estrogen receptor-positive Mcf-7 breast cancer cells. Int J Oncol 33(4):851–859
55. Husain K, Francois RA, Hutchinson SZ et al (2009) Vitamin E Δ-tocotrienol levels in tumor and pancreatic tissue of mice after oral administration. Pharmacology 83(3):157–163
56. Ima-Nirwana S, Fakhrurazi H (2002) Palm vitamin E protects bone against dexamethasone-induced osteoporosis in male rats. Med J Malaysia 57(2):133–141
57. Ima-Nirwana S, Nurshazwani Y, Nazrun AS, Norliza M, Norazlina M (2011) Subacute and subchronic toxicity studies of palm vitamin E in mice. J Pharmacol Toxicol 6:166–173
58. Ima Nirwana S, Kiftiah A, Zainal A, Norazlina M, Abd. Gapor M, Khalid BAK (2000) Palm vitamin E prevents osteoporosis in orchidectomised growing male rats. Nat Prod Sci 6 (4):155–160
59. Ima Nirwana S, Suhaniza S (2004) Effects of tocopherols and tocotrienols on body composition and bone calcium content in adrenalectomized rats replaced with dexamethasone. J Med Food 7(1):45–51
60. Inokuchi H, Hirokane H, Tsuzuki T, Nakagawa K, Igarashi M, Miyazawa T (2003) Anti-angiogenic activity of tocotrienol. Biosci Biotechnol Biochem 67(7):1623–1627
61. Institute of Medicine (2000) Dietary reference intakes for vitamin C, vitamin E, selenium, and carotenoids. The National Academies Press, Washington
62. Iqbal J, Minhajuddin M, Beg ZH (2003) Suppression of 7,12-dimethylbenz[alpha] anthracene-induced carcinogenesis and hypercholesterolaemia in rats by tocotrienol-rich fraction isolated from rice bran oil. Eur J Cancer Prev 12(6):447–453
63. Jiang Q (2014) Natural forms of vitamin E: metabolism, antioxidant, and anti-inflammatory activities and their role in disease prevention and therapy. Free Radic Biol Med 72:76–90
64. Johnell O, Kanis J (2006) An estimate of the worldwide prevalence and disability associated with osteoporotic fractures. Osteoporos Int 17(12):1726–1733
65. Jones MP, Pandak WM, Heuman DM, Chiang JY, Hylemon PB, Vlahcevic ZR (1993) Cholesterol 7 alpha-hydroxylase: evidence for transcriptional regulation by cholesterol or metabolic products of cholesterol in the rat. J Lipid Res 34(6):885–892
66. Kamat JP, Devasagayam TP (1995) Tocotrienols from palm oil as potent inhibitors of lipid peroxidation and protein oxidation in rat brain mitochondria. Neurosci Lett 195(3):179–182
67. Kamat JP, Sarma HD, Devasagayam TP, Nesaretnam K, Basiron Y (1997) Tocotrienols from palm oil as effective inhibitors of protein oxidation and lipid peroxidation in rat liver microsomes. Mol Cell Biochem 170(1–2):131–137
68. Kanis JA, McCloskey EV, Harvey NC, Johansson H, Leslie WD (2015) Intervention thresholds and the diagnosis of osteoporosis. J Bone Miner Res 30(10):1747–1753

69. Kashiwagi K, Harada K, Yano Y et al (2008) A redox-silent analogue of tocotrienol inhibits hypoxic adaptation of lung cancer cells. Biochem Biophys Res Commun 365(4):875–881
70. Kashiwagi K, Virgona N, Harada K et al (2009) A redox-silent analogue of tocotrienol acts as a potential cytotoxic agent against human mesothelioma cells. Life Sci 84(19–20):650–656
71. Kataja-Tuomola MK, Kontto JP, Mannisto S, Albanes D, Virtamo J (2011) Intake of antioxidants and risk of type 2 diabetes in a cohort of male smokers. Eur J Clin Nutr 65 (5):590–597
72. Kawakami Y, Tsuzuki T, Nakagawa K, Miyazawa T (2007) Distribution of tocotrienols in rats fed a rice bran tocotrienol concentrate. Biosci Biotechnol Biochem 71(2):464–471
73. Khor H, Ng T, Rajendran R (2002) Dose-dependent cholesterolemic activity of tocotrienols. Malays J Nutr 8(2):157–166
74. Khor HT, Ng TT (2000) Effects of administration of alpha-tocopherol and tocotrienols on serum lipids and liver Hmg Coa reductase activity. Int J Food Sci Nutr 51(Suppl):S3–S11
75. King AJ (2012) The use of animal models in diabetes research. Br J Pharmacol 166(3):877–894
76. Kuhad A, Bishnoi M, Tiwari V, Chopra K (2009) Suppression of Nf-Kappabeta signaling pathway by tocotrienol can prevent diabetes associated cognitive deficits. Pharmacol Biochem Behav 92(2):251–259
77. Kuhad A, Chopra K (2009) Attenuation of diabetic nephropathy by tocotrienol: involvement of Nfkb signaling pathway. Life Sci 84(9–10):296–301
78. Kuhad A, Chopra K (2009) Tocotrienol attenuates oxidative-nitrosative stress and inflammatory cascade in experimental model of diabetic neuropathy. Neuropharmacology 57(4):456–462
79. Lee SP, Mar GY, Ng LT (2009) Effects of tocotrienol-rich fraction on exercise endurance capacity and oxidative stress in forced swimming rats. Eur J Appl Physiol 107(5):587–595
80. Libby P (2006) Inflammation and cardiovascular disease mechanisms. Am J Clin Nutr 83 (2):456S–460S
81. Lodge JK, Ridlington J, Leonard S, Vaule H, Traber MG (2001) Alpha- and gamma-tocotrienols are metabolized to carboxyethyl-hydroxychroman derivatives and excreted in human urine. Lipids 36(1):43–48
82. Madamanchi NR, Vendrov A, Runge MS (2005) Oxidative stress and vascular disease. Arterioscler Thromb Vasc Biol 25(1):29–38
83. Maniam S, Mohamed N, Shuid AN, Soelaiman IN (2008) Palm tocotrienol exerted better antioxidant activities in bone than α-tocopherol. Basic Clin Pharmacol Toxicol 103(1):55–60
84. Manolagas SC (2010) From Estrogen-Centric to Aging and Oxidative Stress: A Revised Perspective of the Pathogenesis of Osteoporosis. Endocr Rev 31(3):266–300
85. Matough FA, Budin SB, Hamid ZA, Abdul-Rahman M, Al-Wahaibi N, Mohammed J (2014) Tocotrienol-rich fraction from palm oil prevents oxidative damage in diabetic rats. Sultan Qaboos Univ Med J 14(1):e95–e103
86. McAnally JA, Gupta J, Sodhani S, Bravo L, Mo H (2007) Tocotrienols potentiate lovastatin-mediated growth suppression in vitro and in vivo. Exp Biol Med (Maywood) 232:523–531
87. McIntyre BS, Briski KP, Gapor A, Sylvester PW (2008) Antiproliferative and apoptotic effects of tocopherols and tocotrienols on preneoplastic and neoplastic mouse mammary epithelial cells. Proc Soc Exp Biol Med 224(4):292–301
88. McIntyre BS, Briski KP, Tirmenstein MA, Fariss MW, Gapor A, Sylvester PW (2000) Antiproliferative and apoptotic effects of tocopherols and tocotrienols on normal mouse mammary epithelial cells. Lipids 35(2):171–180
89. Mehat M, Shuid A, Mohamed N, Muhammad N, Soelaiman I (2010) Beneficial effects of vitamin E isomer supplementation on static and dynamic bone histomorphometry parameters in normal male rats. J Bone Miner Metab 28(5):503–509
90. Mensink RP, van Houwelingen AC, Kromhout D, Hornstra G (1999) A Vitamin E concentrate rich in tocotrienols had no effect on serum lipids, lipoproteins, or platelet

function in men with mildly elevated serum lipid concentrations. Am J Clin Nutr 69(2):213–219
91. Minhajuddin M, Beg ZH, Iqbal J (2005) Hypolipidemic and antioxidant properties of tocotrienol rich fraction isolated from rice bran oil in experimentally induced hyperlipidemic rats. Food Chem Toxicol 43(5):747–753
92. Miyazawa T, Inokuchi H, Hirokane H, Tsuzuki T, Nakagawa K, Igarashi M (2004) Anti-angiogenic potential of tocotrienol in vitro. Biochemistry (Moscow) 69(1):67–69
93. Miyazawa T, Shibata A, Nakagawa K, Tsuzuki T (2008) Anti-angiogenic function of tocotrienol. Asia Pac J Clin Nutr 17(S1):253–256
94. Miyazawa T, Tsuzuki T, Nakagawa K, Igarashi M (2004) Antiangiogenic potency of vitamin E. Ann N Y Acad Sci 1031:401–404
95. Mizushina Y, Nakagawa K, Shibata A et al (2006) Inhibitory effect of tocotrienol on eukaryotic DNA polymerase Λ and angiogenesis. Biochem Biophys Res Commun 339 (3):949–955
96. Muhammad N, Luke DA, Shuid AN, Mohamed N, Soelaiman IN (2012) Two different isomers of vitamin E prevent bone loss in postmenopausal osteoporosis rat model. Evid Based Complement Altern Med 2012:161527
97. Muhammad N, Razali S, Shuid AN, Mohamed N, Soelaiman IN (2013) Membandingkan Kesan Antara Fraksi-Kaya Tokotrienol, Kalsium Dan Estrogen Terhadap Metabolisme Tulang Tikus Terovariektomi. Sains Malays 42(11):1591–1597
98. Müller M, Cela J, Asensi-Fabado MA, Munné-Bosch S (2012) Tocotrienols in plants: occurrence, biosynthesis, and function. In: Tan B, Watson RR, Preedy VR (eds) Tocotrienols: vitamin E beyond tocopherols. CRC Press, Florida, pp 1–16
99. Mundy GR (2007) Osteoporosis and inflammation. Nutr Rev 65(suppl 3):S147–S151
100. Munteanu A, Ricciarelli R, Massone S, Zingg JM (2007) Modulation of proteasome activity by vitamin E in Thp-1 monocytes. IUBMB Life 59(12):771–780
101. Mustad VA, Smith CA, Ruey PP, Edens NK, DeMichele SJ (2002) Supplementation with 3 compositionally different tocotrienol supplements does not improve cardiovascular disease risk factors in men and women with hypercholesterolemia. Am J Clin Nutr 76(6):1237–1243
102. Naito Y, Shimozawa M, Kuroda M et al (2005) Tocotrienols reduce 25-hydroxycholesterol-induced monocyte-endothelial cell interaction by inhibiting the surface expression of adhesion molecules. Atherosclerosis 180(1):19–25
103. Nakagawa K, Shibata A, Yamashita S et al (2007) In vivo angiogenesis is suppressed by unsaturated vitamin E, tocotrienol. J Nutr 137:1938–1943
104. Nakamura H, Furukawa F, Nishikawa A et al (2001) Oral toxicity of a tocotrienol preparation in rats. Food Chem Toxicol 39(8):799–805
105. Nazrun AS, Luke ·DA, Khalid BAK, Ima Nirwana S (2005) Vitamin E protects from free-radical damage on femur of rats treated with ferric nitrilotriacetate. Curr Topics Pharmacol 9(2):107–115
106. Nesaretnam K, Devasagayam TP, Singh BB, Basiron Y (1993) Influence of palm oil or its tocotrienol-rich fraction on the lipid peroxidation potential of rat liver mitochondria and microsomes. Biochem Mol Biol Int 30(1):159–167
107. Nesaretnam K, Meganathan P, Veerasenan SD, Selvaduray KR (2012) Tocotrienols and breast cancer: the evidence to date. Genes Nutr 7(1):3–9
108. Nesaretnam K, Selvaduray KR, Abdul Razak G, Veerasenan SD, Gomez PA (2010) Effectiveness of tocotrienol-rich fraction combined with tamoxifen in the management of women with early breast cancer: a pilot clinical trial. Breast Cancer Res 12(5):R81
109. Nesaretnam K, Stephen R, Dils R, Darbre P (1998) Tocotrienols inhibit the growth of human breast cancer cells irrespective of estrogen receptor status. Lipids 33(5):461–469
110. Ng LT, Ko HJ (2012) Comparative effects of tocotrienol-rich fraction, alpha-tocopherol and alpha-tocopheryl acetate on inflammatory mediators and nuclear factor kappa B expression in mouse peritoneal macrophages. Food Chem 134(2):920–925
111. Ng MH, Choo YM, Ma AN, Chuah CH, Hashim MA (2004) Separation of vitamin E (tocopherol, tocotrienol, and tocomonoenol) in palm oil. Lipids 39(10):1031–1035

112. Ngah WZW, Jarien Z, San MM et al (1991) Effect of tocotrienols on hepatocarcinogenesis induced by 2-acetylaminofluorene in rats. Am J Clin Nutr 53:1076S–1081S
113. Niki E (2013) Antioxidant action of tocotrienols. In: Tan B, Watson RR, Preedy VR (eds) Tocotrienols: vitamin E beyond tocopherols. CRC Press, Boca Raton, pp 233–240
114. Nikolic K, Agababa D (2009) Design and Qsar study of analogs of Γ-tocotrienol with enhanced antiproliferative activity against human breast cancer cells. J Mol Graph Model 27 (7):777–783
115. Nizar AM, Nazrun AS, Norazlina M, Norliza M, Ima Nirwana S (2011) Low dose of tocotrienols protects osteoblasts against oxidative stress. Clin Ter 162(6):533–538
116. Noguchi N, Hanyu R, Nonaka A, Okimoto Y, Kodama T (2003) Inhibition of Thp-1 cell adhesion to endothelial cells by A-tocopherol and A-tocotrienol is dependent on intracellular concentration of the antioxidants. Free Radic Biol Med 34(12):1614–1620
117. Norazlina M, Hermizi H, Faizah O, Ima-Nirwana S (2010) Vitamin E reversed nicotine-induced toxic effects on bone biochemical markers in male rats. Arch Med Sci 6 (4):505–512
118. Norazlina M, Ima Nirwana S, Abd. Gapor M, Khalid B (2000) Palm vitamin E is comparable to alpha-tocotrienol in maintaining bone mineral density in ovariectomised female rats. Exp Clin Endocrinol Diabetes 108:305–310
119. Norazlina M, Lee P, Lukman H, Nazrun A, Ima-Nirwana S (2007) Effects of vitamin E supplementation on bone metabolism in nicotine-treated rats. Singapore Med J 48(3):195–199
120. O'Byrne D, Grundy S, Packer L et al (2000) Studies of Ldl oxidation following alpha-, gamma-, or delta-tocotrienyl acetate supplementation of hypercholesterolemic humans. Free Radic Biol Med 29(9):834–845
121. Palozza P, Verdecchia S, Avanzi L et al (2006) Comparative antioxidant activity of tocotrienols and the novel chromanyl-polyisoprenyl molecule feaox-6 in isolated membranes and intact cells. Mol Cell Biochem 287(1–2):21–32
122. Parker RA, Pearce BC, Clark RW, Gordon DA, Wright JJ (1993) Tocotrienols regulate cholesterol production in mammalian cells by post-transcriptional suppression of 3-hydroxy-3-methylglutaryl-coenzyme a reductase. J Biol Chem 268(15):11230–11238
123. Patel J, Matnor NA, Iyer A, Brown L (2011) A regenerative antioxidant protocol of vitamin E and alpha-lipoic acid ameliorates cardiovascular and metabolic changes in fructose-fed rats. Evid Based Complement Altern Med 2011:120801
124. Qureshi AA, Pearce BC, Nor RM, Gapor A, Peterson DM, Elson CE (1996) Dietary alpha-tocopherol attenuates the impact of gamma-tocotrienol on hepatic 3-hydroxy-3-methylglutaryl coenzyme a reductase activity in chickens. J Nutr 126(2):389–394
125. Qureshi AA, Peterson DM (2001) The combined effects of novel tocotrienols and lovastatin on lipid metabolism in chickens. Atherosclerosis 156(1):39–47
126. Qureshi AA, Peterson DM, Hasler-Rapacz JO, Rapacz J (2001) Novel tocotrienols of rice bran suppress cholesterogenesis in hereditary hypercholesterolemic swine. J Nutr 131 (2):223–230
127. Qureshi AA, Qureshi N, Hasler-Rapacz JO et al (1991) Dietary tocotrienols reduce concentrations of plasma cholesterol, apolipoprotein B, thromboxane B2, and platelet factor 4 in pigs with inherited hyperlipidemias. Am J Clin Nutr 53(4 Suppl):1042s–1046s
128. Qureshi AA, Qureshi N, Wright JJ et al (1991) Lowering of serum cholesterol in hypercholesterolemic humans by tocotrienols (Palmvitee). Am J Clin Nutr 53(4 Suppl):1021s–1026s
129. Qureshi AA, Reis JC, Papasian CJ, Morrison DC, Qureshi N (2010) Tocotrienols inhibit lipopolysaccharide-induced pro-inflammatory cytokines in macrophages of female mice. Lipids Health Dis 9:143
130. Qureshi AA, Reis JC, Qureshi N, Papasian CJ, Morrison DC, Schaefer DM (2011) Delta-tocotrienol and quercetin reduce serum levels of nitric oxide and lipid parameters in female chickens. Lipids Health Dis 10:39

131. Qureshi AA, Sami SA, Salser WA, Khan FA (2001) Synergistic effect of tocotrienol-rich fraction (Trf(25)) of rice bran and lovastatin on lipid parameters in hypercholesterolemic humans. J Nutr Biochem 12(6):318–329
132. Qureshi AA, Sami SA, Salser WA, Khan FA (2002) Dose-dependent suppression of serum cholesterol by tocotrienol-rich fraction (Trf25) of rice bran in hypercholesterolemic humans. Atherosclerosis 161(1):199–207
133. Qureshi AA, Tan X, Reis JC et al (2011) Inhibition of nitric oxide in Lps-stimulated macrophages of young and senescent mice by delta-tocotrienol and quercetin. Lipids Health Dis 10:239
134. Raederstorff D, Elste V, Aebischer C, Weber P (2002) Effect of either gamma-tocotrienol or a tocotrienol mixture on the plasma lipid profile in hamsters. Ann Nutr Metab 46(1):17–23
135. Rahmat A, Ngah WZW, Top AGM, Khalid BAK (1993) Long term tocotrienol supplementation and glutathione-dependent enzymes during hepatocarcinogenesis in the rat. Asia Pac J Clin Nutr 2:129–134
136. Rasool AH, Yuen KH, Yusoff K, Wong AR, Rahman AR (2006) Dose dependent elevation of plasma tocotrienol levels and its effect on arterial compliance, plasma total antioxidant status, and lipid profile in healthy humans supplemented with tocotrienol rich vitamin E. J Nutr Sci Vitaminol (Tokyo) 52(6):473–478
137. Rasool AHG, Yuen KH, Yusoff K, Wong AR, Rahman ARA (2006) Dose dependent elevation of plasma tocotrienol levels and its effect on arterial compliance, plasma total antioxidant status, and lipid profile in healthy humans supplemented with tocotrienol rich vitamin E. J Nutr Sci Vitaminol 52:473–478
138. Reagan-Shaw S, Nihal M, Ahmad N (2008) Dose translation from animal to human studies revisited. FASEB J 22(3):659–661
139. Rickmann M, Vaquero EC, Malagelada JR, Molero X (2007) Tocotrienols induce apoptosis and autophagy in rat pancreatic stellate cells through the mitochondrial death pathway. Gastroenterology 132(7):2518–2532
140. Sakai M, Okabe M, Tachibana H, Yamada K (2006) Apoptosis induction by Γ-tocotrienol in human hepatoma Hep3b cells. J Nutr Biochem 17(10):672–676
141. Sakai M, Okabe M, Yamasaki A, Tachibana H, Yamada K (2004) Induction of apoptosis by tocotrienol in rat hepatoma Drlh-84 cells. Anticancer Res 24:1683–1688
142. Salman Khan M, Akhtar S, Al-Sagair OA, Arif JM (2011) Protective effect of dietary tocotrienols against infection and inflammation-induced hyperlipidemia: an in vivo and in silico study. Phytother Res PTR 25(11):1586–1595
143. Samant GV, Sylvester PW (2006) Γ-tocotrienol inhibits Erbb3-dependent Pi3k-Akt mitogenic signalling in neoplastic mammary epithelial cells. Cell Prolif 39:563–574
144. Sen CK, Khanna S, Roy S, Packer L (2000) Molecular basis of vitamin E action: tocotrienol potently inhibits glutamate-induced Pp60c-Src kinase activation and death of Ht4 neuronal cells. J Biol Chem 275(17):13049–13055
145. Serbinova E, Kagan V, Han D, Packer L (1991) Free radical recycling and intramembrane mobility in the antioxidant properties of alpha-tocopherol and alpha-tocotrienol. Free Radic Biol Med 10(5):263–275
146. Shah SJ, Sylvester PW (2005) Tocotrienol-induced cytotoxicity is unrelated to mitochondrial stress apoptotic signaling in neoplastic mammary epithelial cells. Biochem Cell Biol 83 (1):86–95
147. Shibata A, Nakagawa K, Shirakawa H et al (2012) Physiological effects and tissue distribution from large doses of tocotrienol in rats. Biosci Biotechnol Biochem 76(9):1805–1808
148. Shibata A, Nakagawa K, Sookwong P et al (2008) Tocotrienol inhibits secretion of angiogenic factors from human colorectal adenocarcinoma cells by suppressing hypoxia-inducible factor-1α. J Nutr 138(11):2136–2142
149. Shuid A, Mehat Z, Mohamed N, Muhammad N, Soelaiman I (2010) Vitamin E exhibits bone anabolic actions in normal male rats. J Bone Miner Metab 28(2):149–156

150. Siddiqui S, Ahsan H, Khan MR, Siddiqui WA (2013) Protective effects of tocotrienols against lipid-induced nephropathy in experimental type-2 diabetic rats by modulation in Tgf-beta expression. Toxicol Appl Pharmacol 273(2):314–324
151. Siddiqui S, Rashid Khan M, Siddiqui WA (2010) Comparative hypoglycemic and nephroprotective effects of tocotrienol rich fraction (Trf) from palm oil and rice bran oil against hyperglycemia induced nephropathy in type 1 diabetic rats. Chem Biol Interact 188 (3):651–658
152. Sies H (1997) Oxidative stress: oxidants and antioxidants. Exp Physiol 82(2):291–295
153. Sies H (2000) What is oxidative stress? In: Keaney J, Jr. (ed) Oxidative stress and vascular disease. Developments in cardiovascular medicine, vol 224. Springer, New York , pp 1–8
154. Soelaiman IN, Ming W, Abu Bakar R et al (2012) Palm tocotrienol supplementation enhanced bone formation in oestrogen-deficient rats. Int J Endocrinol 2012:532862
155. Song BL, DeBose-Boyd RA (2006) Insig-dependent ubiquitination and degradation of 3-hydroxy-3-methylglutaryl coenzyme a reductase stimulated by delta- and gamma-tocotrienols. J Biol Chem 281(35):25054–25061
156. Sookwong P, Nakagawa K, Murata K, Kojima Y, Miyazawa T (2007) Quantitation of tocotrienol and tocopherol in various rice brans. J Agric Food Chem 55(2):461–466
157. Sookwong P, Nakagawa K, Yamaguchi Y et al (2010) Tocotrienol distribution in foods: estimation of daily tocotrienol intake of Japanese population. J Agric Food Chem 58 (6):3350–3355
158. Srivastava JK, Gupta S (2006) Tocotrienol-rich fraction of palm oil induces cell cycle arrest and apoptosis selectively in human prostate cancer cells. Biochem Biophys Res Commun 346(2):447–453
159. Stamler J, Daviglus ML, Garside DB, Dyer AR, Greenland P, Neaton JD (2000) Relationship of baseline serum cholesterol levels in 3 large cohorts of younger men to long-term coronary, cardiovascular, and all-cause mortality and to longevity. JAMA 284(3):311–318
160. Sun W, Xu W, Liu H et al (2009) Γ-tocotrienol induces mitochondria-mediated apoptosis in human gastric adenocarcinoma Sgc-7901 cells. J Nutr Biochem 20(4):276–284
161. Suzuki YJ, Tsuchiya M, Wassall SR et al (1993) Structural and dynamic membrane properties of alpha-tocopherol and alpha-tocotrienol: implication to the molecular mechanism of their antioxidant potency. Biochemistry 32(40):10692–10699
162. Sylvester PW, Nachnani A, Shah S, Briski KP (2002) Role of Gtp-binding proteins in reversing the antiproliferative effects of tocotrienols in preneoplastic mammary epithelial cells. Asia Pac J Clin Nutr 11(Suppl):S452–S459
163. Sylvester PW, Shah S (2005) Intracellular mechanisms mediating tocotrienol-induced apoptosis in neoplastic mammary epithelial cells. Asia Pac J Clin Nutr 14(4):366–373
164. Sylvester PW, Shah SJ (2005) Mechanisms mediating the antiproliferative and apoptotic effects of vitamin E in mammary cancer cells. Front Biosci 10(1–3):699
165. Takahashi K, Loo G (2004) Disruption of mitochondria during tocotrienol-induced apoptosis in Mda-Mb-231 human breast cancer cells. Biochem Pharmacol 67(2):315–324
166. Tan CY, Saw TY, Fong CW, Ho HK (2015) Comparative hepatoprotective effects of tocotrienol analogs against drug-induced liver injury. Redox Biol 4:308–320
167. Tan DT, Khor HT, Low WH, Ali A, Gapor A (1991) Effect of a palm-oil-vitamin E concentrate on the serum and lipoprotein lipids in humans. Am J Clin Nutr 53(4 Suppl):1027s–1030s
168. Theriault A, Wang Q, Gapor A, Adeli K (1999) Effects of gamma-tocotrienol on apob synthesis, degradation, and secretion in Hepg2 cells. Arterioscler Thromb Vasc Biol 19 (3):704–712
169. Tomeo AC, Geller M, Watkins TR, Gapor A, Bierenbaum ML (1995) Antioxidant effects of tocotrienols in patients with hyperlipidemia and carotid stenosis. Lipids 30(12):1179–1183
170. Valko M, Leibfritz D, Moncol J, Cronin MT, Mazur M, Telser J (2007) Free radicals and antioxidants in normal physiological functions and human disease. Int J Biochem Cell Biol 39(1):44–84

171. Vester H, Holzer N, Neumaier M, Lilianna S, Nussler AK, Seeliger C (2014) Green tea extract (Gte) improves differentiation in human osteoblasts during oxidative stress. J Inflamm (Lond) 11:15
172. Wada S, Satomi Y, Murakoshi M, Noguchi N, Yoshikawa T, Nishino H (2005) Tumor suppressive effects of tocotrienol in vivo and in vitro. Cancer Lett 229(2):181–191
173. Wali VB, Bachawal SV, Sylvester PW (2009) Endoplasmic reticulum stress mediates Γ-tocotrienol-induced apoptosis in mammary tumor cells. Apoptosis 14(11):1366–1377
174. Wali VB, Bachawal SV, Sylvester PW (2009) Suppression in mevalonate synthesis mediates antitumor effects of combined statin and Γ-tocotrienol treatment. Lipids 44(10):925–934
175. Wali VB, Sylvester PW (2007) Synergistic antiproliferative effects of Γ-tocotrienol and statin treatment on mammary tumor cells. Lipids 42(12):1113–1123
176. Wan Nazaimoon WM, Khalid BA (2002) Tocotrienols-rich diet decreases advanced glycosylation end-products in non-diabetic rats and improves glycemic control in streptozotocin-induced diabetic rats. Malays J Pathol 24(2):77–82
177. Wang Y, Jiang Q (2013) Gamma-tocotrienol inhibits lipopolysaccharide-induced interlukin-6 and granulocyte colony-stimulating factor by suppressing C/Ebpbeta and Nf-Kappab in macrophages. J Nutr Biochem 24(6):1146–1152
178. Wang Y, Park NY, Jang Y, Ma A, Jiang Q (2015) Vitamin E gamma-tocotrienol inhibits cytokine-stimulated Nf-kappab activation by induction of anti-inflammatory A20 via stress adaptive response due to modulation of sphingolipids. J Immunol 195(1):126–133
179. Watkins T, Lenz P, Gapor A, Struck M, Tomeo A, Bierenbaum M (1993) Gamma-tocotrienol as a hypocholesterolemic and antioxidant agent in rats fed atherogenic diets. Lipids 28(12):1113–1118
180. Weng-Yew W, Selvaduray KR, Ming CH, Nesaretnam K (2009) Suppression of tumor growth by palm tocotrienols via the attenuation of angiogenesis. Nutr Cancer 61(3):367–373
181. Wu SJ, Liu PL, Ng LT (2008) Tocotrienol-rich fraction of palm oil exhibits anti-inflammatory property by suppressing the expression of inflammatory mediators in human monocytic cells. Mol Nutr Food Res 52(8):921–929
182. Xu WL, Liu JR, Liu HK et al (2009) Inhibition of proliferation and induction of apoptosis by Γ-tocotrienol in human colon carcinoma Ht-29 cells. Nutrition 25(5):555–566
183. Yam ML, Abdul Hafid SR, Cheng HM, Nesaretnam K (2009) Tocotrienols suppress proinflammatory markers and cyclooxygenase-2 expression in Raw264.7 macrophages. Lipids 44(9):787–789
184. Yano Y, Satoh H, Fukumoto K et al (2005) Induction of cytotoxicity in human lung adenocarcinoma cells by 6-*O*-carboxypropyl-A-tocotrienol, a redox-silent derivative of A-tocotrienol. Int J Cancer 115(5):839–846
185. Yap SP, Yuen KH, Wong JW (2001) Pharmacokinetics and bioavailability of alpha-, gamma- and delta-tocotrienols under different food status. J Pharm Pharmacol 53(1):67–71
186. Yoshida Y, Hayakawa M, Habuchi Y, Itoh N, Niki E (2007) Evaluation of lipophilic antioxidant efficacy in vivo by the biomarkers hydroxyoctadecadienoic acid and isoprostane. Lipids 42(5):463–472
187. Yoshida Y, Niki E, Noguchi N (2003) Comparative study on the action of tocopherols and tocotrienols as antioxidant: chemical and physical effects. Chem Phys Lipids 123(1):63–75
188. Yu SG, Thomas AM, Gapor A, Tan B, Qureshi N, Qureshi AA (2006) Dose-response impact of various tocotrienols on serum lipid parameters in 5-week-old female chickens. Lipids 41 (5):453–461
189. Yu W, Simmons-Menchaca M, Gapor A, Sanders BG, Kline K (1999) Induction of apoptosis in human breast cancer cells by tocopherols and tocotrienols. Nutr Cancer 33(1):26–32
190. Zaiden N, Yap WN, Ong S et al (2010) Gamma delta tocotrienols reduce hepatic triglyceride synthesis and Vldl secretion. J Atheroscler Thromb 17(10):1019–1032

Chapter 6
Indole-3-Carbinol and Its Role in Chronic Diseases

Barbara Licznerska and Wanda Baer-Dubowska

Abstract Indole-3-carbinol (I3C), a common phytochemical in cruciferous vegetables, and its condensation product, 3,3'-diindolylmethane (DIM) exert several biological activities on cellular and molecular levels, which contribute to their well-recognized chemoprevention potential. Initially, these compounds were classified as blocking agents that increase drug-metabolizing enzyme activity. Now it is widely accepted that I3C and DIM affect multiple signaling pathways and target molecules controlling cell division, apoptosis, or angiogenesis deregulated in cancer cells. Although most of the current data support the role of I3C and DIM in prevention of hormone-dependent cancers, it seems that their application in prevention of the other cancer as well as cardiovascular disease, obesity, and diabetes reduction is also possible. This chapter summarizes the current experimental data on the I3C and DIM activity and the results of clinical studies indicating their role in prevention of chronic diseases.

Keywords Indole-3-carbinol · DIM · Signaling pathways · Chronic diseases · Animal models · Dietary intervention trials

6.1 Introduction

The plant family *Cruciferae*, particularly members of the genus *Brassica*, like cabbage, broccoli, cauliflower, Brussels sprouts, kale, bok choy are rich sources of sulfur-containing glucosinolates. These secondary products of plant metabolism include, among others, glucobrassicin and neoglucobrassicin. When plant tissue is disrupted, an endogenous thioglucosidase (myrosinase) is activated and converts

B. Licznerska · W. Baer-Dubowska (✉)
Department of Pharmaceutical Biochemistry, Poznan University of Medical Sciences, Poznan, Poland
e-mail: baerw@ump.edu.pl

B. Licznerska
e-mail: barlicz@ump.edu.pl

S.C. Gupta et al. (eds.), *Anti-inflammatory Nutraceuticals and Chronic Diseases*,
Advances in Experimental Medicine and Biology 928,
DOI 10.1007/978-3-319-41334-1_6

glucobrassicin and other indolylic glucosinolates to indoles, principally to indole-3-carbinol (I3C) [120].

Since the first reports on possible anti-carcinogenic activity of I3C [122] numerous preclinical studies have confirmed the chemopreventive properties of this compound by preventing, inhibiting, and reversing the progression of cancer. Moreover, preliminary clinical trials have shown that I3C is a promising agent protecting against hormone-dependent as well as hormone-independent human cancers [47].

Thus, it is not surprising that there are many marked diet supplements containing I3C. Several mechanistic studies have been performed in order to elucidate the mechanism of pleiotropic activity of I3C.

This chapter summarizes the current knowledge on the possible interference of I3C with signaling pathways in vitro and in animal models, as well as its application in prevention of chronic diseases.

6.2 Physicochemical Properties and Pharmacokinetics of Indole-3-Carbinol

Among the indoles, generated upon ingestion of cruciferous vegetables, only I3C (IUPAC: 1H-indol-3-ylmethanol) is commercially available as an off-white solid. Basic physical and chemical properties of I3C are summarized in Table 6.1.

I3C is chemically unstable in acidic conditions, in vitro in cell cultures and in vivo in the stomach environment. In such conditions, I3C may rapidly condense into a series of oligomeric products, of which a dimer, 3,3,-diindolylmethane (DIM), is considered the most bioactive product (Fig. 6.1) [2, 115]. Several pharmacokinetics studies, performed mostly in animal models, have been conducted for I3C and its condensation products [5, 6, 34, 39, 105]. When rainbow trout has been administered with radiolabeled [5-^{3}H]-indole-3-carbinol, 40 % of total radioactivity was found in the liver extracts as DIM [34]. Upon oral administration of 250 mg/kg to mice, the I3C was rapidly absorbed and distributed into variety of tissues and body fluids (e.g., liver, kidney, lung, heart, brain, and plasma) with highest concentrations in liver and kidney, but with rapid clearance (concentrations below the limit of detection within 1 hour after administration). In the same experiment, DIM was detected in plasma at 15 min and was still quantifiable after 6 h with a peak at 2 h after I3C dosing [5, 6]. DIM was also found in stomach tissue and contents,

Table 6.1 Physical and chemical properties of I3C (ALOGPS, www.pubchem.com; accessed Dec 26, 2015)

Stability	Off-white powder
Molecular weight	147.17386 g/mol
Melting range	96–99 °C
Storage temperature	2–8 °C
Stability	2–80 °C, considered stable
Water solubility	3.75 mg/ml, mixes with water

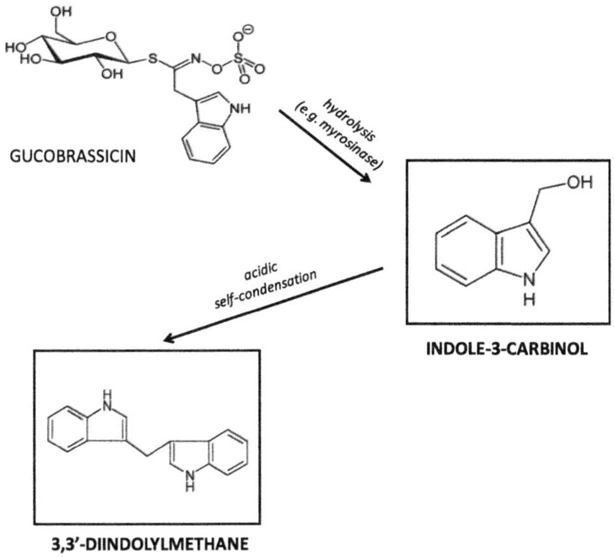

Fig. 6.1 Molecular structure and formation of I3C and DIM

intestines, and liver after 1 h following oral administration of I3C to rats [39]. In human volunteers intervention trial DIM was detected in plasma within 8 h following of 400 mg I3C oral dose [9]. In a phase I clinical trial in women, no I3C was found in the plasma after administration of a single dose of up to 1200 mg or multiple-doses at 400 mg provided twice daily for 4 weeks, and DIM was the only detectable I3C-derived compound in plasma [105]. Fujioka et al. [47] have found that urinary DIM level after uptake of I3C from Brussels sprouts or cabbage is a biomarker of glucobrassicin exposure in humans. All these results support the suggestion that I3C serves as the prodrug rather than the therapeutic agent itself. In this regard, purified I3C as treatment agent used in in vitro models seems to be somewhat contradictory, because there is no certainty that any metabolism of DIM in cells occur. Thus, in this chapter the biological activity and the role in chronic diseases will refer not only to I3C but also to DIM, its major condensation product in humans.

6.3 Modulation of Cell Signaling Pathways by Indole-3-Carbinol

I3C affects multiple signaling pathways and target molecules controlling cell division, apoptosis or angiogenesis deregulated in cancer cells. Figure 6.2 presents the overview of the signaling pathways and possible crosstalks influenced by I3C or DIM. One of the major pathways targeted by I3C is phosphoinositide 3-kinase

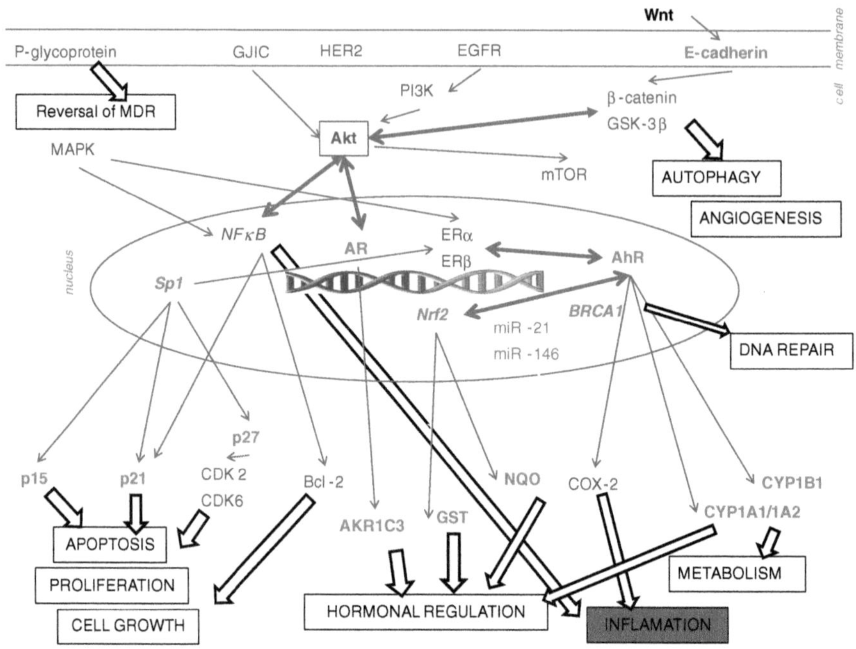

Fig. 6.2 Signaling pathways and proposed crosstalks (↔) affected by I3C/DIM; *red*-inhibition, *green*-induction (AhR-aryl hydrocarbon receptor, AKR-aldo-keto reductase, Akt- protein kinase B, AR-androgen receptor, BRCA-breast cancer tumor suppressor gene, CDK-cyclin-dependent kinase, COX-cyclooxygenase, EGFR-epidermal growth factor receptor, ER-estrogen receptor, GJIC-Gap junctional intracellular communication, GSK-glycogen synthase kinase, GST-glutathione-S-transferases, HER-receptor tyrosine-protein kinase erbB-2, MAPK-mitogen-activated protein kinases, MDR-multidrug resistance, NFκB-nuclear factor kappa-light-chain-enhancer of activated B cells, Nrf2-nuclear transcription factor 2, NQO-NAD (P)H:quinone oxidoreductases, PI3K-phosphoinositide 3-kinase, Sp1-Sp1 transcription factor)

(PI3K)—protein kinase B (Akt)—mammalian target of rapamycin (mTOR) signaling pathway. This pathway is a cascade of events that plays a key role in the broad variety of physiological and pathological processes. PI3K/Akt/mTOR signaling pathway is one of the most frequently affected target in all sporadic human cancers, and it has been estimated that mutations in the individual component of this pathway account for as much as 30 % of all known human cancers [83, 112].

Akt is a serine/threonine protein kinase functioning downstream of PI3K in response to mitogen or growth factor stimulation. The inhibition of phosphorylation and subsequent activation of Akt kinase by I3C or DIM was described in prostate and breast cancer cells. In addition, I3C abrogated epidermal growth factor (EGF)-induced activation of Akt in prostate cancer cells. Furthermore, the known downstream modulators of the Akt/PI3K cell survival pathway, Bcl-x(L), and BAD proteins showed decreased expression after I3C treatment [24, 49]. Several genes that mediate processes involved in carcinogenesis are regulated by transcription factor NF-κB. It plays a central role in general inflammation as well as immune responses, although recent evidences suggest that its role in these processes is more complex [73]. The enhanced activation and expression of NF-κB is linked to development and progression of human cancers as well as in the acquisition of drug-resistant phenotype in highly aggressive malignancies [3, 109].

Activation through Akt is important for many tumorigenic functions of NF-κB. Several studies showed that both indoles inhibited PI3K/Akt/mTOR/NF-κB signaling (reviewed in [4]).

It was also known that there is a crosstalk between Akt and Wnt signaling pathways through the signal communication between glycogen synthase kinase 3 (GSK-3β) and β-catenin, two of the important molecules in Akt and Wnt pathways, respectively [109]. It was found that DIM significantly increased the phosphorylation of β-catenin, and inhibited β-catenin nuclear translocation [77] suggesting that DIM could also downregulate the activation of Wnt signaling.

Mitogen-activated protein kinases (MAPK) are involved in cellular response to a diverse array of stimuli and regulate several cell functions including differentiation, mitosis, cell survival, and apoptosis [100]. Downregulation of the expression of MAP2K3, MAP2K4, MAP4K3, and MAPK3 by I3C and DIM was described suggesting their inhibitory effects on MAPK pathway [76]. It was also reported that the effects of DIM were mediated by crosstalk between protein kinase A and MAPK signaling pathways [75].

Gap junctional intracellular communication (GJIC) also involved in regulating cell proliferation, differentiation and apoptosis is modulated by gap junction channels via broad variety of endogenous and exogenous agents [90]. I3C was reported to prevent H_2O_2-induced inhibition of GJIC by the inactivation of Akt in rat liver epithelial cells [57].

Several studies have focused on the potential effects of I3C and DIM on the proliferation and induction of apoptosis in human prostate or breast cancer cell lines. Cell G_1 cycle arrest of breast cancer cells by I3C was related to inhibition of the expression of cyclin-dependent kinase-6 (CDK6) independently of estrogen receptor signaling [30]. Moreover, the inhibition of CDK6 expression in human MCF7 breast cancer cells was further explained by disrupting Sp1 transcription factor interaction with CDK6 gene promoter [32].

In prostate cancer cell lines, the induction of apoptosis by I3C was p53-independent [94]. The induction of $p21^{WAF1}$ expression by DIM was also independent of p53 status [55]. Pro-apoptotic effect of DIM in HER2/Neu overexpressing breast cancer cells was connected to inhibition of HER2/Neu activity [87]. We have also found a decreased expression of HER2/Neu in estrogen independent MDA-MB-231 breast cancer cells treated with either I3C or DIM (Licznerska et al. unpublished data).

I3C has been known to be a negative regulator of estrogens, while DIM a negative regulator of androgens. I3C inhibited the transcriptional activity of ERα, the estradiol-activated ERα signaling, and the expression of the estrogen-responsive genes [89]. Since I3C and DIM could also inhibit the proliferation of ER-negative breast cancer cells, it is suggested that antitumor activities of indoles could be ER independent. DIM was found to be an antagonist of AR, inhibiting androgen-induced AR translocation to the nucleus [74]. DIM also enhanced expression of aldo-keto reductase 1C3 (AKR1C3), an enzyme responsible for inactivation of 5α-dihydrotestosterone and decreasing estrogen levels in mammary gland and eliminating active androgens from the prostate [92, 101].

Several lines of evidence indicate possible crosstalk between ERα and AhR signaling pathways [96]. It was shown that I3C triggers AhR-dependent ERα protein degradation in MCF7 breast cancer cell line disrupting an ERα-GATA3 transcription factor cross-regulatory loop. This lead to ablation of ERα expression and loss of ERα-responsive proliferation [86].

Our studies showed that both indoles upregulated AhR and downregulated ERα expression in non-tumorigenic MCF10A and tumorigenic MCF7 breast epithelial cells [114]. Upregulation of AhR was also observed in ER-negative MDA-MB-231 cells. This observation is important since increased expression and activation of AhR result in induction of CYPs involved in estrogen metabolism [113].

Both I3C and DIM elicited an inhibition of cell adhesion, migration and invasion in the breast cell lines of different ER status [89]. This appeared to be due, in part, to I3C-induced upregulation of the tumor suppressor gene *BRCA1* and other proteins involved in DNA repair, like RAD51 [105].

Recent studies show that AhR and ERα interact with and modulate the activity of Nrf2 [52]. This transcription factor plays an essential role in cellular protection against electrophiles and oxidative stress by upregulating expression of phase II detoxifying enzymes, including glutathione-S-transferases (GST) and NAD(P)H: quinone oxidoreductases (NQO) [81]. Significant increase of the Nrf2 transcript level in MCF7 and MDA-MB-231 breast cancer cell lines was observed after treatment with I3C. Moreover, increase of Nrf2 expression was correlated with enhanced expression of NQO1 or GSTP in MCF7 cells and MDA-MB-231 cells respectively [114].

Recently, a plethora of evidence has demonstrated that epigenetic alterations, such as DNA methylation, histone modifications, and non-coding miRNAs, consistently contribute to carcinogenesis, and dietary phytochemicals, including glucosinolate derivatives, have the potential to alter a number of these epigenetic events [46, 119].

In this regard, DIM was reported to decrease promoter methylation of Nrf2 in vitro in TRAMP C1 mouse prostate cell line and in vivo in TRAMP mice prostate tumors. This effect was at least in part related to decreased expression and activity of DNA methyltransferases [130]. Moreover, genome-wide promoter methylation in normal and cancer prostate cells showed broad and complex effects on DNA methylation profiles reversing many of the cancer associated methylation alterations, including aberrantly methylated genes that are dysregulated or are highly involved in cancer progression [129].

Histone modifications by DIM were found in several studies. Decreased histone deacetylases (HDACs) protein expression were observed in human colon, breast, and prostate cancer cell lines, human colon cancer xenografts in nude mice and in mouse prostate cells, influencing apoptotic proteins, like p21, p27, and involved in inflammation COX-2 [46].

I3C and DIM were found to downregulate miR-21 and miRNA-146, respectively, in Panc-1 pancreatic cancer cells, which was related to induction of chemosensitivity to gemcitabine in these cells [78, 98]. In another study, I3C reversed the upregulation of miR-21 caused by lung carcinogen—vinyl carbamate in mice [88]. DIM upregulated miR-21 in breast cancer MCF7 cells resulting in reduced proliferation [62], and the let-7 family miRNA leading to inhibition of self-renewal and clonogenic capacity of prostate cancer cells [69, 70].

To sum up, both I3C and its dimer demonstrate pleiotropic effects on cell signaling and subsequently gene expression regulation. Some of these activities are summarized in Table 6.2.

Table 6.2 Summary of the major biological effects of indole-3-carbinol (I3C) and its condensation product—3,3'-diindolylmethane (DIM)

Effect[a]	Target molecules	I3C		DIM	
		In vitro	In vivo	In vitro	In vivo
Induction of phase I enzymes	CYP1A1, CYP1A2, CYP1B1	+	+	+	
Induction of phase II enzymes	GST, NQO	+	+	+	+
Inhibition of DNA adducts formation	CYP1B1		+		
Anti-estrogenic activity	ER, AhR	+	+	+	
Anti-androgenic activity	AR	+		+	
Cell cycle arrest	p21, p27, CDK6	+		+	
Pro-apoptotic	Akt, NFκB, GSK3β, JNK	+		+	
Anti-angiogenic activity	E-cadherin, α-, β-, and γ-catenins, MMP9	+		+	+
Anti-proliferative activity	ERβ/ERα	+	+	+	
DNA repair	BRCA1, RAD51	+	+	+	
Reversal of MDR	P-glycoprotein	+	+		
Epigenetic modifications	DNMTs, HDACs, miRNAs			+	+
Anti-inflammatory activity	NFκB, COX-2	+	+	+	

AhR aryl hydrocarbon receptor, *Akt* protein kinase B, *AR* androgen receptor, *BRCA* breast cancer tumor suppressor gene, *CDK* cyclin-dependent kinase, *DNMT* DNA methyltransferase, ER-estrogen receptor, *GSK* glycogen synthase kinase, *GST* glutathione-S-transferases, *HDAC* histone deacetylases, *JNK* c-Jun N-terminal kinase, *MDR* multidrug resistance, *MMP* matrix metalloproteinase, *NFκB* nuclear factor kappa-light-chain-enhancer of activated B cells, *NQO* NAD(P)H:quinone oxidoreductases

[a]References in the text

6.4 Role of Indole-3-Carbinol in Chronic Diseases

The term “chronic diseases” appear under different names in different contexts. According to WHO this term suggests the following shared features:

- The chronic disease epidemics take decades to become fully established—they have their origins at young age;
- Given their long duration, there are many opportunities for prevention;
- They require a long-term and systematic approach to treatment (WHO Report 2015).

In this context, cardiovascular diseases, chronic respiratory diseases, diabetes along with cancer are mentioned. However, chronic character of cancer is not so obvious as in the case of the other illnesses. The idea of considering cancer as chronic disease emerged recently when it was noted that many cancers, while still very serious could be manageable chronic diseases with ongoing surveillance and/or treatment. While this vision has not yet become a reality for most forms of cancer, the past 10–20 years have brought about a marked acceleration in advance toward this goal. In this regard some types of metastatic breast cancer have become manageable over the long term, perhaps most famously with tamoxifen, which can slow or stop malignant cell growth in many women with estrogen-dependent cancer by blocking hormone receptors on tumor cells. Moreover, a new class of aromatase (*CYP19*) inhibitors that target estrogen production was developed, which seem to provide better results than tamoxifen [127]. I3C can also inhibit the expression of aromatase as well as CYP isoforms involved in estrogen metabolism. Therefore, I3C, as well as its condensation product DIM, appear to be a promising agent for the prevention or recurrence of human tumors, particularly hormone-dependent cancers. There are also data suggesting that I3C or DIM might also be useful for prevention or recurrence of cardiovascular diseases, diabetes, or recurrent respiratory papillomatosis, as well as obesity.

6.4.1 The Role of I3C in Cancer Controlling

It is almost 40 years after Lee Wattenberg and William Loub [122] for the first time reported that I3C inhibited chemically induced breast and forestomach neoplasia in rodents. Since then the antitumor activity of dietary I3C has been widely studied and the inhibition of the development of other cancer types, including liver [95], lung [63], and prostate [110] have been demonstrated.

Breast cancer is the most common and the leading cause of cancer mortality among women worldwide. The preventive efficacy of I3C on mammary carcinoma first observed in animal models, was confirmed in many mechanistic studies in cell cultures and was supported by epidemiological studies with cruciferous vegetables and their extracts or juices [117, 120].

One of the most important risk factor of breast tumors are estrogens, which are classified as carcinogenic in humans [58]. These steroid hormones may contribute to breast cancer development in two ways: (i) acting as promoters by stimulating cell proliferation, (ii) inducing genotoxicity through the reaction of their active metabolites with DNA thus acting as tumor initiators.

Experimental studies in vitro in breast epithelial cell lines showed that I3C, DIM, and cabbage juices induce CYP450 genes *CYP1A1, 1A2, 1B1* encoding the key enzymes of estrogen catabolism. The profile of metabolites was in favor to 2-hydroxyestrogens being noncarcinogenic in comparison to estradiol and 4-hydroxy derivatives [80, 114]. This anti-estrogenic activity of I3C could be explained by the induction of AhR receptor showed in other studies [114].

Moreover, I3C, DIM, and cabbage juices are capable of upregulating phase II detoxifying enzymes, including GST and NQO in breast cancer cell lines [114, 120]. Upregulation of GSTs and NQO1 by I3C was correlated with increased levels of Nrf2, in benign MCF7 and aggressive MDA-MB-231 breast cancer cell lines. Thus, it may be assumed that I3C protects against estrogen-associated carcinogenesis by removal of the genotoxic metabolites of estrogens.

Simultaneously, I3C and DIM influenced in situ production of estrogens in breast epithelial MCF7 cancer cells by reducing the expression of aromatase (*CYP19*), the enzyme that synthesizes estrogens by converting C19 androgens into aromatic C18 estrogenic steroids [80]. Several studies have shown that there is an overexpression of aromatase gene in breast cancer tissue [82]. Interestingly, the potential of I3C to reduce estrogenic activity in the breast cancer cells was confirmed by other mechanisms, particularly via decreasing the AKR1C3 expression mentioned in the previous section. In the mammary gland where enzyme converts androstenedione to testosterone—one of the aromatase substrates [92, 101].

Besides the interference with estrogens metabolism pathways, I3C also affects DNA repair, the cell cycle progression and apoptosis in breast cancer cell lines. In this regard it was shown that I3C induces BRCA1 expression and that both I3C and BRCA1 inhibited estrogen (E2)-stimulated ERα activity in human breast cancer cells [44]. BRCA1 is DNA repair factor involved in repair of DNA double-strand breaks. *BRCA1*gene expression is reduced or completely silenced in a significant proportion of sporadic breast cancer because of hypermethylation of the gene promoter [106, 126]. Thus, I3C-induced BRCA1 expression and inhibition of estrogen-stimulated ERα activity by I3C and BRCA1 showed by some studies could be one of the antitumor activity of the indole [44].

Several lines of evidence suggest I3C ability to arrest cell cycle in breast cancer cells. In this regard I3C was reported to inhibit CDK2 activity in breast cancer MCF7 cell line [48]. Moreover, both I3C and DIM upregulated CDK inhibitors p21 and p27, although in a very high concentration of 200 μM. Activity of this protein is especially critical during the G_1 to S phase transition. Consequently, the ability to arrest G_1 phase by I3C was shown [30]. Other studies suggest the p53 phosphorylation by I3C leading to release p53 and inducing the p21 CDK inhibition and G_1 cell cycle arrest [18, 86]. Importantly, treatment with I3C and tamoxifen ablated expression of the phosphorylated retinoblastoma protein (Rb), an endogenous substrate for the G_1 CDKs, whereas either agent alone only partially inhibited endogenous Rb phosphorylation [31]. Several studies showed that I3C and its derivatives are potent inducers of apoptosis in both ER-positive and ER-negative breast cancer cells[30–32, 50, 80, 103]. Estrogens, particularly estradiol have been also implicated as a cofactors in human papillomavirus (HPV)-mediated cervical cancer, both in animal models and in women using oral contraceptives [72]. Interestingly, it was found that estradiol protects cervical cancer cells treated with DNA-damaging agents such as UVB, mitomycin-C, and cisplatin, from apoptotic death. I3C was able to overcome the anti-apoptotic effect of estradiol but only in higher concentrations. Treatment with I3C resulted in loss of the survival protein Bcl-2. However, the amount of apoptosis versus survival and the level of Bcl-2 depended on the I3C/estradiol ratio [22]. In HPV16-transgenic mice, which develop cervical cancer after chronic estradiol exposure, apoptotic cells were detected in cervical epitheliumonly in mice exposed to estradiol and fed on I3C [20].

Experiments in which cervical cancer HeLa and SiHa cell lines were used, demonstrated that DIM also exerts antitumor effects on these cells through its anti-proliferative and pro-apoptotic roles, especially for SiHa cells. The molecular mechanism for these effects may be related to its regulatory effects on MAPK and PI3K pathway and apoptosis proteins. Thus, DIM may be considered a preventive and therapeutic agent against cervical cancer [135]. The ability of inhibiting spontaneous occurrence of endometrial adenocarcinoma and preneoplastic lesions by I3C was also demonstrated in female Donryu rats. It was suggested that this effect was due to induction by I3C estradiol 2-hydroxylation [68]. On the other hand, promotion of endometrial adenocarcinoma in same strains of rats initiated with N-ethyl-N'-nitro-N-nitrosoguanidine by I3C was described [133]. DIM was also found to have a potent cytostatic effect in cultured human Ishikawa endometrial cancer cells. This effect was related to the stimulation of TGF-α expression and activation of TGF-α signal transduction pathway [75].

Another hormone-dependent cancer, which might be affected by I3C, is prostate cancer, one the most prevalent malignancy in men worldwide and the second leading cause of male death in Western countries [16]. Androgens play a critical role in prostate cancer cells growth and survival. Androgens bind to the androgen receptor (AR), a steroid nuclear receptor, which is translocated into the nucleus and binds to AREs in the promoter regions of target genes to induce cell proliferation and apoptosis. Approximately 80–90 % of prostate cancers are dependent on androgen at initial diagnosis, and endocrine therapy of prostate cancer is directed toward the reduction of plasma androgens and inhibition of AR [37, 54]. It was demonstrated that both I3C and DIM are able to downregulate AR signaling [74], but only DIM was shown to be a strong antagonist of AR and inhibitor of its translocation to the nucleus [30, 74].

Similarly as in the case of breast cancer cells, I3C and its derivatives also affect cell cycle progression and induce apoptosis. In this regard, cell cycle arrest at G_1 checkpoint in different human prostate carcinoma cell lines by I3C and DIM was described [2]. In LNCaP prostate cancer cells I3C selectively inhibited the expression of CDK6 protein and transcripts and stimulated the production of the p16 CDK inhibitor. In vitro protein kinase assays revealed inhibition by I3C CDK2 enzymatic activity and the relatively minor downregulation of CDK4 enzymatic activity [134].

In PC-3 cell line induction of G_1 cell cycle arrest by I3C due to the upregulation of p21(WAF1) and p27(Kip1) CDK inhibitors, followed by their association with cyclin D1 and E and downregulation of CDK6 protein kinase levels and activity was suggested. In addition, I3C inhibited the hyperphosphorylation of the retinoblastoma (Rb) protein in PC-3 cells. Induction of apoptosis was also observed in this cell line when treated with I3C. Thus, it was suggested that I3C inhibits the growth of PC-3 prostate cancer cells by inducing G_1 cell cycle arrest leading to apoptosis, and regulates thc expression of apoptosis-related genes [23]. Further studies showed that I3C-induced apoptosis is partly mediated by the inhibition of Akt activation, resulting in the alterations in the downstream regulatory molecules of Akt activation in PC-3 cells [24]. In the case of DIM an inhibition of a crosstalk between Akt and NF-κB [12], leading to cell cycle arrest and induction of apoptosis was also described. DIM significantly decreased cellular histone deacetylase HDAC2 protein level in androgen sensitive LNCaP and androgen insensitive PC-3 cell lines [10]. In all these studies a formulated DIM (BR-DIM) with higher bioavailability was used and was able to induce apoptosis and inhibit cell growth, angiogenesis, and invasion of prostate cancer cells [21].

The potential protective activity of I3C and DIM against prostate cancer was confirmed by microarray analysis, which showed the modulation of the expression of many genes related to the control of carcinogenesis and cell survival as effect of indoles treatment of PC-3 cells [76]. It was also demonstrated by several groups that I3C and DIM may improve the therapeutic effect of conventional chemotherapy of prostate cancer [44, 71].

Besides the hormone-dependent cancers, both indoles can affect the development of some other cancers. In this regard, it was shown that I3C and DIM induced apoptosis in colorectal cancer cell lines [13, 67, 84]. Interestingly, an effective inhibition of Akt and inactivation of mTOR was observed as a result of combined treatment with I3C and genisteinin HT29 colon cancer cells, leading to induction of apoptosis and autophagy [93].

Anti-carcinogenic activity of I3C was demonstrated in carcinogen-induced lung cancer in mice [63, 64]. Anti-proliferative effects of I3C and DIM in human bronchial epithelial cells (HBEC) and A549 adenocarcinomic human alveolar basal epithelial cells related to marked reductions in the activation of Akt, extracellular signal-regulated kinase and NF-κB were also described [65].

Moreover, upregulation of several miRNAs induced by chemical carcinogen was reversed by I3C in mice and rats lung tumors [46, 59].

The signal transducer and activator of transcription 3 (STAT3) is a latent transcription factor required in proliferation and differentiation. The constitutive activation of STAT3 in human pancreatic carcinoma specimens but not in normal tissues was shown. Activation of STAT3 was also found in pancreatic tumor cell lines and was inhibited by I3C although in relatively high concentration (10 μM) along with induction of apoptosis [79]. Apoptosis in pancreatic cancer cells was also induced by DIM as a result of endoplasmic reticulum stress-dependent upregulation of death receptor 5 [1]. More recent studies showed downregulation of miRNA-21 and miRNA-221 as a result of I3C or DIM treatment of pancreatic cancer cells. As upregulation of these miRNAs is characteristic for more aggressive pancreas cancer, it was suggested that combination of I3C or DIM with conventional chemotherapeutics may increase the chemosensitivity to certain drugs in resistant pancreatic cancer cells [98, 111].

There are also reports showing the anti-proliferative effect, G1 cell cycle and induction of apoptosis in thyroid cancer cells by I3C and DIM [116]. However, earlier reports indicated the enhancement of thyroid gland neoplastic development by I3C in rat medium-term multi-organ carcinogenesis model [66]. UVB-induced mouse skin tumors were reduced in mice fed on I3C [29].

Importantly it was also shown that I3C may overcome multiple drug resistance by downregulation of MDR1-expression in murine melanoma cells and leukemia cells [7, 8, 28].

These observations further support the possible application of I3C or DIM as potential adjuvant therapeutics in conventional chemotherapy of several cancers.

Finally, it must be pointed out that although I3C was shown to have anti-carcinogenic activity in various animal models, at the same time animals studies have also shown a tumor-promoting activity, when animals were exposed to I3C after exposure to carcinogens [131, 133]. This aspect has to be clarified in long-term studies.

6.4.2 Cardiovascular Diseases

Cardiovascular diseases still remain the primary cause of death worldwide. One of the proposed approaches to reduce the high global incidence is the consumption of vegetables and fruits containing biologically active components or phytochemical supplements. Although the most attention was paid to resveratrol, components of cruciferous vegetables, particularly *Brassica oleracea*, were also considered a potential dietary phytochemicals reducing risk of CVDs [97].

In this regard hypocholesterolemic properties of I3C were reported in mice provided with cholesterol-supplemented diet to which I3C were added. Since in vitro experiments revealed that I3C and its condensation products effectively inhibited the enzyme acyl-CoA:cholesterol acyltransferase (ACAT), which is responsible for the conversion of free cholesterol to the cholesteryl ester, the hypocholesterolemic effect of I3C in mice was likely mediated by the inhibition of ACAT [42]. Such mechanism was further confirmed in HepG2 cells. As a result of treatment with I3C the decreased cholesteryl ester synthesis was associated with significantly decreased ACAT gene expression and activity [85].

Moreover, antiplatelet and antithrombotic activity of I3C was shown in in vitro and in vivo studies. I3C significantly inhibited collagen-induced platelet aggregation in human platelet-rich plasma and suppressed the death of mice with pulmonary thrombosis induced by intravenous injection of collagen and epinephrine [99].

The protective activity of I3C in heart failure and vascular proliferative disease was also reported. In this regard, it was shown that I3C can suppress the proliferation of cultured vascular smooth muscle cells and neointima formation in a carotid injury model via the Akt/GSK3β pathway [51]. Vascular smooth muscle cells are the principal cell types involved in the pathogenesis of atheriosclerosis and restenosis after percutaneous coronary intervention [43]. Thus, it was suggested that I3C may be a part of new therapeutic strategy for vascular proliferative diseases as well as heart failure. The latter suggestion was supported by the results of the studies using aortic banding (AB) mouse model, which showed that I3C prevented and reversed cardiac remodeling induced by AB. This effect was mediated by AMPK-α and extracelular signal-regulated kinases 1/2 (ERK1/2) [36]. Since AMPK acts as important energy sensor, attenuation of cardiac remodeling in mice was associated with improved myocardial energy metabolism [36].

6.4.3 Obesity and Diabetes

Chronic inflammatory disease initiated in adipose tissue might lead to obesity-related insulin resistance and may contribute to an increased risk of diabetes [132]. It might be assumed that anti-inflammatory phytochemicals may protect against both diseases. Thus, I3C was also proposed as a potential preventive agent against obesity and metabolic disorders. In this regard, I3C treatment in diet-induced obesity (DIO) mice model decreased body weight and fat accumulation and infiltrated macrophages in epididymal adipose tissue. These effects were associated with improved glucose tolerance and with modulated expression of adipokines and lipogenic-associated gene products, including acetyl coenzyme A carboxylase and peroxisome proliferator-activated receptor-γ (PPARγ) [19]. The reduced level of inflammatory biomarkers was also confirmed in co-culture of adipocytes with macrophages treated with I3C [19].

I3C was also capable to normalize tissue expression of genes related to thermogenesis upregulated by high-fat diet, namely uncoupling proteins 1 and 3, PPARα, PPARγ coactivator 1α [26]. The observed improvement of adipogenesis by I3C could be due to activation of sirtuine SIRT1 [27]. These findings suggest that I3C has a potential benefit in preventing obesity and metabolic disorders, and the action for I3C in vivo may involve multiple mechanisms including decreased adipogenesis and inflammation, along with activated thermogenesis.

Little is known about the possible modulation of different types of diabetes by I3C. Nevertheless, in recent studies with the genetically modified mice (C57BL/6J mice) that closely simulated the metabolic abnormalities of the human disease after the administration of high-fat diet, both I3C and DIM showed a positive modulation of glucose, insulin, hemoglobin and glycated hemoglobin levels. In the same time a decreased levels of different mediators of oxidative stress were noticed, including thiobarbituric acid reactive substances (TBARS), lipid hydroperoxides (LOOH) and conjugated dienes. Simultaneously, in this diabetic mouse model increased levels of antioxidant enzymes and small molecules (SOD, CAT, GPx, vitamin C, vitamin E, GSH) were demonstrated. Interestingly, the antioxidant action was comparable to that of metformin, a standard drug in diabetes 2 treatment [60].

6.5 Biological Activities of Indole-3-Carbinol in Animal Models

Animal models played a crucial role in discovering the cancer chemopreventive activity of cruciferous plants. Initially rodent chemical carcinogenesis models were used to assess anti-carcinogenic activity of minor dietary components, including I3C. Currently genetically modified animals, mentioned in the previous sections, allow to assess detailed mechanisms of their biological activity.

In the very first experiments of Wattenberg and his co-workers, benzo[a]pyrene induced model of lung and forestomach cancer in mice and dimethylbenz[a]anthracene induced breast neoplasia in rats were used. In these models I3C when given prior to carcinogen inhibited the formation of tumors [122]. This effect was linked to modulation of phase I enzymatic systems, namely cytochrome P450 dependent monooxygenases, involved in carcinogens activation [123, 124]. Later, several studies using animals carcinogenesis model of liver, colon, and tongue confirmed the anti-initiating activity of I3C. However, these studies have also provided evidence for promotional activity of I3C. For example, whereas I3C pretreatment and co-treatment with liver carcinogen aflatoxin B_1 (AFB_1) strongly inhibited AFB_1 initiated hepatocarcinogenesis, posttreatment with I3C was strongly promotional [35].

The modulation of cytochromes P450 is also linked with potential protection against breast cancer. On the other hand, the same mechanism is probably responsible for uterine-induced cancer via upregulation of CYP1B1 and increased precancerous 4-hydroxyestrogen concentration [133]. The increase of carcinogenic 4-hydroxyestrogen following oral administration of I3C were documented also by the other studies [56]; reviewed in [15]. These observations led to conclusion that DIM showing higher bioavailability and reducing 4-hydroxyestrogen production should be recommended as an alternative to I3C in potential chemopreventive supplementation [15]. More recent studies have confirmed this suggestion that DIM was more effective in prevention prostate cancer in the transgenic adenocarcinoma mouse prostate (TRAMP) mice model then I3C [25].

Nevertheless, the more recent studies using "traditional" mouse models or transgenic animals documented that I3C has been responsible for a decrease of incidences of carcinogen-induced lung cancer [64, 88, 102], cervical cancer in HPV gene transgenic mice [61], and UV-induced skin cancer [29].

Moreover, it was shown that in rats bearing the 13762 mammary carcinoma, addition of I3C to the diet for 6 days prior to antitumor drug ET-743 (trabectidin) administration almost completely abolished manifestations of hepatotoxicity [41]. These observation further supports the concept that I3C or DIM protecting against specific cancer may be used in adjuvant therapy to overcome side-effects of conventional therapy.

Specific rodent models like mouse carotid artery injury were developed and used to assess I3C or DIM protection against cardiovascular diseases, obesity, or diabetes. As it was described in previous section, generally the results of these studies suggest that I3C has a potential benefit in preventing obesity and metabolic disorders, and the action of I3C in vivo may involve multiple mechanisms including decreased adipogenesis and inflammation, along with activated thermogenesis.

6.6 Biological Activities of Indole-3-Carbinol in Humans

Promising results of the most studies obtained in human cancer cell lines and in animal models prompted the clinical trials dietary intervention studies to evaluate the effect of I3C or DIM in risk group of patients or/and volunteers. A major focus of these trials has been on modulation of hormones metabolism. The urinary estrogen metabolite ratio of 2-hydroxyesterone to 16α-hydroxyestrone was used in most of the trials as the surrogate endpoint biomarker.

The validity of this endpoint biomarker was confirmed in the early randomized clinical trials [14] in which 20 healthy subjects received 400 mg/day of I3C for 3 months. In most of the enrolled subjects I3C increased the 2-hydroxyestrone to estriol (a precursor of 16α-hydroxyestrone) ratio in sustained manner without detectible side-effects, although some individuals were resistant to such change. In another trial women at increased risk for breast cancer were administered with different doses (range 50–400 mg/day) of I3C for 4 weeks. The results of this study suggested that the minimum effective dose schedule of 300 mg/day is optimal for breast cancer prevention, although should be confirmed by long-term breast cancer prevention trial [128].

In subsequent studies by Bradlow group [91] urine samples were collected from healthy subjects before and after oral ingestion of 6–7 mg/kg per day for 1 week (7 men) or 2 months (10 women). Analysis of 13 estrogen profiles supported the hypothesis that I3C induces estrogen 2-hydroxylation resulting in decreased concentrations of metabolites known to activate the estrogen receptor and suggested that I3C may have chemopreventive activity against breast cancer in humans. Later, phase I trial with women with a high-risk breast cancer were enrolled, subjects ingested 400 mg I3C daily for 4 weeks followed by a 4 week period of 800 mg I3C daily [105]. The maximal ratio increase of the urinary 2-hydroxyestrone to 16α-hydroxyestrone was observed with the 400 mg daily dose of I3C, with no further increase found at 800 mg daily. Beside confirmation of the optimal dose of

I3C, these studies showed the induction of CYP1A2 which was mirrored by increase of 2-hydroxyestrone to 16α-hydroxyestrone ratio, and GST.

Cumulative evidence on conversion of I3C to DIM in cell culture, peritoneal and oral use as well as substantial direct activity seen with DIM led to conclusion that there is no longer the case for considering I3C to be directly active, and rather DIM should be considered as a chemopreventive compound of choice [15]. A pilot study on the effect of BR-DIM on urinary hormone metabolites in postmenopausal women with a history of early-stage breast cancer showed a significant increase in levels of 2-hydroxyestrone as result of treatment with only 108 mg DIM/day for 30 days, however, nonsignificant increase (1.46–2.14) of 2-hydroxyestrone to 16α - hydroxyestrone was noted [33]. In another study cohorts of 3–6 patients castrate-resistant, non-metastatic prostate cancer received escalating oral doses twice daily of BR-DIM 75 mg, then 150, 225, and 300 mg. Based on the results of this trial 225 mg BR-DIM dose twice daily was recommended for phase II trial. However, modest efficacy of DIM was demonstrated [53].

Cervical intraepithelial neoplasia (CIN) is a precancerous lesion of cervix. When patients with biopsy proven CIN grade II or III were treated orally with 200, or 400 mg/day of I3C for 12 weeks 50 % of them had complete regression based on their 12-week biopsy. Moreover, 2-hydroxyestrone to 16α-hydroxyestrone ratio have changed in a dose-dependent manner [11]. The significant improvement in confirmed CIN I or II grade was also observed as a result of oral treatment with 2 mg/kg/day of DIM for 12 weeks. Moreover, at median follow-up of 6 months there was no statistically significant difference in any of the measured outcome between the DIM and placebo group [40].

Since the incidence of thyroid cancer is 4–5 times higher in women than in men, estrogens were suggested to contribute the pathogenesis of thyroid proliferative disease (TPD). In limited (7 patients) phase I clinical trial patients with TPD were administered with 300 mg of DIM per day for 14 days. DIM was detectable in thyroid tissue, and the ratio of 2-hydroxyestrone to 16α-hydroxyestrone was increased. These results suggested that DIM can manifest the anti-estrogenic activity in situ to modulate TPD [104].

Although major focus of cancer prevention clinical trials of I3C or DIM has been concentrated on chemoprevention of hormone-dependent cancers, there were also clinical trials performed in order to evaluate indoles effect on pulmonary cancers. In this regard in phase I clinical trial patients with recurrent respiratory papillomatosis (RRP) were treated orally with I3C and had minimum follow-up of 8 months. Thirty-three percent of the study patients had a cession of their papilloma growth and had not required surgery since the start of the study [107]. Subsequent long-term clinical trial performed by the same research group confirmed the preliminary observation indicating that I3C may be a treatment option for RRP [108]. The case of successful use of intralesional and intravenous cidofovir in association with I3C in 8-year-old girl with pulmonary papillomatosis was also reported [38].

As it was mentioned in the previous sections of this chapter, recently a large amount of evidence has demonstrated that epigenetic alterations, such as DNA methylation, histone modifications, and non-coding miRNAs consistently contribute to carcinogenesis, and constituents in the diet, including dietary glucosinolate derivatives, have the potential to alter a number of these epigenetic events [46]. Different studies on cancer also have shown that miRNAs interact with genes in many different cellular pathways, displaying a differential gene expression profile between normal and tumor tissues and between tumor types [17]. Interestingly, interventions including BR-DIM in prostate cancer patients prior to radical prostatectomy showed re-expression of miR-34a, which was consistent with decreased expression of androgen receptor, prostate specific antigen (PSA), and Notch-1 in tissue specimens [70]. These results suggest that BR-DIM could be useful for the inactivation of androgen receptor, critically important during the development and progression of prostate cancer and thus its treatment.

Thus far, seven clinical studies have been registered using I3C and twelve using DIM (www.clinicaltrials.gov; accessed Dec 26, 2015). Four studies registered for I3C treatment have been completed for patients with prostate and breast cancers and one dietary intervention for healthy participants targeting unspecified adult solid tumors. One trial aiming at I3C effects on estrogen metabolism in obese volunteers had to be terminated because of slow accrual in the high BMI group. Among twelve studies registered for DIM, six have been completed for patients with prostate, breast, and cervical cancers as well as healthy volunteers. Trial aiming at new therapy of laryngeal papilloma in children was terminated because of lack of sufficient enrollment. Although the results of these trials have not been published yet, they assure the further extensive prospective studies on chemopreventive and/or chemotherapeutic potential of I3C and its condensation product.

6.7 Summary and Conclusions

It is well known that in populations which consume higher amounts of cruciferous vegetables lower incidence rate of cancer occurs or improved biochemical parameters, such as decreased oxidative stress are noticed [46, 117, 118, 121]. These effects are in part due to the biological activity of I3C and its condensation products, particularly DIM.

A wide range of cellular pathways are regulated by both indoles. Thus, many additional targets for indoles could be identified in the future using in vitro cell cultures and in vivo transgenic animal models and explain a unique anti-inflammatory and endocrine modulating activity of I3C. Although most of current data support the role of I3C and DIM in prevention of hormone-dependent cancers, it seems that their application in prevention of the other cancer as well as cardiovascular diseases, obesity, and diabetes reduction is also possible.

Experimental in vitro and in vivo studies and clinical trials performed so far, showed that I3C is a rather safe dietary supplement. However, since the long-term effects of I3C supplementation in humans are still not clear and due to some contradictory effects of I3C in animal models, the general use of I3C and DIM supplements should be restricted until potential risks and benefits are better characterized. Taking into consideration higher activity of DIM, particularly in BR form, in comparison with I3C in term of potency and time required to obtain the effect, this I3C dimer might be a better alternative as chemopreventive supplement. Important aspect of possible clinical application of both indoles is their drug and radio-sensitization. Emerging new technologies allowing deeper inside in the mechanism of these glucosinolate derivatives activity should help to better explore this aspect.

References

1. Abdelrahim M, Ewman K, Vanderlaag K et al (2006) 3,3'-diindolylmethane (DIM) and its derivatives induce apoptosis in pancreatic cancer cells through endoplasmic reticulum stress-dependent upregulation of DR5. Carcinogenesis 27:717–728
2. Aggarwal BB, Ichikawa H (2005) Molecular targets and anticancer potential of indole-3-carbinol and its derivatives. Cell Cycle 4:1201–1215
3. Ahmad A, Sarkar WA, Rahman KMW (2011) Role of nuclear factor-kappa B signaling in anticancer properties of indole compounds. J Exp Clin Med 3:55–62
4. Ahmad A, Biersack B, Li Y et al (2013) Targeted regulation of PI3 K/Akt/mTOR/NF-κB signaling by indole compounds and their derivatives: mechanistic details and biological implications for cancer therapy. Anticancer Agents Med Chem 13:1002–1013
5. Anderto MJ, Manson MM, Verschoyle RD et al (2004) Pharmacokinetics and tissue disposition of indole-3-carbinol and its acid condensation products after oral administration to mice. Clin Cancer Res 10:5233–5241
6. Anderton MJ, Manson MM, Verschoyle R et al (2004) Physiological modeling of formulated and crystalline 3,3'-diindolylmethane pharmacokinetics following oral administration in mice. Drug Metab Dispos 32:632–638
7. Arora A, Seth K, Kalra N, Shukla Y (2005) Modulation of P-glycoprotein-mediated multidrug resistance in K562 leukemic cells by indole-3-carbinol. Toxicol Appl Pharmacol 202:237–243
8. Arora A, Shukla Y (2003) Modulation of vinca-alkaloid induced P-glycoprotein expression by indole-3-carbinol. Cancer Lett 189:167–173
9. Arneson DW, Hurwitz A, McMahon LM et al (1999) Presence of 3.3'-diindolylmethane in human plasma after oraladministration of indole-3-carbinol. Proc Am Assoc Cancer Res 40:429
10. Beaver LM, Yu TW, Sokolowski EI et al (2012) 3,3'-Diindolylmethane, but notindole-3-carbinol, inhibits histone deacetylase activity in prostate cancer cells. Toxicol Appl Pharmacol 263:345–351
11. Bell MC, Crowley-Nowick P, Bradlow HL et al (2000) Placebo-controlled trial of indole-3-carbinol in the treatment of CIN. Gynecol Oncol 78:123–129
12. Bhuiyan MM, Li Y, Banerjee S et al (2006) Down-regulation of androgen receptor by 3,3′-diindolylmethane contributes to inhibition of cell proliferation and induction of apoptosis in both hormone-sensitive LNCaP and insensitive C4-2B prostate cancer cells. Cancer Res 66:10064–10072
13. Bonnesen C, Eggleston IM, Hayes JD (2001) Dietary indoles and isothiocyanates that are generated from cruciferous vegetables can both stimulate apoptosis and confer protection against DNA damage in human colon cell lines. Cancer Res 61:6120–6130
14. Bradlow HL, Michnovicz JJ, Halper M et al (1994) Long-term responses of women to indole-3-carbinol or a high fiber diet. Cancer Epidemiol Biomarkers Prev 3:591–595

15. Bradlow HL (2008) Review. Indole-3-carbinol as a chemoprotective agent in breast and prostate cancer. In Vivo 22:441–445
16. Bray F, Ren JS, Masuyer E et al (2013) Global estimates of cancer prevalence for 27 sites in the adult population in2008. Int J Cancer 132:1133–1145
17. Brait M, Sidransky D (2011) Cancer epigenetics: above and beyond. Toxicol Mech Methods 21:275–288
18. Brew CT, Aronchik I, Hsu JC et al (2006) Indole-3-carbinol activates the ATM signaling pathway independent of DNA damage to stabilize p53 and induce G1 arrest of human mammary epithelial cells. Int J Cancer 118:857–868
19. Chang HP, Wang ML, Hsu CY et al (2011) Supression of inflammation-associated factors by indole-3-carbinol in mice fed high-fat diets and in isolated, co-cultured macrophages and adipocytes. Int J Obes 35:1530–1538
20. Chen DZ, Qi M, Auborn KJ et al (2001) Indole-3-carbinol and diindolylmethane induce apoptosis of human cervical cancer cells and in murine HPV16-transgenic preneoplasticcervical epithelium. J Nutr 131:3294–3302
21. Chen D, Banerjee S, Cui QC et al (2012) Activation of AMP-activated protein kinase by 3,3'-Diindolylmethane (DIM) is associated with human prostate cancer cell death in vitro and in vivo. PLoS ONE 7:e47186
22. Chen D, Carter TH, Auborn KJ (2004) Apoptosis in cervical cancer cells: implications for adjunct anti-estrogen therapy for cervical cancer. Anticancer Res 24:2649–2656
23. Chinni SR, Li Y, Upadhyay S et al (2001) Indole-3-carbinol (I3C) induced cell growth inhibition, G1 cell cycle arrest and apoptosis in prostate cancer cells. Oncogene 20:2927–2936
24. Chinni SR, Sarkar FH (2002) Akt inactivation is a key event in indole-3-carbinolinduced apoptosis in PC-3 cells. Clin Cancer Res 8:1228–1236
25. Cho HJ, Park SY, Kim EJ et al (2011) 3,3′- diindolylmethane inhibits prostate cancer development in the transgenic adenocarcinoma mouse prostate model. Mol Carcinog 50:100–112
26. Choi Y, Kim Y, Park S et al (2012) Indole-3-carbinolprevents diet-induced obesity through modulation of multiple genes related to adipogenesis, thermogenesis or inflammation in the visceral adipose tissue of mice. J Nutr Biochem 23:1732–1739
27. Choi Y, Um SJ, Park T (2013) Indole-3-carbinol directly targets SIRT1 to inhibit adipocyte differentiation. Int J Obes (Lond) 37:881–884
28. Christensen JG, LeBlanc GA (1996) Reversal of multidrug resistance in vivo by dietary administration of the phytochemical indole-3-carbinol. Cancer Res 56:574–581
29. Cope RB, Loehr C, Dashwood R et al (2006) Ultraviolet radiation-induced non-melanoma skin cancer in the Crl:SKH1:hr-BR hairless mouse: augmentation of tumor multiplicity by chlorophyllin and protection by indole-3-carbinol. Photochem Photobiol Sci 5(5):499–507
30. Cover MC, Hsieh SJ, Tran SH et al (1998) Indole-3-carbinol inhibits the expression of cyclin-dependent kinase-6 and induces a G1 cell cycle arrest of human breast cancer cells independent of estrogen receptor signaling. J Biol Chem 273:3838–3847
31. Cover CM, Hsieh SJ, Cram EJ et al (1999) Indole-3-carbinol and tamoxifen cooperate to arrest the cell cycle of MCF-7 human breast cancer cells. Cancer Res 59:1244–1251
32. Cram EJ, Liu BD, Bjeldanes LF et al (2001) Indole-3-carbinol inhibits CDK6 expression in human MCF-7 breast cancer cells by disrupting Sp1 transcription factor interactions with a composite element in the CDK6 gene promoter. J Biol Chem 276:22332–22340
33. Dalessandri KM, Firestone GL, Fitch MD et al (2004) Pilot study: effect of 3, 3′-diindolylmethane supplements on urinary hormone metabolites in postmenopausal women with a history of early-stage breast cancer. Nutr Cancer 50:161–167
34. Dashwood RH, Fong AT, Arbogast DN et al (1994) Anticarcinogenic activity of indole-3-carbinol acid products: ultrasensitive bioassay by trout embryo microinjection. Cancer Res 54:3617–3619
35. Dashwood RH (1998) Indole-3-carbinol: anticarcinogen or tumor promoter in brassica vegetables? Chem Biol Interact 110:1–5

36. Deng W, Zong J, Bian Z et al (2013) Indole-3-carbinolprotects against pressure overload induced cardiac remodeling via activating AMPK-α. Mol Nutr Food Res 57:1680–1687
37. Denis LJ, Griffiths K (2000) Endocrine treatment in prostate cancer. Semin Surg Oncol 18:52–74
38. de Bilderling G, Bodart E, Lawson G et al (2005) Successful use of intralesional and intravenous Cidofovir in association withindole-3-carbinol in an 8-year-old girl with pulmonary papillomatosis. J Med Virol 75:332–335
39. De Kruif CA, Marsman JW, Venekamp JC et al (1991) Structure elucidation of acid reaction products of indole-3-carbinol: detection in vivo and enzyme induction in vitro. Chem Biol Interact 80:303–315
40. Del Priore G, Gudipudi DK, Montemarano N et al (2010) Oral diindolylmethane (DIM): pilot evaluation of a nonsurgical treatment for cervicaldysplasia. Gynecol Oncol 116:464–467
41. Donald S, Verschoyle RD, Greaves P et al (2004) Dietary agent indole-3-carbinol protects female rats against the hepatotoxicity of the antitumor drug ET-743 (trabectidin) without compromising efficacy in a rat mammary carcinoma. Int J Cancer 111:961–967
42. Dunn SE, LeBlanc GA (1994) Hypocholesterolemic properties of plant indoles. Inhibition of acyl-CoA:cholesterol acyltransferase activity and reduction of serum LDL/VLDL cholesterol levels by glucobrassicin derivatives. BiochemPharmacol 47:359–364
43. Dzau VJ, Braun-Dullaeus RC, Sedding DG (2002) Vascular proliferation and atherosclerosis: new perspectives and therapeutic strategies. Nat Med 8:1249–1256
44. Fan S, Meng Q, Auborn K et al (2006) BRCA1 and BRCA2 as molecular targets for phytochemicals indole-3-carbinol and genistein in breast and prostate cancer cells. Br J Cancer 94:407–426
45. Fares F (2014) The anti-carcinogenic effect of indole-3-carbinol and 3,3'-diindolylmethane and mechanism of action. Med Chem. doi:10.4172/2161-0444.S1-002
46. Fuentes F, Paredes-Gonzalez X, Kong AT (2015) Dietary glucosinolates sulforaphane, phenethyl isothiocyanate, indole-3-carbinol/3,3'-diindolylmethane: anti-oxidative stress/inflammation, nrf2, epigenetics/epigenomics and in vivo cancer chemopreventive efficacy. Curr Pharmacol Rep 1:179–196
47. Fujioka N, Ainslie-Waldman CE, Upadhyaya P et al (2014) Urinary 3,3′-diindolylmethane: a biomarker of glucobrassicin exposure and indole-3-carbinol uptake in humans. Cancer Epidemiol Biomark Prev 23:282–287
48. Garcia HH, Brar GA, Nguyen DH et al (2005) Indole-3-Carbinol (I3C) inhibits cyclin-dependent kinase-2 function in human breast cancer cells by regulating the size distribution, associated cyclin E forms, and subcellular localization of the CDK2 protein complex. J Biol Chem 280:8756–8764
49. Garikapaty VP, Ashok BT, Chen YG et al (2005) Anti-carcinogenic and anti-metastatic properties of indole-3-carbinol in prostate cancer. Oncol Rep 13:89–93
50. Ge X, Fares FA, Yannai S (1999) Induction of apoptosis in MCF-7 cells by indole-3-carbinol is independent of p53 and bax. Anticancer Res 19:3199–3203
51. Guan H, Chen C, Zhu L et al (2013) Indole-3-carbinolblocks platelet-derived growth factor-stimulated vascular smooth muscle cell function and reduces neointima formation in vivo. J NutrBiochem 24:62–69
52. Hayes JD, Dinkova-Kostova AT, McMahon M (2009) Cross-talk between transcription factors AhR and Nrf2: lessons for cancer chemoprevention from dioxin. Toxicol Sci 111:199–201
53. Heath EI, Heilbrun LK, Li J (2010) Phase I dose-escalation study of oral BR-DIM (BioResponse 3,3′- Diindolylmethane) in castrate-resistant, non-metastatic prostate cancer. Am J Transl Res 2:402–411
54. Heinlein CA, Chang C (2004) Androgen receptor in prostate cancer. Endocr Rev 25:276–308
55. Hong C, Kim HA, Firestone GL et al (2002) 3,3'-Diindolylmethane (DIM) induces a G(1) cell cycle arrest in human breast cancer cells that is accompanied by Sp1-mediated activation of p21(WAF1/CIP1) expression. Carcinogenesis 23:1297–1305

56. Horn TL, Reichert MA, Bliss RL (2002) Modulations of P450 mRNA in liver and mammary gland and P450 activities and metabolism of estrogen in liver by treatment of rats with indole-3-carbinol. Biochem Pharmacol 64:393–404
57. Hwang JW, Jung JW, Lee YS et al (2008) Indole-3-carbinol prevents H(2)O(2)-induced inhibition of gap junctional intercellular communication by inactivation of PKB/Akt. J Vet Med Sci 70:1057–1063
58. International Agency for Research on Cancer (1999) Monographs on the evolution of carcinogenic risks to humans: hormonal contraception and postmenopausal hormone therapy, vol 72. IARC, Lyon, France
59. Izzotti A, Calin GA, Steele VE et al (2010) Chemoprevention of cigarette smoke-induced alterations of microRNA expression in rat lungs. Cancer Prev Res 3:62–72
60. Jayakumar P, Pugalendi KV, Sankaran M (2014) Attenuation of hyperglycemia-mediated oxidative stress by indole-3-carbinol and its metabolite 3, 3'- diindolylmethane in C57BL/6 J mice. J Physiol Biochem 70:525–534
61. Jin L, Qi M, Chen DZ et al (1999) Indole-3-carbinol prevents cervical cancer in human papilloma virus type 16 (HPV16) transgenic mice. Cancer Res 59:3991–3997
62. Jin Y (2011) 3,3'-Diindolylmethane inhibits breast cancer cell growth via miR-21-mediated Cdc25A degradation. Mol Cell Biochem 358:345–354
63. Kassie F, Anderson LB, Scherber R et al (2007) Indole-3-carbinol inhibits 4-(methylnitrosamino)-1-(3-pyridyl)-1-butanone plus benzo(a)pyrene-induced lung tumorigenesis in A/J mice and modulates carcinogen-induced alterations in protein levels. Cancer Res 67:6502–6511
64. Kassie F, Kalscheuer S, Matise I et al (2010) Inhibition of vinyl carbamate-induced pulmonary adenocarcinoma by indole-3-carbinol and myo-inositol in A/J mice. Carcinogenesis 31:239–245
65. Kassie F, Melkamu T, Endalew A et al (2010) Inhibition of lungcarcinogenesis and critical cancer-related signaling pathways by N-acetyl-S-(N-2-phenethylthiocarbamoyl)-l-cysteine, indole-3-carbinol and myo-inositol, alone and in combination. Carcinogenesis 31:1634–1641
66. Kim DJ, Han BS, Ahn B et al (1997) Enhancement by indole-3-carbinol of liver and thyroid gland neoplastic development in a rat medium-term multiorgan carcinogenesis model. Carcinogenesis 18:377–381
67. Kim EJ, Park Sy, Shin et al (2007) Activation of caspase-8 contributes to 3,3'-Diindolylmethane-induced apaptosis in colon cancer cells. J Nutr 137:31–36
68. Kojima T, Tanaka T, Mori H (1994) Chemoprevention of spontaneous endometrial cancer in female Donryu rats by dietary indole-3-carbinol. Cancer Res 54:1446–1449
69. Kong D, Heath E, Chen W et al (2012) Loss of let-7 up-regulates EZH2 in prostate cancer consistent with the acquisition of cancer stem cell signatures that are attenuated by BR-DIM. PLoS ONE 7:e33729
70. Kong D, Heath E, Chen W et al (2012) Epigenetic silencing of miR-34a in human prostate cancer cells and tumor tissue specimens can be reversed by BR-DIM treatment. Am J Transl Res 4:14–23
71. Kumi-Diaka J, Merchant K, Haces A et al (2010) Genistein-selenium combination induces growth arrest in prostate cancer cells. J Med Food 13:842–850
72. Kumar MM, Davuluri S, Poojar S et al (2015) Role of estrogen receptor alpha in human cervical cancer-associated fibroblasts: a transcriptomic study. Tumour Biol Oct 24 [Epub ahead of print]
73. Lawrence T (2009) The nuclear factor NF-κB pathway in Inflammation. Cold Spring Harb Perspect Biol 1:a001651. doi:10.1101/cshperspect.a001651
74. Le HT, Schaldach CM, Firestone GL et al (2003) Plant-derived 3,3'-Diindolylmethane is a strong androgen antagonist in human prostate cancer cells. J Biol Chem 278:21136–21145
75. Leong H, Riby JE, Firestone GL et al (2004) Potent ligand-independent estrogen receptor activation by 3,3′-diindolylmethane is mediated by cross talk between the protein kinase A and mitogen-activated protein kinase signaling pathways. Mol Endocrinol 18:291–302

76. Li Y, Li X, Sarkar FH (2003) Gene expression profiles of I3C- and DIM-treated PC3 human prostate cancer cells determined by cDNA microarray analysis. J Nutr 133:1011–1019
77. Li Y, Wang Z, Kong D et al (2007) Regulation of FOXO3a/beta-catenin/GSK-3beta signaling by 3,3'-diindolylmethane contributes to inhibition of cell proliferation and induction of apoptosis in prostate cancer cells. J Biol Chem 282:21542–21550
78. Li Y, VandenBoomII TG, Wang Z et al (2010) miRNA146a suppresses invasion of pancreatic cancer cells. Cancer Res 70:1486–1495
79. Lian JP, Word B, Taylor S et al (2004) Modulation of the constitutive activated STAT3 transcription factor in pancreatic cancer prevention: effects of indole-3-carbinol (I3C) and genistein. Anticancer Res 24:133–137
80. Licznerska BE, Szaefer H, Murias M et al (2013) Modulation of CYP19 expression by cabbage juices and their active components: indole-3-carbinol and 3,3'-diindolylmethane in human breast epithelial cell lines. Eur J Nutr 52:1483–1492
81. Lo R, Matthews J (2013) The aryl hydrocarbon receptor and estrogen receptoralpha differentially modulate nuclear factor erythroid-2-related factor2 transactivation in MCF-7 breast cancer cells. Toxicol Appl Pharmacol 270:139–148
82. Lu Q, Nakmura J, Savinov A et al (1996) Expression of aromatase protein and messenger ribonucleic acid in tumor epithelial cells and evidence of functional significance of locally produced estrogen in human breast cancer. Endocrinology 137:3061–3068
83. Luo J, Manning BD, Cantley LC (2003) Targeting the PI3 K-Akt pathway in human cancer: rationale andpromise. Cancer Cell 4:257–262
84. Lynn A, Collins A, Fuller Z et al (2006) Cruciferous vegetables and colorectal cancer. Proc Nutr Soc 65:135–144
85. Maiyoh GK, Kuh JE, Casaschi A et al (2007) Cruciferous indole-3-carbinol inhibits apolipoprotein B secretion in HepG2 cells. J Nutr 137:2185–2189
86. Marconett CN, Singhal AK, Sundar SN et al (2012) Indole-3-carbinol disrupts estrogen receptor-alpha dependent expression of insulin-like growth factor-1 receptor and insulin receptor substrate-1 and proliferation of human breast cancer cells. Mol Cell Endocrinol 363:74–84
87. McGuire KP, Ngoubilly N, Neavyn M et al (2006) 3,3′-diindolylmethane and paclitaxel act synergistically to promote apoptosis in HER2/Neu human breast cancer cells. J Surg Res 132:208–213
88. Melkamu T, Zhang X, Tan J et al (2010) Alteration of microRNA expression in vinyl carbamate-induced mouse lung tumors and modulation by the chemopreventive agent indole-3-carbinol. Carcinogenesis 31:252–258
89. Meng Q, Qi M, Chen DZ et al (2000) Suppression of breast cancer invasion and migration by indole-3-carbinol: associated with up-regulation of BRCA1 and E-cadherin/catenin complexes. J Mol Med 78:155–165
90. Mesnil M, Crespin S, Avanzo JL et al (2005) Defective gap junctional intercellular communication in the carcinogenic process. Biochim Biophys Acta 1719:125–145
91. Michnovicz JJ, Adlercreutz H, Bradlow HL (1997) Changes in levels of urinary estrogen metabolites after oral indole-3-carbinol treatment in humans. J Natl Cancer Inst 89:718–723
92. Mulvey L, Chandrasekaran A, Liu K et al (2007) Interplay of genes regulated by estrogen and diindolylmethane in breast cancer cell lines. Mol Med 13:69–78
93. Nakamura Y, Yogosawa S, Izutani Y et al (2009) A combination of indol-3-carbinol and genistein synergistically induces apoptosis in human colon cancer HT-29 cells by inhibiting Aktphosphorylation and progression of autophagy. Mol Cancer 8:100. doi:10.1186/1476-4598-8-100
94. Nachshon-Kedmi M, Yannai S, Haj A et al (2003) Indole-3-carbinol and 3,3'-diindolylmethane induce apoptosis in human prostate cancer cells. Food Chem Toxicol 41:745–752
95. Oganesian A, Hendricks JD, Williams DE (1997) Long term dietary indole-3-carbinol inhibits diethylnitrosamine-initiated hepatocarcinogenesis in the infant mouse model. Cancer Lett 118:87–94

96. Ohtake F, Fujii-Kuriyama Y, Kawajiri K et al (2011) Cross-talk of dioxin and estrogen receptor signals through the ubiquitin system. J Steroid Biochem Mol Biol 127:102–107
97. Pagliaro B, Santolamazza C, Simonelli F et al (2015) Phytochemical compounds and protection from cardiovascular diseases: a state of the art. BioMed Res Int. doi:10.1155/2015/918069
98. Paik WH, Kim HR, Park JK et al (2013) Chemosensitivity induced by down-regulation of MicroRNA-21 in gemcitabine-resistant pancreatic cancer cells by indole-3-carbinol. Anticancer Res 33:1473–1482
99. Park MK, Rhee YH, Lee HJ et al (2008) Antiplatelet and antithrombotic activity of indole-3-carbinolin vitro and in vivo. Phytother Res 22:58–64
100. Pearson G, Robinson F, Beers Gibson T et al (2001) Mitogen-activated protein (MAP) kinase pathways: regulation and physiological functions. Endocr Rev 22:153–183
101. Penning TM, Burczynski ME, Jez JM et al (2000) Human 3α-hydroxysteroid dehydrogenase isoforms (AKR1C1-AKR1C4) of the aldo-keto reductase superfamily: functional plasticity and tissue distribution reveals roles in the inactivation and formation of male and female sex hormones. Biochem J 351:67–77
102. Qian X, Melkamu T, Upadhyaya P et al (2011) Indole-3-carbinol inhibited tobacco smokecarcinogen-induced lung adenocarcinoma in A/J mice when administered during the post-initiation or progression phase of lung tumorigenesis. Cancer Lett 311:57–65
103. Rahman KM, Aranha O, Sarkar FH (2003) Indole-3-carbinol (I3C) induces apoptosis in tumorigenic but not in nontumorigenic breast epithelial cells. Nutr Cancer 45:101–112
104. Rajoria S, Suriano R, Parmar PS et al (2011) 3,3'-diindolylmethane modulates estrogen metabolism in patients with thyroid proliferative disease: a pilot study. Thyroid 21:299–304
105. Reed GA, Peterson KS, Smith HJ et al (2005) A phase I study of indole-3-carbinol in women: tolerability and effects. Cancer Epidemiol Biomark Prev 14:1953–1960
106. Rice JC, Ozcelik H, Maxeiner P et al (2000) Methylation of the BRCA1 promoter is associated with decreased BRCA1 mRNA levels in clinical breast cancer specimens. Carcinogenesis 21:1761–1765
107. Rosen CA, Woodson GE, Thompson JW et al (1998) Preliminary results of the use of indole-3-carbinol for recurrent respiratory papillomatosis. Otolaryngol Head Neck Surg 118:810–815
108. Rosen CA, Bryson PC (2004) Indole-3-carbinol for recurrent respiratory papillomatosis: long-term results. J Voice 18:248–253
109. Sarkar FH, Li Y, Wang Z et al (2009) Cellular signaling perturbation by natural products. Cell Signal 21:1541–1547
110. Sarkar FH, Li Y (1997) Indole-3-carbinol and prostate cancer. J Nutr 134:3493S–3498S
111. Sarkar S, Dubaybo H, Ali S et al (2013) Down-regulation of miR-221 inhibits proliferation of pancreatic cancer cells through up-regulation of PTEN, p27(kip1), p57(kip2), and PUMA. Am. J Cancer Res 3:465–477
112. Shaw RJ, Cantley LC (2006) Ras, PI(3)K and mTORsignalling controls tumour cell growth. Nature 441:424–430
113. Singhal R, Shankar K, Badger TM et al (2008) Estrogenic status modulatesaryl hydrocarbon receptor-mediated hepatic gene expression andcarcinogenicity. Carcinogenesis 29:227–236
114. Szaefer H, Krajka-Kuźniak V, Licznerska B (2015) Cabbage juices and indoles modulate the expression profile of AhR, ERα, and Nrf2 in human breast cell lines. Nutr Cancer 67:1342–1345
115. Śmiechowska A, Bartoszek A, Namieśnik J (2008) Cancer chemopreventive agents: Glucosinolates and their decomposition products in white cabbage (Brassica oleracea var. Capitata). Postepy Hig Med Dosw (online) 62:125–140
116. Tadi K, Chang Y, Ashok BT et al (2005) 3,3'-Diidolylmethane, a cruciferous vegetable derived synthetic antiprolifereative compound in thyroid disease. Biochem Biophys Res Commun 337:1019–1025
117. Terry P, Wolk A, Persson I et al (2001) Brassica vegetables and breast cancer risk. JAMA 285:2975–2977

118. van Poppel G, Verhoeven DT, Verhagen H et al (1999) Brassica vegetables and cancer prevention. Epidemiology and mechanisms. Adv Exp Med Biol 472:159–168
119. Vahid F, Zand H, Nosrat-Mirshekarlou E et al (2015) The role dietary of bioactivecompounds on the regulation of histone acetylases and deacetylases: a review. Gene 562:8–15
120. Vang O (2006) Chemopreventive potential of compounds in Cruciferous vegetables. In: Baer-Dubowska W, Bartoszek A, Malejka-Giganti D (eds) Carcinogenic and anticarcinogenic food components. CRC Taylor & Francis, Boca Raton, pp 303–328
121. Verhagen H, Poulsen HE, Loft S et al (1995) Reduction of oxidative DNA-damage in humans by brussels sprouts. Carcinogenesis 16:969–970
122. Wattenberg LW, Loub WD (1978) Inhibition of polycyclic aromatic hydrocarbon-induced neoplasia by naturally occurring indoles. Cancer Res 38:1410–1413
123. Wattenberg LW, Loub WD, Lam LK, Speier JL (1976) Dietary constituents altering the responses to chemical carcinogens. Fed Proc 35:1327–1331
124. Wattenberg LW, Hanley AB, Barany G et al (1985) Inhibition of carcinogenesis by some minor dietary constituents. Princess Takamatsu Symp 16:193–203
125. WHO Report Part II 2015
126. Wilson CA, Ramos L, Villaseñor MR et al (1999) Localization of human BRCA1 and its loss in high-grade, non-inherited breast carcinomas. Nat Genet 21:236–240
127. Witter DC, Le Bas J (2008) Cancer as a chronic disease. Oncology 53:1–3
128. Wong GY, Bradlow L, Sepkovic D et al (1997) Dose-ranging study of indole-3-carbinol for breast cancer prevention. J Cell Biochem Suppl 28–29:111–116
129. Wong CP, Hsu A, Buchanan A et al (2014) Effects of sulforaphane and 3,3′-diindolylmethane on genome-wide promoter methylation in normalprostate epithelial cells and prostate cancer cells. PLoS ONE 9:e86787. doi:10.1371/journal.pone.0086787
130. Wu TY, Khor TO, Su ZY et al (2013) Epigenetic modifications of Nrf2 by 3,3′-diindolylmethanein vitro in TRAMP C1 cell line and in vivo TRAMP prostate tumors. AAPS J 15:864–874
131. Xu M, Orner GA, Bailey GS et al (2001) Post-initiation effects of chlorophyllin and indole-3-carbinol in rats given 1,2-dimethylhydrazine or 2-amino-3- methylimidazo[4, 5-f] quinoline. Carcinogenesis 22:309–314
132. Xu H, Barnes GT, Yang Q et al (2003) Chronic inflammation in fat plays a crucial role in the development of obesity-related insulin resistance. J Clin Invest 112:1821–1830
133. Yoshida M, Katashima S, Ando J et al (2004) Dietary indole-3-carbinol promotes endometrial adenocarcinoma development in rats initiated with N-ethyl-N'-nitro-N-nitrosoguanidine, with induction of cytochrome P450 s in the liver and consequent modulation of estrogen metabolism. Carcinogenesis 25:2257–2264
134. Zhang J, Hsu BAJC, Kinseth BAMA et al (2003) Indole-3-carbinol induces a G1 cell cycle arrest and inhibits prostate-specificantigen production in human LNCaP prostate carcinoma cells. Cancer 98:2511–2520
135. Zhu J, Li Y, Guan C et al (2012) Anti-proliferative and pro-apoptotic effects of 3, 3'-diindolylmethane in human cervical cancer cells. Oncol Rep 28:1063–1068

Chapter 7
Sanguinarine and Its Role in Chronic Diseases

Pritha Basu and Gopinatha Suresh Kumar

Abstract The use of natural products derived from plants as medicines precedes even the recorded human history. In the past few years there were renewed interests in developing natural compounds and understanding their target specificity for drug development for many devastating human diseases. This has been possible due to remarkable advancements in the development of sensitive chemistry and biology tools. Sanguinarine is a benzophenanthridine alkaloid derived from rhizomes of the plant species *Sanguinaria canadensis*. The alkaloid can exist in the cationic iminium and neutral alkanolamine forms. Sanguinarine is an excellent DNA and RNA intercalator where only the iminium ion binds. Both forms of the alkaloid, however, shows binding to functional proteins like serum albumins, lysozyme and hemoglobin. The molecule is endowed with remarkable biological activities and large number of studies on its various activities has been published potentiating its development as a therapeutic agent particularly for chronic human diseases like cancer, asthma, etc. In this article, we review the properties of this natural alkaloid, and its diverse medicinal applications in relation to how it modulates cell death signaling pathways and induce apoptosis through different ways, its utility as a therapeutic agent for chronic diseases and its biological effects in animal and human models. These data may be useful to understand the therapeutic potential of this important and highly abundant alkaloid that may aid in the development of sanguinarine-based therapeutic agents with high efficacy and specificity.

Keywords Benzophenanthridine · Sanguinarine · Nucleic acid binding property · Anticancer · Antimicrobial

---

P. Basu · G.S. Kumar (✉)
Biophysical Chemistry Laboratory, Organic and Medicinal Chemistry Division, CSIR- Indian Institute of Chemical Biology, 4, Raja S. C. Mullick Road, Kolkata 700032, India
e-mail: gskumar@iicb.res.in; gsk.iicb@gmail.com

S.C. Gupta et al. (eds.), *Anti-inflammatory Nutraceuticals and Chronic Diseases*, Advances in Experimental Medicine and Biology 928,
DOI 10.1007/978-3-319-41334-1_7

Fig. 7.1 Molecular structure of sanguinarine

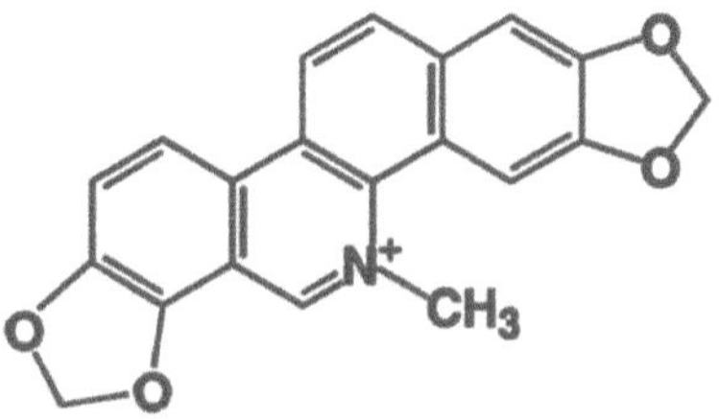

7.1 Introduction

Sanguinarine[13-methyl[1,3]benzodioxolo[5,6-c]-1,3-dioxolo[4,5-i]phenanthridinium] (Fig. 7.1) is the well-known member of the relatively small group of quaternary benzo [c]phenanthridine [QBA] alkaloids. *Sanguinaria canadensis*, also known as bloodroot, is a perennial herbaceous flowering plant of the papaveriaceae family. Bloodroot produces primarily the toxic alkaloid sanguinarine that is largely stored in the rhizome of the plant. From a medicinal perspective, QBAs in general and sanguinarine in particular, have many important properties. They display antimicrobial, antifungal and anti-inflammatory effects in addition to their putative anticancer activity that is widely studied. The molecular action of sanguinarine in expressing its biological activity has been a subject of intense debate; it has been shown to interact with many targets, like nucleic acids, proteins and microtubules, and modify the activities of a wide variety of enzymes. This review summarizes the current state of knowledge on the properties of sanguinarine that are important for their potential use in chronic diseases.

7.2 Physicochemical Properties of Sanguinarine

Sanguinarine occurs either as chloride or sulfate crystalline salts and both are orange-red colored. It is sparingly soluble in aqueous conditions but highly soluble in many organic solvents. Some of the physical properties of sanguinarine are summarized in Table 7.1.

One of the remarkable properties of sanguinarine and other QBAs is their ability to exhibit a pH dependent structural equilibrium between the quaternary iminium form and the 6-hydroxydihydro derivative or the alkanolamine form (Scheme 7.1). The reversible, pH dependent equilibrium between the charged iminium (SGI) and the neutral alkanolamine (SGA) forms in aqueous solution may be represented as follows [76]

$$SG^{+} + OH^{-} \leftrightarrow SGOH$$

The acid–base structural equilibrium of sanguinarine was characterized first by Maiti and colleagues primarily by spectroscopy techniques [56] and confirmed subsequently by others, and was characterized by a pKa value around 8.06 [1, 33,

Table 7.1 Physiochemical properties of sanguinarine

Empirical formula	$C_{20}H_{14}O_4N^+$
Chemical name	13-Methyl-[1,3]-benzodioxolo[5,6-c]-1,3-dioxolo[4,5-i]phenanthridin-13-ium
Molecular weight (ion)	332.33
Polar surface area	40.8 Å^2
Crystal color	Orange-red
Solubility	Water: slightly soluble <0.3 mg mL^{-1}
Melting point (°C)	278–279 °C
Optical rotation $[\alpha]_D$ (solvent)	0 °C (H_2O)
Peak position of absorption spectrum (nm) (In aqueous buffer of pH 6.0)	273, 327, 400, and 470 nm
Molar absorption coefficient (ε) (M^{-1} cm^{-1})	30,700 at 327 nm
Peak position in fluorescence spectrum (nm) (In aqueous buffer of pH 6.0)	Strong, at 570 nm
pKa	8.06
IC_{50} or LD_{50} value (in mice)	19.4 mg kg¯1 of body weight

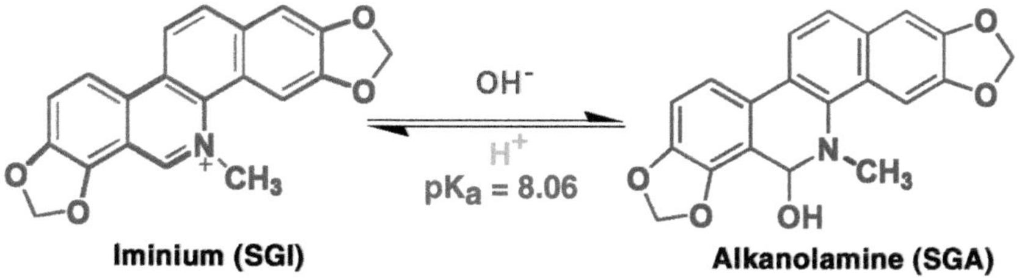

Scheme 7.1 pH dependent structural changes of SGI and SGA forms

36, 39, 42]. These two forms have characteristic absorbance and fluorescence spectra which are presented in Fig. 7.2a, b. Thus, in aqueous solution at physiological pH both forms of the alkaloid are present. The SGI is unsaturated and planar; the SGA has a tilted structure and is essentially nonplanar. The aqueous solubility of the SGI is much higher than that of the SGA. The latter (SGA) form can penetrate the cell membrane increasing its cellular availability. Inside the cell it may be converted partially to the SGI form influenced by pH and other factors. Due to the conjugated aromatic nature of its chromophore sanguinarine has strong spectral bands in the UV–vis region and also exhibits intense fluorescence (Fig. 7.2b). The molecule is, therefore, sensitive to light and can cause adverse phototoxic reactions in the presence of light. The SGA form is known to undergo photo oxidation at the C6 carbon atom to oxysanguinarine in alkaline solutions (Scheme 7.2) [75]. The photo oxidation of sanguinarine was found to be accelerated in the presence of Rose Bengal suggesting the role of singlet molecular oxygen in the reaction mechanism [28].

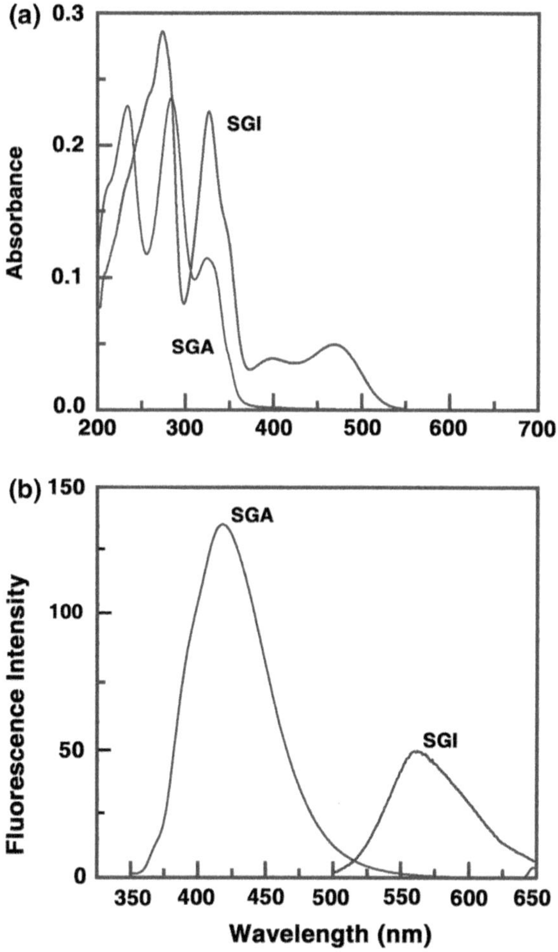

Fig. 7.2 Characteristic absorption (panel A) and fluorescence (panel B) spectra of SGI and SGA forms

The toxicity of sanguinarine has been suggested to be due to its DNA intercalation, inhibition of ion pumps and several thiol dependent proteins, and interaction with cyto skeletal components [24, 86]. Sanguinarine can kill animal cells through a variety of mechanisms. Epidemic dropsy is a form of edema of extremities that results from ingesting argemone oil that contains sanguinarine [73]. Application of sanguinarine to skin may result in tissue damage because of escharotic effect. Phototoxic effect of sanguinarine against mosquito larvae has also been reported [67]. Production of singlet oxygen by sanguinarine is known [6, 54]. Phototoxic action of sanguinarine has also been suggested to be due to the production of H_2O_2 [6, 78]. Reactive oxygen species (ROS) such as superoxide anions (O_2^-) or

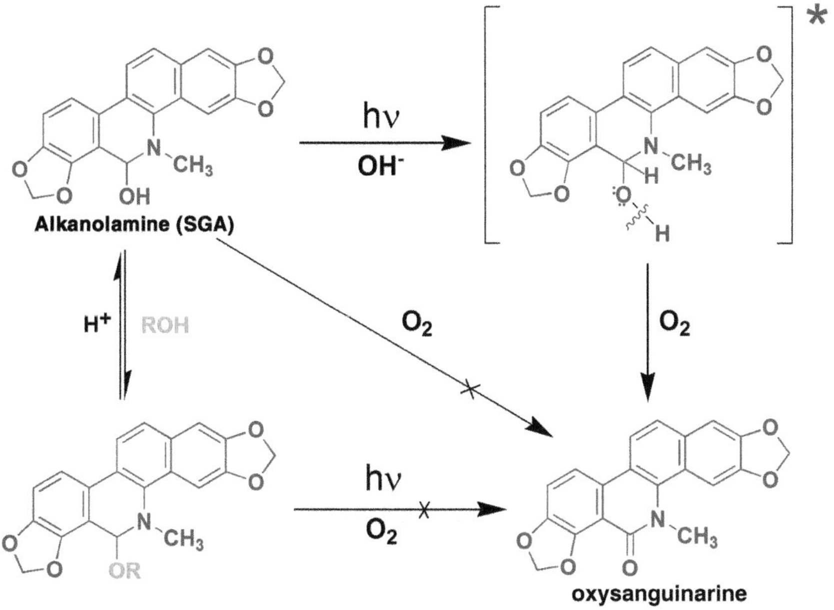

Scheme 7.2 Generation of oxysanguinarine from SGA form in the presence of oxygen by photochemical process. Reprinted from Suresh Kumar et al. 1997 [75] with permission. Copyright Elsevier Science S. A

hydrogen peroxide (H_2O_2) have also been found to be generated in sanguinarine-treated cells [12, 21, 37, 59]. Recent studies have also suggested that sanguinarine inhibited the growth cancer cells and induced their apoptosis through the generation of free radicals [29, 30].

Sanguinarine binds to DNA and RNA in vitro and forms strong intercalation complexes [15, 33, 34, 36, 57, 61, 71, 76]. It has also been proposed that the SGI form intercalates to DNA and RNA. The SGA form does not bind to DNA or RNA but in the presence of large concentration of DNA or RNA the SGA form gets converted to SGI resulting in the binding of the latter [33, 36, 55]. The crystal structure of sanguinarine-DNA oligomer complex has been solved recently [25] (Fig. 7.3) confirming the intercalation model first proposed by Maiti's group [57]. Interestingly both SGI and SGA forms bind to functional proteins like serum albumins, hemoglobin and lysozyme [31, 33, 35, 36, 40]. Kundu and coworkers showed that sanguinarine binds with core histones and induces chromatin aggregation and inhibits important chromatin modifications like acetylation and methylation [70].

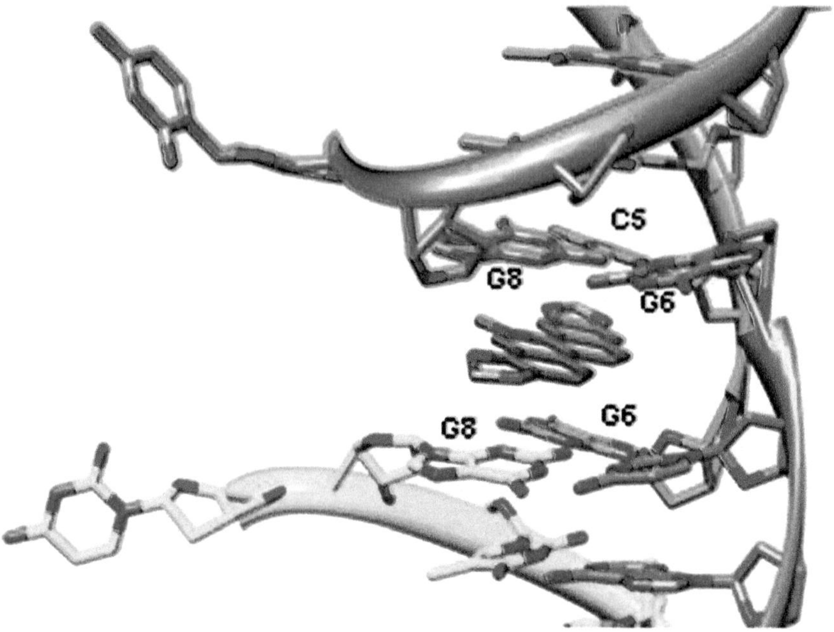

Fig. 7.3 Sanguinarine molecule intercalated at the interface of two "two molecules" DNA units. DNA chains color scheme: A = *orange*, B = *yellow*, C = *green*, D = *blue*. Reprinted from [25] with permission. Copyright The Royal Society of Chemistry 2011

7.3 Modulation of Cell Signaling Pathways by Sanguinarine

Sanguinarine has been reported to induce cell cycle arrest and apoptosis in distinct cancer cells [3, 4, 20, 32, 45, 72, 85]. It modulates multiple signaling pathways causing inhibition of the initiation of cancer, inducing cell cycle arrest, apoptosis, and inhibiting metastasis and angiogenesis in a variety of cancer cells [9, 82] (Fig. 7.4).

One of the first systematic study showing the anticancer effect of sanguinarine was that of Ahmad et al. [4] who showed that sanguinarine treatment resulted in an apoptotic death of human epidermoid carcinoma A431 carcinoma cells and the loss of viability that occurred at much less losses in comparison to normal human epidermal keratinocytes (NHEKs). The DNA cell cycle analysis revealed that sanguinarine treatment did not significantly affect the distribution of cells among the different phases of the cell cycle in A431 cells. It was suggested that the involvement of the NFκB pathway may be a mechanism of sanguinarine-mediated apoptosis [4]. A study by Ding et al. [20] reported that sanguinarine-induced concentration dependent apoptosis with caspase-3 activation and BCD/oncosis without caspase-3 activation suggesting two cell death mechanisms. This suggests

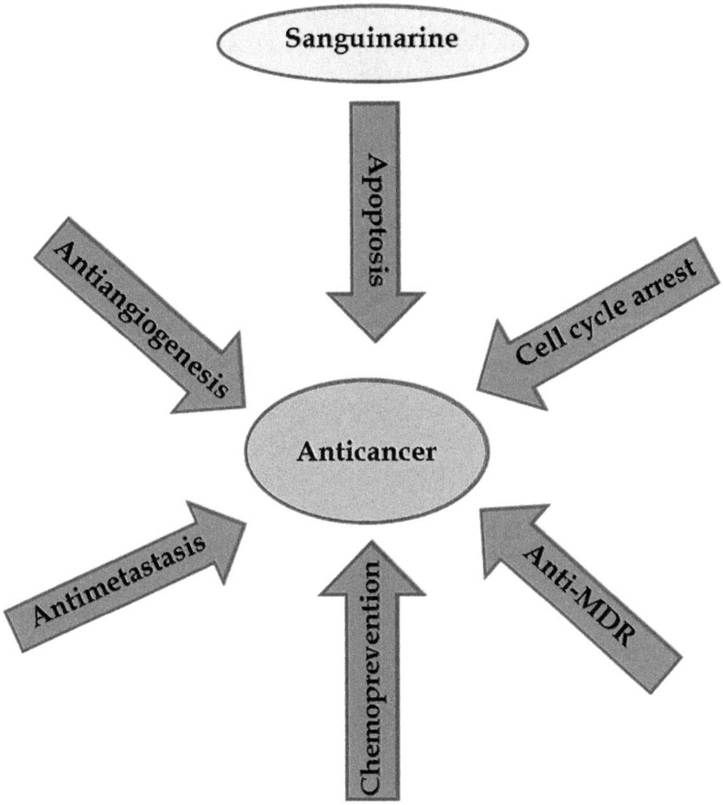

Fig. 7.4 Schematic diagram showing the multiple cell signaling pathway of action of sanguinarine in modulating anticancer activity

the effectiveness of sanguinarine against multidrug resistance being a major obstacle in chemotherapy [20].

Sanguinarine treatment of HaCaT cells was found to inhibit in a dose-dependent manner the cell proliferation and induce apoptosis; significant cleavage of poly (ADP-ribose) polymerase occurred in HaCaT cells. A dose-dependent increase in the level of Bax with a concomitant decrease in Bcl-2 levels and increase in Bax/Bcl-2 ratio was found. A significant increase in the pro-apoptotic members of Bcl-2 family proteins, i.e., B_{ak} and B_{id} was also observed. This was accompanied by increase in (*a*) protein expression of cytochrome *c* and apoptotic protease-activating factor-1 and (*b*) activity and protein expression of caspase-3, caspase-7, caspase-8, and caspase-9. These results showed the involvement of mitochondrial pathway and Bcl-2 family proteins in sanguinarine-mediated apoptosis of immortalized keratiocytes signifying its use in hyper proliferative skin disorders, including skin cancer [2]. Subsequently, the authors showed that sanguinarine imparts anti proliferative effects against androgen-responsive (LNCaP) and androgen-unresponsive (DU145) human prostate cancer cells and that this effect was mediated through deregulation of cell cycle and induction of apoptosis. The involvement of cyclin kinase inhibitors (cki) and cyclin-dependent kinases (cdk), i.e., the cki–cyclin–cdk machinery, during cell cycle arrest and apoptosis of prostate cancer cells by sanguinarine has been suggested [3].

Sanguinarine was found not increase Bax levels in K1735-M2 melanoma cells. A similar result was obtained in human CEM T-leukemia cells [43]. The interesting result was that the absence of Bax over-expression occurred with an increase of p53 protein. Matkar et al. [59] demonstrated that sanguinarine-induced death in human colon cancer cells was p53-independent, although DNA damage was detected in K1735-M2 cells. The results suggested that mitochondrial depolarization induced by sanguinarine is associated with nuclear DNA damage, although it may not exclusively result from pathways activated by the latter event [72].

In vascular smooth muscle cells significant growth inhibition was induced by sanguinarine as a result of G1-phase cell cycle arrest mediated by induction of p27KIP1 expression, and resulted in a down-regulation of the expression of cyclins and cdks. Moreover, sanguinarine-induced inhibition of cell growth appeared to be linked to activation of Ras/ERK through p27KIP1-mediated G1-phase cell cycle arrest. Overall, the unexpected effects of sanguinarine treatment in VSMC provided a theoretical basis for clinical use of therapeutic agents in the treatment of atherosclerosis [49].

Some researches ascribe the pro-apoptotic properties of sanguinarine to production of ROS [29, 30, 43] while others have demonstrated that the effects of sanguinarine are not accompanied by ROS production [19, 60, 81]. Kim et al. [46] reported that the mechanism of sanguinarine-induced apoptosis in human breast cancer MDA-231 cells was due to the generation of ROS. Its ability to directly interact with glutathione (GSH) was thought to lead to depletion of cellular GSH and induction of ROS generation [12, 19, 38, 46]. It was found that the quenching of ROS generation by *N*-acetyl-L-cysteine (NAC), a scavenger of ROS, reversed sanguinarine-induced apoptosis effects. It was also found that sanguinarine-induced rat hepatic stellate T6 cells (HSC-T6 cells) apoptosis was correlated with the generation of increased ROS, leading to decrease in the mitochondrial membrane potential (MMP) and the down-regulation of anti-apoptotic protein Bcl-2 [88].

Sanguinarine is a selective inhibitor of mitogen-activated protein kinase phosphatase 1 (MKP-1), which is over expressed in many tumor cells [79]. The disruption of microtubule assembly dynamics [51], the nucleocytoplasmic trafficking of cyclin D1 and Topisomerase II [32] and the induction of DNA damage [18] allosteric activator of AMP-activated protein kinase [14] also contributed, at least in part to the anticancer effects of sanguinarine [52].

Sanguinarine induces a rapid caspase-dependent cell death in human melanoma cells; partially involving endoplasmic reticulum and mitochondria mediated responses. This cell death is dependent on the generation of reactive oxygen species, and is not prevented by Bcl-XL over expression. The fact that sanguinarine induces a very rapid cell death with apoptotic features in melanoma cells, together with the lack of inhibition by over expressing Bcl-XL, highlight the potent anti-melanoma activity of this isoquinoline alkaloid and suggest its potential in the treatment of skin cancer [9]. Recently Singh et al. [74] identified a number of differentially expressed proteins which are important in the signaling pathways modulated by sanguinarine in its action against pancreatic cancer.

7.4 Role of Sanguinarine in Chronic Diseases

Chronic diseases, like heart disease, COPD, stroke, cancer, respiratory diseases like asthma and metabolic diseases like diabetes are the leading cause of human mortality. Many natural products in general and sanguinarine in particular possess potent activities that have been useful in the treatment of these chronic ailments, and these have also been documented in many studies. Anti proliferative activities have been demonstrated in cells derived from various human carcinomas as reviewed in the previous section. Various mechanisms by which sanguinarine induce apoptosis in cancer cells through various pathways have been described. The therapeutic potential of sanguinarine in cardiovascular disease related to platelet aggregation has been reported by Jeng et al. [41, 53]. Sanguinarine has promising antihypertensive and potent antiplatelet effects; it interferes with renin-angiotensin system and possibly other blood pressure regulating pathways, and also induces calcium mobilization, thromboxane and cAMP production (Scheme 7.3). Many studies on in vitro models are reported to this effect and a recent review summarizes the antihypertensive activity and cardiovascular properties, including hypotensive, antiplatelet, and positive inotropic effects of sanguinarine [53]. Computational bioinformatics analysis has identified sanguinarine as a potential candidate drugs for the treatment of type 2 diabetes [83] but clinical studies are not yet available on this aspect.

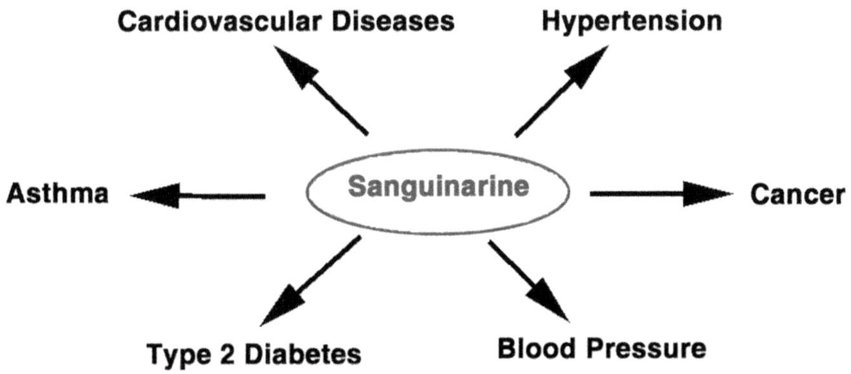

Scheme 7.3 Schematic diagram showing the role of sanguinarine in different chronic diseases

7.5 Biological Activities of Sanguinarine in Animal Models

In the previous sections, we reviewed the effect of sanguinarine in exerting cytotoxic effects or inhibiting cell proliferation in several normal and cancer cell lines, including human gingival fibroblasts [58], rat hepatocytes [16], human promyelocytic leukemia HL-60 cells [80], and human osteosarcoma cells [64]. A number of studies on the effect of sanguinarine have been performed in animal models and the results suggested a complex scenario; both adverse as well as beneficial effects of this alkaloid are reported. Niu et al. [62] examined the anti-inflammatory function of sanguinarine in animal models of acute and chronic inflammation using lipopolysaccharide (LPS)-induced murine peritoneal macrophages. Sanguinarine was found to display significant anti-inflammatory effects both in vitro and in vivo. It was demonstrated that sanguinarine potently inhibited the expression of inflammatory mediators and inflammation in general. Furthermore, it was shown that sanguinarine inhibited the activation of mitogen-activated protein kinase (MAPK), which altered inflammatory mediator synthesis and release in vitro. Anti-inflammatory effects through inhibition of LPS-induced tumor necrosis factor-alpha level, interleukin 6 level, and nitric oxide production in serum was demonstrated for sanguinarine solid lipid nanoparticles in mice endotoxin shock model induced by lipopolysaccharide [50].

Epidemiological studies have suggested that the use of sanguinarine as an oral rinse and in toothpaste effectively suppressed dental plaque formation and reduced gingival inflammation [27, 48, 66] possibly due to its antioxidant, antimicrobial, and anti-inflammatory effects [26]. However, long-term use of oral products containing sanguinarine has also been reported to lead to an increased incidence of leukoplakia of the maxillary vestibule [23]. Sanguinarine has been shown to enhance the skin tumor promoting activity in mouse skin which may have relevance to its carcinogenic potential [5].

Chan et al. had showed that sanguinarine triggers apoptotic processes in mouse blastocysts and impairs early post implantation development in vitro and in vivo [10]. The effect of sanguinarine on early-stage embryo maturation revealed that short-term exposure to sanguinarine at the oocyte stage causes a long-term deleterious impact on subsequent embryonic development leading to retardation of the oocyte maturation, and deleterious effects on IVF and subsequent embryonic development [11].

Chelidonium majus extract in general and sanguinarine in particular were reported to have hERG potassium channel blocking effect. Therefore, in some situations where cardiac repolarization reserve is weak it may increase the risk of potentially fatal ventricular arrhythmias in canines [63].

Sanguinarine has been found to modulate the expression of immune related genes in goldfish and this to some extent was suggested to affect their ability to resist bacterial pathogens [69].

Sanguinarine was demonstrated to markedly induce the expression of HO-1 which leads to a neuro protective response in mouse hippocampus-derived neuronal

HT22 cells from apoptotic cell death induced by glutamate. Sanguinarine significantly attenuated the loss of mitochondrial function and membrane integrity associated with glutamate-induced neurotoxicity. Sanguinarine protected against glutamate-induced neurotoxicity through inhibition of HT22 cell apoptosis. JC-1 staining, a well-established measure of mitochondrial damage, which decreased after treatment with sanguinarine in glutamate-challenged HT22 cells. In addition, sanguinarine diminished the intracellular accumulation of ROS and Ca^{2+}.

Non-cytotoxic concentration of sanguinarine led to a marked protection against glutamate-induced oxidative toxicity in mice through activation of the Nrf2-HO-1 pathway. The antioxidant effect of HO-1 was mainly due to reduction in ROS production and recovery of mitochondrial decay that promoted a decrease in glutamate-trigged apoptosis in HT22 cells [65].

An antidepressant-like effect of sanguinarine in rats was reported through inhibition of mitogen-activated protein kinase phosphatase-1 in rates that enable the use of sanguinarine as anti depressant drug [13]. Radiation protective efficacy of sanguinarine in mice models have also been reported [87].

Recently, sanguinarine treatment was shown to result in reduction of cell migration, a dose-dependent inhibition of cell viability and the induction of cell death by apoptosis in both human (MDA-MB-231 cells) and mouse (A17 cells) in vitro models of basal-like breast cancer (BLBC). Oral administration of sanguinarine reduced the development and growth of A17 transplantable tumors in FVB syngeneic mice. The suppression was correlated with a concurrent up regulation of p27 and down-regulation of cyclin D1 and with the inhibition of STAT3 activation.

The adverse effect, viz., the epidemic dropsy syndrome, is a well-known toxic effect on human health linked to development of glaucoma due to consumption of edible oil adulterated with argemone oil that principally contained sanguinarine. This involves initiation of oxidative stress (ROS formation leading to lipid peroxidation, depletion of GSH and decrease of total antioxidant capacity) and death of red cells via formation of methemoglobin [7, 8, 17]. The detoxification pathway of sanguinarine in animals and in man may be by conversion to dihydrosanguinarine which has been reported in rats [22]. On the other hand, in several European Union nations QBAs and principally sanguinarine are used as feed additives for Pigs. Sangrovit®, a phytogenic feed additive derived from the rhizomes of *Sanguinaria canadensis*, contains high amounts of sanguinarine. This has been shown to increase feed intake and feed conversion in growing pigs, which results in improved growth performance and stimulates anti-inflammatory activity [44]. A study to detect sanguinarine-induced DNA damage has indicated the absence of any DNA adducts in pigs fed with sanguinarine. The observation that the animals remained healthy contradicted the cause of epidemic dropsy syndrome to sanguinarine [47]. Also broilers treated with drinking water containing sanguinarine showed reduced *Salmonella* Enteritidis count [68].

7.6 Biological Activities of Sanguinarine in Humans

Not many studies have been performed in humans on the effect of sanguinarine as such, but herbal preparations containing sanguinarine have been used in folk medicines in small doses for the treatment of many disorders like bronchial problems, asthma, cough and cold remedies, severe throat infections and heart diseases [26]. Benefits have also been reported for leprosy and tuberculosis treatment, antimicrobial treatment for the gastrointestinal system, etc. Sanguinarine, as described in the above section, is traditionally used in tooth pastes and antiseptic mouth rinses due to its ability to suppress dental plaque gingival inflammation and periodontal disease through antimicrobial action and ability to inhibit bacterial adherences [27, 48, 66]. The potential use of sanguinarine in clinical treatment of allergic asthma has also been suggested from an analysis of gene expression profile of asthma patients [84]. Sanguinarine is reported to have hERG potassium channel blocking effect. Therefore, in some situations where cardiac repolarization reserve is weak, it may increase the risk of potentially fatal ventricular arrhythmias in canines [63]. The cardiovascular properties of sanguinarine including hypotensive, antiplatelet and positive inotropic effects have also been described [53]. In a number of human tumor cells sanguinarine treatment resulted in boosting of intra cellular ROS, elevation of mitogen-activated protein kinase p38, triggering caspase 3/7 activation, inhibition of mitogen-activated protein kinase phosphatase 1 (MKP-1), depletion of glutathione and a host of other activities occurred.

7.7 Adverse Effects of Sanguinarine

There are concerns that the use of sanguinarine may cause leukoplakia in the mouth and oral dysplastic lesions. The use of sanguinarine and blood root for periodontal disease abacterially elicited inflammation of the gingival and periodontal tissue is also not based on adequate scientific support. There are unconfirmed reports that suggested that sanguinarine may cause sedation, faintness, vertigo, and possibly impair decision-making and increase response time. Bloodroot was reported to be used to stimulate menstruation and hence it was not advised to be used during pregnancy [77].

7.8 Conclusions

Plants containing sanguinarine were used extensively in traditional medicine in many parts of the world since centuries. Subsequent studies by researchers have found that this molecule has remarkable medicinal relevance. The high medicinal potency of sanguinarine is reported to cover wide spectrum of ailments. Its ability to inhibit bacterial adherence due to its antimicrobic properties potentiates its clinical use in periodontitis treatment and mouth washes. Sanguinarine is used as a dietary supplementation in animal feeds to reduce amino acid degradation, increase feed intake, and promote growth. Sanguinarine is a putative anticancer agent that is reported to arrest the cell cycle and induce apoptosis through various mechanisms that may include binding to DNA and tubilin and inhibiting many enzymes. Specifically, results from several studies reviewed above have indicated that sanguinarine inhibits the proliferation of cancer cells of different origins and apoptosis induction in different malignant cell lines takes place through the activation of cell surface receptors, intrinsic cytochrome *c* release from mitochondria pathways, etc. In spite of a number of studies the precise mechanisms and the diverse pathways by which the anticancer effect of this compound is manifested are still not fully understood. The information reviewed and summarized in this chapter reveals that sanguinarine is a potential cancer drug candidate and detailed studies including further vivo experiments are indispensable to elucidate whether administration of sanguinarine as therapeutics would be safe and effective for the treatment of human diseases.

Acknowledgments GSK acknowledges the Council of Scientific and Industrial Research (CSIR), Govt. of India for funding the research activities through network projects NWP0036 and GenCODE (BSC0123). GSK sincerely thanks Dr. M. Maiti, Ex. Scientist of CSIR-Indian Institute of Chemical Biology, who initiated and introduced him to the research on sanguinarine at the Biophysical Chemistry Laboratory, and also all the graduate students who have contributed to the understanding of the chemistry and biochemistry of the alkaloid. PB is a NET-Senior Research Fellow of the University Grants Commission, Govt. of India.

References

1. Absolínová H, Jančář L, Jančářová I, Vičar J, Kubáň V (2009) Acid–base behaviour of sanguinarine and dihydrosanguinarine. Open Chem 7(4):876–883
2. Adhami VM, Aziz MH, Mukhtar H, Ahmad N (2003) Activation of prodeath Bcl-2 family proteins and mitochondrial apoptosis pathway by sanguinarine in immortalized human HaCaT keratinocytes. Clin Cancer Res 9(8):3176–3182
3. Adhami VM, Aziz MH, Reagan-Shaw SR, Nihal M, Mukhtar H, Ahmad N (2004) Sanguinarine causes cell cycle blockade and apoptosis of human prostate carcinoma cells via modulation of cyclin kinase inhibitor–cyclin–cyclin-dependent kinase machinery. Mol Cancer Ther 3(8):933–940
4. Ahmad N, Gupta S, Husain MM, Heiskanen KM, Mukhtar H (2000) Differential antiproliferative and apoptotic response of sanguinarine for cancer cells versus normal cells. Clin Cancer Res 6(4):1524–1528
5. Ansari KM, Das M (2010) Potentiation of tumour promotion by topical application of argemone oil/isolated sanguinarine alkaloid in a model of mouse skin carcinogenesis. Chem Biol Interact 188(3):591–597
6. Arnason JT, Guèrin B, Kraml MM, Mehta B, Redmond RW, Scaiano JC (1992) Phototoxic and photochemical properties of sanguinarine. Photochem Photobiol 55:35–38
7. Babu CK, Khanna SK, Das M (2006) Safety evaluation studies on argemone oil through dietary exposure for 90 days in rats. Food Chem Toxicol 44:1151–1157

8. Babu CK, Khanna SK, Das M (2007) Adulteration of mustard cooking oil with argemone oil: Do Indian food regulatory policies and antioxidant therapy both need revisitation? Antioxid Redox Signal 9:515–525
9. Burgeiro A, Bento AC, Gajate C, Oliveira PJ, Mollinedo F (2013) Rapid human melanoma cell death induced by sanguinarine through oxidative stress. Eur J Pharmacol 705(1–3):109–118
10. Chan WH (2011) Embryonic toxicity of sanguinarine through apoptotic processes in mouse blastocysts. Toxicol Lett 205(3):285–292
11. Chan WH (2015) Hazardous effects of sanguinarine on maturation of mouse oocytes, fertilization, and fetal development through apoptotic processes. Environ Toxicol 30(8):946–955
12. Chang MC, Chan CP, Wang YJ, Lee PH, Chen LI, Tsai YL, Lin BR, Wang YL, Jeng JH (2007) Induction of necrosis and apoptosis to KB cancer cells by sanguinarine is associated with reactive oxygen species production and mitochondrial membrane depolarization. Toxicol Appl Pharmacol 218:143–151
13. Chen Y, Wang H, Zhang R, Wang H, Peng Z, Sun R, Tan Q (2012) Microinjection of sanguinarine into the ventrolateral orbital cortex inhibits Mkp-1 and exerts an antidepressant-like effect in rats. Neurosci Lett 506(2):327–331
14. Choi J, He N, Sung MK, Yang Y, Yoon S (2011) Sanguinarine is an allosteric activator of AMP-activated protein kinase. Biochem Biophys Res Commun 413(2):259–263
15. Chowdhury SR, Islam MM, Suresh Kumar G (2010) Binding of the anticancer alkaloid sanguinarine to double stranded RNAs: insights into the structural and energetics aspects. Mol BioSyst 6(7):1265–1276
16. Choy CS, Cheah KP, Chiou HY, Li JS, Liu YH, Yong SF, Chiu WT, Liao JW, Hu CM (2008) Induction of hepatotoxicity by sanguinarine is associated with oxidation of protein thiols and disturbance of mitochondrial respiration. J Appl Toxicol 28:945–956
17. Das M, Babu K, Reddy NP, Srivastava LM (2005) Oxidative damage of plasma proteins and lipids in epidemic dropsy patients: alterations in antioxidant status. Biochim Biophys Acta 1722:209–217
18. De Stefano I, Raspaglio G, Zannoni GF, Travaglia D, Prisco MG, Mosca M, Ferlini C, Scambia G, Gallo D (2009) Antiproliferative and antiangiogenic effects of the benzophenanthridine alkaloid sanguinarine in melanoma. Biochem Pharmacol 78(11):1374–1381
19. Debiton E, Madelmont JC, Legault J, Barthomeuf C (2003) Sanguinarine-induced apoptosis is associated with an early and severe cellular glutathione depletion. Cancer Chemother Pharmacol 51:474–482
20. Ding Z, Tang SC, Weerasinghe P, Yang X, Pater A, Liepins A (2002) The alkaloid sanguinarine is effective against multidrug resistance in human cervical cells via bimodal cell death. Biochem Pharmacol 63(8):1415–1421
21. Dong XZ, Zhang M, Wang K, Liu P, Guo DH, Zheng XL, Ge XY (2013) Sanguinarine inhibits vascular endothelial growth factor release by generation of reactive oxygen species in MCF-7 human mammary adenocarcinoma cells. BioMed Res Int 517698
22. Dvorák Z, Simánek V (2007) Metabolism of sanguinarine: the facts and the myths. Curr Drug Metab 8(2):173–176
23. Eversole LR, Eversole GM, Kopcik J (2000) Sanguinaria-associated oral leukoplakia. Comparison with other benign and dysplastic leukoplakic lesions. Oral Surg Oral Med Oral Pathol Oral Radiol Endod 89:455–464
24. Faddeeva MD, Beliaeva TN (1997) Sanguinarine and ellipticine cytotoxic alkaloids isolated from well-known antitumor plants: intracellular targets of their action. Tsitologiia 39:181–208
25. Ferraroni M, Bazzicalupi C, Bilia AR, Gratteri P (2011) X-Ray diffraction analyses of the natural isoquinoline alkaloids berberine and sanguinarine complexed with double helix DNA d (CGTACG). Chem Commun 47(17):4917–4919
26. Frankos VH, Brusick DJ, Johnson EM, Maibach HI, Munro I, Squire RA, Weil CS (1990) Safety of sauguinaria extract as used in commercial tooth- paste and oral rinse products. J Can Dent Assoc 56:41–47

27. Godowski KC, Wolff ED, Thompson DM, Housley CJ, Polson AM, Dunn RL, Duke SP, Stoller NH, Southard GL (1995) Whole mouth microbiota effects following subgingival delivery of sanguinarium. J Periodontol 66(10):870–877
28. Görner H, Miskolczy Z, Megyesi M, Biczók L (2011) Photooxidation of alkaloids: considerable quantum yield enhancement by rose bengal-sensitized singlet molecular oxygen generation. Photochem Photobiol 87(6):1315–1320
29. Han MH, Kim GY, Yoo YH, Choi YH (2013) Sanguinarine induces apoptosis in human colorectal cancer HCT-116 cells through ROS-mediated Egr-1 activation and mitochondrial dysfunction. Toxicol Lett 220:157–166
30. Han MH, Park C, Jin CY, Kim GY, Chang YC, Moon SK, Kim WJ, Choi YH (2013) Apoptosis induction of human bladder cancer cells by sanguinarine through reactive oxygen species-mediated up-regulation of early growth response gene-1. PLoS ONE 8(5):e63425
31. Hazra S, Suresh Kumar G (2014) Structural and thermodynamic studies on the interaction of iminium and alkanolamine forms of sanguinarine with hemoglobin. J Phys Chem B 118 (14):3771–3784
32. Holy J, Lamont G, Perkins E (2006) Disruption of nucleocytoplasmic trafficking of cyclin D1 and topoisomerase II by sanguinarine. BMC Cell Biol 7:13
33. Hossain M, Kabir A, Suresh Kumar G (2012) Binding of the anticancer alkaloid sanguinarine with $tRNA^{phe}$: spectroscopic and calorimetric studies. J Biomol Struct Dyn 30(2):223–234
34. Hossain M, Suresh Kumar G (2009) DNA binding of benzophenanthridine compounds sanguinarine versus ethidium: Comparative binding and thermodynamic profile of intercalation. J Chem Thermodyn 41(6):764–774
35. Hossain M, Khan AY, Suresh Kumar G (2011) Interaction of the anticancer plant alkaloid sanguinarine with bovine serum albumin. PLoS ONE 6(4):e18333
36. Hossain M, Khan AY, Suresh Kumar G (2012) Study on the thermodynamics of the binding of iminium and alkanolamine forms of the anticancer agent sanguinarine to human serum albumin. J Chem Thermodyn 47:90–99
37. Huh J, Liepins A, Zielonka J, Andrekopoulos C, Kalyanaraman B, Sorokin A (2006) Cyclooxygenase 2 rescues LNCaP prostate cancer cells from sanguinarine-induced apoptosis by a mechanism involving inhibition of nitric oxide synthase activity. Cancer Res 66(7):3726–3736
38. Jang BC, Park JG, Song DK, Baek WK, Yoo SK, Jung KH, Park GY, Lee TY, Suh SI (2009) Sanguinarine induces apoptosis in A549 human lung cancer cells primarily via cellular glutathione depletion. Toxicol In Vitro 23(2):281–287
39. Janovská M, Kubala M, Šimánek V, Ulrichová J (2009) Fluorescence of sanguinarine: fundamental characteristics and analysis of interconversion between various forms. Anal Bioanal Chem 395:235–240
40. Jash C, Payghan PV, Ghoshal N, Suresh Kumar G (2014) Binding of the iminium and alkanolamine forms of sanguinarine to lysozyme: spectroscopic analysis, thermodynamics, and molecular modeling studies. J Phys Chem B 118(46):13077–13091
41. Jeng JH, Wu HL, Lin BR, Lan WH, Chang HH, Ho YS, Lee PH, Wang YJ, Wang JS, Chen YJ, Chang MC (2007) Antiplatelet effect of sanguinarine is correlated to calcium mobilization, thromboxane and cAMP production. Atherosclerosis 191(2):250–258
42. Jones RR, Harkrader RJ, Southard GL (1986) The effect of pH on sanguinarine iminium ion form. J Nat Prod 49(6):1109–1111
43. Kaminskyy V, Kulachkovskyy O, Stoika R (2008) A decisive role of mitochondria in defining rate and intensity of apoptosis induction by different alkaloids. Toxicol Lett 177:168–181
44. Kantas D, Papatsiros VG, Tassis PD, Athanasiou LV, Tzika ED (2015) The effect of a natural feed additive (*Macleaya cordata*), containing sanguinarine, on the performance and health status of weaning pigs. Anim Sci J 86(1):92–98
45. Kemény-Beke A, Aradi J, Damjanovich J, Beck Z, Facskó A, Berta A, Bodnár A (2006) Apoptotic response of uveal melanoma cells upon treatment with chelidonine, sanguinarine and chelerythrine. Cancer Lett 237(1):67–75

46. Kim S, Lee TJ, Leem J, Choi KS, Park JW, Kwon TK (2008) Sanguinarine-induced apoptosis: generation of ROS, down-regulation of Bcl-2, c-FLIP, and synergy with TRAIL. J Cell Biochem 104(3):895–907
47. Kosina P, Walterová D, Ulrichová J, Lichnovský V, Stiborová M, Rýdlová H, Vicar J, Krecman V, Brabec MJ, Simánek V (2004) Sanguinarine and chelerythrine: assessment of safety on pigs in ninety days feeding experiment. Food Chem Toxicol 42(1):85–91
48. Laster LL, Lobene RR (1990) New perspectives on sanguinaria clinicals: individual toothpaste and oral rinse testing. J Can Dent Assoc 56(7):19–30
49. Lee B, Lee SJ, Park SS, Kim SK, Kim SR, Jung JH, Kim WJ, Moon SK (2008) Sanguinarine-induced G1-phase arrest of the cell cycle results from increased p27KIP1 expression mediated via activation of the Ras/ERK signaling pathway in vascular smooth muscle cells. Arch Biochem Biophys 471(2):224–231
50. Li W, Li H, Yao H, Mu Q, Zhao G, Li Y, Hu H, Niu X (2014) Pharmacokinetic and anti-inflammatory effects of sanguinarine solid lipid nanoparticles. Inflammation 37(2):632–638
51. Lopus M, Panda D (2006) The benzophenanthridine alkaloid sanguinarine perturbs microtubule assembly dynamics through tubulin binding: a possible mechanism for its antiproliferative activity. FEBS J 273(10):2139–2150
52. Lu JJ, Bao JL, Chen XP, Huang M, Wang YT (2012) Alkaloids isolated from natural herbs as the anticancer agents. Evid Based Complement Altern Med. Article ID 485042
53. Mackraj I, Govender T, Gathiram P (2008) Sanguinarine. Cardiovasc Ther 26(1):75–83
54. Maiti M, Chatterjee A (1995) Production of singlet oxygen by sanguinarine and berberine. Curr Sci 68:734–736
55. Maiti M, Das S, Sen A, Das A, Suresh Kumar G, Nandi R (2002) Influence of DNA structures on the conversion of sanguinarine alkanolamine form to iminium form. J Biomol Struct Dyn 20(3):455–464
56. Maiti M, Nandi R, Chaudhuri K (1983) The effect of pH on the absorption and fluorescence spectra of sanguinarine. Photochem Photobiol 38(2):245–249
57. Maiti M, Nandi R, Chaudhuri K (1982) Sanguinarine: a monofunctional intercalating alkaloid. FEBS Lett 142(2):280–284
58. Malikova J, Zdarilova A, Hlobilkova A, Ulrichova J (2006) The effect of chelerythrine on cell growth, apoptosis, and cell cycle in human normal and cancer cells in comparison with sanguinarine. Cell Biol Toxicol 22:439–453
59. Matkar SS, Wrischnik LA, Hellmann-Blumberg U (2008) Production of hydrogen peroxide and redox cycling can explain how sanguinarine and chelerythrine induce rapid apoptosis. Biochem Biophys 477:43–52
60. Mo S, Xiong H, Shu G, Yang X, Wang J, Zheng C, Xiong W, Mei Z (2013) Phaseoloideside E, a novel natural triterpenoid saponin identified from Entada phaseoloides, induces apoptosis in Ec-109 esophageal cancer cells through reactive oxygen species generation. J Pharmacol Sci 122(3):163–175
61. Nandi R, Chaudhuri K, Maiti M (1985) Effects of ionic strength and pH on the binding of sanguinarine to deoxyribonucleic acid. Photochem Photobiol 42(5):497–503
62. Niu X, Fan T, Li W, Xing W, Huang H (2012) The anti-inflammatory effects of sanguinarine and its modulation of inflammatory mediators from peritoneal macrophages. Eur J Pharmacol 689(1–3):262–269
63. Orvos P, Virág L, Tálosi L, Hajdú Z, Csupor D, Jedlinszki N, Szél T, Varró A, Hohmann J (2015) Effects of Chelidonium majus extracts and major alkaloids on hERG potassium channels and on dog cardiac action potential—a safety approach. Fitoterapia 100:156–165
64. Park H, Bergeron E, Senta H, Guillemette K, Beauvais S, Blouin R, Sirois J, Faucheux N (2010) Sanguinarine induces apoptosis of human osteosarcoma cells through the extrinsic and intrinsic pathways. Biochem Biophys Res Commun 399:446–451
65. Park SY, Jin ML, Kim YH, Kim CM, Lee SJ, Park G (2014) Involvement of heme oxygenase1 in neuroprotection by sanguinarine against glutamate-triggered apoptosis inHT22 neuronal cells. Environ Toxicol Pharmacol 38(3):701–710

66. Parsons LG, Thomas LG, Southard GL, Woodall IR, Jones BJ (1897) Effect of sanguinaria extract on established plaque and gingivitis when supragingivally delivered as a manual rinse or under pressure in an oral irrigator. J Clin Periodontol 14(7):381–385
67. Philogène BJ, Arnason JT, Towers GH, Abramowski Z, Campos F, Champagne D, McLachlan D (1984) Berberine: a naturally occurring phototoxic alkaloid. J Chem Ecol 10:115–123
68. Pickler L, Beirão BCB, Hayashi RM, Durau JF, Lourenço MC, Caron LF, Santin E (2013) Effect of sanguinarine in drinking water on Salmonella control and the expression of immune cells in peripheral blood and intestinal mucosa of broilers. J Appl Poult res 22:430–438
69. Pridgeon JW, Klesius PH, Dominowski PJ, Yancey RJ, Kievit MS (2013) Effects of praziquantel and sanguinarine on expression of immune genes and susceptibility to *Aeromonas hydrophila* in goldfish (*Carassius auratus*) infected with *Dactylogyrus intermedius*. Fish Shellfish Immunol 35:1301–1308
70. Selvi BR, Pradhan SK, Shandilya J, Das C, Sailaja BS, Naga Shankar G, Gadad SS, Reddy A, Dasgupta D, Kundu TK (2009) Sanguinarine interacts with chromatin, modulates epigenetic modifications, and transcription in the context of chromatin. Chem Biol 16(2):203–216
71. Sen A, Maiti M (1994) Interaction of sanguinarine iminium and alkanolamine form with calf thymus DNA. Biochem Pharmacol 48(11):2097–2102
72. Serafim TL, Matos JA, Sardão VA, Pereira GC, Branco AF, Pereira SL, Parke D, Perkins EL, Moreno AJ, Holy J, Oliveira PJ (2008) Sanguinarine cytotoxicity on mouse melanoma K1735-M2 cells–nuclear vs. mitochondrial effects. Biochem Pharmacol 76(11):1459–1475
73. Sharma BD, Malhotra S, Bhatia V, Rathee M (1999) Epidemic dropsy in India. Postgrad Med J 75(889):657–661
74. Singh CK, Kaur S, George J, Nihal M, Hahn MC, Scarlett CO, Ahmad N (2015) Molecular signatures of sanguinarine in human pancreatic cancer cells: a large scale label-free comparative proteomics approach. Oncotarget 6(12):10335–10349
75. Suresh Kumar G, Das A, Maiti M (1997) Photochemical conversion of sanguinarine to oxysanguinarine. J Photochem Photochem A 111:51–56
76. Suresh Kumar G, Hazra S (2014) Sanguinarine, a promising anticancer therapeutic: photochemical and nucleic acid binding properties. RSC Adv 4:56518–56531
77. Wynn SG, Wynn DVM, Fougère B (2007) Veterinary herbal medicine. Mater Med 24:459–672
78. Tuveson RW, Larson RA, Marley KA, Wang GR, Berenbaum MR (1989) Sanguinarine, a phototoxic H_2O_2-producing alkaloid. Photochem Photobiol 50(6):733–738
79. Vogt A, Tamewitz A, Skoko J, Sikorski RP, Giuliano KA, Lazo JS (2005) The benzo[c] phenanthridine alkaloid, sanguinarine, is a selective, cell-active inhibitor of mitogen-activated protein kinase phosphatase-1. J Biol Chem 280(19):19078–19086
80. Vrba J, Dolezel P, Vicar J, Ulrichova J (2009) Cytotoxic activity of sanguinarine and dihydrosanguinarine in human promyelocytic leukemia HL-60 cells. Toxicol In Vitro 23:580–588
81. Vrba J, Hrbac J, Ulrichova J, Modriansky M (2004) Sanguinarine is a potent inhibitor of oxidative burst in DMSO-differentiated HL-60 cells by a non-redox mechanism. Chem Biol Interact 147:35–47
82. Wang L, Cao H, Lu N, Liu L, Wang B, Hu T, Israel DA, Peek RM Jr, Polk BD, Ya F (2013) Berberine inhibits proliferation and down-regulates epidermal growth factor receptor through activation of Cbl in colon tumor cells. PLoS ONE 8(2):e56666
83. Wang Q, Zhao Z, Shang J, Xia W (2014) Targets and candidate agents for type 2 diabetes treatment with computational bioinformatics approach. J Diabetes Res 2014:763936
84. Wang XQ, Wang XM, Zhou TF, Dong LQ (2012) Screening of differentially expressed genes and small molecule drugs of paediatric allergic asthma with DNA microarray. Eur Rev Med Pharmacol Sci 16(14):1961–1966
85. Weerasinghe P, Hallock S, Tang SC, Liepins A (2001) Sanguinarine induces bimodal cell death in K562 but not in high Bcl-2-expressing JM1 cells. Pathol Res Pract 197(11):717–726

86. Wolff J, Knipling L (1993) Antimicrotubule properties of benzophenanthridine alkaloids. Biochemistry 32:13334–13339
87. Xu JY, Zhao L, Chong Y, Jiao Y, Qin LQ, Fan SJ (2014) Protection effect of sanguinarine on whole-body exposure of X radiation in BALB/c mice. Braz J Pharm Sci 50:101–106
88. Zhang DS, Li YY, Chen XJ, Li YJ, Liu ZY, Xie WJ, Sun ZL (2015) BCL2 promotor methylation and miR-15a/16-1 upregulation is associated with sanguinarine-induced apoptotic death in rat HSC-T6 cells. J Pharmacol Sci 127(1):135–144

Chapter 8
Piperine and Its Role in Chronic Diseases

Giuseppe Derosa, Pamela Maffioli and Amirhossein Sahebkar

Abstract Alkaloids include a family of naturally occurring chemical compounds containing mostly basic nitrogen atoms. Piperine is an alkaloid present in black pepper (*Piper nigrum*), one of the most widely used spices, in long pepper (*Piper longum*), and other *Piper* species fruits belonging to the family of Piperaceae. Piperine is responsible for the black pepper distinct biting quality. Piperine has many pharmacological effects and several health benefits, especially against chronic diseases, such as reduction of insulin-resistance, anti-inflammatory effects, and improvement of hepatic steatosis. The aim of this chapter is to summarize the effects of piperine, alone or in combination with other drugs and phytochemicals, in chronic diseases.

G. Derosa (✉) · P. Maffioli
Department of Internal Medicine and Therapeutics, Fondazione IRCCS Policlinico S. Matteo, University of Pavia, P.le C. Golgi 2, 27100 Pavia, Italy
e-mail: giuseppe.derosa@unipv.it

G. Derosa · P. Maffioli
Center for Prevention, Surveillance, Diagnosis and Treatment of Rare Diseases, Fondazione IRCCS Policlinico San Matteo, Pavia, Italy

G. Derosa
Center for the Study of Endocrine-Metabolic Pathophysiology and Clinical Research, University of Pavia, Pavia, Italy

G. Derosa
Laboratory of Molecular Medicine, University of Pavia, Pavia, Italy

P. Maffioli
PhD School in Experimental Medicine, University of Pavia, Pavia, Italy

A. Sahebkar
Biotechnology Research Center, Mashhad University of Medical Sciences, Mashhad, Iran

A. Sahebkar (✉)
Department of Medical Biotechnology, School of Medicine, Mashhad University of Medical Sciences, P.O. Box 91779-48564, Mashhad, Iran
e-mail: sahebkara@mums.ac.ir; amir_saheb2000@yahoo.com

S.C. Gupta et al. (eds.), *Anti-inflammatory Nutraceuticals and Chronic Diseases*,
Advances in Experimental Medicine and Biology 928,
DOI 10.1007/978-3-319-41334-1_8

Keywords Anti-depressant effects · Bioavailability enhancer · Insulin-resistance · Piperine

8.1 Introduction

Alkaloids include a family of naturally occurring chemical compounds containing mostly basic nitrogen atoms. In addition to carbon, hydrogen, and nitrogen, alkaloids may also contain oxygen, sulfur, or, rarely, other elements including chlorine, bromine, and phosphorus [1]. Alkaloids also include some related compounds with neutral, or even weakly acidic properties.

In the recent decades, some alkaloids have been introduced for use in clinical practice: berberine, for example, has been used for long in oriental medicine to treat gastrointestinal infections and diarrhea, but also for its beneficial effects on cardiovascular system. Lately also piperine, formally known as (2E,4E)-5-(1,3-benzodioxol-5-yl)-1-(1-piperidinyl)-2,4-pentadien-1-one with the following formula $C_{17}H_{19}NO_3$ (Fig. 8.1), became very used in clinical practice due to its beneficial properties. Piperine is an alkaloid present in black pepper (*Piper nigrum*), one of the most widely used spices, in long pepper (*Piper longum*), and other Piper species fruits belonging to the family o Piperaceae. Piperine is responsible of black pepper distinct biting quality. Black pepper is used not only in human dietaries, but also for many other purposes such as medicinal, as a preservative, and in perfumery.

8.1.1 Pharmacological Properties of Piperine

Current literature reveals a wide spectrum of biological activities of piperine as it stimulates the digestive enzymes of pancreas, helps in inhibiting oxidation reactions caused by free radicals and enhances the bioavailability of a number of therapeutic drugs. Moreover, piperine proved to have anti-inflammatory activities in models of

Fig. 8.1 piperine structure

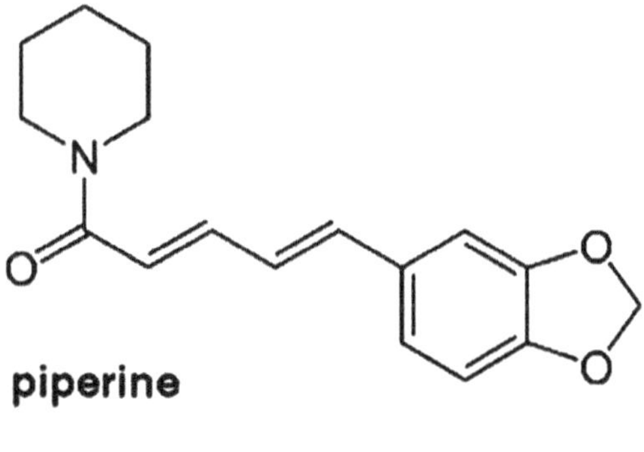

many inflammatory autoimmune diseases, such as inflammatory bowel disease, arthritis, type 1 diabetes as well as cancer [2]. Piperine activates transient receptor potential vanilloid type 1 receptor, and modulates GABAA receptors [3, 4]. At similar levels, piperine inhibits both monoamine oxidases (MAOs), for MAO-A and MAO-B, respectively [5]. Like other natural compounds containing methylenedioxyphenyl substituents, piperine affects cytochrome P450 (CYP) isoforms, inhibiting CYP3A species, and increasing expression of CYP1A and CYP2B in liver [6]. It also has a biphasic effect on P-glycoprotein activity [7]. Piperine is also reported to modulate cell signaling pathways such as NF-kB pathway [8].

Piperine is able to modify supplement and drug metabolism, and it also inhibits drug detoxifying enzymes. This typically increases bioavailability of any compound which would normally be attacked by these enzymes. This can be good to favor positive effects of some compound such as curcumin or resveratrol, or it can be bad by stopping a protective measure against toxic xenobiotics. In fact, piperine inhibits glucuronidation, a process happening in the liver which attaches a molecule (glucuronide) to drugs to signal for their urinary excretion. This process prevents excessive levels of drugs and supplements in the body, but sometimes inhibits all uptake and renders some supplements useless. In the scenario of piperine ingestion, excretion of supplements is hindered and certain drugs and supplements can bypass this regulatory stage (as not all are subject to it). This is good in some cases, as piperine is required to give curcumin to the extremities rather than it getting consumed by glucuronidation in the liver. However, in some other cases, it can lead to elevated levels of certain drugs in the blood. Again, elevated could be good or bad depending on context; regardless, caution should be taken when approaching this compound.

Piperine has many potential benefits in clinical practice; a lot of studies were reported in literature about piperine effects in chronic disease, especially in animals. In vitro studies showed piperine protective effects against oxidative damage by inhibiting or quenching free radicals and reactive oxygen species. Piperine treatment also reduced lipid peroxidation in vivo, and beneficially influenced anti-oxidant molecules and anti-oxidant enzymes in a number of experimental situations of oxidative stress [9]. The aim of this chapter will be to analyze the effects of piperine, alone or in combination, in chronic diseases.

8.2 Role of Piperine in Chronic Diseases

8.2.1 Piperine and Oxidative Stress

Piperine suppresses the accumulation of lipid peroxidation products, enhances the activity of anti-oxidant enzymes and eliminates the accumulation and activation of polymorphonuclear cell. This was showed by Umar et al. [10] that administered piperine at a dose of 100 mg/kg and indomethacin at 1 mg/kg body weight once daily for 21 days in male Wistar rats affected by collagen-induced arthritis (CIA). Piperine was effective in bringing significant changes on all the biochemical and inflammatory and parameters studies, in particular piperine significantly reduced the levels of pro-inflammatory mediators [interleukin-1β (IL-1β), tumor necrosis factor-α (TNF-α), and prostaglandin-2 (PGE2)] and increased level of interleukin-10 (IL-10). The protective effects of piperine against arthritis were also evident from the decrease in arthritis scoring and bone histology. These results clearly indicate that the protective role of piperine was mediated via its anti-oxidant effect through the suppression of lipid peroxidation and boosting the anti-oxidant defense system. Piperine seems to shift the balance of cytokines toward a bone protecting pattern that acts to both lower levels of TNF-a, IL-1β, and raise the levels of IL-10. Part of the beneficial anti-inflammatory and cartilage/bone protective effects of piperine may be mediated through the inhibition of pro-inflammatory cytokines.

8.2.2 Piperine and Inflammation

Piperine proved to have anti-inflammatory effects on Helicobacter pylori-induced gastritis in gerbils, through the suppression of inflammatory factors, such as TNF-α, independent of direct anti-bacterial activities, and may have potential for use in the chemoprevention of Helicobacted pylori-associated gastric carcinogenesis [11]. In vitro studies showed that piperine can induce apoptosis and inhibits the expression of inflammatory cytokines in human cell lines [12, 13].

Piperine also inhibited polyclonal and antigen-specific proliferation of mouse T lymphocytes, as well as cytokine synthesis and the induction of cytotoxic effector cells as reported by Doucette et al. [14]. These actions on T lymphocytes were associated with hypophosphorylation of Akt, extracellular signal-regulated kinase (ERK), and NF-kB components, in particular IκBα, but not ZAP-70, all molecules involved in T lymphocyte activation.

8.2.3 Piperine Effects on Hepatic Steatosis and Insulin-Resistance

Hepatic steatosis is due to an excess of plasma fatty acids, even if de novo lipogenesis is also considered an important contributing factor. Previously published studies showed that AMP-activated protein kinase (AMPK) is thought to regulate hepatic lipogenic gene expression by inhibiting transcription factors [15]. The inhibition of AMPK activates liver X receptor a (LXRa), a major regulator of lipogenesis. In animal models with high-fat diet (HFD)-induced fatty liver, LXRa is transcriptionally upregulated and consequently activates lipogenic target genes, thus exacerbating hepatic steatosis [16]. Piperine plays a role in the transcriptional regulation of LXRa; in particular it antagonized LXRa transcriptional activity by abolishing the interaction of ligand-bound LXRa with the co-activator CREB-binding protein. The effects of piperine on hepatic lipid accumulation were likely regulated via alterations in LXRa-mediated lipogenesis in mice fed a high-fat diet. Piperine positive effects on insulin-resistance and hepatic steatosis were reported by Choi et al. [17]. In this study, Authors examined the effect of piperine on hepatic steatosis and insulin-resistance induced in mice by feeding a high-fat diet (HFD) for 13 weeks. Administration of piperine (50 mg/kg body weight) to mice with HFD-induced hepatic steatosis resulted in a significant increase in plasma adiponectin levels. Also, elevated plasma concentrations of insulin and glucose and hepatic lipid levels induced by feeding a HFD were reversed in mice when they were administered piperine. Piperine reversed HFD-induced downregulation of adiponecitn-AMPK signaling molecules which play an important role in mediating lipogenesis, fatty acid oxidation, and insulin signaling in the livers of mice. Piperine significantly decreased the phosphorylation of insulin receptor substrate-1 (IRS-1) compared with the HFD-fed mice. The positive effects of piperine were confirmed by Rondanelli et al. [18] in humans. They administered a combination of bioactive food ingredients (epigallocatechin gallate, capsaicins, piperine, and L-carnitine) versus placebo, in a randomized, double-blind, 8 weeks trial, involving 86 overweight subjects. Consumption of the dietary supplement was associated with a significantly greater decrease in insulin-resistance, assessed by homeostasis model assessment, leptin/adiponectin ratio, respiratory quotient, LDL-cholesterol. Leptin, ghrelin, C-reactive protein decreased, and resting energy expenditure increased significantly in the supplemented group compared to placebo. These results suggest that piperine, in combination with epigallocatechin gallate, capsaicins, and L-carnitine, could be useful for the treatment of obesity-related inflammatory metabolic dysfunctions.

8.2.4 Piperine and Anti-depressant Effects

Piperine proved to have anti-depressant effects as published by Li et al. [19]: these Authors investigated the anti-depressant-like effect of piperine in mice exposed to chronic mild stress (CMS) procedure, administering piperine for 14 days at the doses of 2.5, 5, and 10 mg/kg. Piperine reversed the CMS-induced changes in sucrose consumption, plasma corticosterone level and open field activity. Furthermore, the decreased proliferation of hippocampal progenitor cells was ameliorated and the level of brain-derived neurotrophic factor (BDNF) in hippocampus of CMS stressed mice was upregulated by piperine treatment in the same time course.

This was further confirmed by Mao et al. [20] who examined the behavioral and biochemical effects of piperine in rats exposed to chronic unpredictable mild stress. The results showed that chronic unpredictable mild stress caused depression-like behavior in rats, as indicated by the significant decrease in sucrose consumption and increase in immobility time in the forced swim test. In addition, it was found that serotonin (5-HT) and BDNF contents in the hippocampus and frontal cortex were significantly decreased in chronic unpredictable mild stress-treated rats. Treating the animals with piperine significantly suppressed behavioral and biochemical changes induced by chronic unpredictable mild stress.

The anti-depressant effects of piperine can be explained throughout upregulation of the progenitor cell proliferation of hippocampus and cytoprotective activity, which may be closely related to the elevation of hippocampal BDNF level. The results indicated that the anti-depressant effects of piperine might be partly related to its modulating in hypothalamic-pituitary-adrenal activity and thereby the resulting neurogenesis. Piperine is a monoamine oxidase inhibitor, and thus can increase the levels of brain monoamines, such as 5-HT or norepinephrine (NE), involved in upregulation of neurogenesis. Also BDNF plays an important role in adult neurogenesis: BDNF can promote cell survival in the subventricular zone in both young and senescent rats [21]. Increase of the 5-HT, NE, and downstream of BDNF level is, at least part, of the mechanism enhancing neurogenesis, cytoprotectivity, and anti-depressant effect of piperine, besides its effects on hypothalamic-pituitary-adrenal axis.

8.2.5 Piperine Analgesic and Anti-pyretic Effects

In literature there are studies about the possible analgesic, and anti-pyretic effects of piperine as reported by Evan Prince et al. [22]. Authors treated mice with piperine (20 and 30 mg/kg) intraperitoneally; hot plate reaction test and acetic acid test were used to determine the analgesic activity of piperine in mice. It was found that piperine has significant analgesic and anti-pyretic activities without ulcerogenic effects. The results were comparable with indomethacin which was used as standard drug for reference. Despite that, further studies are required to elucidate the mechanism of piperine to confirm these activities.

8.2.6 Piperine as a Bioavailability Enhancer

Because of its properties, piperine increases bioavailability of different agents, listed in Table 8.1. Mechanism throughout piperine acts as bioavailability enhancer include: inhibition of a number of enzymes responsible for metabolizing drugs and nutritional substances; stimulation of the activity of amino acid transporters in the intestinal lining, inhibition of P-glycoprotein, the protein that removes substances from cells, decreasing the intestinal production of glucuronic acid, thereby permitting more of the substances to enter the body in active form.

Table 8.1 Compounds with documented bioavailability enhancement upon piperine co-administration

Substances	
Barbiturates	Resveratrol
Pyrazinamide	Thiophylline
Beta-carotene	Propranolol
Rifampicin	Vitamin B-6
Coenzyme Q10	Nalorphine
Selenium	Phyllanthin
Curcumin	

Among agents whose bioavailability is enhanced by piperine is curcumin. Curcumin has been extensively studied for its therapeutic properties, such as anti-oxidant, anti-inflammatory, metabolic, anti-depressant, and neuroprotective activities [23–32]. However, low oral bioavailability of curcumin has been proposed to limit its approval as a therapeutic agent. Studies have reported that curcumin gets reduced through alcohol dehydrogenase, followed by conjugations like sulfation and glucuronidation in liver and intestine [24]. Piperine proved to enhance the bioavailability of curcumin and to potentiate its protective effects against chronic unpredictable stress-induced cognitive impairment and associated oxidative damage in mice [33]. Chronic treatment with curcumin (200 and 400 mg/kg, p.o.) significantly improved behavioral and biochemical alterations induced by chronic unpredictable stress, restored mitochondrial enzyme complex activities, and attenuated increased acetylcholinesterase and serum corticosterone levels. In addition, co-administration of piperine (20 mg/kg; p.o.) with curcumin (100 and 200 mg/kg, p.o.) significantly elevated the protective effect as compared to their effects alone.

This was further demonstrated by Banji et al. [34] that treated Wistar rats with piperine (12 mg/kg) alone, curcumin (40 mg/kg) alone or in combination for a period of 49 days by the oral route with treatment being initiated a week prior to D-galactose (60 mg/kg, i.p.). A control group, D-galactose alone and naturally aged control were also evaluated. The results suggested a superior response to combination therapy compared to monotherapy as evidenced by improved spatial memory, reduced oxidative burden, reduced accumulation of lipofuscin, improvement in signaling, increase in hippocampal volume and protection of hippocampal neurons. The powerful anti-oxidant nature of both, augmented response of curcumin in the presence of piperine and enhanced serotoninergic signaling was responsible for improved cognition and prevention in senescence.

Piperine combined with curcumin also proved to have a better anti-genotoxic effect compared to single treatment against benzo(a)pyrene (BaP)-induced DNA damage in lungs and livers of mice [35]. Authors administered curcumin (100 mg/kg body weight) and piperine (20 mg/kg body weight) separately as well as in combination orally in corn oil to swiss albino mice for 7 days as pretreatments and subsequently, 2 h after, BaP was administered orally in corn oil (125 mg/kg body weight). Pretreatments of curcumin and curcumin plus piperine before administration of single dose of BaP significantly decreased the levels of 8-oxo-dG content and percentage of DNA in the comet tail in both the tissues. Moreover, the genoprotective potential of curcumin plus piperine was significantly higher as compared to curcumin alone against BaP-induced DNA damage.

The anti-cancer property of curcumin is attributed to its anti-oxidant properties that inhibit free radicals from mediating peroxidation of membrane lipids or oxidative DNA damage as both are important initiators of cancer development. The enhanced anti-genotoxic potential of curcumin plus piperine may be due to increase bioavailability of curcumin thanks to piperine.

The synergic effect of piperine in combination with curcuminoid was confirmed also in humans by a meta-analysis conducted by Panahi et al. [36]: in this meta-analysis Authors evaluated the effectiveness of supplementation with a bioavailable curcuminoid preparation on measures of oxidative stress and inflammation in patients with metabolic syndrome. Authors concluded that short-term supplementation with curcuminoid-piperine combination significantly improves oxidative and inflammatory status in patients with metabolic syndrome. Also in this case piperine has been shown to overcome several pharmacokinetic drawbacks of curcuminoids, reducing the activity of glucuronidase enzymes both at the site of intestinal brush border and liver, resulting in improved absorption of curcuminoids. Increased intestinal perfusion and enterocyte permeability are additional mechanisms whereby piperine improves the bioavailability of curcuminoids [37].

The same authors also conducted a randomized controlled trial on the effects of a combination of piperine with curcuminoids on lipid profile, showing that curcuminoids-piperine combination is an efficacious adjunctive therapy in patients with metabolic syndrome and can modify serum lipid concentrations beyond what is achieved with standard of care [38].

This was also reported by Neyrinck et al. [39]: they fed mice with either a control diet, a high-fat diet or a high-fat diet containing *Curcuma longa* extract (0.1 % of curcumin in the high-fat diet) associated with white pepper (0.01 %) which contains piperine for 4 weeks. The co-supplementation in *Curcuma* extract and white pepper decreased high-fat-induced pro-inflammatory cytokines expression in the subcutaneous adipose tissue, an effect independent of adiposity, immune cells recruitment, angiogenesis, or modulation of gut bacteria controlling inflammation.

Piperine also acts as enhancer of quercitin, this was reported by Rinwa et al. [40]. They evaluated the efficacy of a combination of quercitin with piperine against chronic unpredictable stress-induced behavioral and biochemical alterations. They administered quercitin (20, 40, and 80 mg/kg, p.o.), piperine (20 mg/kg, p.o.) and their combinations daily 30 min before chronic unpredictable stress procedure to Laca mice for a period of 28 days. Chronic unpredictable stress increased brain oxidative stress markers and neuro-inflammation (TNF-a) in placebo groups treated with piracetam (100 mg/kg, i.p.). This was coupled with marked rise in acetylcholinesterase and serum corticosterone levels. Co-administration of piperine with quercitin significantly elevated their potential to restore these behavioral, biochemical, and molecular changes associated with mouse model of chronic unpredictable stress. Co-administration of quercitin (20 mg/kg) with piperine (20 mg/kg) significantly lowered TNF-α level which was significant as compared to their effects alone. These results suggest that piperine enhances the neuroprotective effects of quercitin against chronic unpredictable stress-induced oxidative stress, neuro-inflammation and memory deficits.

Piperine also enhanced phyllanthin bioavailability as published by Sethiya et al. [41]. These Authors evaluated the hepato-protective effects of phyllanthin along with piperine in a mixed micellar lipid formulation (MMLF). Authors compared phyllanthin (30 mg/kg p.o.), a complex phosphatidylcholine formulation of phyllanthin (CP–PC) (30 mg/kg p.o.), phyllanthin + piperine (CP–P–PC) (30 mg/kg p. o.), and the reference drug silymarin (100 mg/kg, p.o.) administered daily to rats for 10 days, followed by liver damage by administering a 1:1 (v/v) mixture of $CCl4$ and olive oil (1 ml/kg, i.p.) for 7 days from day 4 to day 10. The degree of protection was evaluated by determining the level of marker enzymes (SGOT and SGPT), bilirubin, and total proteins.

CP–P–PC (30 mg/kg p.o.) showed significant hepato-protective effect by reducing the levels of serum marker enzymes (SGOT, SGPT, and bilirubin), whereas, elevated the levels of depleted total protein, lipid peroxidation and anti-oxidant marker enzyme activities such as, glutathione, superoxide dismutase, catalase, glutathione peroxidase, and glutathione reductase. The complex MMLF normalized adverse conditions of rat livers more efficiently than the non-formulated phyllanthin, confirming, again, the effects of piperine in enhancing low bioavailability of phyllanthin.

Piperine can be used also in combination with resveratrol to enhance its bioavailability [42]: in this study Authors evaluated if co-supplementation of piperine with resveratrol affects the bioavailability and efficacy of resveratrol with regard to cognition and cerebral blood flow. In this randomized, double-blind, placebo-controlled, within-subjects study, 23 adults were given placebo, trans-resveratrol (250 mg) and trans-resveratrol with 20 mg piperine on separate days at least a week apart. The results indicated that when co-supplemented, piperine, and resveratrol significantly augmented cerebral blood flow during task performance in comparison with placebo and resveratrol alone. Cognitive function, mood, and blood pressure were not affected.

8.3 Conclusions

In conclusion, piperine has several important roles that can be useful in clinical practice, in particular for reduction of insulin-resistance, inflammation, and hepatic steatosis. However, the most far-reaching attribute of piperine is its inhibitory effect on enzymatic drug biotransformation reactions in the liver. Piperine strongly inhibits hepatic and intestinal aryl hydrocarbon hydroxylase and UDP-glucuronyl transferase, thus enhancing the bioavailability of a number of therapeutic drugs as well as phytochemicals. Piperine's bioavailability-enhancing property is also partly attributed to increased absorption as a result of its effect on the ultrastructure of intestinal brush border. This promising effect of piperine has been extensively employed to increase the bioavailability and pharmacological effects of several drugs and phytopharmaceuticals.

References

1. Manske RHF (1965) The alkaloids. Chemistry and physiology, vol VIII. Academic Press, New York, p 673
2. Selvendiran K, Sakthisekaran D (2004) Chemopreventive effect of piperine on modulating lipid peroxidation and membrane bound enzymes in benzo(a)pyrene induced lung carcinogenesis. Biomed Pharmacother 58:264–267
3. McNamara FN, Randall A, Gunthorpe MJ (2005) Effects of piperine, the pungent component of black pepper, at the human vanilloid receptor (TRPV1). Br J Pharmacol 144(6):781–790
4. Schöffmann A, Wimmer L, Goldman D et al (2014) Efficient modulation of γ-aminobutyric acid type A receptors by piperine derivatives. J Med Chem 57(37):5602–5619
5. Lee SA, Hong SS, Han XH et al (2005) Piperine from the fruits of *Piper longum* with inhibitory effect on monoamine oxidase and antidepressant-like activity. Chem Pharm Bull (Tokyo) 53(7):832–835
6. Murray M (2012) Toxicological actions of plant-derived and anthropogenic methylenedioxyphenyl-substituted chemicals in mammals and insects. J Toxicol Environ Health B Crit Rev 15(6):365–395
7. Najar IA, Sachin BS, Sharma SC et al (2010) Modulation of P-glycoprotein ATPase activity by some phytoconstituents. Phytother Res 24(3):454–458
8. Vaibhav K, Shrivastava P, Javed H, Khan A, Ahmed ME, Tabassum R, Khan MM, Khuwaja G, Islam F, Siddiqui MS, Safhi MM, Islam F (2012) Piperine suppresses cerebral ischemia-reperfusion-induced inflammation through the repression of COX-2, NOS-2, and NF-κB in middle cerebral artery occlusion rat model. Mol Cell Biochem 367(1–2):73–84
9. Srinivasan K (2007) Black pepper and its pungent principle-piperine: a review of diverse physiological effects. Crit Rev Food Sci Nutr 47(8):735–748
10. Umar S, Golam Sarwar AH, Umar K, Ahmad N, Sajad M, Ahmad S, Katiyar CK, Khan HA (2013) Piperine ameliorates oxidative stress, inflammation and histological outcome in collagen induced arthritis. Cell Immunol 284(1–2):51–59
11. Toyoda T, Shi L, Takasu S, Cho YM, Kiriyama Y, Nishikawa A, Ogawa K, Tatematsu M, Tsukamoto T (2015) Anti-Inflammatory effects of capsaicin and piperine on helicobacter pylori-induced chronic gastritis in mongolian gerbils. Helicobacter. doi:10.1111/hel.12243
12. Cai XZ, Huang WY, Qiao Y, Du SY, Chen Y, Chen D, Yu S, Che RC, Liu N, Jiang Y (2013) Inhibitory effects of curcumin on gastric cancer cells: a proteomic study of molecular targets. Phytomedicine 20:495–505
13. Xia Y, Khoi PN, Yoon HJ, Lian S, Joo YE, Chay KO, Kim KK, Jung YD (2015) Piperine inhibits IL-1b-induced IL-6 expression by suppressing p38 MAPK and STAT3 activation in gastric cancer cells. Mol Cell Biochem 398:147–156
14. Doucette CD, Rodgers G, Liwski RS, Hoskin DW (2015) Piperine from black pepper inhibits activation-induced proliferation and effector function of T lymphocytes. J Cell Biochem 116 (11):2577–2588
15. Nafisi S, Adelzadeh M, Norouzi Z, Sarbolouki MN (2009) Curcumin binding to DNA and RNA. DNA Cell Biol 28:201–208
16. Hwahng SH, Ki SH, Bae EJ, Kim HE, Kim SG (2009) Role of adenosine monophosphate activated protein kinase-p70 ribosomal S6 kinase-1 pathway in repression of liver X receptor-alpha-dependent lipogenic gene induction and hepatic steatosis by a novel class of dithiolethiones. Hepatology 49:1913–1925

17. Choi S, Choi Y, Choi Y, Kim S, Jang J, Park T (2013) Piperine reverses high fat diet-induced hepatic steatosis and insulin resistance in mice. Food Chem 141(4):3627–3635
18. Rondanelli M, Opizzi A, Perna S, Faliva M, Solerte SB, Fioravanti M, Klersy C, Cava E, Paolini M, Scavone L, Ceccarelli P, Castellaneta E, Savina C, Donini LM (2013) Improvement in insulin resistance and favourable changes in plasma inflammatory adipokines after weight loss associated with two months' consumption of a combination of bioactive food ingredients in overweight subjects. Endocrine 44(2):391–401
19. Li S, Wang C, Wang M, Li W, Matsumoto K, Tang Y (2007) Antidepressant like effects of piperine in chronic mild stress treated mice and its possible mechanisms. Life Sci 80 (15):1373–1381
20. Kirschenbaum B, Goldman SA (1995) Brain-derived neurotrophic factor promotes the survival of neurons arising from the adult rat forebrain subependymal zone. Proc Natl Acad Sci USA 92(1):210–214
21. Mao QQ, Huang Z, Zhong XM, Xian YF, Ip SP (2014) Piperine reverses chronic unpredictable mild stress-induced behavioral and biochemical alterations in rats. Cell Mol Neurobiol 34(3):403–408
22. Evan Prince S, Aayesha N, Mahima V, Mahaboobkhan R (2013) Analgesic, antipyretic and ulcerogenic effects of piperine: an active ingredient of pepper. J Pharm Sci Res 5(10):203–206
23. Motterlini R, Foresti R, Bassi R, Green CJ (2000) Curcumin, an antioxidant and anti-inflammatory agent, induces heme oxygenase-1 and protects endothelial cells against oxidative stress. Free Radic Biol Med 28:1303–1312
24. Wahlstrom B, Blennow GA (1978) Study on the fate of curcumin in the rat. Acta Pharm Toxicol 43:86–92
25. Sahebkar A, Chew GT, Watts GF (2014) Recent advances in pharmacotherapy for hypertriglyceridemia. Prog Lipid Res 56:47–66
26. Panahi Y, Badeli R, Karami GR, Sahebkar A (2015) Investigation of the efficacy of adjunctive therapy with bioavailability-boosted curcuminoids in major depressive disorder. Phytother Res 29(1):17–21
27. Panahi Y, Rahimnia AR, Sharafi M, Alishiri G, Saburi A, Sahebkar A (2014) Curcuminoid treatment for knee osteoarthritis: a randomized double-blind placebo-controlled trial. Phytother Res 28(11):1625–1631
28. Panahi Y, Saadat A, Beiraghdar F, Sahebkar A (2014) Adjuvant therapy with bioavailability-boosted curcuminoids suppresses systemic inflammation and improves quality of life in patients with solid tumors: a randomized double-blind placebo-controlled trial. Phytother Res 28(10):1461–1467
29. Sahebkar A (2014) Are curcuminoids effective C-reactive protein-lowering agents in clinical practice? Evidence from a meta-analysis. Phytother Res 28(5):633–642
30. Sahebkar A, Mohammadi A, Atabati A, Rahiman S, Tavallaie S, Iranshahi M, Akhlaghi S, Ferns GA, Ghayour-Mobarhan M (2013) Curcuminoids modulate pro-oxidant-antioxidant balance but not the immune response to heat shock protein 27 and oxidized LDL in obese individuals. Phytother Res 27:1883–1888
31. Mohammadi A, Sahebkar A, Iranshahi M, Amini M, Khojasteh R, Ghayour-Mobarhan M, Ferns GA (2013) Effects of supplementation with curcuminoids on dyslipidemia in obese patients: a randomized crossover trial. Phytother Res 27(3):374–379
32. Panahi Y, Ghanei M, Bashiri S, Hajihashemi A, Sahebkar A (2015) Short-term curcuminoid supplementation for chronic pulmonary complications due to sulfur mustard intoxication: Positive results of a randomized double-blind placebo-controlled trial. Drug Res (Stuttg) 65 (11):567–573
33. Rinwa P, Kumar A (2012) Piperine potentiates the protective effects of curcumin against chronic unpredictable stress-induced cognitive impairment and oxidative damage in mice. Brain Res 1488:38–50
34. Banji D, Banji OJ, Dasaroju S, Annamalai AR (2013) Piperine and curcumin exhibit synergism in attenuating D-galactose induced senescence in rats. Eur J Pharmacol 703(1–3):91–99

35. Sehgal A, Kumar M, Jain M, Dhawan DK (2011) Combined effects of curcumin and piperine in ameliorating benzo(a)pyrene induced DNA damage. Food Chem Toxicol 49(11): 3002–3006
36. Panahi Y, Hosseini MS, Khalili N, Naimi E, Majeed M, Sahebkar A (2015) Antioxidant and anti-inflammatory effects of curcuminoid-piperine combination in subjects with metabolic syndrome: A randomized controlled trial and an updated meta-analysis. Clin Nutr. doi:10.1016/j.clnu.2014.12.019
37. Atal CK, Dubey RK, Singh J (1985) Biochemical basis of enhanced drug bioavailability by piperine: evidence that piperine is a potent inhibitor of drug metabolism. J Pharmacol Exp Ther 232:258–262
38. Panahi Y, Khalili N, Hosseini MS, Abbasinazari M, Sahebkar A (2014) Lipid-modifying effects of adjunctive therapy with curcuminoids-piperine combination in patients with metabolic syndrome: results of a randomized controlled trial. Complement Ther Med 22 (5):851–857
39. Neyrinck AM, Alligier M, Memvanga PB, Névraumont E, Larondelle Y, Préat V, Cani PD, Delzenne NM (2013) Curcuma longa extract associated with white pepper lessens high fat diet-induced inflammation in subcutaneous adipose tissue. PLoS ONE 8(11):e81252
40. Rinwa P, Kumar A (2013) Quercetin along with piperine prevents cognitive dysfunction, oxidative stress and neuro-inflammation associated with mouse model of chronic unpredictable stress. Arch Pharm Res. doi:10.1007/s12272-013-0205-4
41. Sethiya NK, Shah P, Rajpara A, Nagar PA, Mishra SH (2015) Antioxidant and hepatoprotective effects of mixed micellar lipid formulation of phyllanthin and piperine in carbon tetrachloride-induced liver injury in rodents. Food Funct. doi:10.1039/c5fo00947b
42. Wightman EL, Reay JL, Haskell CF, Williamson G, Dew TP, Kennedy DO (2014) Effects of resveratrol alone or in combination with piperine on cerebral blood flow parameters and cognitive performance in human subjects: a randomised, double-blind, placebo-controlled, cross-over investigation. Br J Nutr 112(2):203–213

Chapter 9
Therapeutic Potential and Molecular Targets of Piceatannol in Chronic Diseases

Young-Joon Surh and Hye-Kyung Na

Abstract Piceatannol (3,3′,4,5′-tetrahydroxy-*trans*-stilbene; PIC) is a naturally occurring stilbene present in diverse plant sources. PIC is a hydroxylated analog of resveratrol and produced from resveratrol by microsomal cytochrome P450 1A11/2 and 1B1 activities. Like resveratrol, PIC has a broad spectrum of health beneficial effects, many of which are attributable to its antioxidative and anti-inflammatory activities. PIC exerts anticarcinogenic effects by targeting specific proteins involved in regulating cancer cell proliferation, survival/death, invasion, metastasis, angiogenesis, etc. in tumor microenvironment. PIC also has other health promoting and disease preventing functions, such as anti-obese, antidiabetic, neuroptotective, cardioprotective, anti-allergic, anti-aging properties. This review outlines the principal biological activities of PIC and underlying mechanisms with special focus on intracellular signaling molecules/pathways involved.

Keywords Piceatannol · Astringin · *trans*-Stilbene · Resveratrol

9.1 Introduction

Piceatannol (3,3′,4,5′-tetrahydroxy-*trans*-stilbene; PIC) is a naturally occurring stilbene found in a variety of plant sources including grapes, rhubarb, peanuts, sugarcane, white tea, and the seeds of passion fruit (*Passiflora edulis*). Astringin, a PIC glucoside, is found in red wine. PIC was identified as a selective inhibitor of

Y.-J. Surh (✉)
Department of Molecular Medicine and Biopharmaceutical Sciences,
Research Institute of Pharmaceutical Sciences, College of Pharmacy,
Seoul National University, Seoul 151-742, South Korea
e-mail: surh@snu.ac.kr

H.-K. Na (✉)
Department of Food and Nutrition, College of Human Ecology,
Sungshin Women's University, Seoul 142-732, South Korea
e-mail: nhkdec28@gmail.com

S.C. Gupta et al. (eds.), *Anti-inflammatory Nutraceuticals and Chronic Diseases*,
Advances in Experimental Medicine and Biology 928,
DOI 10.1007/978-3-319-41334-1_9

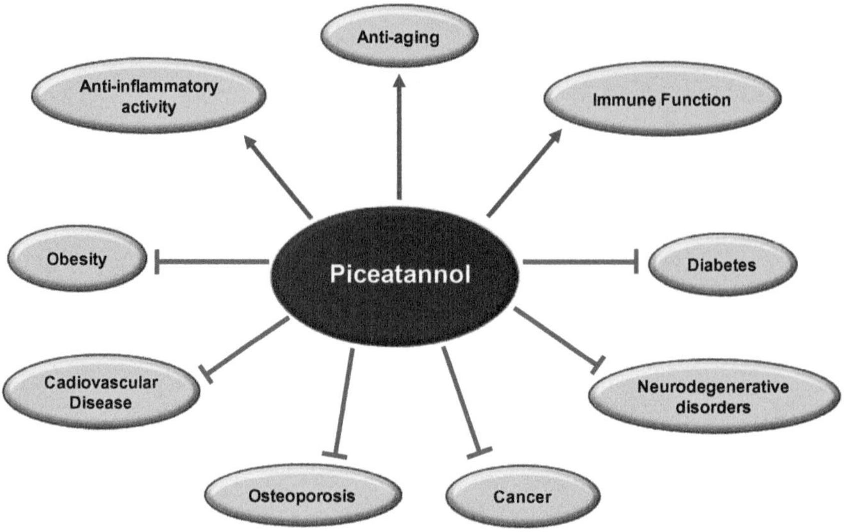

Fig. 9.1 Health beneficial and therapeutic effects of PIC

non-receptor spleen tyrosine kinase (Syk) which plays a critical role in the regulation of not only immune and inflammatory responses of hematopoietic cells, but also general physiological functions in a wide variety of non-hematopoietic cells [1].

As a hydroxylated analog and a metabolite of resveratrol (3,5,4′-trihydroxy-*trans*-stilbene), PIC has multiple biological functions, including antioxidative, anti-inflammatory, anticancer, antidiabetic, cardioprotective, neuroprotective, and immunomodulatory properties (Fig. 9.1). PIC has structural similarity to resveratrol and both compounds share a spectrum of biological activities [2, 3]. This review summarizes the updated research findings regarding the cancer chemopreventive/anticarcinogenic and other health promoting effects of PIC and underlying mechanisms.

9.2 Chemopreventive/Anticarcinogenic Effects

In an early study, PIC was shown to inhibit the development of 7,12-dimethylbenz(*a*)anthracene-induced preneoplastic lesions in a mouse mammary organ culture model [4]. In addition, the chemotherapeutic effects of PIC have been recently highlighted [5]. The anticarcinogenic and cancer chemopreventive effects of PIC are summarized below based on its action mechanisms (Fig. 9.2). The majority of studies on the anticarcinogenic and chemopreventive effects of PIC were done in cultured cells, and only few animal as well as human data are available. This may partly be due to the limited availability of relatively large amount of pure PIC needed for in vivo studies and resulting high cost.

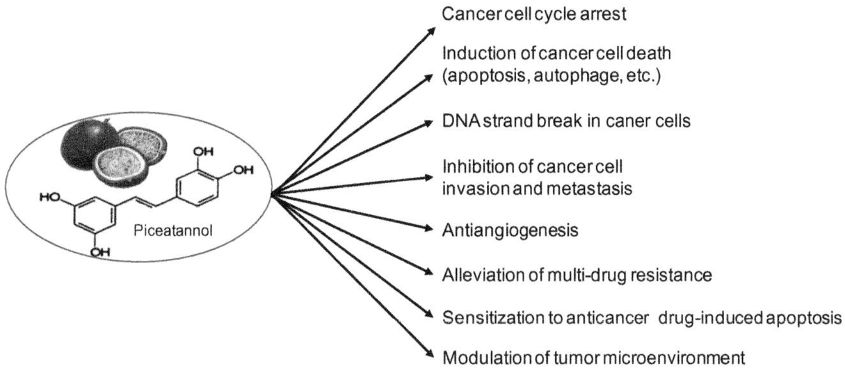

Fig. 9.2 Mechanisms of anticarcinogenic and cancer chemopreventive effects of PIC

9.2.1 Cell Cycle Arrest

Treatment of the human colon carcinoma Caco-2 cell line with PIC resulted in the reduced cell proliferation without influencing the differentiation [6]. Flow cytometric analysis of cell cycle distribution revealed an accumulation of cells in the S phase. Immunoblot analysis demonstrated that cyclin-dependent kinases (CDK) 2 and 6 as well as cdc2 were expressed at steady-state levels, whereas the expression of cyclin D1, cyclin B1, and CDK 4 was downregulated. The level of $p27^{KIP1}$ was also reduced, whereas that of cyclin E was enhanced. Similar changes were also observed in studies with HCT-116 colon cancer cells [6].

PIC also inhibits cell cycle progression in the DU145 human prostate cancer cell line. PIC treatment enhanced the percentage of cells in the G_1 phase and decreased [^{3}H]thymidine incorporation as well as expression of cyclin A, cyclin D1, CDK2, and CDK4. PIC suppressed CDK4 and CDK2 activities as well, but had no effect on the levels of $p21^{WAF1/CIP1}$ or $p27^{KIP1}$ [7]. PIC inhibited the proliferation of T24 and HT1376 human bladder cancer cells by blocking cell cycle progression in the G_0/G_1 phase and induced apoptosis. The G_0/G_1 phase arrest was attributed to an increased expression of $p21^{WAF1/CIP1}$. An enhancement in Fas/APO-1 and membrane-bound Fas ligand might be responsible for the apoptotic effect induced by PIC in the aforementioned bladder cancer cells [8].

9.2.2 Induction of Apoptosis

9.2.2.1 Hematologic Tumor Cells

Multiple Myeloma (MM) and Lymphoma

MM is a clonal B cell cancer characterized by proliferation of malignant plasma cells in the bone marrow. Although the introduction of immunomodulatory drugs like bortezomib or lenalidomide has improved patient survival, MM is still incurable, and new treatment options are needed. Treatment of MM cell lines (AMO-1, U266, and RPMI8226) as well as primary MM cells with PIC reduced proliferation and stromal cell-derived factor-1 alpha induced migration [9]. PIC induced apoptosis of MM cells, as revealed by reduced expression of procaspase 3, increased cleavage of poly(ADP-ribose) polymerase(PARP)-1 and enhanced release of cytochrome *c* (cyt *c*). The anti-proliferative and proapoptotic activities of PIC in MM cells appear to be mediated through suppression of Syk [9].

Aberrant activation of Wnt/β-catenin signaling promotes development and progression of various malignant neoplasms. The Wnt signaling pathway is constitutively activated in MM, which exaggerates cell proliferation. PIC inhibited Wnt/β-catenin signaling in murine plasmocytoma MPC11 cells as well as human MM (OPM-2, RPMI-8226, and U-266) cells. PIC induced apoptosis and suppressed the proliferation of these cells [10]. The combination of PIC with ethacrynic acid or ciclopirox olamine had a significant additive effect on the vitality of MM cells compared to single-agent application, while healthy cells remained unaffected [11].

PIC induced apoptosis in BJAB Burkitt-like lymphoma cells as evidenced by activation of caspase-3 and perturbation of mitochondrial permeability transition [12]. The antileukemic properties of PIC were also assessed using primary, leukemic lymphoblasts from 21 patients suffering from childhood lymphoblastic leukemia. PIC was found to be a very efficient inducer of apoptosis in this ex vivo assay as well [12].

Leukemia

PIC and other stilbenes were investigated for their tumor-specific cytotoxicity and apoptosis-inducing activity, using four human tumor cell lines (squamous cell carcinoma HSC-2, HSC-3, submandibular gland carcinoma HSG and promyelocytic leukemia HL-60) and three normal human oral cell lines (gingival fibroblast HGF, pulp cell HPC, periodontal ligament fibroblast HPLF). Among the seven cell lines, HL-60 and HSC-2 cells were the most sensitive to the cytotoxic action of these compounds. PIC induced internucleosomal DNA fragmentation and activation of caspases-3, -8, and -9 in HL-60 cells. [13].

PIC treatment to the human leukemia cell line U937 induced the formation of apoptotic bodies, DNA fragmentation, and the accumulation of the sub-G_1 phase [14]. The proapoptotic effect of PIC was associated with downregulation of anti-apoptotic Bcl-2 and cIAP-2, proteolytic activation of caspase-3, and the degradation/cleavage of PARP. z-DEVD-fmk, a caspase-3-specific inhibitor, attenuated the proapoptotic activity of PIC in U937 cells [14]. PIC-induced apoptotic death of human leukemia U937 cells was accompanied by an increase in the intracellular Ca^{2+} concentration ($[Ca^{2+}]_i$), inactivation of extracellular signal-regulated kinase (ERK), activation of p38 mitogen-activated protein kinase (MAPK), degradation of procaspase-8 and production of t-Bid [15]. PIC treatment increased the levels of Fas and FasL and their mRNA transcripts. Downregulation of FADD blocked PIC-induced procaspase-8 degradation and rescued viability of

PIC-treated cells [15]. PIC induced tumor necrosis factor-α (TNF-α)-related apoptosis-inducing ligand (TRAIL)-mediated leukemia cell death which was associated with significantly elevated expression of DR5, a death receptor of TRAIL [16]. Further, PIC-enhanced DR5 promoter activity via Sp1 activation. The DR5 chimera antibodies significantly suppressed PIC-mediated apoptosis in human monocytic leukemia cells by inactivating TRAIL signaling [16].

9.2.2.2 Solid Tumor Cells

PIC inhibited the growth of the androgen receptor-negative prostate PC3 cancer cell line which was associated with accumulation of endogenous ceramide [17]. In another study, the effects of PIC on proliferation of androgen-dependent LNCaP and androgen-independent DU145 and PC-3 prostate cancer cells were investigated [18]. PIC exerted anti-proliferative effects, which was accompanied by cell cycle blockade in G_1/S and S phases in LNCaP and PC-3 cells and induction of apoptosis in DU145 cells [18]. PIC induced apoptosis of DU145 cells was evidenced by cleavage of caspase 3 and apoptosis inducing factor AIF and an increase in total cyt *c*. The apoptotic changes occurred in concordance with DNA damage, as revealed by increased phosphorylation of histone H2AX at Ser139. Treatment of different-stage prostate cancer cells with PIC also resulted in cell type-specific downregulation of the mammalian target of rapamycin (mTOR), a kinase involved in growth control of eukaryotic cells [18]. PIC also increased the protein levels of cleaved caspase-8, -9, -7, and -3 and cleaved PARP in DU145 cells, thereby inducing apoptosis [19]. PIC induced mitochondrial outer membrane permeability changes, resulting in cyt *c* release from the mitochondria to the cytosol. PIC treatment enhanced the levels of truncated Bid, Bax, Bik, and Bok with a concomitant decrease in the levels of Mcl-1 and Bcl-xL [19]. These results indicate that PIC induces apoptosis via the activation of the death receptor and mitochondrial-dependent pathways in prostate cancer cells.

PIC induced HCT116 and HT29 colon cancer cell apoptosis by promoting expression of microRNA-129, and suppressing expression of Bcl-2, a known target of microRNA-129. Moreover, knock down of microRNA-129 reversed the reduction of cell viability induced by PIC in these cells [20]. PIC exerted anti-proliferative activities in prostate cancer cell lines. The anti-tumorigenic effects of PIC was determined in LNCaP-Luc-xenografts. Two-week pretreatment with PIC diminished cell colonization, tumor volume, and tumor growth in the xenografts [21]. Treatment of MDA-MB-231 human breast cancer cells with PIC caused a rapid release of calcium from the endoplasmic reticulum. This elevation of intracellular calcium modulates the activity of p53 and the subsequent transcription of several genes encoding proapoptotic proteins [22]. Nanomolar concentration of PIC induced c-Myc expression and activated survival signaling in MCF-7 human breast cancer cells, leading to accelerated cell proliferation [23]. In contrast, PIC at the concentrations in the micromolar range suppressed c-Myc expression and induced apoptosis.

9.2.3 Induction of Autophage

Environmental conditions or chemical agents can interfere with the function of the endoplasmic reticulum (ER), and the resultant ER stress can be toxic to the cell if it is not relieved. Agents that cause ER stress in cancer cells can elicit anticancer activity. PIC was identified as one of the potent inducers of ER stress. In the HT1080 reporter cells treated with PIC, there were both splicing of XBP1 and induction of the ATF4 target gene product CCAAT-enhancer-binding protein homologous protein (CHOP), leading to ER stress [24]. This was accompanied by a modest increase in LC3 processing, indicative of a mild autophagic response.

The health beneficial effect of resveratrol may be associated, at least in part, with its capacity to promote autophagy by activating the NAD^+-dependent deacetylase sirtuin 1 [25]. PIC is a weak activator of sirtuin 1, and its induction of autophage is independent of this enzyme. Resveratrol and PIC, in combination, induced autophagy and stimulated the deacetylation of cytoplasmic proteins more efficiently than either compound alone. These findings suggest that both compounds, through different mechanisms, may synergize in inducing autophagy [25].

9.2.4 DNA Strand Break

Resveratrol is recognized as a naturally occurring antioxidant but it also catalyzes oxidative DNA degradation in a test tube reaction in the presence of transition metal ions such as copper. PIC was found to be a more efficient DNA-cleaving agent than resveratrol in the presence of Cu(II) as assessed by the conversion of supercoiled pBR322 plasmid into linear forms [26]. In this study, *trans*-stilbene, which lacks any hydroxyl group, failed to induce DNA cleavage in the presence of Cu(II). PIC plus Cu(II) also caused DNA damage in lymphocytes isolated from human peripheral blood to a greater extent than resveratrol in the presence of Cu(II) as measured by the Comet assay. Based on these findings, it is hypothesized that anticancer properties of various plant-derived polyphenols including PIC may involve mobilization of endogenous copper and the consequent prooxidant action [26].

9.2.5 Anti-metastatic Effects

Cancer invasion and metastasis are two main causes of treatment failure and cancer-related mortality. Several studies have demonstrated that matrix metalloproteinases (MMPs) are critical for tumor invasion and metastasis. PIC inhibited MMP-2 activity and manifestation of the invasive phenotype of MCF10A human breast epithelial cells harboring mutated H-*ras* (H-*ras* MCF10A cells) more effectively than resveratrol [27]. PIC attenuated the H-*ras*-induced phosphorylation of Akt in a time- and dose-dependent manner, whereas resveratrol, at the same concentrations, did not exert an inhibitory effect. In vitro kinase assays demonstrated that PIC significantly inhibited phosphatidylinositol 3-kinase (PI3K) activity and suppressed phosphatidylinositol (3,4,5)-trisphosphate expression in the H-*ras* MCF10A cells. Interestingly, PIC directly binds to PI3K, thereby inhibiting its catalytic activity. Data from molecular docking suggested that PIC is a more tight-binding inhibitor of PI3K than resveratrol due to the additional hydrogen bond between the hydroxyl group and the backbone amide group of Val882 located in the ATP-binding pocket of PI3K [27].

The anti-invasive and anti-metastatic effects of PIC were investigated in MDA-MB-231 human breast cancer cells. PIC significantly reduced serum-induced cell invasion and migration as well as adhesion without affecting the viability of these cells [28]. Furthermore, PIC markedly inhibited the activity of MMP-9 and its expression at both protein and mRNA levels. PIC attenuated PI3K and phosphorylation of AKT and mTOR, whereas the protein level of the PI3K inhibitor, PTEN (Phosphatase and Tensin Homolog Deleted on Chromosome Ten) was increased. Moreover, PIC inhibited transcriptional activity of nuclear factor κB (NF-κB) and its binding to DNA harboring an MMP-9 promoter consensus sequence. In addition, PIC diminished NF-κB nuclear translocation by blocking IκBα phosphorylation in the cytoplasm [28].

In order to evaluate the anti-metastatic property of PIC, the lung metastasis of MAT-Ly-Lu (MLL) rat prostate cancer cells expressing luciferase were injected into the tail veins of male nude mice [29]. The oral administration of PIC (20 mg/kg) significantly inhibited the accumulation of MLL cells in the lung of these mice [29]. In the cell culture studies, PIC inhibited the basal and epidermal growth factor (EGF)-induced migration of DU145, MLL, PC3, and TRAMP-C2 prostate cancer cells. In addition, PIC attenuated invasion of DU145 cells in the absence and presence of EGF [29]. In DU145 cells, PIC reduced secretion and messenger RNA levels of MMP-9, urokinase-type plasminogen activator (uPA), and vascular endothelial growth factor (VEGF), while increasing the protein levels of tissue inhibitor of MMP-2. Additionally, PIC inhibited the phosphorylation of signal transducer and activator of transcription (STAT) 3. Furthermore, PIC reduced both basal and EGF-induced interleukin (IL)-6 secretion. PIC also inhibited IL-6-induced increases in the secretion of uPA and VEGF, STAT3 phosphorylation and the migration of DU145 cells. [29]. PIC also suppressed the expression of MMP-9 in DU145 human prostate cancer cells treated with TNF-α. In addition, PIC reduced the TNF-α-induced invasion of DU145 cells. PIC attenuated MMP-9 gene expression via the suppression of NF-κB activity. Furthermore, TNF-α-induced Akt phosphorylation was significantly attenuated in the presence of PIC [30].

PIC suppressed both the proliferation and invasion of cultured AH109A hepatoma cells [31]. PIC, at lower concentrations (25–50 μM), induced cell cycle arrest at G2/M phase, while it caused apoptosis at a higher concentration (100 μM). PIC suppressed invasive capacity of hepatoma cells by scavenging reactive oxygen species (ROS). PIC also suppressed the tumor growth and metastasis in hepatoma-bearing rats [31].

9.2.6 Multidrug Resistance (MDR) Modulation

The identification of compounds that overcome the resistance to cancer cell apoptosis that frequently accompanies MDR is of great therapeutic importance. PIC effectively inhibited the multidrug resistance-associated protein, MRP1 as assessed by its ability to suppress the efflux of the fluorescent MRP1 substrate (BCECF) from human erythrocytes [32].

9.2.7 Modulation of Tumor Microenvironment

Chronic lymphocytic leukemia (CLL) is characterized by the progressive accumulation of clonal B lymphocytes. Proliferation occurs in lymphoid tissues upon interaction of leukemic cells with a supportive microenvironment [33]. Therefore, the mobilization of tissue-resident CLL cells into the circulation is a useful therapeutic strategy to minimize the reservoir of tumor cells within survival niches. The exit of normal lymphocytes from lymphoid tissues depends on the presence of sphingosine-1 phosphate (S1P) and the expression of S1P receptor-1 (S1PR1). Activated CLL cells displayed reduced expression of S1PR1 and the migratory response toward S1P. PIC enhanced S1PR1 expression in CLL cells and their migratory response toward S1P [33].

4T1 mammary carcinoma cells were injected into the mammary fat pad of syngeneic female BALB/c mice. PIC treatment reduced tumor growth. In tumors from PIC-treated groups, there was reduced expression of transcription factors P-NF-κB, P-STAT3, and HIF-1α and multiple proteins involved in regulation of cell cycle progression (Ki67, cyclin D1, cyclin A, CDK2, and CDK4), angiogenesis (VEGF-A, VEGFR-2, VE-cadherin, and CD31), and lymphangiogenesis (VEGF-C and LYVE-1), as well as macrophage infiltration [34]. PIC administration also significantly increased the number of apoptotic cells and expression of both Bax and cleaved caspase-3 but reduced anti-apoptotic Bcl-2 expression in tumor tissues. In addition, PIC reduced the number and the volume of pulmonary tumor nodules and expression of MMP-9 in the tumor tissues. It also lowered tissue levels of cytokines/chemokines, including macrophage colony-stimulating factor (M-CSF) and macrophage chemoattractant protein (MCP-1). PIC inhibited migration of 4T1 mouse mammary cancer cells and monocytes, as well as secretion of MCP-1 and M-CSF by 4T1 cells. These results indicate that alteration in tumor microenvironment is an important mechanism by which PIC inhibits tumor proliferation, angiogenesis, and lymphangiogenesis, leading to suppression of mammary tumor growth and metastasis [34].

9.2.8 Potentiation of Cytotoxic Effects of Chemotherapeutic Agents

The potential synergistic effect of PIC on gemcitabine cytotoxicity was investigated in the human non-small cell lung cancer, A459 cell line. Gemcitabine alone induced the expression of the proapoptotic proteins Bad and Bak, and pretreatment with PIC further enhanced Bak expression, leading to an increased number of cells undergoing late apoptosis. PIC can hence potentiate the cytotoxic effects of gemcitabine by upregulating the proapoptotic protein expression [35].

PIC was found to sensitize the ovarian cancer cells to cisplatin-induced cytotoxicity, and this effect was achieved through modulation of several major determinants of chemoresistance [36]. PIC enhanced p53-mediated expression of the proapoptotic protein NOXA, XIAP degradation via the ubiquitin-proteasome pathway, and caspase-3 activation. This response was associated with an increase in Drp1-dependent mitochondrial fission, leading to more effective induction of apoptosis. In vivo studies using a murine model of ovarian cancer also revealed apoptotic changes in association with a greater overall reduction in tumor weight when mice were co-treated with both PIC and cisplatin, in comparison to treatment with either agent alone [36].

Arabinofuranosyl cytidine (Ara-C) is a chemotherapeutic agent used mainly in the treatment of hematological malignancies, such as acute myeloid leukemia and non-Hodgkin lymphoma. It inhibits cancer cell growth by interfering with DNA synthesis. Incubation of human HL-60 leukemia cells with PIC induced apoptosis and caused an arrest in the G_2/M phase of the cell cycle [37]. PIC depleted intracellular dCTP and dGTP pools, and thereby inhibited the incorporation of [^{14}C]-labeled cytidine into DNA. PIC significantly abolished all NTP pools, and sequential treatment with PIC and Ara-C yielded synergistic growth inhibitory effects [37]. PIC or myricetin alone induced apoptotic cell death in HL-60 cells, but combined treatment further enhanced the proportion of apoptotic cells [38].

9.2.9 Miscellaneous Effects

It has been reported that glypican-3 (GPC3) is significantly elevated in human hepatocellular carcinoma compared with benign liver lesions or normal liver. In the human hepatocellular carcinoma cell lines, GPC3 expression was consistently observed, and was mainly located in the cell membrane and cytoplasm. PIC increased the expression of GPC3 [39]. The Cbl family of proteins are evolutionarily conserved negative regulators of signaling cascades involving receptor and non-receptor tyrosine kinases. PIC caused the loss of the Cbl family of proteins [40]. It is likely that the oxidative conversion of the catechol ring of PIC into a highly reactive *o*-benzoquinoneis required for the PIC-induced Cbl loss.

9.3 Other Pharmacological Effects

9.3.1 Anti-obesity Effects

Obesity is associated with an increased risk of several metabolic diseases, such as type 2 diabetes, high blood pressure, and cardiovascular disorders as well as cancer. The differentiation of preadipocytes to adipocytes, a process called adipogenesis, is essential for expansion of the fat tissue. Dysfunction of adipogenesis is a hallmark of obesity, and elucidation of underlying mechanisms is essential for identifying targets for pharmacological and nutritional intervention. CHOP, as an adipocyte repressor, inhibits the differentiation of preadipocytes. PIC induced CHOP expression and thereby blocked differentiation of human liposarcoma (LiSa-2) preadipocytes as characterized by reduced fat droplet formation and VEGF production [41]. In another study, PIC inhibited adipogenesis of 3T3-L1 preadipocytes [42]. In the early phase of adipogenesis, PIC-treated preadipocytes displayed a delayed cell cycle entry into G_2/M phase at 24 h after initiation of adipogenesis. Furthermore, the PIC-induced expression of mitotic clonal expansion was accompanied by reduced activation of insulin signaling. PIC directly binds to insulin receptor and inhibits insulin receptor kinase activity which may account for its capability to inhibit adipogenesis [42].

The effects of PIC on obesity-associated complications in Zucker obese rats were measured after a 6-week supplementation. While PIC tended to improve lipid handling, it did not mitigate hyperinsulinemia and cardiac hypertrophy. However, it did increase cardiac expression of ephrin-B1, a membrane protein involved in maintaining cardiomyocyte architecture. Thus, PIC did not exhibit strong slimming capacities but could limit several obesity complications [43].

9.3.2 Antidiabetic Effects

As a hydroxylated analog of resveratrol, PIC may have similar or distinct protective/preventive effects on the metabolic disorders. Resveratrol has been known to ameliorate diet-induced obesity and insulin resistance [44]. Intragastric administration of PIC suppressed significantly the increases in the fasting blood glucose levels in genetically diabetic *db/db* mice without affecting body weights and food intake [45]. In addition, PIC significantly suppressed the rises in the blood glucose levels in *db/db* mice given glucose after 12-h fasting. These findings indicate that PIC administration represses the rises in blood glucose levels at early stages while it can exert a remedial effect on impaired glucose tolerance at late stages of diabetes in *db/db* mice [45].

Similar antidiabetic effects of PIC have been observed in C57BL/6Jjcl mice fed high-fat diet [46]. PIC did not affect high-fat diet-induced body weight gain or visceral fat gain in these animals, but lowered fasting blood glucose levels. In agreement with the observation in the previous study by Minakawa et al. [45], a single intragastric administration of PIC reduced the blood glucose levels in *db/db* mice [46]. In skeletal muscle cells, glucose uptake occurs mainly through glucose transporter 4 (GLUT4) in response to insulin. 5′-Adenosine monophosphate-activated protein kinase (AMPK) is known as a GLUT4 translocation promoter, and AMPK activators, hence have a potential to overcome insulin resistance in the diabetic state. PIC increased glucose uptake in L6 myotubes by promoting GLUT4 translocation to plasma membrane via AMPK activation [45].

The hypoglycemic effect of PIC was examined after intravascular administration to healthy rats. Intravascularly administered PIC reduced the blood glucose concentrations during both fasting and the glucose tolerance test [47]. Furthermore, PIC increased the insulinogenic index during glucose tolerance tests but had no influence on insulin sensitivity. Based on these observations, it is likely that PIC given orally enhances glucose tolerance, and this effect is mediated by intact PIC itself, not its metabolite, by stimulating early phase secretion of insulin.

PIC effectively mitigated the inhibitory effects of palmitic acid on the insulin-mediated phosphorylation of insulin receptor substrate-1 in human umbilical vein endothelial cells (HUVECs). The protective effect of PIC against palmitic acid-induced impairment of insulin signaling was mediated by heme oxygenase-1 (HO-1) activity [48].

9.3.3 Neuroprotective Effects

9.3.3.1 Alzheimer Disease (AD)

β-Amyloid (Aβ), a key protein involved in the pathogenesis of AD, is a major component of senile plaques formed in the brain of AD patients. Apoptotic cell death caused by ROS has been implicated in the Aβ-induced neurotoxicity. PIC inhibited the formation of Aβ fibrils [49]. Notably, the choroid plexus secretes transthyretin, a protein that has been shown to inhibit Aβ aggregation and that may hence be critical to the maintenance of normal learning capacities in aging. The misfolding of transthyretin is implicated in amyloid diseases. It is worthwhile determining whether PIC can inhibit misfolding of this particular protein in exerting its inhibitory effects on formation and neurotoxicity of Aβ fibrils [49].

PIC treatment attenuated the accumulation of ROS and inhibited apoptosis in rat pheochromocytoma PC12 cells treated with Aβ [50]. PIC exerted much stronger protective effects than did resveratrol [50]. 4-Hydroxynonenal (4-HNE) is a major lipid peroxidation product produced by oxidative stress, and its level is elevated in the AD brain. PIC protected PC12 cells from 4-HNE-induced apoptosis as revealed by attenuation of nuclear condensation, PARP cleavage and downregulation of anti-apoptotic Bcl-2 expression. PIC also inhibited the phosphorylation of c-Jun N-terminal kinase (JNK), which is a key regulator of apoptotic cell death [51]. Similar increased cell viability, a decreased apoptosis rate and reduced intracellular

ROS accumulation were observed after PIC treatment to PC12 cells [52]. PIC significantly promoted activation of anti-apoptotic Bad and Akt through phosphorylation, while it reduced the Bcl-2/Bax ratio and cleavage of caspase-9, caspase-3, and PARP.

9.3.3.2 Glutamate-Induced Neurotoxicity

Oxidative cell death is a common mechanism underlying pathogenesis of not only AD, but also a variety of other neural diseases. The amino acid glutamate at high concentrations causes depletion of reduced glutathione (GSH) by inhibiting the glutamate/cystine antiporter system, with a concomitant increase in intracellular accumulation of ROS. This leads to oxidative stress-induced neuronal cell death. PIC reduced glutamate-induced ROS formation and cytotoxicity in cultured HT22 neuronal cells [53]. PIC also increased the expression of HO-1 via activation of nuclear factor-erythroid 2 (NF-E2) p45-related factor 2 (Nrf2), a master transcription factor responsible for regulating transcription of many antioxidant/anti-inflammatory and other cytoptotective genes. Interestingly, the neuroprotective effect of PIC was partly abolished by either downregulation of HO-1 expression or blockade of HO-1 activity [53].

9.3.3.3 Ischemic Stroke

Inflammation occurs in the ischemic brain, which consists of various types of cells, such as neurons, endothelial cells, and immune cells. Macrophage-inducible C-type lectin (Mincle, CLEC4E) receptor is involved in neuroinflammation in cerebral ischemia and traumatic brain injury. Mincle, its ligand SAP130, and its downstream tyrosine kinase Syk were upregulated in the brain after ischemia, and participate in the pathogenesis of ischemic stroke by initiating inflammation [1]. In mice treated with PIC intraperitoneally before ischemia and just after reperfusion, the cerebral ischemic injury was ameliorated. The protective effects of PIC against ischemic brain injury were attributed to its inhibition of Syk [1]. Subarachnoid hemorrhage (SAH) accounts for 5–7 % of all strokes. PIC reduced brain edema and ameliorated neurological deficits after SAH in a rat stroke model [54].

9.3.3.4 Neuroinflammation

Prostaglandin E_2 (PGE_2), nitric oxide (NO), and proinflammatory cytokines, such as IL-1β, IL-6, and TNF-α, play pivotal roles in brain injuries. PIC significantly inhibited the release of NO, PGE_2, and proinflammatory cytokines in LPS-stimulated BV2 microglia [55]. PIC also attenuated the expression of inducible NO synthase (iNOS) and cyclooxygenase-2 (COX-2) at both transcriptional and translational levels. PIC exhibits anti-inflammatory properties by suppressing the transcription of proinflammatory cytokine genes through inhibition of the NF-κB signaling pathway [55].

Prion diseases are a group of transmissible fatal neurodegenerative disorders of humans and animals, including bovine spongiform encephalopathy, scrapie, and Creutzfeldt–Jakob disease. Microglia, the resident macrophages of the central nervous system, are exquisitely sensitive to pathological tissue alterations. CD36, a class B scavenger receptor expressed on the surface of microglia, is involved in microglial activation induced by a neurotoxic prion protein fragment, $PrP_{106-126}$. PIC was found to abrogate CD36-mediated iNOS expression induced by neurotoxic prion peptides in BV2 microglial cells [56].

9.3.4 Cardioprotective Effects

Cardiovascular disease (CVD) is a global health problem. Due to high morbidity and mortality rates, CVD accounts for an enormous socioeconomic burden. Consumption of dietary supplements or functional foods for reducing the risk of CVDs has also gained wide recognition by the general public. PIC is one such candidate with a potential to prevent CVD-associated disorders, such as hypercholesterolemia, arrhythmia, and atherosclerosis. It also has vasorelaxation and antioxidant activities [57].

Reperfusion is associated with potentially lethal arrhythmias that occurs within seconds of the onset of reflow. Presumably due to its additional hydroxyl group, PIC has more potent free radical scavenging activity than resveratrol in association with antiarrhythmic and cardioprotective activities in ischemic and ischemic-reperfused rat hearts [58]. PIC also exerted antiarrhythmic activity in isolated rat hearts subjected to ischemia–reperfusion (I/R) injury [59]. Ischemic tissue injury is caused by the adhesion of polymorphonuclear neutrophils to the lining of the vascular endothelium. Administration of albumin nanoparticles loaded with PIC detached the adherent neutrophils and thereby facilitated their release into the circulation [60].

Atherosclerosis is a major risk factor for CVD, in which inflammation plays a prominent role in its pathogenesis. Eotaxin, a newly discovered C-C motif chemokine (CCL11), has been shown to increase coronary artery endothelial cell permeability and is involved in endothelial inflammation and vascular smooth muscle cell migration. Release as well as expression of ecotaxin-1 and its gene promoter activity were increased in human coronary artery endothelial cells stimulated with IL-13 and TNF-α, and this was effectively inhibited by PIC as well as resveratrol [61].

PIC pretreatment suppressed cardiac hypertrophy induced by isoproterenol in mice as assessed by the heart weight/body weight ratio, cross-sectional area, and expression of hypertrophic markers. The anti-hypertrophic effect of PIC was also verified in cultured rat neonatal cardiomyocytes, and the underlying mechanism appears to involve the modulation of the transcription factor GATA binding factor 6 [62].

9.3.5 Vascular Endothelial Function/Protection

Glucose-induced oxidative stress is involved in endothelial dysfunction. Dimethylarginine dimethylaminohydrolase (DDAH) is a regulator of the endothelial NO synthase (eNOS). DDAH activity and expression were decreased in bovine aortic endothelial cells challenged with 25 mM glucose as compared to control cells. DDAH inhibition led to intracellular accumulation of asymmetric dimethylarginine (ADMA), a natural inhibitor of eNOS. PIC restored the basal DDAH activity and the ADMA level [63].

Arginase competitively inhibits NOS by use of the common substrate L-arginine. Arginase II has been reported as a novel therapeutic target for the treatment of CVDs, such as atherosclerosis. PIC-3′-*O*-beta-D-glucopyranoside (PG) inhibited the activity of arginase I and II prepared from mouse liver and kidney lysates, respectively [64]. Incubation of HUVECs with PG also blocked arginase activity and increased NO production.

P-selectin glycoproteinligand-1 (PSGL-1) not only functions as an anchor molecule to capture monocytes and other leukocytes to endothelial cells in ischemic tissues through its interaction with P-selectin, but also transduces signals to initiate firm adhesion. Endothelial progenitor cells are derived from monocytes and play an important role in neovascularization. When transfected with human PSGL-1 gene, endothelial progenitor cells exhibited higher affinity for activated HUVECs or recombined P-selectin/intercellular adhesion molecule 1 (ICAM-1) monolayer. The overexpression of PSGL-1 enhanced expression of beta2-integrin expression on the surface of endothelial progenitor cells and their adherence affinity, and these effects were abolished by PIC through suppression of Syk [65].

PIC induced a relaxation in aortic preparations precontracted with phenylephrine. The PIC-induced vascular relaxation in rat aorta appears to be mediated by an endothelium-dependent NO signaling pathway, at least partially, through the activation of large conductance Ca^{2+}-activated K^{+} channels [66].

9.3.6 Antiallergic Effects

Mast cells and basophils are major effector cells in the immunoglobulin E (IgE)-dependent allergic reactions as well as in the innate immunity. Upon allergen exposure, these cells are stimulated via the high affinity IgE receptor (FcepsilonRI) to release several proinflammatory chemical mediators, such as leukotrienes, immunoregulatory cytokines, and histamine. FcepsilonRI-mediated signaling is initiated upon tyrosine phosphorylation of this receptor by the Src family kinase Lyn, which is followed by an activation of Syk. PIC, as a classical Syk kinase inhibitor, can modulate the FcepsilonRI-mediated signaling in mast cells, and has a potential for use in the treatment of inflammatory and allergy diseases [67].

Histamine is one of the key chemical mediators that play an important role in allergic inflammation. PIC 4′-β-glucoside formed in cultured *Phytolacca Americana* treated with PIC showed the strong inhibitory effects on histamine release from rat peritoneal mast cells [68]. Compound 48/80 (8 mg/kg) was used to induce a systemic fatal allergic reaction in mice. Intraperitoneal administration of PIC inhibited the compound 48/80-induced systemic anaphylaxis and serum histamine release [69]. PIC treatment also ameliorated local allergic reactions in an IgE-mediated passive cutaneous anaphylaxis model [70]. The rat basophilic leukemia RBL-2H3 cell line exhibits phenotypic characteristics of mucosal mast cells. After stimulation with antigens cells release histamine and β-hexosaminidase, a marker of mast cell degranulation. PIC pretreatment strongly suppressed histamine release and degranulation in the RBL-2H3 cells stimulated with phorbol 12-myristate 13-acetate (PMA) and the calcium ionophore A23187 [69]. PIC treatment of the human mast cell line HMC-1 reduced PMA plus A23187-induced mRNA expression and release of the proinflammatory cytokines (TNF-α and IL-8).

9.3.7 Effects on Immune Cell Functions

Chronic inflammatory diseases are characterized by neutrophil infiltration in inflamed tissues. Neutrophils are able to release cytotoxic substances and inflammatory mediators, which have a potential to maintain persistent inflammation. Apoptosis is an important process for successful removal of recruited neutrophils. Neutrophils from healthy volunteers were incubated in vitro with PIC and some other stilbenoids, including resveratrol. Neutrophils treated with resveratrol and PIC underwent apoptosis [71]. The ability of PIC to reduce the toxic action of neutrophils was verified in another study [72]. It elevated the percentage of early apoptotic neutrophils, inhibited the activity of protein kinase C, the main regulatory enzyme in neutrophils, and reduced phosphorylation of protein kinase C isoforms α, β II, and δ on their catalytic region. PIC may hence be useful as a complementary medicine in states associated with persisting neutrophil activations [72]. The anticancer drug arsenic trioxide is known to be toxic for human mononuclear and neutrophil cell populations. PIC inhibited the arsenic trioxide-induced phagocytic ability of neutrophils and degranulation by inhibiting Syk kinase [73].

The effect of PIC on T cell activation, proliferation, and differentiation was assessed using murine splenic T cells isolated from C57BL/6 mice. PIC treatment inhibited surface expression of CD4 and CD8 T cell activation markers CD25 and CD69, reduced production of cytokines IFNγ, IL-2, and IL-17, and suppressed proliferation of activated T cells. Moreover, PIC treatment significantly inhibited differentiation of $CD4^+$ $CD25^-$ $CD62L^+$ naïve CD4 T cells into Th1, Th2, and Th17 cells, presumably due to inhibition of TcR signaling [74].

9.3.8 Modulation of Bone Metabolism

Decreases in new bone formation, followed by estrogen deficiency are implicated in postmenopausal osteoporosis. PIC was found to stimulate osteoblast maturation and differentiation required for bone mass increases. These effects were ascribed to overproduction of bone morphogenetic protein-2 by PIC [75]. Osteoclast formation occurs when bone marrow macrophages derived from hematopoietic stem cells are stimulated by osteoclastogenic factors, including receptor activator of nuclear factor-κB ligand (RANKL). Increased osteoclast formation is responsible for excess bone resorption, leading to the bone loss seen in osteoporosis, and inflammation-induced bone destruction [76]. PIC has been reported to inhibit osteoclast function and formation through upregulation of HO-1 expression. PIC reduced the production of microRNA-183 and consequently increased HO-1 expression, leading to attenuation of osteoclastogenesis [76].

Prostate cancer primarily metastasizes to bone, and the interaction of cancer cells with bone cells results in a local activation of bone formation and/or bone resorption. When the cells were grown in the presence of conditioned medium from osteolytic PC-3 prostate cancer cells, matrix mineralization was largely reduced, suggesting the suppression of osteoblast differentiation by PC-3-secreted molecules [77]. Treatment of primary murine osteoblasts with conditioned medium from osteolytic PC-3 prostate cancer cells led to a marked induction of several cytokine genes, including Cxcl5, Cxcl12, and Tnfsf11, the latter one encoding for the osteoclast differentiation factor RANKLl. PIC abrogated transcription of these genes in osteoblasts stimulated with PC-3-conditioned medium. Similarly, PIC inhibited the expression of Cxcl5 and Tnfs11 genes in primary human osteoblasts co-incubated with the PC-3 conditioned medium [77].

9.3.9 Anti-aging Effects

9.3.9.1 Expansion of Life Span

Cellular senescence is characterized by cellular hypertrophy in which cells grow without division. The genes that regulate this process can be activated or inactivated by numerous plant polyphenols, including resveratrol [78]. The anti-aging potential of resveratrol has been subjects of numerous research endeavors [2]. Resveratrol has been shown to prolong the lifespan of experimental animals, and the main mechanism involves the activation of Sirtuins (Sir [invertebrates] or Sirt [vertebrates]). A recent study has demonstrated that both resveratrol and PIC enhance the expression levels of SIRT1 and its mRNA transcript in THP-1 monocytic cells. An extract of passion fruit seeds, which is rich in PIC, has also been found to upregulate sirtuin 1 (SIRT1) mRNA expression [79].

9.3.9.2 Melanogenesis

The effects of passion fruit on melanin inhibition and collagen synthesis were studied using cultured human melanoma and fibroblast cells [80]. Treatment of melanoma cells with the seed part of passion fruit resulted in inhibition of melanogenesis. The production of total soluble collagen in cultured dermal fibroblast cells was also elevated. PIC is speculated as the major component responsible for the passion fruit effects on melanogenesis and collagen synthesis [80]. The skin lightening potential of PIC was investigated in terms of its ability to inhibit melanogenesis [81]. PIC strongly inhibited tyrosinase activity involved in melanin biosynthesis and lowered the melanin content in cultured B16F10 melanoma cells. The antioxidative property is closely linked to the melanogenic activity. PIC reduced the ROS accumulation and the ratio of GSH to its oxidized form GSSG in these cells [81].

9.3.9.3 Photoaging and Skin Inflammation

The use of naturally occurring botanicals with substantial antioxidant activity to prevent photoaging has received increasing attention. The passion fruit seed extract and its principal component PIC elevated the GSH levels in human keratinocytes, while suppressing the ultraviolet (UV)B-induced generation of ROS in these cells [82]. In addition, the transfer of the medium from the UVB-irradiated keratinocytes to nonirradiated fibroblasts enhanced MMP-1 activity, and this induction was reduced when the keratinocytes were pretreated with PIC [82].

In order to identify inhibitors of ultraviolet UV-induced cytotoxicity, more than 50 plant extracts were screened, using cultured normal human epidermal keratinocytes (NHEK). Among them, fruit of rose myrtle (*Rhodomyrtus tomentosa*) displayed the most potent effects on UVB-induced cytotoxicity [83]. Both PIC and the rose myrtle extract reduced the production of UVB-induced cyclobutane pyrimidine dimers and enhanced the activity of the DNA polymerases in UVB-irradiated NHEK cells. In addition, the secretion of the inflammatory mediator, PGE_2 was decreased [83].

Pretreatment of hairless mouse skin topically with PIC attenuated PMA-induced expression of COX-2 and iNOS [84]. PIC also diminished nuclear translocation and DNA binding of NF-κB, a major transcription factor known to regulate these proinflammatory gene expression, through the blockade of phosphorylation and subsequent degradation of IκBα. Likewise, the catalytic activity of IKKβ and the phosphorylation of MAPKs in PMA-treated mouse skin were inhibited by topically applied PIC. In addition, PIC decreased PMA-induced expression of c-Fos and the DNA binding of AP-1, another transcription factor that plays an important role in inflammatory signaling [84].

9.3.10 *Anti-colitic Effects*

Inflammatory tissue injury is considered to be implicated in tumor promotion and progression. For instance, inflammatory bowel diseases (IBD), such as ulcertative colitis and Crohn's disease, have been considered to increase the risk of colon cancer. The potential protective effect of PIC on IBD was investigated in a dextran sulfate sodium (DSS)-induced murine colitis model that mimics human IBD. Administration of DSS (2.5 %) in drinking water for 7 days to male ICR mice resulted in colitis and elevated expression of iNOS and activation of NF-κB [85]. Phosphorylation of ERK and STAT3 was also enhanced after DSS treatment. Oral administration of PIC (10 mg/kg body weight each) for 7 constitutive days attenuated the DSS-induced inflammatory injury, upregulation of iNOS expression, and activation of NF-κB, STAT3, and ERK [85]. Similarly, PIC administration blunted the weight loss and clinical signs of intestinal inflammation caused by 5 % DSS in the BALB/c mice. This was associated with remarkable amelioration of the disruption of the colonic architecture, significant reduction in colonic myeloperoxidase activity and decreased the production of inflammatory mediators, such as NO, PGE_2, and proinflammatory cytokines [86].

PIC undergoes extensive phase II hepatic metabolism, which lowers its bioavailability. To overcome such limitation, a special capsule containing PIC for colon-targeted delivery was formulated. The anti-colitic effects of PIC in a colon-targeted capsule were compared with those of PIC in a conventional gelatin capsule in a trinitrobenzene sulfonic acid-induced rat colitis, another animal model of human IBD [87]. Colon-targeted PIC elicited greatly enhanced recovery of the colonic inflammation. When treated to human colon carcinoma HCT116 cells, PIC inhibited NF-κB signaling while activating the anti-inflammatory transcription factor, Nrf2. Colon-targeted PIC, but not conventional PIC, modulated production of the target gene products of these transcription factors in the inflamed colonic mucosa [87].

9.3.11 *Miscellaneous Effects*

9.3.11.1 Septic Shock

Interferon regulatory factor 3 (IRF3) mediates the transcriptional induction of interferon-stimulated genes in response to viral and bacterial infections. PIC inhibited the LPS-mediated activation of IRF3 and subsequent interferon-stimulated gene expression [88]. Furthermore, the LPS-mediated induction of tissue factor, a cell surface protein responsible for initiating the coagulation cascade, was also inhibited by PIC. The effectiveness of PIC in blocking both the inflammatory response and the coagulation pathway is likely to be associated with its protection against LPS-induced septic shock in a murine model [88].

9.3.11.2 Retinal/Ocular Protection

Inflammatory response has a critical role in neuronal damage after retinal I/R injury, and is regulated tightly by TLR4. The expression of TLR4 was upregulated after I/R [89]. TLR4 knockout (KO) mice were much less susceptible to the histologic damage causedby I/R compared to wild-type mice. The phosphorylation level of NF-κB after I/R in TLR4 KO mice was decreased compared to that in wild-type mice. The expression of phosphorylated Syk was upregulated after I/R, and this was blunted in TLR4 KO mice. PIC inhibited the histologic and functional retinal damage, and reduced the phosphorylation level of NF-κB induced by I/R [89].

Pre- or post-treatment of PIC significantly blocked the LPS-induced ocular inflammation in rats [90]. Further, PIC also suppressed the expression of COX-2 and iNOS and activation of NF-κB in the ciliary bodies as well as retina, and also in primary human non-pigmented ciliary epithelial cells treated with LPS. Similarly, PIC diminished the LPS-induced production of NO and PGE_2 in these cells [90].

9.4 Metabolic Formation of PIC

Microsomal preparation of the human cytochrome P450 (CYP)1B1 and recombinant human CYP1B1 expressed in *E. coli* catalyze conversion of resveratrol to PIC [91]. Of interest, CYP1B1 is overexpressed in a wide variety of human tumors, and this observation implies that the anticarcinogenic effects of resveratrol are, at least in part, mediated by PIC formed by CYP1B1 activity in the cancer cells. In this context, CYP1B1 in tumors may function to suppress the growth of cancer cells. In addition, resveratrol was metabolized to PIC by recombinant human CYP1A1 and CYP1A2 as well as by CYP1B1 [92]. Incubation of *trans*-resveratrol with human microsomes produced PIC as a major metabolite, and this was markedly diminished by CYP1A2 inhibitors, α-naphthoflavone, and furafylline. Likewise, an antibody raised against CYP1A2 suppressed the formation of PIC from resveratrol [92].

CYP102A1 from the bacterium *Bacillus megaterium* was found to metabolize various drugs through reactions similar to those catalyzed by human CYP enzymes [93]. Resveratrol is oxidized to PIC by human P4501A2. The formation of PIC from resveratrol by human and bacterial CYPs is schematically illustrated in Fig. 9.3.

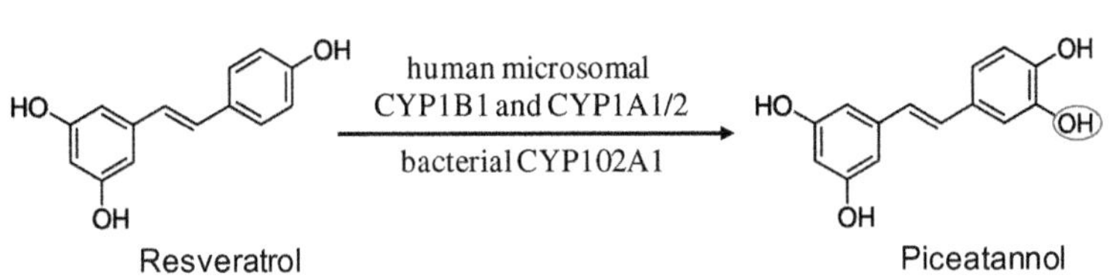

Fig. 9.3 Formation of PIC from resveratrol by human microsomal/recombinant CYP1B1 and CYP1A1/2 activities. The bacterial CYP101A1 also catalyzes the formation of PIC

9.5 Absorption and Biotransformation

PIC is rapidly metabolized in the liver and is converted mainly to a glucuronide or sulfate conjugate. The absorption and metabolism of PIC were investigated following intragastric administration to rats [79, 94]. PIC and isorhapontigenin (3,4′,5-trihydroxy-3′-methoxystilbene), an *O*-methyl PIC metabolite detected in the plasma, upregulated SIRT1 expression in THP-1 human monocytes [79].

The pharmacokinetics of PIC were investigated in male Sprague-Dawley rats after single intravenous doses of 10 mg/kg body weight. PIC was extensively glucuronidated, and predominantly eliminated via non-urinary routes. The estimates of oral bioavailability characterize PIC as a poorly bioavailable compound [95]. Incubation of PIC with human liver microsomes as well as using a panel of 12 recombinant UDP-glucuronosyltransferase isoforms produced distinct glucuronide conjugates [96]. Similarly, sulfation of PIC was investigated in human liver cytosol as well as using a panel of recombinant sulfotransferase isoforms. In the presence of the sulfate donor, 3′-phosphoadenosine-5′-phosphosulfate, mono- and disulfate conjugates of PIC were produced [97].

Although *trans*-resveratrol can be biotransformed to PIC by human CYP1A1 and CYP1A2, it also inhibit reactions catalyzed by these enzymes [98]. Aryl hydrocarbon receptor (AhR), following ligand-dependent activation, translocates to the nucleus where it forms a dimer with aryl hydrocarbon receptor nuclear translocator (ARNT). The AhR/ARNT complex then binds to AhR response elements located in regulatory regions of some xenobiotic metabolizing enzymes including CYP1A1 and CYP1B1. Resveratrol has been shown to inhibit dioxin-induced AhR activation and expression of CYP1A1 and CYP1B1 in cultured human mammary epithelial MCF10A cells [99] and T-47D human breast carcinoma cells [100]. Likewise, PIC treatment to T-47D breast cancer cells inhibited CYP1A1 and CYP1B1 mRNA expression induced by a low (1 nM) concentration of dioxin [100]. Moreover, PIC also inhibited dioxin-induced recruitment of AhR and ARNT to *CYP1A1* and *CYP1B1* enhancer regions. These data show that PCI is an inhibitor of AhR-dependent transcription and suggest that it may contribute to the prolonged inhibition of AHR-dependent gene expression following resveratrol treatment [100]. PIC, as well as its parent compound *trans*-resveratrol, decreased the in vitro catalytic activity of rat CYP1A1 and CYP1A2 by mixed inhibition [101]. PIC was a weak inhibitor of mouse hepatic microsomal CYP1A2 activity [102].

Secretion of dehydroepiandrosterone, testosterone, and cortisol was markedly decreased by a nontoxic dose of [103]. In contrast, secretion of rogesterone and aldosterone was enhanced. This steroid secretion pattern can be explained by the demonstrated inhibition of CYP17A1, a key enzyme in the androgen biosynthesis and a target for prostate cancer therapy. Treatment of cells with PIC caused increased estradiol levels, which was attributed to its inhibition of estrogen sulfate conjugation catalyzed by SULT1E1 [103].

9.6 Conclusions and Future Perspectives

As a naturally occurring hydroxylated derivative or a metabolite of well-known stilbene resveratrol, PIC has a spectrum of biological activity similar to resveratrol although the relative potency varies depending on the experimental system and dosage. PIC has a catechol moiety and hence can undergo redox cycling to produce an electrophilic quinone metabolite capable of interacting with cellular nucleophiles. While the number of publications on the health benefits of PIC is growing, few human studies on this stilbenoid have been performed. A comprehensive review of PIC concludes that the compound has the health promoting and disease preventive potential. However, low water-solubility and bioavailability of PIC limit its pharmaceutical application and also use in functional foods. In this context, it is noticeable that β-cyclodextrin was found to improve the bioavailability, the solubility and the stability of PIC [104]. Nanoparticle encapsulated PIC may be considered as an alternative innovative formulation. Derivatives of PIC with enhanced bioavailability as well as therapeutic efficacy might also be considered for future human intervention trials.

References

1. Suzuki Y, Nakano Y, Mishiro K, Takagi T, Tsuruma K, Nakamura M, Yoshimura S, Shimazawa M, Hara H (2013) Involvement of Mincle and Syk in the changes to innate immunity after ischemic stroke. Sci Rep 3:3177
2. Kasiotis KM, Pratsinis H, Kletsas D, Haroutounian SA (2013) Resveratrol and related stilbenes: their anti-aging and anti-angiogenic properties. Food Chem Toxicol 61:112–120
3. Piotrowska H, Kucinska M, Murias M (2012) Biological activity of piceatannol: leaving the shadow of resveratrol. Mutat Res 750:60–82
4. Waffo-Teguo P, Hawthorne ME, Cuendet M, Merillon JM, Kinghorn AD, Pezzuto JM, Mehta RG (2001) Potential cancer-chemopreventive activities of wine stilbenoids and flavans extracted from grape (*Vitis vinifera*) cell cultures. Nutr Cancer 40:173–179
5. Seyed MA, Jantan I, Bukhari SN, Vijayaraghavan K (2016) A comprehensive review on the chemotherapeutic potential of piceatannol for cancer treatment, with mechanistic insights. J Agric Food Chem 64:725–737
6. Wolter F, Clausnitzer A, Akoglu B, Stein J (2002) Piceatannol, a natural analog of resveratrol, inhibits progression through the S phase of the cell cycle in colorectal cancer cell lines. J Nutr 132:298–302
7. Lee YM, do Lim Y, Cho HJ, Seon MR, Kim JK, Lee BY, Park JH (2009) Piceatannol, a natural stilbene from grapes, induces G1 cell cycle arrest in androgen-insensitive DU145 human prostate cancer cells via the inhibition of CDK activity. Cancer Lett 285:166–173
8. Kuo PL, Hsu YL (2008) The grape and wine constituent piceatannol inhibits proliferation of human bladder cancer cells via blocking cell cycle progression and inducing Fas/membrane bound Fas ligand-mediated apoptotic pathway. Mol Nutr Food Res 52:408–418
9. Koerber RM, Held SA, Heine A, Kotthoff P, Daecke SN, Bringmann A, Brossart P (2015) Analysis of the anti-proliferative and the pro-apoptotic efficacy of Syk inhibition in multiple myeloma. Exp Hematol Oncol 4:21

10. Schmeel FC, Schmeel LC, Kim Y, Schmidt-Wolf IG (2014) Piceatannol exhibits selective toxicity to multiple myeloma cells and influences the Wnt/beta-catenin pathway. Hematol Oncol 32:197–204
11. Schmeel LC, Schmeel FC, Kim Y, Endo T, Lu D, Schmidt-Wolf IG (2013) Targeting the Wnt/beta-catenin pathway in multiple myeloma. Anticancer Res 33:4719–4726
12. Wieder T, Prokop A, Bagci B, Essmann F, Bernicke D, Schulze-Osthoff K, Dorken B, Schmalz HG, Daniel PT, Henze G (2001) Piceatannol, a hydroxylated analog of the chemopreventive agent resveratrol, is a potent inducer of apoptosis in the lymphoma cell line BJAB and in primary, leukemic lymphoblasts. Leukemia 15:1735–1742
13. Chowdhury SA, Kishino K, Satoh R, Hashimoto K, Kikuchi H, Nishikawa H, Shirataki Y, Sakagami H (2005) Tumor-specificity and apoptosis-inducing activity of stilbenes and flavonoids. Anticancer Res 25:2055–2063
14. Kim YH, Park C, Lee JO, Kim GY, Lee WH, Choi YH, Ryu CH (2008) Induction of apoptosis by piceatannol in human leukemic U937 cells through down-regulation of Bcl-2 and activation of caspases. Oncol Rep 19:961–967
15. Liu WH, Chang LS (2010) Piceatannol induces Fas and FasL up-regulation in human leukemia U937 cells via Ca^{2+}/p38alpha MAPK-mediated activation of c-Jun and ATF-2 pathways. Int J Biochem Cell Biol 42:1498–1506
16. Kang CH, Moon DO, Choi YH, Choi IW, Moon SK, Kim WJ, Kim GY (2011) Piceatannol enhances TRAIL-induced apoptosis in human leukemia THP-1 cells through Sp1- and ERK-dependent DR5 up-regulation. Toxicol In Vitro 25:605–612
17. Sala G, Minutolo F, Macchia M, Sacchi N, Ghidoni R (2003) Resveratrol structure and ceramide-associated growth inhibition in prostate cancer cells. Drugs Exp Clin Res 29:263–269
18. Hsieh TC, Lin CY, Lin HY, Wu JM (2012) AKT/mTOR as Novel targets of polyphenol piceatannol possibly contributing to inhibition of proliferation of cultured prostate cancer cells. ISRN Urol 2012:272697
19. Kim EJ, Park H, Park SY, Jun JG, Park JH (2009) The grape component piceatannol induces apoptosis in DU145 human prostate cancer cells via the activation of extrinsic and intrinsic pathways. J Med Food 12:943–951
20. Zhang H, Jia R, Wang C, Hu T, Wang F (2014) Piceatannol promotes apoptosis via up-regulation of microRNA-129 expression in colorectal cancer cell lines. Biochem Biophys Res Commun 452:775–781
21. Dias SJ, Li K, Rimando AM, Dhar S, Mizuno CS, Penman AD, Levenson AS (2013) Trimethoxy-resveratrol and piceatannol administered orally suppress and inhibit tumor formation and growth in prostate cancer xenografts. Prostate 73:1135–1146
22. van Ginkel PR, Yan MB, Bhattacharya S, Polans AS, Kenealey JD (2015) Natural products induce a G protein-mediated calcium pathway activating p53 in cancer cells. Toxicol Appl Pharmacol 288:453–462
23. Vo NT, Madlener S, Bago-Horvath Z, Herbacek I, Stark N, Gridling M, Probst P, Giessrigl B, Bauer S, Vonach C, Saiko P, Grusch M, Szekeres T, Fritzer-Szekeres M, Jager W, Krupitza G, Soleiman A (2010) Pro- and anticarcinogenic mechanisms of piceatannol are activated dose dependently in MCF-7 breast cancer cells. Carcinogenesis 31:2074–2081
24. Papandreou I, Verras M, McNeil B, Koong AC, Denko NC (2015) Plant stilbenes induce endoplasmic reticulum stress and their anti-cancer activity can be enhanced by inhibitors of autophagy. Exp Cell Res 339:147–153
25. Pietrocola F, Marino G, Lissa D, Vacchelli E, Malik SA, Niso-Santano M, Zamzami N, Galluzzi L, Maiuri MC, Kroemer G (2012) Pro-autophagic polyphenols reduce the acetylation of cytoplasmic proteins. Cell Cycle 11:3851–3860
26. Azmi AS, Bhat SH, Hadi SM (2005) Resveratrol-Cu(II) induced DNA breakage in human peripheral lymphocytes: implications for anticancer properties. FEBS Lett 579:3131–3135

27. Song NR, Hwang MK, Heo YS, Lee KW, Lee HJ (2013) Piceatannol suppresses the metastatic potential of MCF10A human breast epithelial cells harboring mutated H-ras by inhibiting MMP-2 expression. Int J Mol Med 32:775–784
28. Ko HS, Lee HJ, Kim SH, Lee EO (2012) Piceatannol suppresses breast cancer cell invasion through the inhibition of MMP-9: involvement of PI3K/AKT and NF-kappaB pathways. J Agric Food Chem 60:4083–4089
29. Kwon GT, Jung JI, Song HR, Woo EY, Jun JG, Kim JK, Her S, Park JH (2012) Piceatannol inhibits migration and invasion of prostate cancer cells: possible mediation by decreased interleukin-6 signaling. J Nutr Biochem 23:228–238
30. Jayasooriya RG, Lee YG, Kang CH, Lee KT, Choi YH, Park SY, Hwang JK, Kim GY (2013) Piceatannol inhibits MMP-9-dependent invasion of tumor necrosis factor-alpha-stimulated DU145 cells by suppressing the Akt-mediated nuclear factor-kappaB pathway. Oncol Lett 5:341–347
31. Kita Y, Miura Y, Yagasaki K (2012) Antiproliferative and anti-invasive effect of piceatannol, a polyphenol present in grapes and wine, against hepatoma AH109A cells. J Biomed Biotechnol 2012:672416
32. Wesolowska O, Wisniewski J, Duarte N, Ferreira MJ, Michalak K (2007) Inhibition of MRP1 transport activity by phenolic and terpenic compounds isolated from Euphorbia species. Anticancer Res 27:4127–4133
33. Borge M, Remes Lenicov F, Nannini PR, de los Rios Alicandu MM, Podaza E, Ceballos A, Fernandez Grecco H, Cabrejo M, Bezares RF, Morande PE, Oppezzo P, Giordano M, Gamberale R (2014) The expression of sphingosine-1 phosphate receptor-1 in chronic lymphocytic leukemia cells is impaired by tumor microenvironmental signals and enhanced by piceatannol and R406. J Immunol 193:3165–3174
34. Song H, Jung JI, Cho HJ, Her S, Kwon SH, Yu R, Kang YH, Lee KW, Park JH (2015) Inhibition of tumor progression by oral piceatannol in mouse 4T1 mammary cancer is associated with decreased angiogenesis and macrophage infiltration. J Nutr Biochem 26:1368–1378
35. Xu B, Tao ZZ (2015) Piceatannol enhances the antitumor efficacy of gemcitabine in human A549 non-small cell lung cancer cells. Oncol Res 22:213–217
36. Farrand L, Byun S, Kim JY, Im-Aram A, Lee J, Lim S, Lee KW, Suh JY, Lee HJ, Tsang BK (2013) Piceatannol enhances cisplatin sensitivity in ovarian cancer via modulation of p53, X-linked inhibitor of apoptosis protein (XIAP), and mitochondrial fission. J Biol Chem 288:23740–23750
37. Fritzer-Szekeres M, Savinc I, Horvath Z, Saiko P, Pemberger M, Graser G, Bernhaus A, Ozsvar-Kozma M, Grusch M, Jaeger W, Szekeres T (2008) Biochemical effects of piceatannol in human HL-60 promyelocytic leukemia cells—synergism with Ara-C. Int J Oncol 33:887–892
38. Morales P, Haza AI (2012) Selective apoptotic effects of piceatannol and myricetin in human cancer cells. J Appl Toxicol JAT 32:986–993
39. Suzuki M, Sugimoto K, Tanaka J, Tameda M, Inagaki Y, Kusagawa S, Nojiri K, Beppu T, Yoneda K, Yamamoto N, Ito M, Yoneda M, Uchida K, Takase K, Shiraki K (2010) Up-regulation of glypican-3 in human hepatocellular carcinoma. Anticancer Res 30:5055–5061
40. Klimowicz AC, Bisson SA, Hans K, Long EM, Hansen HC, Robbins SM (2009) The phytochemical piceatannol induces the loss of CBL and CBL-associated proteins. Mol Cancer Ther 8:602–614
41. Huang X, Ordemann J, Muller JM, Dubiel W (2012) The COP9 signalosome, cullin 3 and Keap1 supercomplex regulates CHOP stability and adipogenesis. Biol Open 1:705–710
42. Kwon JY, Seo SG, Heo YS, Yue S, Cheng JX, Lee KW, Kim KH (2012) Piceatannol, natural polyphenolic stilbene, inhibits adipogenesis via modulation of mitotic clonal expansion and insulin receptor-dependent insulin signaling in early phase of differentiation. J Biol Chem 287:11566–11578

43. Hijona E, Aguirre L, Perez-Matute P, Villanueva-Millan MJ, Mosqueda-Solis A, Hasnaoui M, Nepveu F, Senard JM, Bujanda L, Aldamiz-Echevarria L, Llarena M, Andrade F, Perio P, Leboulanger F, Hijona L, Arbones-Mainar JM, Portillo MP, Carpene C (2016) Limited beneficial effects of piceatannol supplementation on obesity complications in the obese Zucker rat: gut microbiota, metabolic, endocrine, and cardiac aspects. J Physiol Biochem 72:567–582
44. Baur JA, Pearson KJ, Price NL, Jamieson HA, Lerin C, Kalra A, Prabhu VV, Allard JS, Lopez-Lluch G, Lewis K, Pistell PJ, Poosala S, Becker KG, Boss O, Gwinn D, Wang M, Ramaswamy S, Fishbein KW, Spencer RG, Lakatta EG, Le Couteur D, Shaw RJ, Navas P, Puigserver P, Ingram DK, de Cabo R, Sinclair DA (2006) Resveratrol improves health and survival of mice on a high-calorie diet. Nature 444:337–342
45. Minakawa M, Miura Y, Yagasaki K (2012) Piceatannol, a resveratrol derivative, promotes glucose uptake through glucose transporter 4 translocation to plasma membrane in L6 myocytes and suppresses blood glucose levels in type 2 diabetic model db/db mice. Biochem Biophys Res Commun 422:469–475
46. Uchida-Maruki H, Inagaki H, Ito R, Kurita I, Sai M, Ito T (2015) Piceatannol lowers the blood glucose level in diabetic mice. Biol Pharm Bull 38:629–633
47. Oritani Y, Okitsu T, Nishimura E, Sai M, Ito T, Takeuchi S (2016) Enhanced glucose tolerance by intravascularly administered piceatannol in freely moving healthy rats. Biochem Biophys Res Commun 470:753–758
48. Jeong SO, Son Y, Lee JH, Cheong YK, Park SH, Chung HT, Pae HO (2015) Resveratrol analog piceatannol restores the palmitic acid-induced impairment of insulin signaling and production of endothelial nitric oxide via activation of anti-inflammatory and antioxidative heme oxygenase-1 in human endothelial cells. Mol Med Rep 12:937–944
49. Bastianetto S, Dumont Y, Han Y, Quirion R (2009) Comparative neuroprotective properties of stilbene and catechin analogs: action via a plasma membrane receptor site? CNS Neurosci Ther 15:76–83
50. Kim HJ, Lee KW, Lee HJ (2007) Protective effects of piceatannol against beta-amyloid-induced neuronal cell death. Ann N Y Acad Sci 1095:473–482
51. Jang YJ, Kim JE, Kang NJ, Lee KW, Lee HJ (2009) Piceatannol attenuates 4-hydroxynonenal-induced apoptosis of PC12 cells by blocking activation of c-Jun N-terminal kinase. Ann N Y Acad Sci 1171:176–182
52. Fu Z, Yang J, Wei Y, Li J (2016) Effects of piceatannol and pterostilbene against beta-amyloid-induced apoptosis on the PI3K/Akt/Bad signaling pathway in PC12 cells. Food Funct 7:1014–1023
53. Son Y, Byun SJ, Pae HO (2013) Involvement of heme oxygenase-1 expression in neuroprotection by piceatannol, a natural analog and a metabolite of resveratrol, against glutamate-mediated oxidative injury in HT22 neuronal cells. Amino Acids 45:393–401
54. He Y, Xu L, Li B, Guo ZN, Hu Q, Guo Z, Tang J, Chen Y, Zhang Y, Tang J, Zhang JH (2015) Macrophage-inducible C-type lectin/spleen tyrosine kinase signaling pathway contributes to neuroinflammation after subarachnoid hemorrhage in rats. Stroke 46:2277–2286
55. Jin CY, Moon DO, Lee KJ, Kim MO, Lee JD, Choi YH, Park YM, Kim GY (2006) Piceatannol attenuates lipopolysaccharide-induced NF-kappaB activation and NF-kappaB-related proinflammatory mediators in BV2 microglia. Pharmacol Res 54:461–467
56. Zhang S, Yang L, Kouadir M, Tan R, Lu Y, Chang J, Xu B, Yin X, Zhou X, Zhao D (2013) PP2 and piceatannol inhibit PrP106-126-induced iNOS activation mediated by CD36 in BV2 microglia. Acta Biochim Biophys Sin 45:763–772
57. Tang YL, Chan SW (2014) A review of the pharmacological effects of piceatannol on cardiovascular diseases. Phytother Res PTR 28:1581–1588
58. Hung LM, Chen JK, Lee RS, Liang HC, Su MJ (2001) Beneficial effects of astringinin, a resveratrol analogue, on the ischemia and reperfusion damage in rat heart. Free Radic Biol Med 30:877–883

59. Chen WP, Hung LM, Hsueh CH, Lai LP, Su MJ (2009) Piceatannol, a derivative of resveratrol, moderately slows I(Na) inactivation and exerts antiarrhythmic action in ischaemia-reperfused rat hearts. Brit J Pharmacol 157:381–391
60. Wang Z, Li J, Cho J, Malik AB (2014) Prevention of vascular inflammation by nanoparticle targeting of adherent neutrophils. Nat Nanotechnol 9:204–210
61. Yang CJ, Lin CY, Hsieh TC, Olson SC, Wu JM (2011) Control of eotaxin-1 expression and release by resveratrol and its metabolites in culture human pulmonary artery endothelial cells. Am J Cardiovasc Dis 1:16–30
62. Kee HJ, Park S, Kang W, Lim KS, Kim JH, Ahn Y, Jeong MH (2014) Piceatannol attenuates cardiac hypertrophy in an animal model through regulation of the expression and binding of the transcription factor GATA binding factor 6. FEBS Lett 588:1529–1536
63. Frombaum M, Therond P, Djelidi R, Beaudeux JL, Bonnefont-Rousselot D, Borderie D (2011) Piceatannol is more effective than resveratrol in restoring endothelial cell dimethylarginine dimethylaminohydrolase expression and activity after high-glucose oxidative stress. Free Radic Res 45:293–302
64. Woo A, Min B, Ryoo S (2010) Piceatannol-3'-*O*-beta-D-glucopyranoside as an active component of rhubarb activates endothelial nitric oxide synthase through inhibition of arginase activity. Exp Mol Med 42:524–532
65. Cao L, Li L, Yang H, Yin H (2010) Overexpression of P-selectin glycoprotein ligand-1 enhances adhesive properties of endothelial progenitor cells through Syk activation. Acta Biochim Biophys Sin 42:507–514
66. Oh KS, Ryu SY, Kim YS, Lee BH (2007) Large conductance Ca^{2+}-activated K^{+} (BKCa) channels are involved in the vascular relaxations elicited by piceatannol isolated from *Rheum undulatum* rhizome. Planta Med 73:1441–1446
67. Luskova P, Draber P (2004) Modulation of the Fcepsilon receptor I signaling by tyrosine kinase inhibitors: search for therapeutic targets of inflammatory and allergy diseases. Curr Pharm Des 10:1727–1737
68. Sato D, Shimizu N, Shimizu Y, Akagi M, Eshita Y, Ozaki S, Nakajima N, Ishihara K, Masuoka N, Hamada H, Shimoda K, Kubota N (2014) Synthesis of glycosides of resveratrol, pterostilbene, and piceatannol, and their anti-oxidant, anti-allergic, and neuroprotective activities. Biosci Biotechnol Biochem 78:1123–1128
69. Ko YJ, Kim HH, Kim EJ, Katakura Y, Lee WS, Kim GS, Ryu CH (2013) Piceatannol inhibits mast cell-mediated allergic inflammation. Int J Mol Med 31:951–958
70. Matsuda H, Tomohiro N, Hiraba K, Harima S, Ko S, Matsuo K, Yoshikawa M, Kubo M (2001) Study on anti-Oketsu activity of rhubarb II. Anti-allergic effects of stilbene components from Rhei undulati Rhizoma (dried rhizome of Rheum undulatum cultivated in Korea). Biol Pharm Bull 24:264–267
71. Perecko T, Drabikova K, Nosal R, Harmatha J, Jancinova V (2012) Involvement of caspase-3 in stilbene derivatives induced apoptosis of human neutrophils in vitro. Interdiscip Toxicol 5:76–80
72. Jancinova V, Perecko T, Nosal R, Svitekova K, Drabikova K (2013) The natural stilbenoid piceatannol decreases activity and accelerates apoptosis of human neutrophils: involvement of protein kinase C. Oxid Med Cell Longev 2013:136539
73. Antoine F, Ennaciri J, Girard D (2010) Syk is a novel target of arsenic trioxide (ATO) and is involved in the toxic effect of ATO in human neutrophils. Toxicol In Vitro 24:936–941
74. Kim DH, Lee YG, Park HJ, Lee JA, Kim HJ, Hwang JK, Choi JM (2015) Piceatannol inhibits effector T cell functions by suppressing TcR signaling. Int Immunopharmacol 25:285–292
75. Chang JK, Hsu YL, Teng IC, Kuo PL (2006) Piceatannol stimulates osteoblast differentiation that may be mediated by increased bone morphogenetic protein-2 production. Eur J Pharmacol 551:1–9
76. Ke K, Sul OJ, Rajasekaran M, Choi HS (2015) MicroRNA-183 increases osteoclastogenesis by repressing heme oxygenase-1. Bone 81:237–246

77. Schulze J, Albers J, Baranowsky A, Keller J, Spiro A, Streichert T, Zustin J, Amling M, Schinke T (2010) Osteolytic prostate cancer cells induce the expression of specific cytokines in bone-forming osteoblasts through a Stat3/5-dependent mechanism. Bone 46:524–533
78. Cherniack EP (2010) The potential influence of plant polyphenols on the aging process. Forschende Komplementarmedizin 17:181–187
79. Kawakami S, Kinoshita Y, Maruki-Uchida H, Yanae K, Sai M, Ito T (2014) Piceatannol and its metabolite, isorhapontigenin, induce SIRT1 expression in THP-1 human monocytic cell line. Nutrients 6:4794–4804
80. Matsui Y, Sugiyama K, Kamei M, Takahashi T, Suzuki T, Katagata Y, Ito T (2010) Extract of passion fruit (*Passiflora edulis*) seed containing high amounts of piceatannol inhibits melanogenesis and promotes collagen synthesis. J Agric Food Chem 58:11112–11118
81. Yokozawa T, Kim YJ (2007) Piceatannol inhibits melanogenesis by its antioxidative actions. Biol Pharm Bull 30:2007–2011
82. Maruki-Uchida H, Kurita I, Sugiyama K, Sai M, Maeda K, Ito T (2013) The protective effects of piceatannol from passion fruit (*Passiflora edulis*) seeds in UVB-irradiated keratinocytes. Biol Pharm Bull 36:845–849
83. Shiratake S, Nakahara T, Iwahashi H, Onodera T, Mizushina Y (2015) Rose myrtle (*Rhodomyrtus tomentosa*) extract and its component, piceatannol, enhance the activity of DNA polymerase and suppress the inflammatory response elicited by UVB induced DNA damage in skin cells. Mol Med Rep 12:5857–5864
84. Liu L, Li J, Kundu JK, Surh YJ (2014) Piceatannol inhibits phorbol ester-induced expression of COX-2 and iNOS in HR-1 hairless mouse skin by blocking the activation of NF-kappaB and AP-1. Inflamm Res 63:1013–1021
85. Youn J, Lee JS, Na HK, Kundu JK, Surh YJ (2009) Resveratrol and piceatannol inhibit iNOS expression and NF-kappaB activation in dextran sulfate sodium-induced mouse colitis. Nutr Cancer 61:847–854
86. Kim YH, Kwon HS, Kim DH, Cho HJ, Lee HS, Jun JG, Park JH, Kim JK (2008) Piceatannol, a stilbene present in grapes, attenuates dextran sulfate sodium-induced colitis. Int Immunopharmacol 8:1695–1702
87. Yum S, Jeong S, Lee S, Nam J, Kim W, Yoo JW, Kim MS, Lee BL, Jung Y (2015) Colon-targeted delivery of piceatannol enhances anti-colitic effects of the natural product: potential molecular mechanisms for therapeutic enhancement. Drug Des Dev Therapy 9:4247–4258
88. Dang O, Navarro L, David M (2004) Inhibition of lipopolysaccharide-induced interferon regulatory factor 3 activation and protection from septic shock by hydroxystilbenes. Shock 21:470–475
89. Ishizuka F, Shimazawa M, Inoue Y, Nakano Y, Ogishima H, Nakamura S, Tsuruma K, Tanaka H, Inagaki N, Hara H (2013) Toll-like receptor 4 mediates retinal ischemia/reperfusion injury through nuclear factor-kappaB and spleen tyrosine kinase activation. Invest Ophthalmol Vis Sci 54:5807–5816
90. Kalariya NM, Shoeb M, Reddy AB, Sawhney R, Ramana KV (2013) Piceatannol suppresses endotoxin-induced ocular inflammation in rats. Int Immunopharmacol 17:439–446
91. Potter GA, Patterson LH, Wanogho E, Perry PJ, Butler PC, Ijaz T, Ruparelia KC, Lamb JH, Farmer PB, Stanley LA, Burke MD (2002) The cancer preventative agent resveratrol is converted to the anticancer agent piceatannol by the cytochrome P450 enzyme CYP1B1. Brit J Cancer 86:774–778
92. Piver B, Fer M, Vitrac X, Merillon JM, Dreano Y, Berthou F, Lucas D (2004) Involvement of cytochrome P450 1A2 in the biotransformation of trans-resveratrol in human liver microsomes. Biochem Pharmacol 68:773–782
93. Kim DH, Ahn T, Jung HC, Pan JG, Yun CH (2009) Generation of the human metabolite piceatannol from the anticancer-preventive agent resveratrol by bacterial cytochrome P450 BM3. Drug Metab Dispos 37:932–936
94. Setoguchi Y, Oritani Y, Ito R, Inagaki H, Maruki-Uchida H, Ichiyanagi T, Ito T (2014) Absorption and metabolism of piceatannol in rats. J Agric Food Chem 62:2541–2548

95. Roupe KA, Yanez JA, Teng XW, Davies NM (2006) Pharmacokinetics of selected stilbenes: rhapontigenin, piceatannol and pinosylvin in rats. J Pharm Pharmacol 58:1443–1450
96. Miksits M, Maier-Salamon A, Vo TP, Sulyok M, Schuhmacher R, Szekeres T, Jager W (2010) Glucuronidation of piceatannol by human liver microsomes: major role of UGT1A1, UGT1A8 and UGT1A10. J Pharm Pharmacol 62:47–54
97. Miksits M, Sulyok M, Schuhmacher R, Szekeres T, Jager W (2009) In-vitro sulfation of piceatannol by human liver cytosol and recombinant sulfotransferases. J Pharm Pharmacol 61:185–191
98. Chun YJ, Kim MY, Guengerich FP (1999) Resveratrol is a selective human cytochrome P450 1A1 inhibitor. Biochem Biophys Res Commun 262:20–24
99. Chen ZH, Hurh YJ, Na HK, Kim JH, Chun YJ, Kim DH, Kang KS, Cho MH, Surh YJ (2004) Resveratrol inhibits TCDD-induced expression of CYP1A1 and CYP1B1 and catechol estrogen-mediated oxidative DNA damage in cultured human mammary epithelial cells. Carcinogenesis 25:2005–2013
100. Macpherson L, Matthews J (2010) Inhibition of aryl hydrocarbon receptor-dependent transcription by resveratrol or kaempferol is independent of estrogen receptor alpha expression in human breast cancer cells. Cancer Lett 299:119–129
101. Chang TK, Chen J, Yu CT (2007) In vitro inhibition of rat CYP1A1 and CYP1A2 by piceatannol, a hydroxylated metabolite of trans-resveratrol. Drug Metab Lett 1:13–16
102. Mikstacka R, Rimando AM, Szalaty K, Stasik K, Baer-Dubowska W (2006) Effect of natural analogues of trans-resveratrol on cytochromes P4501A2 and 2E1 catalytic activities. Xenobiotica 36:269–285
103. Oskarsson A, Spatafora C, Tringali C, Andersson AO (2014) Inhibition of CYP17A1 activity by resveratrol, piceatannol, and synthetic resveratrol analogs. Prostate 74:839–851
104. Messiad H, Amira-Guebailia H, Houache O (2013) Reversed phase high performance liquid chromatography used for the physicochemical and thermodynamic characterization of piceatannol/beta-cyclodextrin complex. J Chromatogr B Analyt Technol Biomed Life Sci 926:21–27

Chapter 10
Fisetin and Its Role in Chronic Diseases

Harish C. Pal, Ross L. Pearlman and Farrukh Afaq

Abstract Chronic inflammation is a prolonged and dysregulated immune response leading to a wide variety of physiological and pathological conditions such as neurological abnormalities, cardiovascular diseases, diabetes, obesity, pulmonary diseases, immunological diseases, cancers, and other life-threatening conditions. Therefore, inhibition of persistent inflammation will reduce the risk of inflammation-associated chronic diseases. Inflammation-related chronic diseases require chronic treatment without side effects. Use of traditional medicines and restricted diet has been utilized by mankind for ages to prevent or treat several chronic diseases. Bioactive dietary agents or "Nutraceuticals" present in several fruits, vegetables, legumes, cereals, fibers, and certain spices have shown potential to inhibit or reverse the inflammatory responses and several chronic diseases related to chronic inflammation. Due to safe, nontoxic, and preventive benefits, the use of nutraceuticals as dietary supplements or functional foods has increased in the Western world. Fisetin (3,3′,4′,7-tetrahydroxyflavone) is a dietary flavonoid found in various fruits (strawberries, apples, mangoes, persimmons, kiwis, and grapes), vegetables (tomatoes, onions, and cucumbers), nuts, and wine that has shown strong anti-inflammatory, anti-oxidant, anti-tumorigenic, anti-invasive, anti-angiogenic, anti-diabetic, neuroprotective, and cardioprotective effects in cell culture and in animal models relevant to human diseases. In this chapter, we discuss the beneficial pharmacological effects of fisetin against different pathological conditions with special emphasis on diseases related to chronic inflammatory conditions.

H.C. Pal · R.L. Pearlman · F. Afaq (✉)
Department of Dermatology, University of Alabama at Birmingham,
Volker Hall, Room 501, 1670 University Blvd., Birmingham, AL 35294, USA
e-mail: farrukhafaq@uabmc.edu

F. Afaq
Comprehensive Cancer Center, University of Alabama at Birmingham,
Birmingham, AL, USA

S.C. Gupta et al. (eds.), *Anti-inflammatory Nutraceuticals and Chronic Diseases*,
Advances in Experimental Medicine and Biology 928,
DOI 10.1007/978-3-319-41334-1_10

Keywords Fisetin · Inflammation · Chronic diseases · Cytokines · Transcription factors · Nutraceuticals · Neurological diseases · Cardiovascular diseases · Pulmonary diseases · Diabetes · Obesity · Allergy · Cancer

Abbreviations

AChE	Acetylcholinesterase
CAT	Catalase
COX	Cyclooxygenase
EMT	Epithelial-to-mesenchymal transition
EPCR	Endothelial cell protein C receptor
ERK	Extracellular signal-regulated kinase
$GABA_A$	Gamma-aminobutyric acid A
GLUT4	Glucose transporter type 4
GR	Glutathione reductase
GSH	Glutathione
GSH-Px	Glutathione peroxidase
GST	Glutathione S-transferase
HDL	High density lipoprotein
HMGB1	High mobility group box 1
IL	Interleukin
iNOS	Inducible nitrogen oxide synthase
LDL	Low-density lipoprotein
LOX	Lipoxygenase
MAPKs	Mitogen-activated protein kinases
MMP	Matrix metalloproteinase
MPO	Myeloperoxidase
mTOR	Mammalian target of rapamycin
NFκB	Nuclear factor-kappa B
NO	Nitric oxide
Nrf2	Nuclear factor erythroid-2-related factor 2
PECAM-1	Platelet endothelial cell adhesion molecule 1
PGE_2	Prostaglandin E_2
PI3K	Phosphatidylinositol 3-kinase
PPARγ	Peroxisome proliferator-activated receptor gamma
SCD-1	Stearoyl-CoA desaturase-1
SCEM	Small Clot Embolism Model
SOD	Superoxide dismutase
$SREBP_{1C}$	Sterol-regulatory-element-binding protein-1c
STAT	Signal transducer and activator of transcription
TARC	Thymus and activation regulated chemokine
TLR4	Toll-like receptor 4
TSLP	Thymic stromal lymphopoietin
VLDL	Very-low-density lipoprotein

10.1 Introduction

Inflammation is a powerful and highly complex adaptive component of the body's immune response that helps to repair damaged tissue and protects against a variety of harmful stimuli, such as pathogens, dead cells, or chemical or physical irritants. In response to harmful stimuli, initiation of the inflammatory reaction, progression of inflammation, termination of harmful events followed by resolution of inflammation are major coordinated series of events [1, 2]. These inflammatory responses attract and activate phagocytic cells such as neutrophils, monocytes, and macrophages to destroy pathogens, limit tissue damage, and spread of pathogens by constructing a physical barrier to repair and heal the damaged tissues. Stage of inflammation is governed by inflammatory mediators, inflammatory cytokines, and pro-inflammatory transcription factors. Production of these inflammatory regulators further recruits inflammatory cells to amplify inflammatory condition [3, 4]. The end point of acute inflammation is usually favorable. However, there is a fine line between the beneficial and harmful effects of inflammation. Acute inflammation is generally a short-term immune response that diminishes after healing or elimination of pathogens. Inadequate immune response or insufficient inflammation may lead to delayed wound repair and persistent infection of pathogens. However, the beneficial and harmful outcome of inflammation depends on precisely controlled response. Uncontrolled acute immune response can result in allergic response or fatal anaphylactic shock. On the other hand, prolonged and dysregulated chronic inflammation leads to development of various chronic conditions such as neurological abnormalities, cardiovascular diseases, diabetes, obesity, pulmonary diseases, immunological diseases, cancers, and other life-threatening inflammatory diseases (Fig. 10.1) [5]. Thus, modulating inflammatory response is of preventive and therapeutic interest, and approaches targeting inflammation are used to treat a wide variety of illnesses. Although acute inflammatory conditions can be effectively managed by steroidal anti-inflammatory drugs (SAID) and nonsteroidal anti-inflammatory drugs (NSAIDs), long-term treatment of chronic inflammatory conditions by these drugs is associated with severe adverse effects. A growing body of evidence has demonstrated that long-term use of NSAIDs results in severe adverse effects in the gastrointestinal tract and also results in liver toxicities [6, 7]. Therefore, inflammation-related chronic diseases require chronic treatment without side effects [8].

Use of traditional medicines and restricted diet has been utilized by mankind for ages to prevent or treat several chronic diseases. The term "nutraceuticals" consists of "nutrition" and "pharmaceutical" and thus is defined as "a food (or part of a food) that provides medical or health benefits, including the prevention and/or treatment of a disease" [9]. Bioactive dietary agents (i.e., nutraceuticals) present in several fruits, vegetables, legumes, cereals, fibers, and certain spices have shown potential to inhibit or reverse the inflammatory responses and several chronic diseases related to chronic inflammation [10, 11]. Bioactive foods containing natural anti-inflammatory agents are gaining attention due to their potential nutritional value, low toxicity, low

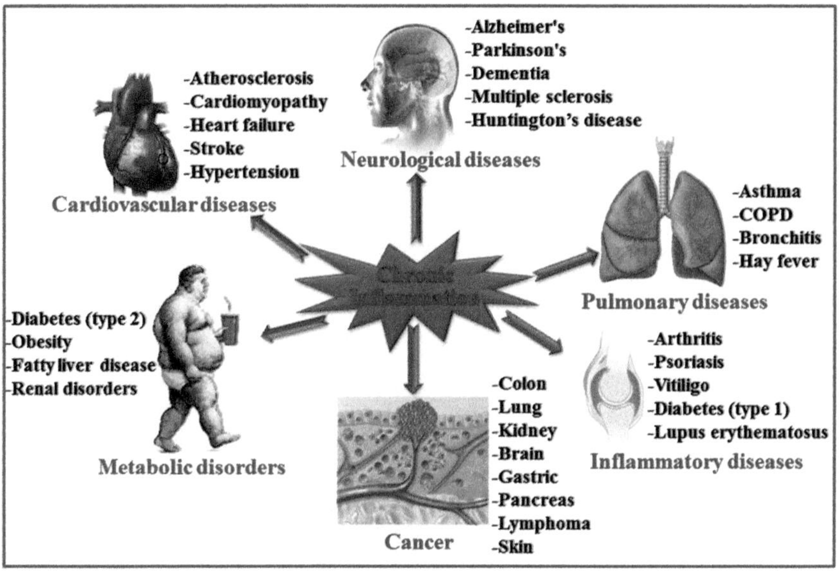

Fig. 10.1 Inflammation-related chronic disease

cost, oral bioavailability, and preventive/therapeutic effects. Nutraceuticals have demonstrated several health benefits by preventing or delaying the onset of chronic diseases; therefore, use of nutraceuticals as dietary supplements or functional foods has also increased in the Western world [8, 12].

Fisetin (3,3′,4′,7-tetrahydroxyflavone) (Fig. 10.2) is one such dietary flavonoid found in various fruits (strawberries, apples, persimmons, mangoes, kiwis, and grapes), vegetables (tomatoes, onions, and cucumbers), nuts, and wine (Fig. 10.3). Concentration of fisetin in these sources ranged from 2 to 160 μg/g of the material [13]. The highest amount of fisetin has been found to be present in strawberries, apples, and persimmon. Fisetin average daily intake has been estimated to be 0.4 mg [13, 14]. It is also abundantly present in various acacias trees and shrubs belonging to Fabaceae family such as *Acacia greggii*, *Acacia berlandieri*, *Gleditschia triacanthow*, Anacardiaceae family members such as the parrot tree (*Butea fronds*), the honey locust (*Gleditsia triacanthos*). In addition, fisetin can be

Fig. 10.2 Structure of fisetin

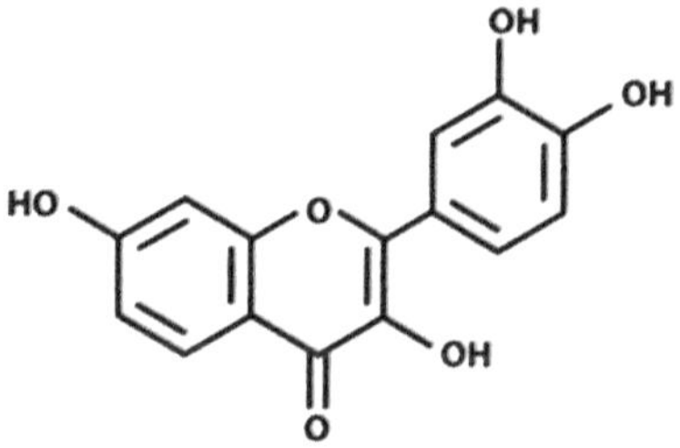

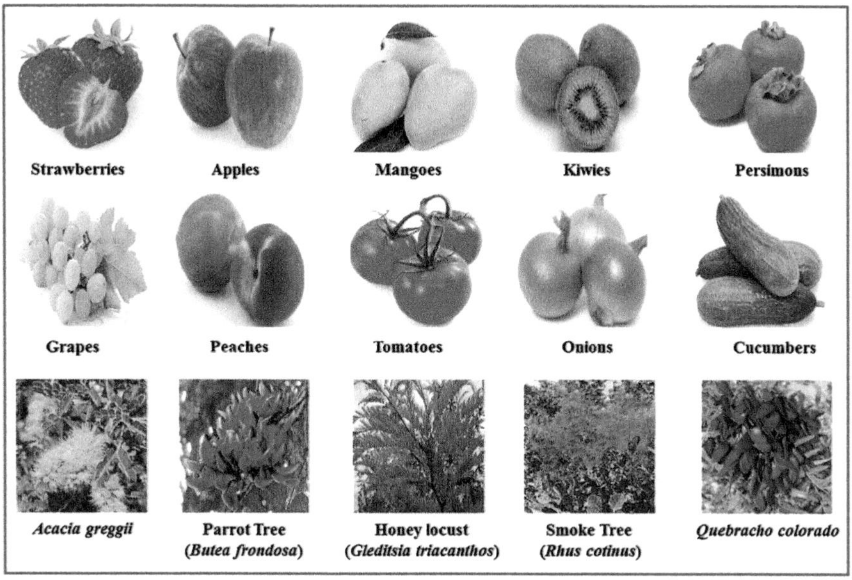

Fig. 10.3 Source of fisetin

found in the *Quebracho colorado* and *Rhus cotinus*, lac tree (*Rhus vemiciflua* Stokes) extract, smoke tree (*Cotinus coggygria*), *Pinopyta* species like *Callitropsis nootkatensis* (yellow cypress) and other trees and shrubs (Fig. 10.3) [15]. Fisetin is a potent antioxidant and free radical scavenger. It has shown potential to inhibit cell proliferation, growth, and survival of various cancer cells via different mechanisms [16–21]. Its anti-invasive and anti-angiogenic effects were also recently reported [22–24]. A growing body of evidence has demonstrated that fisetin has potential to prevent and/or inhibit various chronic inflammation-related conditions [25–30]. Neuroprotective, cardioprotective, and anti-diabetic potentials of fisetin have been established by employing cell culture studies and animal models relevant to human diseases [26, 31–37]. More importantly, treatment of these animals with fisetin was devoid of any sign of measurable toxicity. Using experimental animals, studies have demonstrated that fisetin was readily absorbed and distributed to the blood vessels [38]. Moreover, studies have demonstrated that after 40 min of oral administration, fisetin can be detected within the blood vessels of the brain for 2 h suggesting that it is well absorbed and bioavailable in the distal organs [38]. Due to low toxicity and a wide range of beneficial pharmacological effects, fisetin has been accepted as a nutraceutical and nutritional dietary supplement for neuroprotection.

As the medical sciences progress, we are beginning to understand with greater detail the mechanisms by which inflammation, cancer, and chronic disease progress. Despite having our greater understanding, many chronic disease processes continue to evade and defy modern therapies. For this reason, novel approaches to the management of chronic disease are necessary. Fisetin is a natural compound that

Table 10.1 Effects of fisetin on inflammation-related chronic diseases

Chronic diseases	Effects of fisetin	References
Neurological disorders	Inhibits progression of Parkinson's, Alzheimer's, Multiple sclerosis, and Huntington's disease	[31, 35–37, 53]
	Enhances memory, object recognition, and learning	[34, 48, 58]
	Reduces ROS and LPO	[26, 52, 62, 63, 67, 68]
	Enhances SOD, CAT, GSH, GST, and AChe	[63–66].
	Reduces TNFα, IL-1β, COX-2, LOX, TXB, iNOS, NO, and MMPs	[31, 47, 59, 60, 63–66]
	Downregulates NFκB and MAPK pathways	[35, 36,59, 60]
	Enhances neuronal differentiation and survival	[32, 54, 59, 62]
	Enhances serotonin and noradrenalin	[61]
	Protects from $AlCl_3$ neurotoxicity	[63]
	Inhibits invasion of glioblastoma	[67, 68]
Diabetes	Reduces plasma glucose levels and gluconeogenesis	[69, 70]
	Enhances glycolysis and glycogen storage	[69, 70]
	Restores hexokinase, pyruvate kinase, and lactate dehydrogenase enzyme activities	[69]
	Inhibits gluconeogenic enzymes	[69]
	Activates glycogenesis enzymes	[69]
	Reduces histone acetylation and histone acetyltransferases	[71].
	Reduces TNFα, IL6, and NFκB	[26, 71]
	Reduces vascular permeability	[26]
	Reduces expression of ICAM-1, VCAM-1, and E-selectin	[26]
	Reduces ROS generation	[26, 73, 74]
	Reduces kidney hypertrophy and albuminuria	[35, 36]
	Reduces severity of cataracts and delays onset of cataracts	[72]
	Reduces neuropathic pain by targeting $GABA_A$ receptors	[73, 74]

(continued)

Table 10.1 (continued)

Chronic diseases	Effects of fisetin	References
Obesity	Reduces high-fat diet-induced weight gain	[75]
	Inhibits proliferation and differentiation of adipocytes	[75, 76]
	Reduces phosphorylation of mTORC1, AKT, and S6K1	[75]
	Inhibits cyclin A, cyclin D1, and cdk 4 expression	[76]
	Upregulates p27 expression	[76]
	Reduces total cholesterol, LDL, VLDL, and HDL	[77, 78]
	Normalizes bile acid metabolism and reduces hepatic abundance of CYP7A1	[65, 66, 77, 78]
	Reduces lipogenesis and inhibits PRAPγ, $SREBP_{1C}$ and SCD-1	[77, 78]
	Reduces fatty acid synthesis and ATP citrate lyase	[77, 78]
	Inhibits high-fat diet-induced expression of miR-378	[79]
	Decreases hepatic fat accumulation	[79]
Atherosclerosis	Inhibits atherosclerosis	[88]
	Reduces LDL, VLDL, and enhances HDL	[88, 89]
	Inhibits oxidation of LDLs by macrophages	[90]
	Inhibits CD36 expression in macrophages	[90, 91]
	Inhibits ROS generation in endothelial cells	[90]
Cancers	Reduces cell proliferation, induces cell cycle arrest and apoptosis by intrinsic and extrinsic pathways	[16,19, 21, 22, 44, 100, 103, 104, 107–110, 117, 118].
	Inhibits cell invasion, EMT, and angiogenesis	[23, 24, 46, 67, 68, 105, 106, 117]
	Inhibits PI3 K/AKT/mTOR, Wnt/β-catenin, NFκB, MAPKs, AP-1, and other signaling pathways	[16, 18, 21, 22, 24, 46, 93, 104, 106, 109, 122–124]
	Protects from UVB-induced DNA damage and inflammation	[18, 92, 93]
	Inhibits infiltration of inflammatory cells	[18, 92, 93]
	Inhibits inflammatory mediators (COX-2, PGE_2, EP receptors, MPO, MMPs, NO, and iNOS)	[18, 92, 93, 109]
	Inhibits inflammatory cytokines (TNFα, IL-1β, IL-6, and IL-8)	[18, 92, 93, 122, 123]

(continued)

Table 10.1 (continued)

Chronic diseases	Effects of fisetin	References
Other inflammatory diseases	Reduces allergic reaction and inhibits atopic dermatitis	[25]
	Inhibits IgE production and allergic inflammation	[25]
	Reduces TNFα, IFNγ, IL-1β, IL-4, IL-5, IL-6, IL-8, IL-13, and hexoaminidase production	[29, 125, 126, 128]
	Inhibits production of COX-2, NO, and iNOS	[28, 130]
	Inhibits NFκB, MAPKs, Src, and Syk levels in immune cells	[25, 26, 28, 30, 129, 130]

has evoked a great amount of research interest in recent years, demonstrating potent anti-inflammatory, anti-tumorigenic, and anti-oxidant properties. In this chapter, we discuss various pharmacological effects of fisetin against different pathological conditions with special emphasis on diseases related to chronic inflammatory conditions (Table 10.1).

10.2 Physciochemical Properties of Fisetin

Fisetin is a yellow bioactive pigment with molecular formula $C_{15}H_{10}O_6$ [IUPAC Name: 2-(3,4-dihydroxyphenyl)-3,7-dihydroxychromen-4-one)] and molecular weight of 286.2363 g/mol. Fisetin has a density of 1.688 g/ml and melting point of 330 °C. Its topological polar surface area is 107 Å with low lipophilicity (CLogP = 1.24). It has four hydrogen bond donors, 6 hydrogen bond acceptors, and one rotatable bond with one covalently bonded unit count. Fisetin is a rare flavone without 5-hydroxy substitution and has four hydroxyl groups in its structure. Fisetin is partly soluble in aqueous buffer. Its solubility in ethanol is approximately 5 mg/ml while in DMSO it is highly soluble (approximately 30 mg/ml) at 25 °C and gives a yellow color.

10.3 Modulation of Cell Signaling Pathways by Fisetin

Studies have demonstrated that fisetin inhibits proliferation of various cancer cells in vitro and in vivo. Fisetin at lower doses targets Aurora B kinase by inhibiting kinetochore and centromere localization leading to immature segregation of chromosomes and premature cessation of mitosis without cytokinesis resulting in aneuploidy [39]. However at higher doses, fisetin inhibited DNA replication enzymes topoisomerase I and II resulting in chromosomal breakage [40, 41]. In addition, fisetin inhibited cell cycle progression by targeting cyclins and cyclin-dependent kinases (cdks) [42, 43]. Fisetin also induced apoptosis in different cancer cell lines by modulating expression and translocation of Bcl-2 family proteins involved in the intrinsic apoptotic pathway. In addition, fisetin induced apoptosis *via* the extrinsic pathway by enhancing expression of cell surface death receptors and their ligands such as death receptor 5 (DR5), Fas ligand, and tumor necrosis factor (TNF)-related apoptosis-inducing ligand (TRAIL) in various cancer cell lines [44]. Higher affinity of fisetin for androgen receptors (AR) than dihydrotestosterone suggested that fisetin inhibits AR-mediated transactivation of target genes in prostate cancer [45]. Moreover, fisetin inhibited cell proliferation and survival by dual inhibition of PI3 K/AKT and mTOR signaling. At molecular levels, fisetin inhibited expression of PI3 K, phosphorylation of AKT and expression and phosphorylation of mTOR. Fisetin also inhibited mTOR kinase activity and CAP-dependent protein translation by inhibiting mTOR complex formation [20, 46]. Fisetin exerted its apoptotic effects by suppressing the phosphorylation of p38, ERK1/2, and AKT [22, 46]. Fisetin treatment also inhibited NFκB DNA binding activity and activation of NFκB in different cancer cells. In melanoma cells, fisetin treatment induced apoptosis by targeting PI3 K and Wnt/β-catenin signaling pathways [21, 22]. Furthermore, it inhibited cell invasion and metastasis by targeting PI3 K, MAPK, and NFκB signaling pathways and downregulated angiogenesis by reducing MMP and VEGF expression [22–24]. Fisetin also inhibited inflammatory responses by reducing NFκB signaling, pro-inflammatory mediators (such as COX-2/PGE_2, NO, iNOS, and MPO), and inflammatory cytokines (such as TNFα, IL-1β, IL-6, and IL-8) in UVB-induced SKH-1 hairless mice [18].

In addition to its antitumor activity, fisetin is a well-known protector of cerebrovascular and neurodegenerative diseases by inducing neurite outgrowth and neuronal differentiation via ERK1/2 activation. Fisetin also suppressed lipopolysaccharides (LPS)-induced neuroinflammation by inhibiting activation of NFκB and MAPKs pathways and by reducing pro-inflammatory mediators and inflammatory cytokines in cell culture as well as in brain microglia of neuroprotective murine models [31, 35, 36, 47, 48].

10.4 Role of Fisetin in Chronic Diseases

10.4.1 Fisetin and Neurological Diseases

Various neurological pathologies such as stroke, trauma, Alzheimer's, and Parkinson's have been implicated with oxidative stress-induced nerve cell death. Epidemiological and experimental studies have shown that flavonoids have potential to protect the brain due to their ability to modulate intracellular signals promoting cellular survival [49–51]. Fisetin effectively protected central nervous system-derived nerve cells (HT-22 cells) and rat primary neurons from glutamate toxicity, hypoglycemia, and oxidative injuries by altering glutathione (GSH) metabolism. In addition, fisetin blocked hydrogen peroxide (H_2O_2)-induced neuronal death by reactive oxygen species (ROS) scavenging effects [52]. Fisetin also inhibited in vitro myelin phagocytosis by macrophages responsible for secretion of inflammatory mediators, suggesting the potential to reduce the risk of a chronic inflammatory disease of central nervous system called multiple sclerosis leading to neurological deficits [53]. In addition, fisetin treatment significantly reduced ROS production without affecting the viability of macrophage cells. Upon in vitro experimental evaluation of a variety of flavonoids using a well-studied model system of neuronal differentiation PC-12 cells expressing nerve growth factor (NGF) derived from rat embryonic origin from the neural crest, Sagara et al. [54] found that fisetin was the most effective neuroprotective flavonoid. Employing an extensive mechanistic approach, it was found that fisetin most effectively induced neurite outgrowth and PC-12 cell differentiation by activation of the Ras-ERK cascade, particularly by ERK activation [32, 54].

It was also shown that fisetin promotes nerve cell survival by enhancement of proteasome activity after neurotrophic factor withdrawal, suggesting that it can also act as neurotrophic factor [55]. Most importantly, Maher et al. [34] found that fisetin treatment enhances memory in experimental rats by activation of ERK and induction of cAMP response element-binding protein (CREB) phosphorylation in rats hippocampal slices. Moreover, intraperitoneal administration of a single dose of liposomal preparation containing 30 mg/kg dose of fisetin resulted in detection of 8.23 ng fisetin per gram of brain tissue and exerted protective effects demonstrated by recovery of the cytoarchitecture in ischemic areas of striatum and cortex in rats. However, a similar dose of fisetin went undetected in the brain when administered in aqueous preparation [56]. Similarly, intravenous injection of 50 mg/kg fisetin initiated after 5 min of embolizaion resulted in significant protection in Rabbit Small Clot Embolism Model (SCEM) [55]. Moreover, oral administration of 5–25 mg/kg of fisetin resulted in dose-dependent enhancement in long-term memory in mice [34]. Furthermore, feeding of mice for 10 months with diet containing fisetin (500 mg/kg of food) resulted in substantial improvement in learning compared to age-matched mice fed on a fisetin-free diet. Moreover, feeding of fisetin-containing diet to these mice resulted in significantly improved memory in the morris water maze (MWM) test relative to age-matched mice fed on a fisetin-free diet [48]. In addition, studies have demonstrated that feeding of 14.8 gm of dried aqueous strawberry extract (a major source of fisetin) per kilogram of diet for 8 weeks to 19-months old rats indicated that fisetin-containing strawberry extract reversed age-related deficits and improved memory in the MWM compared to control diet fed rats [57]. Feeding of strawberry extract containing diet to rats demonstrated better protection against spatial deficits caused by irradiation with 1.5 Gy of 1 GeV/n ^{56}Fe particles. The results from this study provided evidence that strawberry extract fed animals were better able to retain place information (a hippocampally mediated behavior) compared to control [58]. These studies clearly demonstrated that fisetin has potential to protect and enhance survival of nerve cells, induce differentiation and enhance long-term memory.

Pathogenesis of chronic neurodegenerative diseases such as Alzheimer's, Parkinson's, Huntington's disease, multiple sclerosis, and HIV-associated dementia is highly associated with neuroinflammation. Inflammation-mediated neurotoxicity is governed by microglia, which are the primary immune effector cells in the central nerves system (CNS). Upon stimulation by LPS, interferon γ(IFNγ) or β-amyloid activated microglia secrete various pro-inflammatory cytokines (such as TNFα, PGE_2, IL-1, and IL-6) and free radicals like nitric oxide (NO) and superoxide anion. Secretion of these pro-inflammatory mediators leads to neuroinflammatory diseases. Fisetin treatment of LPS-stimulated BV-2 microglia cells and primary microglia cultures greatly reduced secretion of TNFα, $PGE_{2,}$ and NO [59]. LPS-induced stimulation of TNFα, IL-1β, COX-2, and iNOS were inhibited both at the mRNA and protein levels after fisetin treatment [47, 59]. Furthermore, fisetin treatment inhibited the activation of NFκB, a central regulator of inflammation by reducing IκB degradation and nuclear translation of NFκB/p65 subunit in LPS-stimulated BV-2 microglia cells. Fisetin treatment also inhibited phosphorylation of p38 in these cells. Moreover, fisetin protected B35 neuroblastoma cells from toxicity induced by activated BV-2 microglia cells in coculture [59]. In mice, intraperitoneal administration of fisetin (10 and 20 mg/kg) improved neuroinflammation by reducing IL-1β and inhibiting microglial activation. Fisetin treatment to mice enhanced the level of heme-oxygenase-1(HO-1) expression, an enzyme associated with endogenous antioxidative activities. In BV-2 microglial cells induction of HO-1 expression after fisetin treatment was associated with increase in p38 and AKT phosphorylation [47].

Overexpression of pro-inflammatory markers, COX-2, and MMP-9, from brain tumor cells and associated microvascular endothelial cells has been linked to increased disruption of the blood–brain barrier (BBB) and neuroinflammation as well as enhanced tumor invasion. The production of COX-2, MMP-9, and other inflammatory markers is regulated by NFκB signaling [60]. Treatment of human brain microvascular endothelial cells (HBMECs) with fisetin (30 μM) inhibited capillary-like structure formation in vitro. By employing zymography, immunoblotting, and qRT-PCR techniques, Tahanian et al. [60] demonstrated that fisetin treatment inhibited activity, protein expression, and mRNA levels of COX-2 and MMP-9 in HBMECs induced by phorbol 12-myristate 13-acetate (PMA) exposure. Furthermore, this study also demonstrated that fisetin-inhibited PMA induced IκB phosphorylation and activation of NFκB.

Huntington's disease is a fatal neurodegenerative disorder characterized by disturbed psychiatric, cognitive, and motor functions. It is a late-onset and progressive disease involving MAPKs, particularly Ras-ERK signaling cascade. Studies have demonstrated that activation of ERK provides neuroprotection in Htt-expressing mutant nerve cells, whereas inhibition of ERK promotes nerve cell death. Ponasterone treatment has been shown to induce death in $\sim$45 % cells within 72 h by inducing Htt (Httex1-103QP-EGFP) mutation in PC12/Htt^{Q103} cells.

Studies have demonstrated that treatment of PC12/Htt^{Q103} cells with 2.5–10 μM fisetin increased cell survival by inducing ERK activation in ponasterone-treated cells without affecting the formation of Httex1-103QP aggregates or the overall level of Httex1-103QP-EGFP expression [35]. In addition, fisetin treatment reduced JNK activation in PC12/Htt^{Q103} cells in which Httex1-103QP-induced JNK phosphorylation leads to nerve cell death by caspase-3 activation. Furthermore, feeding of 1–300 μM fisetin-containing diet to Drosophila flies expressing pathogenic human Htt(w elav:Gal4/w; P{UAS-Httex1p Q93}/+) Httex1p Q93) in neuronal cells suppressed Huntington's disease like symptoms by enhanced ERK phosphorylation and activation. Feeding of fisetin-containing diet demonstrated the least neurodegeneration with rescue of ~25 % flies with enhanced survival of up to 77 % at 300 μM concentration of fisetin. Moreover, feeding of 0.05 % fisetin-containing diet to ~6 weeks old transgenic R6/2 mouse (a mammalian model of Huntington's disease) for 1 week or 7 weeks showed improved performance on the rotorod with ~30 % increase in life span as compared to wild-type littermates [35]. Furthermore, fisetin administration (5, 10, and 20 mg/kg, via gavage, p.o.) to male ICR mice evaluated for despair tests demonstrated anti-depressant effects. Neurochemical examination showed that fisetin administration enhanced serotonin and noradrenalin production in the frontal cortex and hippocampus and inhibited monoamine oxidase activity [61].

Moreover, a human case study revealed that consumption of a low-fat diet rich in fisetin and hexacosanol for 6 months resolved the clinical symptoms of Parkinson's disease such as cogwheel rigidity, bradykinesia, dystonia, micrographia, hypomimia, constricted arm swing with gait, and retropulsion. However, only little improvement in tremor or seborrhea was observed [37]. Studies have also demonstrated that fisetin (20–80 μM) treatment protected hippocampal neuronal HT22 and osteoblast-like MC3T3-E1 cells from neurotoxin fluoride, dexamethasone-induced cytotoxicity, and apoptosis by inhibiting ROS production [62]. Furthermore, aluminum is a potent environmental neurotoxin that affects cerebral functions by activating astrocytes, microglia, and associated inflammatory events. Administration of aluminum chloride ($AlCl_3$) has been associated with increased lipid peroxidation(LPO), reduction of SOD, CAT, GSH, and GST and compromised acetylcholine esterase (AChE) activity leading to neurodegenerative disorders and neuroinflammation by production of pro-inflammatory cytokines such as TNFα, IL-1β, and iNOS. Mice studies have demonstrated that co-treatment of $AlCl_3$ and fisetin orally at a dosage of 15 mg/kg b.wt. attenuated $AlCl_3$ induced neurotoxicity [63]. This study demonstrated that pre- and co-treatment of fisetin reversed $AlCl_3$ impaired recognition memory and discrimination of the object. Fisetin administration enhanced production of endogenous antioxidants such as SOD, CAT, GST, and GSH levels in the brain tissues (cortex and hippocampi) of mice with reduction in LPO. Fisetin treatment also inhibited activation of astrocytic and microglial as a result of inhibition of $AlCl_3$-induced production of pro-inflammatory cytokines such as TNFα, IL-1β, and iNOS in cortex and hippocampus of mice. Furthermore, fisetin ameliorated morphological abnormalities due to neurotoxicity and neuroinflammation induced by $AlCl_3$ [63]. Studies have demonstrated that flavonoid-rich methanolic extract of Rhus verniciflua containing fisetin as one of the ten flavonoids possesses neuroprotective and anti-inflammatory activities. Isolated fisetin from this extract significantly protected HT22 cells from glutamate-induced neurotoxicity. Fisetin treatment also protected antioxidative defense system against glutamate-induced oxidative stress by maintaining activities of different enzymes such as SOD, GSH, GSH-Px, and GR. Fisetin treatment also inhibited LPS-induced production of NO, iNOS, and COX-2 in BV2 cells [64–66].

Expression of cytosolic phospholipase A2 (cPLA2), COXs, and LOX is enhanced in hippocampi of Alzheimer's mice and these are associated with neuroinflammation. Studies employing this mouse model showed that oral feeding of fisetin in diet (0.05 % of feed, i.e., equivalent to 25 mg/kg of daily dose) restored cPLA2 levels in the hippocampi to levels similar to that of control. Expression of COXs and 12-LOX were also reduced by fisetin treatment. Feeding of fisetin to these mice inhibited production of the pro-inflammatory thromboxanes TXB1 and TXB2, which are increased in this mouse model. Furthermore, levels of the pro-inflammatory primary metabolites of 5-LOX and 12-LOX were reduced in fisetin-treated mice. Levels of multiple monohydroxy docosahexaenoic acids that are the metabolites of decosahexaenoic acid (DHA) generated by either auto-oxidation of DHA or metabolized by LOX pathways were also strongly reduced by fisetin treatment in Alzheimer's mice [31]. Long-term feeding of fisetin to mice was safe as no significant difference in body weight was observed. Furthermore, no toxicity was observed in the pathologic evaluation of lungs, liver, spleen, kidneys, heart, stomach, intestine, or reproductive organs. In acute toxicity testing, no toxicity was observed at doses up to 2 g/kg, and Ames test was negative [31].

In a recent important study, Krasieva et al. [38] using label-free two-photon microscopy of intrinsic fisetin fluorescence, demonstrated that only fisetin (no other structurally related flavonols such as 3,3′,4′-trihydroxyflavone and quercetin (3,5,7,3′,4′-pentahydroxyflavone) localized to the nucleoli in living nerve cells suggesting that the key targets of fisetin reside in the nucleus. Furthermore, fisetin was rapidly distributed to the blood vessels of the brain followed by a slower dispersion into the brain parenchyma of living mice after intraperitoneal injection and oral administration. After 8 min of intraperitoneal injection of 74 mg/kg of fisetin, it was observed within the blood vessels of the brain and continued until 15 min before diffusing to adjacent parenchyma. More importantly, after oral administration of 25 mg/kg fisetin, it was readily detectable within the blood vessels of the brain after 40 min and continued until 2 h in blood vessels and parenchyma along with more localized areas suggestive of individual neuronal cell uptake [38].

Fisetin treatment inhibited invasion of glioblastoma GBM8401 cells. Treatment with fisetin suppressed the expression of multifunctional gene family, ADAM (a disintegrin and metalloproteinase) involved in myogenesis, neurogenesis, tumorigenesis, angiogenesis, and activation of growth factors/cytokines related to inflammation. The anti-invasive effect of fisetin was associated with induction of ERK phosphorylation in these cells [67, 68]. Furthermore, studies have demonstrated that fisetin protected PC-12 cells from enhanced ROS generation induced by cobalt dichloride. Fisetin treatment increased hypoxiainducible factor 1α (HIF-1α), its nuclear accumulation and the hypoxia-response element (HRE)-driven transcriptional activation. These effects were the results of fisetin-induced phosphorylation of ERK, p38, and AKT proteins in PC-12 cells [68].

10.4.2 Fisetin and Diabetes

Diabetes mellitus is a widespread, chronic illness characterized by persistent hyperglycemia due to destruction of pancreatic β-islet cells or acquired insulin resistance of peripheral cells throughout the body. According to the United States Center for Disease Control, approximately 9.3 % of the United States population has been diagnosed with diabetes or about 9.3 million people. Fisetin may have a role to play in diabetes management as a naturopathic option with fewer side effects than current diabetes therapies. Studies have demonstrated several potential roles for fisetin in the modulation of diabetes mellitus.

Fisetin has been found to decrease plasma glucose levels in diabetic animal models by potentiating glycolysis, inhibiting gluconeogenesis, and increasing glycogen storage. Administration of oral fisetin to diabetic rats over the course of one month significantly decreased blood glucose levels, increased insulin and reduced glycosylation of red blood cells [69, 70]. Oral administration of fisetin to rats demonstrated similar metabolic changes to rats that receive gliclazide, a known oral hypoglycemic agent. Fisetin achieved these effects via modulation of enzymes involved in carbohydrate metabolism. In liver and kidney tissues, fisetin supplementation restored the activity of glycolytic pathway enzymes hexokinase, pyruvate kinase, and lactate dehydrogenase to near-normal levels. In contrast, treatment with fisetin inhibited the activity of gluconeogenic enzymes glucose-6-phosphatase, fructose-1,6-bisphosphatase, and glucose-6-phosphate dehydrogenase. Fisetin treatment also affected intrahepatic glycogen metabolism in diabetic rats via increased concentration of glycogen, activation of glycogen synthase, and inhibition of glycogen phosphorylase [69].

Evidence suggests that fisetin may have a role in the regulation of hyperglycemia-induced inflammatory responses. Innate and secondary immune cells synthesize and release inflammatory cytokines under hyperglycemic conditions. In human monocytic THP-1 cells, culture in hyperglycemic environments activates NFκB, and induces synthesis of IL-6 and TNFα. Treatment with fisetin reduced expression of these pro-inflammatory cytokines and reduced activation and translocation of NFκB [26, 71]. Fisetin exerted its anti-inflammatory effects via epigenetic regulation. Changes in expression of inflammatory cytokines were likely due to a decrease in histone acetylation via inhibition of histone acetyltransferases [71].

In addition to modulation of pro-inflammatory cytokines, fisetin has been found to decrease hyperglycemic vascular inflammation. Recent studies show that fisetin can affect several pathophysiologic processes that promote vascular inflammation including vascular permeability, leukocyte adhesion, and migration, and ROS generation. Data from *in vivo* studies suggested that pretreatment with fisetin prevents hyperglycemia-induced increases in vascular permeability of albumin. These findings were confirmed in murine models. In addition, pretreatment with fisetin inhibited hyperglycemia-induced overexpression of intercellular adhesion molecule 1 (ICAM-1), vascular cell adhesion molecule 1 (VCAM-1) and E-selectin in endothelial cells; this reduction results in decreased THP-1 adhesion to hyperglycemia-activated human umbilical vein endothelial cells (HUVECs) [26]. Vascular inflammation in diabetes patients promotes atherosclerosis and thrombosis, and fisetin treatments may be a viable option for reducing the potential for long-term cardiovascular sequelae.

Fisetin may also play a role in alleviating or reducing common complications related to diabetes mellitus. There is a well-established link between diabetes mellitus and abnormalities of lipoprotein metabolism. A recent study demonstrated that fisetin treatment of rats with streptozotocin-induced diabetes returned serum LDL and VLDL levels to normal range. Additionally, HDL levels were increased in fisetin-treated rats compared to controls [70].

Diabetes patients also frequently experience complications due to macromolecular glycosylation and hyperglycemia in multiple organ systems. Fisetin has been shown to potentiate removal of methylglyoaxal from macromolecules increase synthesis of glutathione. Activation of glyoxalase 1 by fisetin reduces the number of proteins glycated by methylgoyoxal. In Akita mice modes, this effect was linked to a reduction of kidney hypertrophy and albuminuria, both reduced by fisetin treatment [36]. Ophthalmic complications often include cataracts. A recent study demonstrated that fisetin treatment of mice with streptozotocin-induced diabetes reduced the severity of cataracts and delayed onset of late stage cataracts [72]. Moreover, antinociceptive effects of fisetin against diabetic neuropathic pain targeting spinal γ-aminobutyric acid A ($GABA_A$) receptors in mice with type 1 diabetes have been reported [73, 74]. Chronic treatment of streptozotocin-induced diabetic rats with 5–45 mg/kg body weight of fisetin administered orally twice per day for two weeks, delayed development of thermal hyperplasia and mechanical allodynia. Furthermore, fisetin treatment reduced oxidative stress in tissues of spinal cord, dorsal root ganglion, and peripheral nerves. The analgesic effect of fisetin was further potentiated by combination of fisetin with ROS scavenger phenyl-N-tert-butylnitrone.

10.4.3 *Fisetin and Obesity*

In the United States, obesity is one of the greatest public health concerns of the twenty-first century. Several mechanisms have been suggested by which fisetin treatment may mitigate the pathogenesis of diet-induced obesity. Preliminary evidence suggests that fisetin supplementation may reduce the risk of developing obesity by decreasing differentiation and proliferation of adipocytes. Undifferentiated fibroblasts, or preadipocytes, have been identified as a potential target of fisetin treatment. Recent studies have demonstrated that differentiation of 3T3-L1 undifferentiated fibroblasts into adipocytes is reduced by fisetin [75, 76]. One study found that fisetin treatment reduced phosphorylation of mTORC1 and upstream promoters of mTORC1 signaling including AKT and S6K1. In vivo experiments confirmed these findings; in murine models fed high-fat diets; fisetin supplementation reduced weight gains and accumulation of white adipose tissue via suppression of mTORC1 signaling and reduced differentiation of preadipocytes [75]. Another study suggested that fisetin treatment decreased adipocyte differentiation and proliferation by suppressing mitotic clonal expansion. Fisetin treatment reduced expression of several key cell cycle promoters including cyclin A, cyclin D1, and cdk4. In addition, fisetin upregulated the cell cycle inhibitor p27, promoting a sustained G_0 phase [76].

Fisetin may play a role in obesity treatment or prevention by modulating cholesterol homeostasis. In Sprague-Dawley hypercholesterolemic rat models, treatment with fisetin reduced several critical markers of obesity risk. The blood lipid profile of rats on a high-fat diet was improved by fisetin treatment; total cholesterol, LDL, HDL, and hepatic cholesterol levels were all reduced. The hepatic abundance of CYP7A1 was reduced to near control levels after fisetin treatment, suggesting a return to normal bile acid metabolism. Another possible mechanism by which fisetin may regulate obesity pathogenesis is by reducing hepatic lipogenesis. In Sprague-Dawley rats fed with high-fat diets, fisetin reduced expression of hepatic mRNA associated with lipogenesis including PPARγ, $SREBP_{1C}$, and SCD-1 compared to controls. Expression of gene products associated with fatty acid synthesis including fatty acid synthase and ATP citrate lyase were also markedly reduced by fisetin treatment. In addition, fisetin-induced expression of GLUT4 in 3T3-L1 differentiated adipose cells, decreasing concentrations of serum glucose [77, 78]. Another study found that fisetin treatment inhibited high-fat diet-induced expression of miR-378 and PGC-1B resulting in decreased hepatic fat accumulation and reversal of metabolic enzyme dysregulation [79]. These data indicate that fisetin treatment may attenuate obesity by reducing hepatic lipid biosynthesis.

10.4.4 Fisetin and Atherosclerosis

Atherosclerosis is a chronic disease of the arteries and considered a leading cause of mortality and morbidity associated with cardiovascular disease. Initially, atherosclerosis was believed to be a disease of lipid accumulation in the arterial wall; however, a growing body of evidence has demonstrated that dysregulated lipid metabolism is not the only cause of atherosclerosis, but maladaptive chronic inflammatory responses also play a critical role in the initiation and progression of atherosclerosis [80–82]. Accumulation of lipid-laden macrophages in the subendothelial area of the arterial wall is considered a hallmark of atherosclerosis. In addition, results from recent studies have demonstrated that neutrophils also modulate the pathogenesis of arthrosclerosis [83, 84]. Moreover, the role of IL-1β, IL-6, TNFα, P-selectin, and 5-LOX is well documented in the promotion of atherosclerosis. Experimental and preclinical studies have demonstrated that anti-inflammatory and immune-modulatory therapies reduced the risk of cardiovascular disease and atherosclerosis [85–87].

In vitro studies have suggested that fisetin treatment may be a potent inhibitor of a key step in atherosclerosis pathogenesis. Uptake of LDLs by macrophages results in the formation of foam cells, and the accumulation of foam cells promotes atherosclerotic plaque development. Studies have found that fisetin inhibits oxidation of LDLs by macrophages. Fisetin preserves the antioxidant properties of α-tocopherol associated with LDLs and prevents oxidation of this critical compound [88, 89]. In addition, fisetin inhibits copper ion-dependent LDL oxidation and subsequently blocks binding of oxidized-LDLs to the Class-B scavenger receptor CD36 on macrophages, which has been associated with atherosclerotic lesions [90, 91]. Inhibition of CD36 receptor expression in macrophages by fisetin is achieved by decreasing mRNA expression [90]. Although these in vitro findings are promising, in vivo studies demonstrating these effects have not yet emerged.

10.4.5 Fisetin and Skin Cancer

Basal cell carcinomas (BCCs) and squamous cell carcinomas (SCCs) are the most frequently diagnosed non-melanoma skin cancers (NMSCs). Ultraviolet (UV) irradiation is considered the most important extrinsic factor contributing to inflammation and skin cancer. Consumption of nontoxic dietary flavonoids to potentially prevent skin cancers has drawn a great deal of attention. Treatment of human epidermoid carcinoma A431 cells with fisetin resulted in decease in cell proliferation. Fisetin treatment enhanced G_2/M cell population and induced apoptosis through disruption of mitochondrial membrane potential and modulation in Bcl-2 family proteins. Fisetin treatment also promoted release of cytochrome c and

Smac/DIABLO proteins from mitochondria to cytosol, inducing activation of caspases, and PARP cleavage [19]. Studies have demonstrated that the expression of COX-2, PGE_2, MMPs, and other inflammatory mediators increases after UVB exposure. Fisetin treatment of UVB-irradiated human fibroblasts inhibited the expression of COX-2, PGE_2, and MMPs as well as collagen degradation. Fisetin treatment also inhibited UVB-induced intracellular ROS and NO production [92]. UVB-induced phosphorylation of MAPKs was inhibited by fisetin treatment. In addition, fisetin suppressed NFκB activation and translocation of p65 subunit to the nucleus along with the inhibition of phosphorylation of cAMP response element-binding protein (CREB) at Ser^{133} [92].

Oxidative damage and inflammation are key factors in the pathogenesis of skin cancers. Studies have shown that fisetin treatment to HaCaT cells induced nuclear factor erythroid-2-related factor 2 (Nrf2)-related HO-1 protein and mRNA expression. HO-1 is known to inhibit inflammatory responses by inhibiting neutrophil trafficking. HO-1 is a member of antioxidant response element (ARE)-related expression of phase 2 detoxifying genes regulated by Nrf2 and work as a rate-limiting enzyme in heme catabolism during UV light- or hypoxia-induced inflammatory responses. Fisetin treatment inhibited TNFα-induced expression of iNOS and COX-2, production of NO, PGE_2, IL-1β, IL-6, and activation of NFκB in HaCaT cells by inducing nuclear translocation of Nrf2 [93]. Furthermore, topical application of fisetin inhibited UVB-induced cell proliferation, hyperplasia, and infiltration of inflammatory cells in SKH-1 hairless mouse skin [18]. Fisetin treatment also reduced UVB-induced DNA damage evidenced by accelerated removal of cyclobutane pyrimidine dimers and enhanced expression of p53 and p21 proteins. Moreover, topical application of fisetin resulted in inhibition of UVB-induced inflammatory mediators (such as COX-2 and PGE_2), their receptors (EP1–EP4), and MPO activity, along with reduction in inflammatory cytokines (such as TNFα, IL-1β, and IL-6). Fisetin treatment also inhibited UVB-induced activation of PI3 K/AKT and NFκB signaling pathways [18].

Melanoma, is the least common but most lethal form of skin cancer. Due to its metastatic potential, melanoma accounts for approximately 80 % of all skin cancer-related deaths. The incidence of melanoma is increasing worldwide at an alarming rate. The global incidence rate of melanoma is 12–25 per 100,000 individual populations. Incidence rates are highest in Australia and New Zealand with ~60 cases per 100,000 inhabitants per year. The incidence rates in the United States and Europe are ~30 and ~20 cases per 100,000 per year, respectively. According to an estimate, 73,870 new cases of cutaneous melanoma and 9940 deaths due to cutaneous melanoma have been projected to occur in the United States in 2015 [94, 95]. Exposure to solar UV radiation is still considered one of the major risk factors for melanoma development. White populations with fair skin are at higher risk for developing melanoma than pigmented populations. Moreover, detection of cyclin-dependent kinase inhibitor 2A (*CDKN2A*) and *CDK4* germline alterations in families have demonstrated a genetic inheritance pattern of melanoma. In addition, gain of oncogenic functional mutations in *BRAF*, NRAS, and KIT have been observed in the majority of melanomas. Furthermore, evidence has demonstrated the cooperation between these oncogenic mutations and PI3 K/AKT/mTOR, and PTEN signaling pathways supports melanoma development. In addition, the cytokine/chemokine spectrum of melanoma tumor microenvironment significantly overlaps with chemoattractant and inflammatory mediators produced by neutrophils and macrophages at the site of inflammation. Moreover, tumor growth, angiogenesis, and metastasis are enhanced by inflammatory tumor microenvironment [96–98]. An accumulating body of evidence has demonstrated that human melanoma cells produce various cytokines such as IL-6, IL-8, CXCL1–3 (MGSA-GROa-c), CCL5 (RANTES), and monocyte chemotactic protein-1 (MCP-1, also known as CCL2) that are regulated by IL-1β, suggesting that IL-1β may be a potential link between inflammation and melanoma [99].

Studies have demonstrated that fisetin inhibits melanoma cell growth and induces apoptosis. Fisetin treatment to human melanoma 451Lu cells induced G1-phase cell cycle arrest and downregulated cell cycle regulatory cdks (2, −4, and −6) protein expression. Fisetin treatment resulted in downregulation of Wnt5a protein expression and its coreceptor (Frizzled/LRP6). Moreover, these treatments stimulated cytosolic degradation of β-catenin, resulting in decreased nuclear localization of β-catenin. Furthermore, fisetin treatment downregulated the protein levels of c-myc, Brn2, and Mitf, which are positively regulated by the β-catenin/TCF complex. These data demonstrated that fisetin interfered with the functional cooperation between TCF-2 and β-catenin in melanoma cells [21]. Fisetin also induced apoptosis in melanoma cells through induction of ER stress and activation of extrinsic and intrinsic apoptotic pathways [100]. Employing silico modeling and cell-free competition assays, it has been demonstrated that fisetin inhibits human melanoma cell growth through direct binding to p70S6 K and mTOR [101]. Moreover, treatment of BRAF-mutant, NRAS-mutant, and wild-type melanoma cells with fisetin (5–20 μM) resulted in a significant decrease in cell invasion. The anti-invasive effect of fisetin was also observed in three-dimensional skin equivalents consisting of human melanoma A375 cells. Furthermore, fisetin treatment modulated the expression of epithelial-to-mesenchymal transition (EMT) proteins. The anti-invasive and anti-EMT effects of fisetin were associated with a decrease in the phosphorylation of MEK1/2 and ERK1/2 and reduction in the activation of the NFκB signaling pathway [24]. In addition, oral administration of fisetin (45 mg/kg b.wt.) inhibited melanoma xenograft tumor growth in nude mice implanted with BRAF mutated melanoma cells. Melanoma growth inhibition and pro-apoptotic effects of fisetin were observed due to reduction in MAPK and PI3 K/AKT/mTOR signaling pathways [22]. Moreover, analysis of tumor xenograft tissues revealed that fisetin inhibited EMT progression by reducing the expression of EMT-related transcription factors such as Snail1, Twist1, ZEB1, and Slug. Fisetin treatment also inhibited angiogenesis and lung colonization of melanoma cells injected intravenously in the tail vein of athymic nude mice [23].

10.4.6 Fisetin and Prostate Cancer

Prostate cancer is one of the most common cancers and leading causes of death in men [95, 102]. Consumption of flavonoid-rich diets in East Asian countries such as China and Japan has been associated with a 60- to 80-fold lower incidence and reduced mortality of prostate cancer [103]. Fisetin has been found to be effective against prostate cancer. In vitro studies using fisetin have demonstrated that fisetin inhibits cell proliferation and induces cell cycle arrest and apoptosis in androgen-sensitive human prostate LNCaP and CWR22Rυ1 cells as well as in androgen receptor (AR)-negative prostate cancer PC-3 cells [103, 104]. Furthermore, fisetin treatment inhibited viability and colony formation of a P-glycoprotein-overexpressing multi-drug resistant cancer cell line NCI/ADR-RE [105]. Importantly, fisetin exhibited minimal cytotoxic effects on normal prostate epithelial cells (PrECs). Fisetin treatment induced cell cycle arrest at G_2/M phase in PC-3 cells; whereas LNCaP cells were arrested at G1 phase of cell cycle. G1-phase cell cycle arrest in LNCaP cells induced by fisetin treatment was associated with reduced protein expression of cyclins D1, D2, and E. Fisetin treatment also reduced the protein expression of cdks 2, 4, and 6 with simultaneous increase in protein expression of WAF1/p21 and KIP1/p27. Furthermore, fisetin treatment induced apoptosis in LNCaP cells through induction of pro-apoptotic proteins (Bax, Bak, Bad, and Bid) and inhibition of anti-apoptotic proteins (Bcl-2 and Bcl-xL), cytochrome c release, activation of caspases (3, 8, and 9) and cleavage of PARP. In addition, fisetin treatment also reduced protein expression of upstream regulators of apoptosis such as PI3 K and decreased the phosphorylation of AKT at Ser^{473} and Thr^{308}, which are involved in cell proliferation and survival [104]. Fisetin induced PC3 cell death by induction of autophagy, as observed by an increase in LC3 II protein expression. Fisetin treatment of PC-3 cells resulted in inhibition of mTOR kinase activity, basal expression of mTOR and autophosphorylation of mTOR at Ser^{2481}. It also inhibited formation of mTORC1/2 complexes via downregulation of Raptor, Rictor, PRAS40, and GβL protein expression. Fisetin treatment also inhibited the activation of p70-S6 kinase (S6K70) and increased expression of eukaryotic translation initiation factor 4E-binding protein 1(4EBP1) by its dephosphorylation from hyperphosphorylated γ form to the hypo- or non-phosphorylated α form. Furthermore, fisetin treatment of PC-3 cells disrupted assembly of translation complex by increasing eIF4E bound 4EBP1 and simultaneous reduction in eIF4G binding to eIF4E [20].

Studies have demonstrated that combination of fisetin with TRAIL resulted in enhanced apoptosis of TRAIL-resistant androgen-dependent LNCaP cells and the androgen-independent DU145 and PC-3 cells [44]. In TRAIL-resistant LNCaP cells, fisetin treatment increased the expression of TRAIL-R1 and reduced NFκB activity. Moreover, studies have demonstrated that fisetin (5–20 μM) inhibited adhesion, migration, and invasion of highly metastatic PC-3 cells [46, 105]. Fisetin treatment significantly reduced protein expression as well as mRNA expression of MMP-2 and MMP-9 involved in the degradation of ECM to facilitate invasion and migration of tumor cells. Activation of JNK1/2 was suppressed due to decreased phosphorylation of JNK1/2 in PC-3 after fisetin treatment; however, phosphorylation of ERK1/2 and p38 was not affected in these cells. Furthermore, fisetin treatment inhibited expression of PI3 K and phosphorylation of AKT and decreased the protein expression and DNA binding activities of NFκB and AP-1 (c-Fos, and c-Jun) involved in transcriptional and translational regulation of MMP-2 and MMP-9 expression, which are required for invasion and migration of prostate cancer cells [46]. In addition, studies have demonstrated that fisetin promoted an epithelial phenotype cellular morphology in the two prostate cell lines DU145 and C4-2 and decreased migration. Fisetin treatment inhibited EMT in prostate cancer cells by inducing mRNA and protein levels of E-cadherin while downregulating mRNA and protein levels of vimentin and slug. Moreover, fisetin treatment reduced EGF-induced YB-1 phosphorylation (required for EMT progression) at Ser^{102} both in vitro and in vivo by interacting with the cold shock domain (CSD) domain of YB-1 [106]. Surface plasmon resonance and computational docking studies suggested that fisetin binds to β-tubulin and stabilizes microtubules by upregulating microtubule associated proteins (MAP)-2 and -4 [105].

10.4.7 Fisetin and Colon Cancer

In Western countries, colon cancer remains one of the leading causes of cancer-related deaths. Modification of life style and diet habits, including consumption of vegetables and fruits can reduce the risk of colon cancer. Dietary flavonoid fisetin inhibited cell growth and clonogenicity of human colon cancer cells. Fisetin inhibited cell cycle progression in HT-29 cells by G_2/M phase arrest. Fisetin treatment suppressed cdk2 and cdk4 activities resulting in a decrease in the level of cyclin E and D1 with an increase in p21 levels. Fisetin particularly targeted cdk4 activity in cell-free system, indicating that cdk4 may be the direct target of fisetin. In addition, fisetin treatment resulted in reduced phosphorylation (from hyperphosphorylated to hypophosphorylated) of retinoblastoma (Rb) proteins [107]. Moreover, cdc2 and cdc25c kinase protein expression and kinase activity of cdc2 were reduced in HT-29 cells after fisetin treatment. Induction of tumor suppressor gene p53 by fisetin contributes to apoptosis in human colon cancer HCT-116 cells harboring the wild-type *p53* gene [108]. Fisetin-induced apoptosis was accompanied by reduction in expression of anti-apoptotic Bcl-2 and Bcl-xL proteins with concomitant increase in pro-apoptotic Bak and Bim proteins. Fisetin-induced mitochondrial translocation of Bax protein resulted in increased mitochondrial membrane permeability and release of cytochrome c and Smac/DIABLO from mitochondria to cytosol. In addition, fisetin treatment resulted in caspase-3 and PARP cleavage [108, 109]. Moreover, fisetin treatment inhibited protein expression and activity of COX-2 in HT-29 cells (COX-2 overexpressing colon cancer cell line), which are known to play a crucial role in colon carcinogenesis. However, fisetin treatment did not affect COX1 expression in HT-29 cells.

Fisetin treatment also inhibited activation and translocation of NFκB, which are required for stimulation of COX-2 expression. PGE_2 secretion was also reduced as a consequence of COX-2 inhibition by fisetin in HT-29 cells. Fisetin did not affect EP-2 and EP-4 expression, suggesting that fisetin inhibits COX-2/PGE_2 signaling through regulating ligand availability. Moreover, fisetin treatment also inhibited phosphorylation of EGFR at the Tyr^{1068} residue in HT-29 cells as a consequence of PGE_2 inhibition, which is a known transactivator of EGFR leading to promotion of tumor growth and invasion [109]. Furthermore, depletion of Securin expression (also known as pituitary tumor transforming gene and acts as a marker of invasiveness in colon cancers) sensitized human colon cancer cells to fisetin-induced apoptosis. Phosphorylation of p53 and cleavage of caspase-3 and PARP were enhanced in HCT116 securin-null cells or in wild-type cells in which securin was knock down [110]. Studies have also demonstrated that the apoptotic effect of fisetin on colon cancer cells (COLO205, HCT-116, HT-29, and HCT-15) is enhanced with N-Acetyl-L-Cysteine treatment, suggesting that fisetin-induced apoptosis in colon cancer cells is independent of ROS induction [111, 112].

10.4.8 Fisetin and Lung Cancer

Lung cancer is the most deadly cancer in the United States and worldwide. Tobacco smoking is considered as the most important risk factor for lung cancer development. Results from clinical and epidemiologic studies have demonstrated a strong association between chronic inflammation and lung cancer [113, 114]. A growing body of evidence has demonstrated that tobacco smoke exposure induces carcinogenic inflammatory responses and mutagenic effects in the lungs. Infiltration of inflammatory cells in the lungs is the initial pathological hallmark of smoking. These inflammatory macrophages and neutrophils produce pro-inflammatory mediators and cytokines to further enhance the inflammatory condition and promote tumor growth [115, 116]. Fisetin treatment significantly inhibited lung cancer cell proliferation but had minimal toxic effects on normal human embryonic epithelial cells at physiologically achievable concentration [16, 117]. Fisetin treatment induced intracellular ROS production, mitochondrial membrane depolarization, and apoptosis in NSCLC cells with an increase in Sub-G1 cell population. Fisetin treatment resulted in reduced expression of Bcl-2 and enhanced expression of Bax, as well as activation of caspase-3 and -9 [118]. Relatively nontoxic concentrations of fisetin inhibited adhesion, invasion, and migration of A549 cells. Gelatin and casein zymography experiments demonstrated that fisetin inhibited MMP-2 and u-PA at protein and mRNA levels. In addition, fisetin decreased ERK1/2 phosphorylation, however it did not affect the phosphorylation of JNK1/2 and p38. Moreover, fisetin inhibited DNA binding activities of transcription factors NFκB and AP-1 (c-Fos, and c-Jun) in A549 cells [117]. Furthermore, fisetin treatment to lung cancer cells inhibited the expression of regulatory (p85) and catalytic (p110) subunits of PI3 K and phosphorylation of

AKT both at Ser^{473} and Thr^{308} moieties. Fisetin treatment also activated PTEN, a negative regulator of PI3 K signaling, and increased phosphorylation of AMPKα kinase thus inhibiting protein translation by mTOR. Fisetin treatment also inhibited the phosphorylation of mTOR at Ser^{2448} as a consequence of inhibition of AKT phosphorylation [16].

In experimental lung carcinogenesis, fisetin inhibited benzo(a)pyrene-induced lung cancer development in Swiss albino mice [119]. Histological evaluation of lungs revealed that fisetin treatment significantly reduced the degree of histological lesions with reduced cell proliferation. Biochemical analysis demonstrated that fisetin treatment restored enzymatic and nonenzymatic antioxidants. Furthermore, evaluation of mitochondrial specific enzymes and tumor markers demonstrated that fisetin treatment inhibited production of isocitrate dehydrogenase, α-ketoglutarate dehydrogenase, succinate dehydrogenase, malate dehydrogenase and carcinogenic embryonic tumor antigen in benzo(a)pyrene-induced lung carcinogenesis [120]. In addition, fisetin treatment resulted in release of cytochrome c and activation of caspase-3. Furthermore, fisetin treatment inhibited viability of Lewis lung carcinoma (LLC) and endothelial cells (EAhy 926), with minimum effect on normal NIH 3T3 cells. NIH3T3 cells were five times less sensitive to fisetin than either LLC or endothelial cells, demonstrating that fisetin specifically targets cancer cells and endothelial cells involved in tumor angiogenesis [121]. Fisetin treatment to LLC cells induced apoptosis and accumulation of cells in G2/M phase with concomitant decrease in G1 phase. Endothelial cells (EAhy 926) were more sensitive to fisetin treatment with increase in sub-G1cells and decrease in G1, S, and G2/M cells. Fisetin treatment also inhibited migration and capillary-like structure-forming abilities of endothelial cells and inhibited tumor growth and angiogenesis in vivo as demonstrated by reduced expression of PECAM-1. Moreover, antitumor activity of fisetin was enhanced in combination with cyclophosphamide [121].

Intraperitoneal administration of 1 or 3 mg/kg fisetin in BALB/c mice inhibited ovalbumin-induced allergic asthma, which is a chronic disease of lung inflammation, airway hyper-responsiveness and mucus overproduction associated with the bronchial epithelium, mucus-secreting glands and lung parenchyma [122, 123]. Treatment of fisetin in experimental asthma mouse model resulted in inhibition of lung inflammation, goblet cell hyperplasia, and airway hyper-responsiveness. These effects were associated with a decrease in eosinophils and lymphocytes in bronchoalveolar lavage fluid. In addition, fisetin treatment reduced expression of eotaxin-1 and thymic stromal lymphopoietin (TSLP) (key initiators of allergic airway inflammation), IL-4, IL-5, and IL-13 (Th2-associated cytokines) production in lungs. Fisetin treatment also inhibited mRNA expression of adhesion molecules, chitinase, IL-17, IL-33, Muc5ac, and iNOS, as wells as eosinophilia and airway mucus production in lung tissue induced by ovalbumin. In addition, fisetin treatment also inhibited expression of Th2-predominant transcription factor GATA-3 and cytokines in thoracic lymph node cells and splenocytes. Moreover, in TNFα-stimulated bronchial epithelial cells and OVA-stimulated lung tissues, fisetin inhibited activation of NFκB by blocking nuclear translocation of subunit p65 and DNA binding activity [122, 123]. A recent study demonstrated that fisetin inhibits

LPS-induced acute lung injury by downregulation of TLR4-mediated NFκB signaling pathway in rats [124]. The results of this study demonstrated that LPS-induced increase of neutrophil, MPO activity and macrophage infiltration in lung tissues were attenuated by fisetin treatment via inhibition of TLR4 and NFκB [124].

10.4.9 Fisetin and Other Inflammatory Diseases

Consumption of flavonoid-rich fruits and vegetables has been associated with reduced risk of other chronic inflammatory conditions. Generally, cross-linking of the cell-bound specific antigens with mast cell and basophils leads to release of inflammatory mediators, histamine, leukotrienes and cytokines (such as IL-4, IL-5, and IL-13) related to IgE production, TH2 differentiation and allergic inflammation. Pro-inflammatory cytokines derived from activated mast cells play an important role in the development of acute- and late-phase allergic inflammatory reactions. Studies have demonstrated that fisetin treatment inhibited allergic inflammation by reduction in mRNA expression and secretion of IL-4, IL-5, and IL-13 in allergen stimulated KU812 cells and basophils [125, 126]. In addition, among the 13 flavonoids tested, fisetin was the most potent inhibitor of hexosaminidase secretion from allergen stimulated RBL-2H3 cells [127]. Furthermore, treatment of fisetin to PMA plus calcium ionophore A23187 (PMACI) stimulated human mast cells (HMC-1) suppressed the gene expression and production of inflammatory cytokines TNFα, IL-1β, IL-4, IL-6, and IL-8 [29, 128]. Moreover, fisetin treatment inhibited activation of MAPKs by reducing phosphorylation of p38, ERK, and JNK. In addition, fisetin treatment inhibited PMACI-induced transcriptional activation of NFκB, NFκB/DNA binding and enhanced phosphorylation and degradation of IκBα [29, 128]. Further studies on mast cell (HMC-1) by activated T cell membrane demonstrated that fisetin inhibited mast cell activation by inhibition of cell-to-cell interactions, reduction in the amount of cell surface antigen CD40 and ICAM-1 and down regulation of NFκB and MAPKs pathways [129].

Animal studies employing 2,4-Dinitrofluorobenzene (DNFB)-induced allergic contact dermatitis mouse model demonstrated that Bark of *Rhus verniciflua* Stokes containing fisetin as its major constituent and isolated fisetin inhibited TNFα, IL-6 and iNOS production mediated through NFκB signaling pathway [28]. Atopic dermatitis is a relapsing and pruritic inflammatory skin disease in which infiltration of inflammatory cells and production of inflammatory cytokines in the skin lesions is enhanced. Enhanced cutaneous hyper-sensitivity to immunoglobulin E (IgE)-mediated sensitization promotes development of intense pruritus, edema, erythematous, scaly and lichenified lesions in the skin [25]. During acute response, production of inflammatory cytokines (such as IL-4, IL-5 and IL-13) and IgEis increased by infiltratory eosinophil and mast cells (Th2 cells). Fisetin treatment has been associated with reduced production of these inflammatory mediators from eosinophils and mast cells. Whereas, in chronic atopic dermatitis, dermal thickening and tissue remodeling by excessive collagen accumulation due to IFNγ and IL-2 (Th1-dominat immune response) is associated with delayed-type hyper-sensitivity. A recent study by Kim et al. [25] demonstrated that oral administration of fisetin at 20 or 50 mg/kg daily from days 8 to 15, significantly inhibited DNFB-induced atopic dermatitis-like clinical symptoms such as erythema, edema, oozing, and excoriation in NC/Nga mice. Fisetin treatment also inhibited DNFB-induced epidermal thickness and infiltration of eosinophils, mast cells, $CD4^+$ T and $CD8^+$ T cells in ear and dorsal skin. Moreover, fisetin treatment also reduced expression of Th2 cytokines IL-5, IL-13, TNFα, thymus, and activation regulated chemokine (TARC) and TSLP mRNA expression produced by dermal leukocytes and keratinocytes. Furthermore, fisetin treatment suppressed production of IFNγ and IL-4 by the activated lymph node $CD4^+$ T cells with increased production of IL-10. In addition, fisetin inhibited activation of NFκB by reducing levels of phosphorylated p65 [25].

Studies on HUVECs and septic mice have demonstrated that fisetin inhibited sepsis-related mortality. Fisetin treatment inhibited hyperpermeability and leukocyte migration in septic mice induced by LPS and cecal ligation and puncture (CLP)-mediated release of high mobility group box 1 (HMGB1) protein. In addition, fisetin treatment greatly inhibited PMA and CLP-induced expression of endothelial cell protein C receptor involved in vascular inflammation. Furthermore, fisetin treatment also inhibited production of TNFα and IL-1β as well as activation of AKT, NFκB, and ERK1/2 in HUVEC cells induced by HMGB1 [30]. In addition, in vitro and in vivo studies have demonstrated that fisetin inhibited high glucose-induced vascular inflammation, vascular permeability, leukocyte adhesion, and migration, cell adhesion molecule expression, ROS formation and NFκB activation [26].

A recent study by Kim et al. [130] demonstrated that fisetin suppresses macrophage-mediated inflammation by blocking Src and Syk, the major NFκB regulatory protein tyrosine kinases. Fisetin treatment of RAW264.7 cells inhibited LPS-induced production of NO, transcriptional activation of inflammatory genes (iNOS, COX-2, and TNFα) and activation of NFκB without any cytotoxic effect on these cells. Moreover, the autophosphorylation levels of Src and Syk were significantly suppressed without decreasing total levels of Src and Syk [130].

10.5 Conclusions

Fisetin has demonstrated various health-promoting effects by acting as an anti-inflammatory, antioxidant, and antitumorigenic agent. Fisetin exhibits beneficial neurologic effects by improving behaviors, learning capabilities, and memory enhancement in animals. These properties make fisetin a candidate for future therapies to manage Alzheimer's, Huntington's, and other neurological diseases. Other chronic diseases including diabetes, atherosclerosis, obesity, and lipid dysregulation continue to harm patient health and burden healthcare systems with exorbitant costs. Similarly, despite great advances in treatment options, effective treatments for advanced cancers continue to challenge clinicians. For these reasons, alternative approaches to the management of chronic conditions require innovative adjuvant and monotherapies to improve patient outcomes. Fisetin has shown potential to prevent inflammation in in vitro systems and animal models relevant to chronic inflammation-related life-threatening diseases. However, in-depth clinical trials are needed to scientifically validate fisetin's role in inflammation-related chronic diseases and to translate potential health benefits into clinical application.

Acknowledgments The work highlighted from the author's laboratory was supported by NIH Grant R21CA173043.

References

1. Krishnamoorthy S, Honn KV (2006) Inflammation and disease progression. Cancer Metastasis Rev 25(3):481–491
2. Libby P (2007) Inflammatory mechanisms: the molecular basis of inflammation and disease. Nutr Rev 65(12 Pt 2):S140–S146
3. Aggarwal BB (2004) Nuclear factor-kappaB: the enemy within. Cancer Cell 6(3):203–208
4. Ahn KS, Aggarwal BB (2005) Transcription factor NF-kappaB: a sensor for smoke and stress signals. Ann N Y Acad Sci 1056:218–233
5. Tabas I, Glass CK (2013) Anti-inflammatory therapy in chronic disease: challenges and opportunities. Science 339(6116):166–172
6. Lanza FL, Chan FK, Quigley EM (2009) Practice Parameters Committee of the American College of Gastroenterology. Guidelines for prevention of NSAID-related ulcer complications. Am J Gastroenterol 104(3):728–738
7. Sinha M, Gautam L, Shukla PK, Kaur P, Sharma S, Singh TP (2013) Current perspectives in NSAID-induced gastropathy. Mediators Inflamm 2013:258209
8. Prasad S, Aggarwal BB (2014) Chronic diseases caused by chronic inflammation require chronic treatment: anti-inflammatory role of dietary spices. J Clin Cell Immunol 5:4. doi:10.4172/2155-9899.1000238
9. Brower V (1998) Nutraceuticals: poised for a healthy slice of the healthcare market? Nat Biotechnol 16(8):728–731
10. Cencic A, Chingwaru W (2010) The role of functional foods, nutraceuticals, and food supplements in intestinal health. Nutrients 2(6):611–625
11. Gupta SC, Kim JH, Prasad S, Aggarwal BB (2010) Regulation of survival, proliferation, invasion, angiogenesis, and metastasis of tumor cells through modulation of inflammatory pathways by nutraceuticals. Cancer Metastasis Rev 29(3):405–434
12. Gupta SC, Tyagi AK, Deshmukh-Taskar P, Hinojosa M, Prasad S, Aggarwal BB (2014) Downregulation of tumor necrosis factor and other proinflammatory biomarkers by polyphenols. Arch Biochem Biophys 559:91–99
13. Arai Y, Watanabe S, Kimira M, Shimoi K, Mochizuki R, Kinae N (2000) Dietary intakes of flavonols, flavones and isoflavones by Japanese women and the inverse correlation between quercetin intake and plasma LDL cholesterol concentration. J Nutr 130(9):2243–2250
14. Kimira M, Arai Y, Shimoi K, Watanabe S (1998) Japanese intake of flavonoids and isoflavonoids from foods. J Epidemiol 8(3):168–175
15. Jash SK, Mondal S (2014) Bioactive flavonoid fisetin—a molecule of pharmacological interest. J Org Biomol Chem 2:89–128. Article ID 010314, 40 pp. ISSN:2321- 4163 http://signpostejournals.com

16. Khan N, Afaq F, Khusro FH, Mustafa Adhami V, Suh Y, Mukhtar H (2012) Dual inhibition of phosphatidylinositol 3-kinase/Akt and mammalian target of rapamycin signaling in human nonsmall cell lung cancer cells by a dietary flavonoid fisetin. Int J Cancer 130(7):1695–1705
17. Khan N, Afaq F, Mukhtar H (2008) Cancer chemoprevention through dietary antioxidants: progress and promise. Antioxid Redox Signal 10(3):475–510
18. Pal HC, Athar M, Elmets CA, Afaq F (2015) Fisetin inhibits UVB-induced cutaneous inflammation and activation of PI3 K/AKT/NFκB signaling pathways in SKH-1 hairless mice. Photochem Photobiol 91(1):225–234
19. Pal HC, Sharma S, Elmets CA, Athar M, Afaq F (2013) Fisetin inhibits growth, induces G_2/M arrest and apoptosis of human epidermoid carcinoma A431 cells: role of mitochondrial membrane potential disruption and consequent caspases activation. Exp Dermatol 22 (7):470–475
20. Suh Y, Afaq F, Khan N, Johnson JJ, Khusro FH, Mukhtar H (2010) Fisetin induces autophagic cell death through suppression of mTOR signaling pathway in prostate cancer cells. Carcinogenesis 31(8):1424–1433
21. Syed DN, Afaq F, Maddodi N, Johnson JJ, Sarfaraz S, Ahmad A, Setaluri V, Mukhtar H (2011) Inhibition of human melanoma cell growth by the dietary flavonoid fisetin is associated with disruption of Wnt/β-catenin signaling and decreased Mitf levels. J Invest Dermatol 131(6):1291–1299
22. Pal HC, Baxter RD, Hunt KM, Agarwal J, Elmets CA, Athar M, Afaq F (2015) Fisetin, a phytochemical, potentiates sorafenib-induced apoptosis and abrogates tumor growth in athymic nude mice implanted with BRAF-mutated melanoma cells. Oncotarget. 6 (29):28296–28311
23. Pal HC, Diamond AC, Strickland LR, Kappes JC, Katiyar SK, Elmets CA, Athar M, Afaq F (2016) Fisetin, a dietary flavonoid, augments the anti-invasive and anti-metastatic potential of sorafenib in melanoma. Oncotarget. 7(2):1227–1241.
24. Pal HC, Sharma S, Strickland LR, Katiyar SK, Ballestas ME, Athar M, Elmets CA, Afaq F (2014) Fisetin inhibits human melanoma cell invasion through promotion of mesenchymal to epithelial transition and by targeting MAPK and NFκB signaling pathways. PLoS ONE 9(1): e86338
25. Kim GD, Lee SE, Park YS, Shin DH, Park GG, Park CS (2014) Immunosuppressive effects of fisetin against dinitrofluorobenzene-induced atopic dermatitis-like symptoms in NC/Nga mice. Food Chem Toxicol 66:341–349
26. Kwak S, Ku SK, Bae JS (2014) Fisetin inhibits high-glucose-induced vascular inflammation in vitro and in vivo. Inflamm Res 63(9):779–787
27. Lee JD, Huh JE, Jeon G, Yang HR, Woo HS, Choi DY, Park DS (2009) Flavonol-rich RVHxR from Rhus verniciflua Stokes and its major compound fisetin inhibits inflammation-related cytokines and angiogenic factor in rheumatoid arthritic fibroblast-like synovial cells and in vivo models. Int Immunopharmacol 9(3):268–276
28. Park DK, Lee YG, Park HJ (2013) Extract of *Rhus verniciflua* bark suppresses 2,4-dinitrofluorobenzene-induced allergic contact dermatitis. Evid Based Complement Alternat 2013:879696
29. Park HH, Lee S, Oh JM, Lee MS, Yoon KH, Park BH, Kim JW, Song H, Kim SH (2007) Anti-inflammatory activity of fisetin in human mast cells (HMC-1). Pharmacol Res 55 (1):31–37
30. Yoo H, Ku SK, Han MS, Kim KM, Bae JS (2014) Anti-septic effects of fisetin in vitro and in vivo. Inflammation. 37(5):1560–1574
31. Currais A, Prior M, Dargusch R, Armando A, Ehren J, Schubert D, Quehenberger O, Maher P (2014) Modulation of p25 and inflammatory pathways by fisetin maintains cognitive function in Alzheimer's disease transgenic mice. Aging Cell 13(2):379–390
32. Maher P (2006) A comparison of the neurotrophic activities of the flavonoid fisetin and some of its derivatives. Free Radic Res 40(10):1105–1111
33. Maher P (2008) The flavonoid fisetin promotes nerve cell survival from trophic factor withdrawal by enhancement of proteasome activity. Arch Biochem Biophys 476(2):139–144

34. Maher P, Akaishi T, Abe K (2006) Flavonoid fisetin promotes ERK-dependent long-term potentiation and enhances memory. Proc Natl Acad Sci USA 103(44):16568–16573
35. Maher P, Dargusch R, Bodai L, Gerard PE, Purcell JM, Marsh JL (2011) ERK activation by the polyphenols fisetin and resveratrol provides neuroprotection in multiple models of Huntington's disease. Hum Mol Genet 20(2):261–270
36. Maher P, Dargusch R, Ehren JL, Okada S, Sharma K, Schubert D (2011) Fisetin lowers methylglyoxal dependent protein glycation and limits the complications of diabetes. PLoS ONE 6(6):e21226
37. Renoudet VV, Costa-Mallen P, Hopkins E (2012) A diet low in animal fat and rich in N-hexacosanol and fisetin is effective in reducing symptoms of Parkinson's disease. J Med Food 15(8):758–761
38. Krasieva TB, Ehren J, O'Sullivan T, Tromberg BJ, Maher P (2015) Cell and brain tissue imaging of the flavonoid fisetin using label-free two-photon microscopy. Neurochem Int 89:243–248
39. Gollapudi P, Hasegawa LS, Eastmond DA (2014) A comparative study of the aneugenic and polyploidy-inducing effects of fisetin and two model Aurora kinase inhibitors. Mutat Res, Genet Toxicol Environ Mutagen 767:37–43
40. Lopez-Lazaro M, Willmore E, Austin CA (2010) The dietary flavonoids myricetin and fisetin act as dual inhibitors of DNA topoisomerases I and II in cells. Mutat Res 696(1):41–47
41. Olaharski AJ, Mondrala ST, Eastmond DA (2005) Chromosomal malsegregation and micronucleus induction in vitro by the DNA topoisomerase II inhibitor fisetin. Mutat Res 582 (1–2):79–86
42. Salmela AL, Pouwels J, Varis A, Kukkonen AM, Toivonen P, Halonen PK, Perälä M, Kallioniemi O, Gorbsky GJ, Kallio MJ (2009) Dietary flavonoid fisetin induces a forced exit from mitosis by targeting the mitotic spindle checkpoint. Carcinogenesis 30(6):1032–1040
43. Sung B, Pandey MK, Aggarwal BB (2007) Fisetin, an inhibitor of cyclin-dependent kinase 6, down-regulates nuclear factor-kappaB-regulated cell proliferation, antiapoptotic and metastatic gene products through the suppression of TAK-1 and receptor-interacting protein-regulated IkappaBalpha kinase activation. Mol Pharmacol 71(6):1703–1714
44. Szliszka E, Helewski KJ, Mizgala E, Krol W (2011) The dietary flavonol fisetin enhances the apoptosis-inducing potential of TRAIL in prostate cancer cells. Int J Oncol 39(4):771–779
45. Khan N, Asim M, Afaq F, Abu Zaid M, Mukhtar H (2008) A novel dietary flavonoid fisetin inhibits androgen receptor signaling and tumor growth in athymic nude mice. Cancer Res 68 (20):8555–8563
46. Chien CS, Shen KH, Huang JS, Ko SC, Shih YW (2010) Antimetastatic potential of fisetin involves inactivation of the PI3 K/Akt and JNK signaling pathways with downregulation of MMP-2/9 expressions in prostate cancer PC-3 cells. Mol Cell Biochem 333(1–2):169–180
47. Chuang JY, Chang PC, Shen YC, Lin C, Tsai CF, Chen JH, Yeh WL, Wu LH, Lin HY, Liu YS, Lu DY (2014) Regulatory effects of fisetin on microglial activation. Molecules 19 (7):8820–8839
48. Maher P (2009) Modulation of multiple pathways involved in the maintenance of neuronal function during aging by fisetin. Genes Nutr 4(4):297–307
49. Dajas F, Rivera F, Blasina F, Arredondo F, Echeverry C, Lafon L, Morquio A, Heinzen H (2003) Cell culture protection and in vivo neuroprotective capacity of flavonoids. Neurotox Res 5(6):425–432
50. Dajas F, Rivera-Megret F, Blasina F, Arredondo F, Abin-Carriquiry JA, Costa G, Echeverry C, Lafon L, Heizen H, Ferreira M, Morquio A (2003) Neuroprotection by flavonoids. Braz J Med Biol Res 36(12):1613–1620
51. Echeverry C, Arredondo F, Martínez M, Abin-Carriquiry JA, Midiwo J, Dajas F (2015) Antioxidant activity, cellular bioavailability, and iron and calcium management of neuroprotective and nonneuroprotective flavones. Neurotox Res 27(1):31–42
52. Ishige K, Schubert D, Sagara Y (2001) Flavonoids protect neuronal cells from oxidative stress by three distinct mechanisms. Free Radic Biol Med 30(4):433–446

53. Hendriks JJ, de Vries HE, van der Pol SM, van den Berg TK, van Tol EA, Dijkstra CD (2003) Flavonoids inhibit myelin phagocytosis by macrophages; a structure–activity relationship study. Biochem Pharmacol 65(5):877–885
54. Sagara Y, Vanhnasy J, Maher P (2004) Induction of PC12 cell differentiation by flavonoids is dependent upon extracellular signal-regulated kinase activation. J Neurochem 90 (5):1144–1155
55. Maher P, Salgado KF, Zivin JA, Lapchak PA (2007) A novel approach to screening for new neuroprotective compounds for the treatment of stroke. Brain Res 1173:117–125
56. Rivera F, Urbanavicius J, Gervaz E, Morquio A, Dajas F (2004) Some aspects of the in vivo neuroprotective capacity of flavonoids: bioavailability and structure-activity relationship. Neurotox Res 6(7–8):543–553
57. Joseph JA, Shukitt-Hale B, Denisova NA, Bielinski D, Martin A, McEwen JJ, Bickford PC (1999) Reversals of age-related declines in neuronal signal transduction, cognitive, and motor behavioral deficits with blueberry, spinach, or strawberry dietary supplementation. J Neurosci 19(18):8114–8121
58. Shukitt-Hale B, Carey AN, Jenkins D, Rabin BM, Joseph JA (2007) Beneficial effects of fruit extracts on neuronal function and behavior in a rodent model of accelerated aging. Neurobiol Aging 28(8):1187–1194
59. Zheng LT, Ock J, Kwon BM, Suk K (2008) Suppressive effects of flavonoid fisetin on lipopolysaccharide-induced microglial activation and neurotoxicity. Int Immunopharmacol 8 (3):484–494
60. Tahanian E, Sanchez LA, Shiao TC, Roy R, Annabi B (2011) Flavonoids targeting of IκB phosphorylation abrogates carcinogen-induced MMP-9 and COX-2 expression in human brain endothelial cells. Drug Des Devel Ther 5:299–309
61. Zhen L, Zhu J, Zhao X, Huang W, An Y, Li S, Du X, Lin M, Wang Q, Xu Y, Pan J (2012) The antidepressant-like effect of fisetin involves the serotonergic and noradrenergic system. Behav Brain Res 228(2):359–366
62. Inkielewicz-Stepniak I, Radomski MW, Wozniak M (2012) Fisetin prevents fluoride- and dexamethasone-induced oxidative damage in osteoblast and hippocampal cells. Food Chem Toxicol 50(3–4):583–589
63. Prakash D, Gopinath K, Sudhandiran G (2013) Fisetin enhances behavioral performances and attenuates reactive gliosis and inflammation during aluminum chloride-induced neurotoxicity. NeuroMol Med 15(1):192–208
64. Cho N, Choi JH, Yang H, Jeong EJ, Lee KY, Kim YC, Sung SH (2012) Neuroprotective and anti-inflammatory effects of flavonoids isolated from Rhus verniciflua in neuronal HT22 and microglial BV2 cell lines. Food Chem Toxicol 50(6):1940–1945
65. Cho N, Lee KY, Huh J, Choi JH, Yang H, Jeong EJ, Kim HP, Sung SH (2013) Cognitive-enhancing effects of Rhus verniciflua bark extract and its active flavonoids with neuroprotective and anti-inflammatory activities. Food Chem Toxicol 58:355–361
66. Cho Y, Chung JH, Do HJ, Jeon HJ, Jin T, Shin MJ (2013) Effects of fisetin supplementation on hepatic lipogenesis and glucose metabolism in Sprague–Dawley rats fed on a high fat diet. Food Chem 139(1–4):720–727
67. Chen CM, Hsieh YH, Hwang JM, Jan HJ, Hsieh SC, Lin SH, Lai CY (2015) Fisetin suppresses ADAM9 expression and inhibits invasion of glioma cancer cells through increased phosphorylation of ERK1/2. Tumour Biol 36(5):3407–3415
68. Chen PY, Ho YR, Wu MJ, Huang SP, Chen PK, Tai MH, Ho CT, Yen JH (2015) Cytoprotective effects of fisetin against hypoxia-induced cell death in PC12 cells. Food Funct. 6(1):287–296
69. Prasath GS, Subramanian SP (2011) Modulatory effects of fisetin, a bioflavonoid, on hyperglycemia by attenuating the key enzymes of carbohydrate metabolism in hepatic and renal tissues in streptozotocin-induced diabetic rats. Eur J Pharmacol 668(3):492–496
70. Prasath GS, Subramanian SP (2014) Antihyperlipidemic effect of fisetin, a bioflavonoid of strawberries, studied in streptozotocin-induced diabetic rats. J Biochem Mol Toxicol 28 (10):442–449

71. Kim HJ, Kim SH, Yun JM (2012) Fisetin inhibits hyperglycemia-induced proinflammatory cytokine production by epigenetic mechanisms. Evid Based Complement Alternat Med 2012:639469
72. Kan E, Kiliçkan E, Ayar A, Colak R (2014) Effects of two antioxidants; α-lipoic acid and fisetin against diabetic cataract in mice. Int Ophthalmol [Epub ahead of print] PubMed PMID: 25488016
73. Zhao X, Li XL, Liu X, Wang C, Zhou DS, Ma Q, Zhou WH, Hu ZY (2015) Antinociceptive effects of fisetin against diabetic neuropathic pain in mice: engagement of antioxidant mechanisms and spinal GABA(A) receptors. Pharmacol Res 102:286–297
74. Zhao X, Wang C, Cui WG, Ma Q, Zhou WH (2015) Fisetin exerts antihyperalgesic effect in a mouse model of neuropathic pain: engagement of spinal serotonergic system. Sci Rep 5:9043
75. Jung CH, Kim H, Ahn J, Jeon TI, Lee DH, Ha TY (2013) Fisetin regulates obesity by targeting mTORC1 signaling. J Nutr Biochem 24(8):1547–1554
76. Lee Y, Bae EJ (2013) Inhibition of mitotic clonal expansion mediates fisetin-exerted prevention of adipocyte differentiation in 3T3-L1 cells. Arch Pharm Res 36(11):1377–1384
77. Jin T, Kim OY, Shin MJ, Choi EY, Lee SS, Han YS, Chung JH (2014) Fisetin up-regulates the expression of adiponectin in 3T3-L1 adipocytes via the activation of silent mating type information regulation 2 homologue 1 (SIRT1)-deacetylase and peroxisome proliferator-activated receptors (PPARs). J Agric Food Chem 62(43):10468–10474
78. Kwon O, Eck P, Chen S, Corpe CP, Lee JH, Kruhlak M, Levine M (2007) Inhibition of the intestinal glucose transporter GLUT2 by flavonoids. FASEB J 21(2):366–377
79. Jeon TI, Park JW, Ahn J, Jung CH, Ha TY (2013) Fisetin protects against hepatosteatosis in mice by inhibiting miR-378. Mol Nutr Food Res 57(11):1931–1937
80. Lima LCF, Braga VA, do Socorro de França Silva M, Cruz JC, Sousa Santos SH, de Oliveira Monteiro MM, Balarini CM (2015) Adipokines, diabetes and atherosclerosis: an inflammatory association. Front Physiol 6:304
81. Viola J, Soehnlein O (2015) Atherosclerosis—a matter of unresolved inflammation. Semin Immunol 27(3):184–193
82. Wong BW, Meredith A, Lin D, McManus BM (2012) The biological role of inflammation in atherosclerosis. Can J Cardiol 28(6):631–641
83. Chistiakov DA, Bobryshev YV, Orekhov AN (2015) Neutrophil's weapons in atherosclerosis. Exp Mol Pathol 99(3):663–671
84. Pende A, Artom N, Bertolotto M, Montecucco F, Dallegri F (2015) Role of Neutrophils in atherogenesis: an update. Eur J Clin Invest [Epub ahead of print]. doi:10.1111/eci.12566
85. Back M, Hansson GK (2015) Anti-inflammatory therapies for atherosclerosis. Nat Rev Cardiol 12(4):199–211
86. Khan R, Spagnoli V, Tardif JC, L'Allier PL (2015) Novel anti-inflammatory therapies for the treatment of atherosclerosis. Atherosclerosis. 240(2):497–509
87. Yamashita T, Sasaki N, Kasahara K, Hirata K (2015) Anti-inflammatory and immune-modulatory therapies for preventing atherosclerotic cardiovascular disease. J Cardiol 66(1):1–8
88. de Whalley CV, Rankin SM, Hoult JR, Jessup W, Leake DS (1990) Flavonoids inhibit the oxidative modification of low density lipoproteins by macrophages. Biochem Pharmacol 39 (11):1743–1750
89. Podrez EA (2010) Anti-oxidant properties of high-density lipoprotein and atherosclerosis. Clin Exp Pharmacol Physiol 37(7):719–725
90. Lian TW, Wang L, Lo YH, Huang IJ, Wu MJ (2008) Fisetin, morin and myricetin attenuate CD36 expression and oxLDL uptake in U937-derived macrophages. Biochim Biophys Acta 1781(10):601–609
91. Podrez EA, Abu-Soud HM, Hazen SL (2000) Myeloperoxidase-generated oxidants and atherosclerosis. Free Radic Biol Med 28(12):1717–1725
92. Chiang HM, Chan SY, Chu Y, Wen KC (2015) Fisetin ameliorated photodamage by suppressing the mitogen-activated protein kinase/matrix metalloproteinase pathway and nuclear factor-κB pathways. J Agric Food Chem 63(18):4551–4560

93. Seo SH, Jeong GS (2015) Fisetin inhibits TNF-α-induced inflammatory action and hydrogen peroxide-induced oxidative damage in human keratinocyte HaCaT cells through PI3 K/AKT/Nrf-2-mediated heme oxygenase-1 expression. Int Immunopharmacol 29 (2):246–253
94. Schadendorf D, Fisher DE, Garbe C, Gershenwald JE, Grob JJ, Halpern A, Herlyn M, Marchetti MA, McArthur G, Ribas A, Roesch A, Hauschild A (2015) Melanoma. Nature Reviews Disease Primers. Article number: 15003, Published online: 23 April 2015
95. Siegel RL, Miller KD, Jemal A (2015) Cancer statistics, 2015. CA Cancer J Clin 65(1):5–29
96. Melnikova V, Bar-Eli M (2007) Inflammation and melanoma growth and metastasis: the role of platelet-activating factor (PAF) and its receptor. Cancer Metastasis Rev 26(3–4):359–371
97. Melnikova VO, Bar-Eli M (2009) Inflammation and melanoma metastasis. Pigment Cell Melanoma Res. 22(3):257–267
98. Richmond A, Yang J, Su Y (2009) The good and the bad of chemokines/chemokine receptors in melanoma. Pigment Cell Melanoma Res 22(2):175–186
99. Dunn JH, Ellis LZ, Fujita M (2012) Inflammasomes as molecular mediators of inflammation and cancer: potential role in melanoma. Cancer Lett 314(1):24–33
100. Syed DN, Lall RK, Chamcheu JC, Haidar O, Mukhtar H (2014) Involvement of ER stress and activation of apoptotic pathways in fisetin induced cytotoxicity in human melanoma. Arch Biochem Biophys 563:108–117
101. Syed DN, Chamcheu JC, Khan MI, Sechi M, Lall RK, Adhami VM, Mukhtar H (2014) Fisetin inhibits human melanoma cell growth through direct binding to p70S6 K and mTOR: findings from 3-D melanoma skin equivalents and computational modeling. Biochem Pharmacol 89(3):349–360
102. Torre LA, Bray F, Siegel RL, Ferlay J, Lortet-Tieulent J, Jemal A (2015) Global cancer statistics, 2012. CA Cancer J Clin 65(2):87–108
103. Haddad AQ, Venkateswaran V, Viswanathan L, Teahan SJ, Fleshner NE, Klotz LH (2006) Novel antiproliferative flavonoids induce cell cycle arrest in human prostate cancer cell lines. Prostate Cancer Prostatic Dis 9(1):68–76
104. Khan N, Afaq F, Syed DN, Mukhtar H (2008) Fisetin, a novel dietary flavonoid, causes apoptosis and cell cycle arrest in human prostate cancer LNCaP cells. Carcinogenesis 29 (5):1049–1056
105. Mukhtar E, Adhami VM, Sechi M, Mukhtar H (2015) Dietary flavonoid fisetin binds to β-tubulin and disrupts microtubule dynamics in prostate cancer cells. Cancer Lett 367 (2):173–183
106. Khan MI, Adhami VM, Lall RK, Sechi M, Joshi DC, Haidar OM, Syed DN, Siddiqui IA, Chiu SY, Mukhtar H (2014) YB-1 expression promotes epithelial-to-mesenchymal transition in prostate cancer that is inhibited by a small molecule fisetin. Oncotarget. 5(9):2462–2474
107. Lu X, Ji Jung, Cho HJ, Lim DY, Lee HS, Chun HS, Kwon DY, Park JH (2005) Fisetin inhibits the activities of cyclin-dependent kinases leading to cell cycle arrest in HT-29 human colon cancer cells. J Nutr 135(12):2884–2890
108. do Lim Y, Park JH (2009) Induction of p53 contributes to apoptosis of HCT-116 human colon cancer cells induced by the dietary compound fisetin. Am J Physiol Gastrointest Liver Physiol 296(5):G1060–G1068
109. Suh Y, Afaq F, Johnson JJ, Mukhtar H (2009) A plant flavonoid fisetin induces apoptosis in colon cancer cells by inhibition of COX2 and Wnt/EGFR/NF-kappaB-signaling pathways. Carcinogenesis 30(2):300–307
110. Yu SH, Yang PM, Peng CW, Yu YC, Chiu SJ (2011) Securin depletion sensitizes human colon cancer cells to fisetin-induced apoptosis. Cancer Lett 300(1):96–104
111. Wu MS, Lien GS, Shen SC, Yang LY, Chen YC (2013) HSP90 inhibitors, geldanamycin and radicicol, enhance fisetin-induced cytotoxicity via induction of apoptosis in human colonic cancer cells. Evid Based Complement Alternat Med 2013:987612
112. Wu MS, Lien GS, Shen SC, Yang LY, Chen YC (2014) *N*-Acetyl-L-cysteine enhances fisetin-induced cytotoxicity via induction of ROS-independent apoptosis in human colonic cancer cells. Mol Carcinog 53(Suppl 1):E119–E129

113. Cho WC, Kwan CK, Yau S, So PP, Poon PC, Au JS (2011) The role of inflammation in the pathogenesis of lung cancer. Expert Opin Ther Targets 15(9):1127–1137
114. O'Callaghan DS, O'Donnell D, O'Connell F, O'Byrne KJ (2010) The role of inflammation in the pathogenesis of non-small cell lung cancer. J Thorac Oncol 5(12):2024–2036
115. Bremnes RM, Al-Shibli K, Donnem T, Sirera R, Al-Saad S, Andersen S, Stenvold H, Camps C, Busund LT (2011) The role of tumor-infiltrating immune cells and chronic inflammation at the tumor site on cancer development, progression, and prognosis: emphasis on non-small cell lung cancer. J Thorac Oncol 6(4):824–833
116. Gomes M, Teixeira AL, Coelho A, Araújo A, Medeiros R (2014) The role of inflammation in lung cancer. Adv Exp Med Biol 816:1–23
117. Liao YC, Shih YW, Chao CH, Lee XY, Chiang TA (2009) Involvement of the ERK signaling pathway in fisetin reduces invasion and migration in the human lung cancer cell line A549. J Agric Food Chem 57(19):8933–8941
118. Kang KA, Piao MJ, Hyun JW (2015) Fisetin induces apoptosis in human nonsmall lung cancer cells via a mitochondria-mediated pathway. Vitro Cell Dev Biol Anim 51(3):300–309
119. Ravichandran N, Suresh G, Ramesh B, Siva GV (2011) Fisetin, a novel flavonol attenuates benzo(a)pyrene-induced lung carcinogenesis in Swiss albino mice. Food Chem Toxicol 49 (5):1141–1147
120. Ravichandran N, Suresh G, Ramesh B, Manikandan R, Choi YW, Vijaiyan Siva G (2014) Fisetin modulates mitochondrial enzymes and apoptotic signals in benzo(a)pyrene-induced lung cancer. Mol Cell Biochem 390(1–2):225–234
121. Touil YS, Seguin J, Scherman D, Chabot GG (2011) Improved antiangiogenic and antitumour activity of the combination of the natural flavonoid fisetin and cyclophosphamide in Lewis lung carcinoma-bearing mice. Cancer Chemother Pharmacol 68(2):445–455
122. Goh FY, Upton N, Guan S, Cheng C, Shanmugam MK, Sethi G, Leung BP, Wong WS (2012) Fisetin, a bioactive flavonol, attenuates allergic airway inflammation through negative regulation of NF-κB. Eur J Pharmacol 679(1–3):109–116
123. Wu MY, Hung SK, Fu SL (2011) Immunosuppressive effects of fisetin in ovalbumin-induced asthma through inhibition of NF-κB activity. J Agric Food Chem 59(19):10496–10504
124. Feng G, Jiang ZY, Sun B, Fu J, Li TZ (2015) Fisetin alleviates lipopolysaccharide-induced acute lung injury via TLR4-Mediated NF-κB signaling pathway in rats. Inflammation [Epub ahead of print] PubMed PMID: 26272311
125. Higa S, Hirano T, Kotani M, Matsumoto M, Fujita A, Suemura M, Kawase I, Tanaka T (2003) Fisetin, a flavonol, inhibits TH2-type cytokine production by activated human basophils. J Allergy Clin Immunol 111(6):1299–1306
126. Hirano T, Higa S, Arimitsu J, Naka T, Shima Y, Ohshima S, Fujimoto M, Yamadori T, Kawase I, Tanaka T (2004) Flavonoids such as luteolin, fisetin and apigenin areinhibitors of interleukin-4 and interleukin-13 production by activated human basophils. Int Arch Allergy Immunol 134(2):135–140
127. Morimoto Y, Yasuhara T, Sugimoto A, Inoue A, Hide I, Akiyama M, Nakata Y (2003) Anti-allergic substances contained in the pollen of *Cryptomeria japonica* possess diverse effects on the degranulation of RBL-2H3 cells. J Pharmacol Sci 92(3):291–295
128. Park HH, Lee S, Son HY, Park SB, Kim MS, Choi EJ, Singh TS, Ha JH, Lee MG, Kim JE, Hyun MC, Kwon TK, Kim YH, Kim SH (2008) Flavonoids inhibit histamine release and expression of proinflammatory cytokines in mast cells. Arch Pharm Res. 31(10):1303–1311
129. Nagai K, Takahashi Y, Mikami I, Fukusima T, Oike H, Kobori M (2009) The hydroxyflavone, fisetin, suppresses mast cell activation induced by interaction with activated T cell membranes. Br J Pharmacol 158(3):907–919
130. Kim JH, Kim MY, Kim JH, Cho JY (2015) Fisetin suppresses macrophage-mediated inflammatory responses by blockade of Src and Syk. Biomol Ther (Seoul) 23(5):414–420

Chapter 11
Honokiol, an Active Compound of *Magnolia* Plant, Inhibits Growth, and Progression of Cancers of Different Organs

Ram Prasad and Santosh K. Katiyar

Abstract Honokiol ($C_{18}H_{18}O_2$) is a biphenolic natural product isolated from the bark and leaves of *Magnolia* plant *spp*. During the last decade or more, honokiol has been extensively studied for its beneficial effect against several diseases. Investigations have demonstrated that honokiol possesses anti-carcinogenic, anti-inflammatory, anti-oxidative, anti-angiogenic as well as inhibitory effect on malignant transformation of papillomas to carcinomas in vitro and in vivo animal models without any appreciable toxicity. Honokiol affects multiple signaling pathways, molecular and cellular targets including nuclear factor-κB (NF-κB), STAT3, epidermal growth factor receptor (EGFR), cell survival signaling, cell cycle, cyclooxygenase and other inflammatory mediators, etc. Its chemopreventive and/or therapeutic effects have been tested against chronic diseases, such as cancers of different organs. In this chapter, we describe and discuss briefly the effect of honokiol against cancers of different organs, such as melanoma, non-melanoma, lung, prostate, breast, head and neck squamous cell carcinoma, urinary bladder cancer, gastric cancer, and neuroblastoma, etc. and describe its mechanism of action including various molecular and cellular targets. Although more rigorous in vivo studies are still needed, however it is expected that therapeutic effects and activities of honokiol may help in the development and designing of clinical trials against chronic diseases in human subjects.

R. Prasad · S.K. Katiyar (✉)
Department of Dermatology, University of Alabama at Birmingham,
1670, University Boulevard, Volker Hall 557, Birmingham, AL 35294, USA
e-mail: skatiyar@uab.edu

S.K. Katiyar
Comprehensive Cancer Center, University of Alabama at Birmingham,
Birmingham, AL 35294, USA

S.K. Katiyar
Nutrition Obesity Research Center, University of Alabama at Birmingham,
Birmingham, AL 35294, USA

S.K. Katiyar
Birmingham Veterans Affairs Medical Center, Birmingham, AL 35233, USA

S.C. Gupta et al. (eds.), *Anti-inflammatory Nutraceuticals and Chronic Diseases*,
Advances in Experimental Medicine and Biology 928,
DOI 10.1007/978-3-319-41334-1_11

Keywords Honokiol · Ultraviolet radiation · Cancer of different organs · Cell cycle regulation · Inflammatory mediators · Tumor cell migration

Abbreviations

BCC	Basal cell carcinomas
CDK	Cyclin dependent kinases
CHS	Contact hypersensitivity
COX-2	Cyclooxygenase-2
EGFR	Epidermal growth factor receptor
EMT	Epithelial-mesenchymal transition
HNSCC	Head and neck squamous cell carcinoma
IL	Interleukin
iNOS	Inducible nitric oxide synthase
MMP	Matrix metalloproteinase
NF-κB	Nuclear factor-kappa B
NSCLC	Non-small cell lung cancer
PCNA	Proliferating cell nuclear antigen
PG	Prostaglandin
PGE_2	Prostaglandin E2
SCC	Squamous cell carcinomas
TNF-α	Tumor necrosis factor-alpha
UVR	Ultraviolet radiation

11.1 Introduction

Honokiol, a biphenolic and bioactive small molecule phytochemical (Fig. 11.1), is isolated from the bark and leaves of *Magnolia* plant species (*Magnolia officinalis*), and has been widely used in the traditional Japanese medicine Saiboku-to for the treatment of various ailments due to its anxiolytic, antithrombotic, anti-depressant, anti-emetic, and antibacterial properties [1]. Since long, the barks and leaves from the *Magnolia* plant also have been used in traditional Chinese system of medicine,

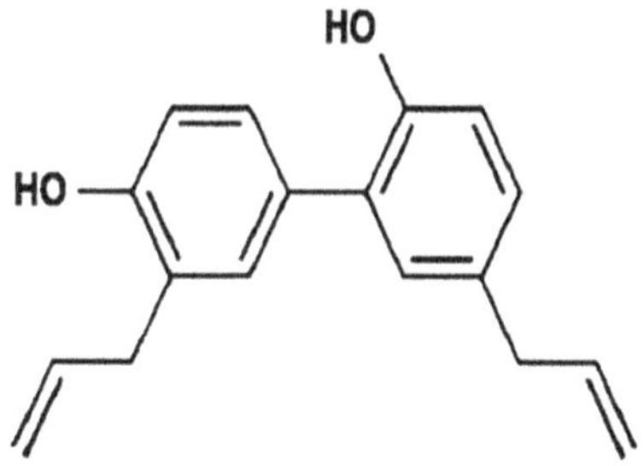

Fig. 11.1 Molecular structure of honokiol, a phytochemical from *Magnolia spp.*

therefore, in the recent past, honokiol achieved a great deal of research interest due to its diverse biologic and pharmacologic activities that include antibacterial, anti-inflammatory, anti-fungal, anti-oxidative, and anti-carcinogenic effects [1–8]. Chemically, honokiol is hydrophobic in nature but soluble in organic solvents, such as acetone. Therefore, to avoid the use of organic solvents in some topical applications and formulation, which may cause deleterious effects, the research laboratory of Dr. Katiyar has developed a topical formulation by mixing it in a hydrophilic cream, and this cream-based topical formulation is ready and easy-to-use for experimental purposes [8].

The protective and therapeutic effect of phytochemicals such as honokiol may be associated with their antioxidant activity, as overproduction of reactive oxygen and nitrogen species in the human body is involved in the pathogenesis of many chronic diseases including cancer. To provide better understanding of the use of honokiol in prevention and treatment of chronic diseases such lung cancer, prostate cancer, head and neck cancer, gastric cancer, prostate cancer, urinary bladder cancer and neuroblastoma, etc., we are summarizing and explaining the investigations conducted in vitro and in vivo animal models. It is well documented that many diseases occur or initiated due to chronic and sustained inflammation in animals as well as in humans, which includes cancer of several organs and aging processes, etc. Inflammation is a localized reaction of tissue to infection, irritation, or other injury, e.g., exposure of the skin to solar ultraviolet (UV) radiation. The key features of inflammation are redness or erythema, warmth, swelling, pain, etc. Inflammation, considered as a necessary response to clear viral infection, repair tissue insults and suppress tumor initiation and progression. However, when inflammation is chronic and persists, diseases may develop, including cancer. Importantly, inflammation involves in all the three stages of tumor development: initiation, promotion/progression, and metastasis. During the initiation phase, inflammation induces the release of a variety of cytokines and chemokines (mostly pro-inflammatory) that promote the activation of inflammatory cells. These conditions change the tissue microenvironment, which resulted in the favor of increased cell survival and proliferation. Clinical and epidemiological evidences suggest a connection between inflammation and a predisposition for the development of cancer. Here, we summarize and discuss the therapeutic effects and mechanisms of action of honokiol against cancers of some specific organs with particular emphasis on ultraviolet (UV) radiation-induced skin cancer development.

11.2 Effect of UVR Exposure on the Skin: Inflammation and Immune Suppression

Exposure of the skin to solar UV radiation, specifically UVB (290–320 nm) spectrum, induces inflammatory mediators and generates oxidative stress, which all together have been implicated in various skin diseases including the initiation and progression of non-melanoma and melanoma skin cancers [9–13]. UVB-induced inflammatory responses are characterized by the development of edema, erythema, hyperplastic responses, increases in the expression levels of inducible cyclooxygenase-2 (COX-2) and production of prostaglandin (PG) metabolites [9]. UV-induced inflammation is considered as an early and important event in tumor promotion and the growth of skin tumors, and is associated with all the three stages of tumor development, i.e., initiation, promotion and progression [9]. The prostaglandin (PG) metabolites have been implicated in UVB-induced immunosuppression as well as implicated in the development of melanoma and non-melanoma skin cancers. This involvement has been supported by the facts that nonsteroidal anti-inflammatory drugs exert their effects through COX-2 inhibition and can reverse the immunosuppressive effects of UV radiation [14, 15]. Among different PG metabolites, PGE_2 is produced abundantly by keratinocytes in UVB-exposed skin. It is a major and most effective metabolite generated by COX-2 activity and considered as a potent mediator of inflammatory responses. The role of PGE_2 in UV-induced immunosuppression is supported by the evidence that COX-2-deficient mice are resistant to UVB-induced suppression of contact hypersensitivity (CHS) response, whereas the treatment of UVB-exposed COX-2-deficient mice with PGE_2 resulted in suppression of CHS response, thus suggesting the role of PGE_2 in UVB-induced immunosuppression [16]. CHS response is considered as a prototype of T-cell mediated immune reaction/response. Hence, the regulation of UVB-induced inflammatory responses has been considered as an important strategy in reducing the risk of skin cancer. To determine the anti-inflammatory effect of honokiol, studies have been conducted using in vivo mouse models and subsequently its effect on UVB radiation-induced skin tumor development.

11.3 Treatment of Honokiol Inhibits UVB-Induced Inflammatory Mediators in the Skin

A characteristic response of skin keratinocytes to UVB irradiation is enhanced COX-2 expression and a subsequent increase in the production of PG metabolites in the skin [9, 16, 17]. The exposure of the skin to UV radiation triggers the release of PGs, such as PGD_2, $PGF_{2\alpha}$, and PGE_2, which are produced from arachidonic acid by the action of COX-2 [17, 18]. Vaid et al. [8] have shown that chronic exposure of the mouse skin to UVB radiation resulted in greater expression of COX-2 as compared with the skin of the non-UVB-exposed normal skin. Topical treatment of mice with honokiol, whether applied before or after UVB-irradiation, resulted in a suppression of COX-2 expression as compared to the expression in non-honokiol-treated UVB-irradiated mouse skin. The levels of PG metabolites in the skin with a particular emphasis on PGE_2 were also analyzed. The levels of PGE_2 in UVB-irradiated skin were significantly greater as compared with the skin of the non-UVB-irradiated mouse skin, however, the levels of

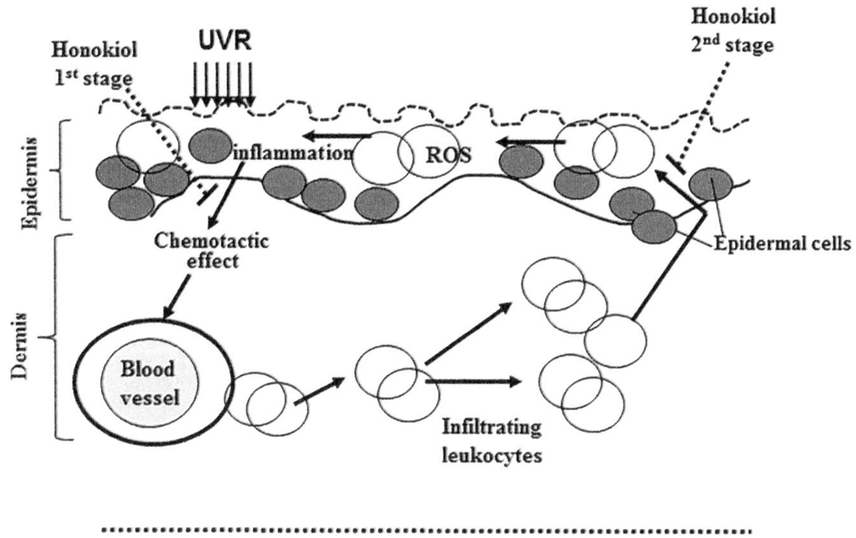

Fig. 11.2 This generalized schematic diagram depicts the mechanism of UVR-induced inflammation in the skin. UVR exposure induces inflammatory responses, including overexpression of COX-2 and PGs production and reactive oxygen species (ROS) generation at early time points (within few hours) of irradiation. Inflammatory mediators and ROS act as chemotactic factors and stimulate the infiltration of leukocytes, particularly activated macrophages and neutrophils, at UV irradiated skin site. Peak time of infiltration is in between 48 and 72 h after UV irradiation of the skin. Activated infiltrating leukocytes are the major source of inflammatory mediators as well as ROS. Topical treatment of the skin with honokiol inhibits UVR-induced effects both at 1st stage (early stage), and 2nd stage (48–72 h after UV) through inhibition of leukocyte infiltration. Inhibition of UVR-induced inflammatory mediators as well as ROS by honokiol treatment contributes to the prevention of UVR-induced skin tumor development

PGE_2 were significantly lower in the UVB-irradiated mouse skin, which was treated with honokiol. Skin exposure to UV radiation induces infiltration of inflammatory leukocytes in the skin, and most prominently are the activated macrophages and neutrophils. These infiltrating leukocytes (majority of them are $CD11b^+$ cell subset) have a role in UV-induced immune suppression, and are the major source of inflammatory mediators, such as prostaglandins and pro-inflammatory cytokines at the UV-exposed site, as demonstrated in Fig. 11.2. In addition, these infiltrating $CD11b^+$ leukocytes have been shown to have suppressive effects on immune system. UVB irradiation also induces production of pro-inflammatory cytokines, such as tumor necrosis factor-alpha (TNF-α), interleukin (IL)-1β, IL-6, etc., in the skin. Topical treatment of mouse skin with honokiol resulted in a significant reduction in UVB-induced production of TNF-α, IL-1β, IL-6 as compared to non-honokiol-treated UVB-exposed mouse skin.

11.4 Honokiol Inhibits UVB-Enhanced Expression of Proliferating Cell Nuclear Antigen (PCNA) in the Skin

Chronic inflammation caused by UV irradiation promotes cellular proliferation in skin cells, and it is commonly measured by determining the levels of PCNA in the skin. Treatment of the skin with honokiol inhibited UVB-induced expression of PCNA in skin. Uncontrolled cellular proliferation may give rise to tumor growth and its development. Based on the above information, it can be suggested that honokiol acts as an anti-inflammatory agent, which is an initial step of skin carcinogenesis.

11.5 Honokiol Treatment Inhibits UV Radiation-Induced Skin Tumor Development and Malignant Progression of Papillomas to Carcinomas in Mice

Non-melanoma skin cancer (NMSC) is the most common cancer in the United States. The majority of NMSCs is environmentally induced and caused by excessive exposure to solar UVB radiation which induces inflammation, oxidative stress, suppression of immune system, and DNA damage. NMSC is composed of two types of skin cancer; basal cell carcinomas (BCCs), and squamous cell carcinomas (SCCs). The incidence of SCC has increased approximately 200 % over the past three decades, and represents about 20 % of NMSC [19, 20]. As topical treatment of honokiol prevents UVB-induced inflammation and their mediators in the mouse skin, the effect of honokiol was assessed against UVB-induced skin tumor development in SKH-1 hairless mouse model [8]. To induce tumors, mice were exposed to UVB radiation (180 mJ/cm^2) 3 times a week for 24 weeks. It was observed that topical treatment of honokiol significantly inhibits UVB-induced initiation and progression of skin tumors [8]. Honokiol treatment also increased the latency period of skin tumor development. The tumor multiplicity and tumor size were significantly reduced in the group of UVB-irradiated mice that were treated with honokiol than in the control group of mice that were UVB-irradiated but not treated with honokiol. When data were compared in terms of average tumor volume/tumor bearing mouse between honokiol-treated and non-honokiol-treated groups, a significant reduction was observed after the treatment of honokiol. Similar observations were also noted by Chilampalli et al. [21] wherein chemopreventive effect of honokiol was determined on UVB-induced skin carcinogenesis. However, these investigators have determined the chemopreventive effect of topical treatment of honokiol at lower dose (30 μg/200 ml acetone/mouse) as well as lower dose of UVB exposure (30 mJ/cm^2). This study also concluded that honokiol treatment affords photoprotection in terms of tumor multiplicity. In addition to the inhibition of skin tumor development in UVB-exposed mouse skin, the malignant progression of papillomas to carcinomas were also significantly prevented by the topical treatment of honokiol in mice. Histochemical analysis revealed that most of the carcinomas were identified as kerato-acanthomas and squamous cell carcinomas [8].

11.5.1 Honokiol Controls Cell Cycle Regulators in UVB-Induced Skin Tumors

Enhanced expression of cell cycle regulatory proteins such as cyclin-dependent kinases (CDKs) and cyclins or decreased expression of CDK inhibitors have been implicated in UV-induced skin carcinogenesis [22, 23]. The cell cycle deregulation affects skin carcinogenesis under the influence of UV-induced inflammatory mediators. Regulation of cyclin-CDK complexes plays a key role in cell cycle progression at different phases in which CDKs are negatively regulated by a group of functionally related proteins known as CDK inhibitors, such as Kip/Cip family members [24, 25]. Cip1/p21 is a universal CDK inhibitor, and binds with PCNA to inhibit PCNA function in DNA replication process [26], while Kip1/p27 is upregulated in response to anti-proliferative signals. The expression levels of cyclins (cyclin D1, D2, and E) and CDKs (CDK2, CDK4, and CDK6) were considerably higher in UVB-induced skin tumors compared with non-UVB-irradiated normal skin from age-matched control mice. However, treatment of the skin with honokiol resulted in inhibition of UVB-induced expression levels of cyclins (cyclins D1, D2, and E) and CDKs in skin tumors compared to skin tumors obtained from non-honokiol-treated mice. Further, tumor suppressor genes or proteins are also involved in tumor development. Cip1/p21 also act as tumor suppressor, and regulates cell cycle progression. Treatment of honokiol enhances the levels of Cip1/p21 in skin tumors compared with non-honokiol-treated skin tumors. Cell cycle arrest in tumor cells could lead to the reduction in proliferation potential of cells as observed by a decrease in the levels of PCNA in UVB-exposed skin and skin tumors. Thus, the modulation in cell cycle progression and inhibition of cell proliferation could be one of the possible mechanisms through which honokiol inhibits UVB-induced skin tumor development [8]. Kip1/p27 is another important CDK inhibitor that regulates CDK-cyclin activity at G1-S transition of cell cycle [22]. The level of Kip1/p27 was also upregulated in the skin tumors obtained from honokiol-treated mice. These observations reflect the molecular mechanism through which honokiol acts as an anti-inflammatory and anti-skin carcinogenic agent.

11.5.2 Honokiol Inhibits Cell Survival Signals/Pathways in UVB-Induced Skin Tumors

The risk of UVB radiation-induced skin tumor development increases through various signaling pathways including the activation of the cell survival kinases, such as PI3K/Akt [27, 28]. Studies revealed that the levels of both the catalytic (p110) and regulatory (p85) subunits of PI3K were enhanced in the UVB-induced skin tumors as compared with the non-UVB-exposed normal mouse skin; however, the levels of the p85 and p110 subunits were greatly reduced in the UV-induced skin tumors from honokiol-treated mice compared to the skin tumors of non-honokiol-treated mice. Most of the biological effects of PI3K are mediated through the activation of the downstream target Akt. Akt is a serine/threonine kinase, which has been identified as an important component of pro-survival signaling pathways [29]. It was observed that the treatment of honokiol resulted in reduction of UVB-induced phosphorylation of Akt (Ser^{473}) as compared to the skin tumors of non-honokiol-treated group. Further, cell survival signals have been associated with cellular proliferation and carcinogenesis [30–32]. The skin tumors augment UVB radiation-induced activation of PI3K and phospho-Akt as compared to the non-UVB-exposed mouse skin. The PI3K/Akt signaling pathway regulates the activity of the transcriptional factor, NF-κB, which in turn known to regulate several well-known markers of tumor promotion and tumor cell proliferation, e.g., COX-2, inducible nitric oxide synthase (iNOS) and PCNA [33, 34]. Thus, the inhibition of PI3K/p-Akt pathway in skin tumors by honokiol may have a role in inhibition of UVB-induced skin tumor growth in mouse model.

11.6 Honokiol Inhibits Metastatic Potential of Melanoma Cells

Melanoma is a leading cause of skin cancer-related deaths due to its propensity to metastasize at distant organs of the body, and the average survival of patients with advanced stage melanoma is less than 1 year. The American Cancer Society indicated that the incidence of melanoma is increasing, and increasing particularly in children [35]. The oxidative stress plays a significant role in cancer cell progression and migration. Nox1 is a multi-protein complex that consists of cytosolic ($p47^{phox}$, $p40^{phox}$, and $p67^{phox}$) and membrane-bound proteins ($p22^{phox}$, $gp91^{phox}$) that when assembled becomes activated, and initiates respiratory bursts or generation of oxidative stress [36, 37]. A recent study by Prasad et al. [38] reported that honokiol treatment inhibits the migration capacity of melanoma cells and this effect was associated with the inhibition of Nox1 expression and NADPH oxidase activity in melanoma cells. Honokiol not only reduces the NADPH oxidase activity, but also reduces oxidative bursts in melanoma cells. Treatment of melanoma cells with honokiol blocks the interaction between membrane-bound and cytosolic-bound proteins. The $p22^{phox}$ protein is the binding partner of $p47^{phox}$ [39, 40], the subunits required for oxidase assembly. Failure of this interaction between membrane-bound and cytosolic-bound proteins would lead to the inactivation of Nox in melanoma cells, and that would result in the reduction of oxidative stress, which is responsible for invasive or metastatic phenotype of melanoma cells. The inhibitory effect of honokiol on migratory potential of melanoma cells was supported by an action of diphenyleneiodonium chloride, a Nox 1 inhibitor, in melanoma cells. The treatment of melanoma cells with diphenyleneiodonium chloride also blocked or reduced melanoma cell migration. Activation of matrix metalloproteinases (MMPs), especially MMP-2 and MMP-9, plays crucial roles in tissue matrix degradation, and thus, paves the way for cell migration. Prasad et al. [38] also found that honokiol treatment reduces the expression of MMP-2 and MMP-9 in Hs294t and SK-Mel28 melanoma cells, thus suggesting a mechanism of action by honokiol.

11.7 Honokiol Promotes Cell Death of Neuroblastoma Cells

In children, several childhood cancers such as leukemia, neuroblastoma, Wilms tumor, lymphoma, rhabdomyosarcoma, retinoblastoma, bone cancer including osteosarcoma and Ewing sarcoma are the leading cause of deaths [35]. Among various tumor types diagnosed in children, neuroblastomas are the most common solid cancer and develop from neural crest elements of the sympathetic nervous system [41]. Based on severity of disease, neuroblastomas are classified into three risk categories as low, intermediate, and high. Unfortunately, neuroblastomas diagnosed in children, belongs to high-risk category [42], and it is a severe problem in pediatric oncology. Children with neuroblastoma achieve a long-term treatment, and which usually causes other serious complications such hearing loss, cardiac dysfunction, infertility, and secondary malignancies after therapy [43]. Studies indicated that honokiol has beneficial effect against neuroblastoma as it can pass through blood brain barrier and kill neuroblastoma cells without affecting too much viability of normal brain cells [44]. Autophagy is a self-degradative physiological process in the body that deals with cell's destruction and maintains homeostasis or normal functioning. Studies have shown that honokiol induces autophagy in various types of tumor cells including neuroblastoma via diverse mechanisms [45–48]. DNA fragmentation and cell cycle arrest at the sub-G1 phase are two typical characteristics that indicate that cells are undergoing apoptosis. In human neuroglioma H4 cells, honokiol have been reported to cause cell cycle arrest and induce apoptosis through an activation of p53 [49]. The mammalian target of rapamycin (mTOR) signaling is a negative regulator of cellular autophagy [50]. Following phosphorylation, mTOR inhibits activation of downstream protein kinases, including ULK1 and ATG13, and subsequently suppress cellular autophagy. The study by Yeh et al. [45] revealed that treatment of neuroblastoma cells with honokiol caused significant downregulation of mTOR phosphorylation which leads to induction of autophagy of neuroblastoma cells.

11.8 Honokiol Inhibits the Growth of Head and Neck Squamous Cell Carcinoma

Head and neck squamous cell carcinoma (HNSCC) is a commonly occurring malignancy worldwide and account approximately 20,000 deaths in the United States annually [51, 52]. In addition to several other factors, the over expression of epidermal growth factor receptor (EGFR) has been commonly reported and observed in more than 90 % cases of HNSCC. Overexpression of EGFR is associated with poor clinical outcomes of HNSCC [53–55]. Therefore, EGFR is considering as a promising target for the treatment of patients suffering from HNSCC. Honokiol treatment significantly decreased the cell viability and induced apoptosis in various HNSCC cell lines, such as derived from tongue, larynx, oral cavity, and pharynx, and suggests that honokiol possesses broad therapeutic effect on this malignancy. A recent study published by Singh et al. [56] reported that honokiol targets EGFR signaling to inhibit HNSCC growth. Treatment of HNSCC cell lines with honokiol decreases the expression levels of total EGFR as well as p-EGFR and its downstream target mTOR signaling. An activation of mTOR signaling has been shown to contribute in tumor growth and progression. To confirm the findings, authors further verified the inhibition of mTOR and its downstream targets using rapamycin, an inhibitor of mTOR, and its effect on cell viability. It was found that treatment of cells with rapamycin results in significant inhibition of cell viability of HNSCC cells as well as decrease in the levels of mTOR and its downstream targets. Based on these observations, it appears that honokiol acts as an antagonist and/or causes increased turnover of EGFR, thus accounting for decreased expression of EGFR in HNSCC cells. The iNOS is involved in tumorigenesis [57]. Studies reported that honokiol treatment not only inhibits HNSCC cell proliferation, but also induced apoptosis in HNSCC cell lines through decreasing the expression level of iNOS at the protein as well as mRNA levels. NO is an important regulator of various MMPs, which are over expressed in metastatic cancers and promote cancer cell migration [58]. Studies also indicated that honokiol treatment reduces metastatic potential of HNSCC cells by targeting MMPs and inhibiting nuclear translocation of NF-κB [59]. A proteomic study based on LC-MS/MS analysis revealed that out of 181 identified proteins, 96 proteins were differentially expressed in honokiol-treated HN22 cells. Cho et al. [59] list the biological functions of several identified proteins. The endoplasmic reticulum protein 44 (ERp44) acts as an anchoring protein for ER-resident proteins that lack an ER retention signal and in many instances, a family of ER oxidoreductases including ERp44 catalyzes oxidative protein folding. The treatment of honokiol significantly reduces ERp44 expression in HNSCC cell lines. After ERp44 degradation, ER calcium ion flows into the cytoplasm. ERp44 is a key regulator of protein secretion, calcium signaling and redox regulation via interaction with IP3R1 in a calcium ion, redox and pH dependent manner [60]. In pathologic conditions, excessive influx of cytosolic calcium ion into the mitochondria triggers dysfunction of the mitochondrial membrane permeabilization with mitochondrial ROS induction [61]. Studies have identified that honokiol treatment induced a significant release of cytochrome c from the mitochondria, followed by an increase in mitochondrial Bax and a significant decrease in the expression levels of the pro-apoptotic proteins Bid, Bcl-xL that results in death of HNSCC cells.

11.9 Protective Effect of Honokiol in Breast Cancer

There has been growing emphasis on the importance of epithelial to mesenchymal transition (EMT), an essential normal physiological process for embryonic development, tissue remodeling, wound healing, and in cancer progression. An oncogenic EMT not only derives tumors to gain a mesenchymal phenotype but also facilitate in migration and invasion potential of cancer cells. The adoption of mesenchymal characteristics not only promotes separation of cancer cells from primary tumor sites but also provides favorable microenvironment such as increase in tumor-initiating cell characteristics including self-renewal, multi potency and resistance to conventional therapeutics [62–64]. Recent study by Avtanski et al. [65] indicates that honokiol effectively inhibits EMT in breast cancer cells as evident from morphological changes and molecular alterations of mesenchymal and epithelial genes. Breast tumors treated with honokiol also showed reduced expression of mesenchymal markers, and provide convincing evidence to support the efficacy of honokiol as a potent inhibitor of EMT. An inactivation of serine–threonine kinase liver kinase B1 (LKB1; also known as STK11), a known tumor suppressor, is correlated with poor prognosis of breast carcinoma [66], and its knockdown increases motility and invasiveness of cancer cells, through induction in the expression of many mesenchymal marker proteins indicating its possible role in EMT [67, 68]. SIRT1 and SIRT3 have been shown to deacetylate LKB1 leading to an increase in its cytoplasmic localization, binding with STRAD and MO25 and activation of kinase function. Avtanski et al. [65] have found that honokiol increases the expressions of SIRT1 and SIRT3, which leads to increase in the cytoplasmic localization of LKB1 in breast cancer cells. The miRNAs play essential roles in various biological processes, including cell proliferation, survival, and differentiation. The loss of miR-34a expression has been reported in many cancer types including breast cancer [69]. Treatment of honokiol enhances miR-34a expression and inhibits mesenchymal markers while enhancing the expression of epithelial markers in breast cancer cells. These changes may result in suppression of cell viability of breast cancer cells.

11.10 Growth Inhibitory Effect of Honokiol in Urinary Bladder Cancer

Urinary bladder cancer is one of the most common urogenital malignant cancer with an estimated 74,690 new cases and 15,580 deaths occurring in USA during 2014 [70]. Recent studies reported that cancer stem cells might account for chemotherapy failure, which are enriched after therapy and have the ability to generate all types of differentiated cells to repopulate tumors and eventually lead to metastasis [71–73]. Histone modifications through polycomb repressive complexes also play an essential role for normal and malignant cell stemness maintenance. Deregulation of Enhancer of Zeste Homologue 2 (EZH2), an important component of polycomb repressive complex 2, is frequently detected in a variety of cancer along with urinary bladder cancer [74–76]. Activation EZH2 specifically represses the transcription of differentiation-related genes throughout the cell cycle to maintain the stemness of cells, and this make it a promising therapeutic target for cancer. Zhang et al. [77] have found that depletion of EZH2 by honokiol treatment inhibited cell proliferation and clonogenicity of urinary bladder cancer cells.

11.11 Anti-Tumorigenic Activity of Honokiol in Prostate Cancer

Prostate cancer is the most frequently diagnosed cancer and the second leading cause of cancer-related death in males after skin cancer in economically developed countries [70]. The major cause of mortality in prostate cancer is associated with metastasis. Approximately, 90 % of deaths from solid tumors are caused by metastasis [78]. Studies have shown that honokiol induces autophagy in cancer cells [79, 80]. An induction of autophagy with different functional consequences has been described for a number of structurally divergent naturally occurring anticancer agents. Studies have implicated that mTOR is a negative regulator of autophagy. A study published by Hahm et al. [48] reported the suppression of mTOR and Akt phosphorylation by honokiol treatment in prostate cancer cells (PC-3). An induction of apoptosis by natural agents is significantly attenuated by antioxidants because of reduced activation of multi domain Bcl-2 family member Bax. Hahm et al. [48] also found that treatment of honokiol induced apoptosis in PC-3 and LNCaP cells, which was associated with induction of Bax and Bak, and claimed that honokiol may be effective in prevention and therapy of prostate cancer.

11.12 Honokiol Inhibits Metastatic Potential and Tumor Growth of Gastric Cancer

Gastric cancer is also a leading cause of cancer-related death worldwide, and the majority of patients exhibit a high incidence of lymph node metastases. Emerging evidence suggests that EMT leads to increased tumor formation, tissue invasiveness, and tumor dissemination [81]. Recent studies have shown a close relation between EMT and gastric cancer progression. A number of signaling pathways, including developmental transcriptional factors, are involved in regulating the motile-invasion phenotype of tumor cells [82]. The decreased expression of epithelial marker E-cadherin in gastric cancer has established the potential role of EMT in gastric cancer metastasis [83, 84]. Tumor progression locus 2 (Tpl2) is a serine-threonine kinase, regulates the activation of the mitogen-activated protein kinase, and critically involved in inflammation, oncogenic events, and tumor progression [85, 86]. Pan et al. [87] have shown that honokiol treatment regulates Tpl2 mediated mesenchymal markers and significantly down regulates Snail, vimentin, N-cadherin expression, and upregulates cytokeratin-18 and E-cadherin expression. Tumor growth in gastric cancer has been associated with Tpl2 [88, 89]. Pan et al. [87] also reported that honokiol treatment reduces growth of gastric tumor through an inhibition of Tpl2 expression. Honokiol significantly inhibited tumor angiogenesis as indicated by reduced microvessel density in tumor mass [87]. Cell cycle regulation is an important regulatory mechanism to control cell growth, and activation of p53, a tumor suppressor protein, is involved in the regulation of cell cycle arrest and apoptosis. The phosphorylation of cell cycle regulatory proteins is involved in arresting effect of gastric carcinoma cells on the cell cycle at G2/M phase [90, 91]. Yen et al. [92] investigated the anticancer mechanism of honokiol in human gastric carcinoma using MGC-803 cells and investigated that honokiol induces apoptosis in gastric carcinoma cells, and the underlying mechanism was mediated through downregulation of CDC2/cdc25C and upregulation of p53. These studies provide evidence of anticancer activity of honokiol against human gastric carcinoma.

11.13 Honokiol Inhibits Migratory Potential of Lung Cancer Cells

Lung cancer is a major cause of cancer-related deaths in the United States as well as worldwide each year and thus have a tremendous impact on human health and health care expenditures. Non-small-cell lung cancer (NSCLC) accounts for approximately 80 % of all types of lung cancer. COX-2 is frequently over express in lung cancer and associated with excessive production of PGE_2, which promotes tumor cell survival, invasion and metastasis [93–96]. Therefore, COX-2 inhibitors have shown potential in treatment of lung cancer. Singh and Katiyar [97] reported the use of honokiol as an inhibitor of COX-2 expression to inhibit migratory potential of lung cancer cells and supported their findings by the evidence that treatment of the NSCLC cells with celecoxib, a potent COX-2 inhibitor, resulted in a reduction in cell migration. The β-catenin signaling is downstream target of

COX-2 and played important roles in tumor progression as well as cell migration. β-catenin forms a dynamic link between E-cadherin and cytoskeleton [98, 99], and this cell-to-cell adhesion may prevent the migration of tumor cells. In contrast, the breaking of cell-to-cell adhesion due to activation of β-catenin and its nuclear accumulation may increase the migration potential of tumor cells. Singh and Katiyar [97] also reported that honokiol induced degradation of β-catenin or reduces nuclear accumulation, which leads to inhibition of lung cancer cell migration.

11.14 Honokiol Inhibits Pancreatic Cancer Growth

Pancreatic cancer is one of the most lethal malignancies with increasing incidence in the United States [33]. Due to its asymptomatic progression, pancreatic cancer is diagnosed at later stage, when it has already metastasized or locally advanced. The NF-κB is constitutively activated in a variety of hematologic and solid malignancies, including pancreatic cancer and controls the expression of an array of genes involved in cell proliferation and survival through direct and indirect mechanisms [100]. Arora et al. [101, 102] examined the effect of honokiol against pancreatic cancer and reported that honokiol showed growth inhibitory potential for pancreatic cancer lines (such as, Miapaca and PANC-1), which may result of cell cycle arrest and induction of apoptosis. Furthermore, to explore the underlying mechanism, these authors have tested the effect of honokiol on NF-κB signaling in this system. Treatment of honokiol to pancreatic cancer cells inhibited transcriptional activity of NF-κB, and decrease protein expression in the nuclear fraction and suppresses constitutive activation of NF-κB in pancreatic cancer cells and thus induce cell death.

11.15 Conclusion and Future Prospects

Honokiol, a small molecule phytochemical, has been shown to have significant chemopreventive and therapeutic effects against cancers of various organs in vitro and in vivo animal models. Honokiol targets distinct signaling pathways, molecular and cellular targets and leads to inhibition of growth and progression of tumors of various organs (Fig. 11.3). Importantly, development of cancers are considered as chronic disease. Therefore, it has significant potential to serve as a novel agent for prevention and therapy of chronic diseases, like cancers. This small molecule from *Magnolia spp*. may be of significant interest for attenuation of the adverse effects of environmental factors, such as solar UV radiation, on human skin. The use of honokiol in combination with already available cancer therapeutic drugs may offer an enhanced ability to attack other cancer-related targets, reduce toxicity and resistance to the cancer drugs and may improve the therapeutic efficacy of the existing cancer drugs.

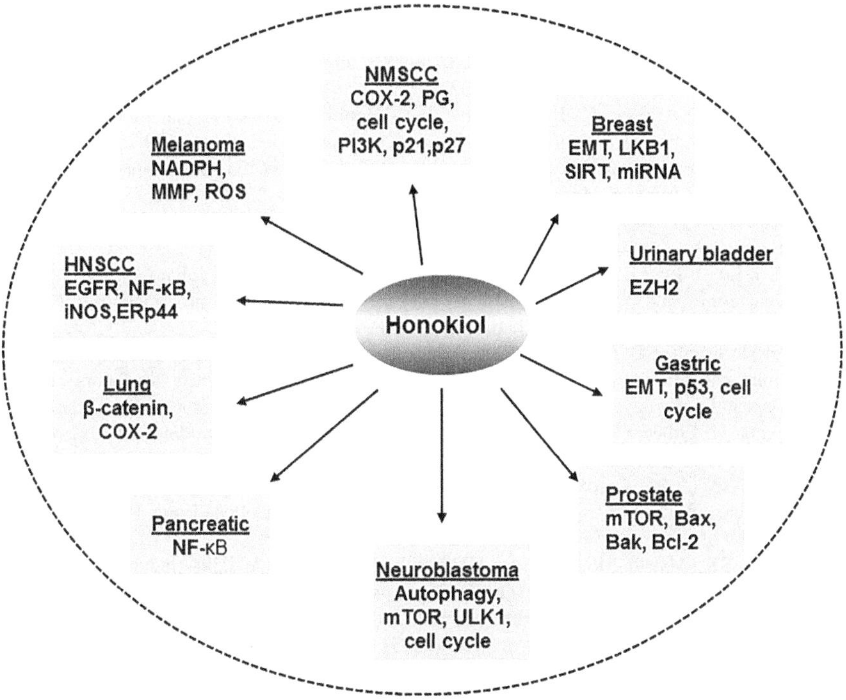

Fig. 11.3 The schematic diagram reflects the preventative and therapeutic effect of honokiol on cancers of different organs. Various molecular and cellular targets in cancers of different organs are affected by the treatment of honokiol in vitro and in vivo models. Inflammation and inflammatory mediators are the main targets of honokiol in prevention or treatment of cancers. *Underline words* indicate the name of organ-specific cancer

Acknowledgments The work reported from Dr. Katiyar's research laboratory was financially supported from the funds from National Cancer Institute/NIH (CA183869) and Veterans Administration Merit Review Award (1I01BX001410). The content of this communication does not necessarily reflect the views or policies of the funding agencies.

Conflict of interest The author has declared no conflict of interest.

References

1. Li TSC (2002) Chinese and related North American herbs: Phytopharmacology and therapeutic values. CRC Press, Boca Raton, FL
2. Hahm ER, Arlotti JA, Marynowski SW, Singh SV (2008) Honokiol, a constituent of oriental medicinal herb magnolia officinalis, inhibits growth of PC-3 xenografts in vivo in association with apoptosis induction. Clin Cancer Res 14:1248–1257

3. Bai X, Cerimele F, Ushio-Fukai M, Waqas M, Campbell PM, Govindarajan B, Der CJ, Battle T, Frank DA, Ye K, Muradm E, Dubiel W, Soff G, Arbiser JL (2003) Honokiol, a small molecular weight natural product, inhibits angiogenesis in vitro and tumor growth in vivo. J Biol Chem 278:35501–35507
4. Munroe ME, Arbiser JL, Bishop GA (2007) Honokiol, a natural plant product, inhibits inflammatory signals and alleviates inflammatory arthritis. J Immunol 179:753–763
5. Pyo MK, Lee Y, Yun-Choi HS (2002) Anti-platelet effect of the constituents isolated from the barks and fruits of *Magnolia obovata*. Arch Pharm Res 25:325–328
6. Clark AM, El-Feraly FS, Li WS (1981) Antimicrobial activity of phenolic constituents of *Magnolia grandiflora* L. J Pharm Sci 70:951–952
7. Park J, Lee J, Jung E, Park Y, Kim K, Park B, Jung K, Park E, Kim J, Park D (2004) In vitro antibacterial and anti-inflammatory effects of honokiol and magnolol against *Propionibacterium* spp. Eur J Pharmacol 496:189–195
8. Vaid M, Sharma SD, Katiyar SK (2010) Honokiol, a phytochemical from the Magnolia plant, inhibits photocarcinogenesis by targeting UVB-induced inflammatory mediators and cell cycle regulators: development of topical formulation. Carcinogenesis 11:2004–2011
9. Mukhtar H, Elmets CA (1996) Photocarcinogenesis: mechanisms, models and human health implications. Photochem Photobiol 63:355–447
10. Katiyar SK (2006) Oxidative stress and photocarcinogenesis: strategies for prevention. In: Singh KK (ed) Oxidative stress, disease and cancer. Imperial College Press, London, pp 933–964
11. Katiyar SK, Matsui MS, Mukhtar H (2000) Kinetics of UV light- induced cyclobutane pyrimidine dimers in human skin in vivo: an immunohistochemical analysis of both epidermis and dermis. Photochem Photobiol 72:788–793
12. Meeran SM, Akhtar S, Katiyar SK (2009) Inhibition of UVB-induced skin tumor development by drinking green tea polyphenols is mediated through DNA repair and subsequent inhibition of inflammation. J Invest Dermatol 129:1258–1270
13. Rivas JM, Ullrich SE (1994) The role of IL-4, IL-10, and TNF-alpha in the immune suppression induced by ultraviolet radiation. J Leukoc Biol 56:769–775
14. Hart PH, Townley SL, Grimbaldeston MA, Khalil Z, Finlay-Jones JJ (2002) Mast cells, neuropeptides, histamine, and prostaglandins in UV-induced systemic immunosuppression. Methods 28:79–89
15. Chung HT, Burnham DK, Robertson B, Roberts LK, Daynes RA (1986) Involvement of prostaglandins in the immune alterations caused by the exposure of mice to ultraviolet radiation. J Immunol 137:2478–2484
16. Prasad R, Katiyar SK (2013) Prostaglandin E2 promotes ultraviolet radiation induced immune suppression through DNA hypermethylation. Neoplasia 15:795–804
17. Beissert S, Granstein RD (1996) UV-induced cutaneous photobiology. Crit Rev Biochem Mol Biol 31:381–404
18. Fischer SM (2002) Is cyclooxygenase-2 important in skin carcinogenesis? J Environ Pathol Toxicol Oncol 21:183–191
19. Karia PS, Han J, Schmults CD (2012) Cutaneous squamous cell carcinoma: estimated incidence of disease, nodal metastasis, and deaths from disease in the United States. J Am Acad Dermatol 68:957–966
20. Christenson LJ, Borrowman TA, Vachon CM, Tollefson MM, Otley CC, Weaver AL, Roenigk RK (2005) Incidence of basal cell and squamous cell carcinomas in a population younger than 40 years. JAMA 294:681–690
21. Chilampalli S, Zhang X, Fahmy H, Kaushik RS, Zeman D, Hildreth MB, Dwivedi C (2010) Chemopreventive effects of honokiol on UVB-induced skin cancer development. Anticancer Res 30:777–783
22. Meeran SM, Katiyar SK (2008) Cell cycle control as a basis for cancer chemoprevention through dietary agents. Front Biosci 13:2191–2202

23. Graña X, Reddy EP (1995) Cell cycle control in mammalian cells: role of cyclins, cyclin dependent kinases (CDKs), growth suppressor genes and cyclin-dependent kinase inhibitors (CKIs). Oncogene 11:211–219
24. Sherr CJ, Roberts JM (1999) CDK inhibitors: positive and negative regulators of G1-phase progression. Genes Dev 13:1501–1512
25. Morgan DO (1995) Principles of CDK regulation. Nature 374:131–134
26. Fotedar R, Bendjennat M, Fotedar A (2004) Role of p21WAF1 in the cellular response to UV. Cell Cycle 3:134–137
27. Luo J, Manning BD, Cantley LC (2003) Targeting the PI3K-Akt pathway in human cancer: rationale and promise. Cancer Cell 4:257–262
28. Nomura M, Kaji A, Ma WY, Zhong S, Liu G, Bowden GT, Miyamoto KI, Dong Z (2001) Mitogen- and stress-activated protein kinase 1 mediates activation of Akt by ultraviolet B irradiation. J Biol Chem 276:25558–25567
29. Downward J (1998) Mechanisms and consequences of activation of protein kinase B/Akt. Curr Opin Cell Biol 10:262–267
30. Tyrrell RM (1996) Activation of mammalian gene expression by the UV component of sunlight-from models to reality. BioEssays 18:139–148
31. Osaki M, Kase S, Adachi K, Takeda A, Hashimoto K, Ito H (2004) Inhibition of the PI3K-Akt signaling pathway enhances the sensitivity of Fas-mediated apoptosis in human gastric carcinoma cell line, MKN-45. J Cancer Res Clin Oncol 130:8–14
32. Saleem M, Afaq F, Adhami VM, Mukhtar H (2004) Lupeol modulates NF-kappaB and PI3K/Akt pathways and inhibits skin cancer in CD-1 mice. Oncogene 23:5203–5214
33. Carpenter CL, Cantley LC (1996) Phosphoinositide kinases. Curr Opin Cell Biol 8:153–158
34. Callejas NA, Casado M, Bosca L, Martin-Sanz P (1999) Requirement of nuclear factor kappaB for the constitutive expression of nitric oxide synthase-2 and cyclooxygenase-2 in rat trophoblasts. J Cell Sci 18:3147–3155
35. American Cancer Society. Cancer facts and figures. http://www.cancer.org/research/cancerfactsfigures/. Accessed July 2014
36. Lewis EM, Sergeant S, Ledford B, Stull N, Dinauer MC, McPhail LC (2010) Phosphorylation of $p22^{phox}$ on threonine 147 enhances NADPH oxidase activity by promoting $p47^{phox}$ binding. J Biol Chem 285:2959–2967
37. Sheppard FR, Kelher MR, Moore EE, McLaughlin NJ, Banerjee A, Silliman CC (2005) Structural organization of the neutrophil NADPH oxidase: phosphorylation and translocation during priming and activation. J Leukoc Biol 78:1025–1042
38. Prasad R, Kappes JC, Katiyar SK (2016) Inhibition of NADPH oxidase 1 activity and blocking the binding of cytosolic and membrane-bound proteins by honokiol inhibit migratory potential of melanoma cells. Oncotarget 7:7899–7912
39. Ambasta RK, Kumar P, Griendling KK, Schmidt HH, Busse R, Brandes RP (2004) Direct interaction of the novel Nox proteins with $p22^{phox}$ is required for the formation of a functionally active NADPH oxidase. J Biol Chem 279:45935–45941
40. Sumimoto H, Hata K, Mizuki K, Ito T, Kage Y, Sakaki Y, Fukumaki Y, Nakamura M, Takeshige K (1996) Assembly and activation of the phagocyte NADPH oxidase. Specific interaction of the N-terminal Src homology 3 domain of $p47^{phox}$ with $p22^{phox}$ is required for activation of the NADPH oxidase. J Biol Chem 271:22152–22158
41. Hoehner JC, Gestblom C, Hedborg F, Sandstedt B, Olsen L, Pahlman S (1996) A developmental model of neuroblastoma: differentiating stroma-poor tumors' progress along an extra-adrenal chromaffin lineage. Lab Invest 75:659–675
42. Park JR, Eggert A, Caron H (2008) Neuroblastoma: biology, prognosis, and treatment. Pediatr Clin North Am 55:97–120
43. Zage PE, Kletzel M, Murray K, Marcus R, Castleberry R, Zhang Y, London WB, Kretschmar C, Children's Oncology Group (2008) Outcomes of the POG 9340/9341/9342 trials for children with high-risk neuroblastoma: a report from the Children's Oncology Group. Pediatr Blood Cancer 51:747–753

44. Lin JW, Chen JT, Hong CY, Lin YL, Wang KT, Yao CJ, Lai GM, Chen RM (2012) Honokiol traverses the blood-brain barrier and induces apoptosis of neuroblastoma cells via an intrinsic Bax-mitochondrion-cytochrome c-caspase protease pathway. Neuro Oncol 14:302–314
45. Yeh PS, Wang W, Chang YA, Lin CJ, Wang JJ, Chen RM (2016) Honokiol induces autophagy of neuroblastoma cells through activating the PI3K/Akt/mTOR and endoplasmic reticular stress/ERK1/2 signaling pathways and suppressing cell migration. Cancer Lett 370:66–77
46. Lv X, Liu F, Shang Y, Chen SZ (2015) Honokiol exhibits enhanced antitumor effects with chloroquine by inducing cell death and inhibiting autophagy in human non-small cell lung cancer cells. Oncol Rep 34:1289–1300
47. Kaushik G, Venugopal A, Ramamoorthy P, Standing D, Subramaniam D, Umar S, Jensen RA, Anant S, Mammen JM (2014) Honokiol inhibits melanoma stem cells by targeting notch signaling. Mol Carcinog 54:1710–1721
48. Hahm ER, Sakao K, Singh SV (2014) Honokiol activates reactive oxygen species mediated cytoprotective autophagy in human prostate cancer cells. Prostate 74:1209–1221
49. Guo YB, Bao XJ, Xu SB, Zhang XD, Liu HY (2015) Honokiol induces cell cycle arrest and apoptosis via p53 activation in H4 human neuroglioma cells. Int J Clin Exp Med 15:7168–7175
50. Kim KC, Guan KL (2015) mTOR: a pharmacologic target for autophagy regulation. J Clin Invest 125:25–32
51. Hunter KD, Parkinson EK, Harrison PR (2005) Profiling early head and neck cancer. Nat Rev Cancer 5:127–135
52. Casiglia J, Woo SB (2001) A comprehensive review of oral cancer. Gen Dent 49:72–82
53. Grandis JR, Melhem MF, Barnes EL, Tweardy DJ (1996) Quantitative immunohistochemical analysis of transforming growth factor-α and epidermal growth factor receptor in patients with squamous cell carcinoma of the head and neck. Cancer 78:1284–1292
54. He Y, Zeng Q, Drenning SD, Melhem MF, Tweardy DJ, Huang L, Grandis JR (1998) Inhibition of human squamous cell carcinoma growth in vivo by epidermal growth factor receptor antisense RNA transcribed from the U6 promoter. J Natl Cancer Inst 90:1080–1087
55. Grandis JR, Melhem MF, Gooding WE, Day R, Holst VA, Wagener MM, Drenning SD, Tweardy DJ (1998) Levels of TGF-α and EGFR protein in head and neck squamous cell carcinoma and patient survival. J Natl Cancer Inst 90:824–832
56. Singh T, Gupta NA, Xu S, Prasad R, Velu SE, Katiyar SK (2015) Honokiol inhibits the growth of head and neck squamous cell carcinoma by targeting epidermal growth factor receptor. Oncotarget 6:21268–21282
57. Crowell JA, Steele VE, Sigman CC, Fay JR (2003) Is inducible nitric oxide synthase a target for chemoprevention? Mol Cancer Ther 2:815–823
58. Choi BD, Jeong SJ, Wang G, Park JJ, Lim DS, Kim BH, Cho YI, Kim CS, Jeong MJ (2011) Secretory leukocyte protease inhibitor is associated with MMP-2 and MMP-9 to promote migration and invasion in SNU638 gastric cancer cells. Int J Mol Med 28:527–534
59. Cho JH, Jeon YJ, Park SM, Shin JC, Lee TH, Jung S, Park H, Ryu J, Chen H, Dong Z, Shim JH, Chae JI (2015) Multifunctional effects of honokiol as an anti-inflammatory and anticancer drug in human oral squamous cancer cells and xenograft. Biomaterials 53:274–284
60. Higo T, Hattori M, Nakamura T, Natsume T, Michikawa T, Mikoshiba K (2005) Subtype-specific and ER lumenal environment-dependent regulation of inositol1,4,5-trisphosphate receptor type 1 by ERp44. Cell 120:85–98
61. Armstrong JS (2006) Mitochondrial membrane permeabilization: the sine qua non for cell death. BioEssays 28:253–260
62. Mani SA, Guo W, Liao MJ, Eaton EN, Ayyanan A, Zhou AY, Brooks M, Reinhard F, Zhang CC, Shipitsin M, Campbell LL, Polyak K, Brisken C, Yang J, Weinberg RA (2008) The epithelial-mesenchymal transition generates cells with properties of stem cells. Cell 133:704–715

63. Morel AP, Lievre M, Thomas C, Hinkal G, Ansieau S, Puisieux A (2008) Generation of breast cancer stem cells through epithelial-mesenchymal transition. PLoS ONE 3:e2888
64. Santisteban M, Reiman JM, Asiedu MK, Behrens MD, Nassar A, Kalli KR, Haluska P, Ingle JN, Hartmann LC, Manjili MH, Radisky DC, Ferrone S, Knutson KL (2009) Immune-induced epithelial to mesenchymal transition in vivo generates breast cancer stem cells. Cancer Res 69:2887–2895
65. Avtanski DB, Nagalingam A, Bonner MY, Arbiser JL, Saxena NK, Sharma D (2015) Honokiol activates LKB1-miR-34a axis and antagonizes the oncogenic actions of leptin in breast cancer. Oncotarget 6:29947–29962
66. Shen Z, Wen XF, Lan F, Shen ZZ, Shao ZM (2002) The tumor suppressor gene LKB1 is associated with prognosis in human breast carcinoma. Clin Cancer Res 8:2085–2090
67. Li J, Liu J, Li P, Mao X, Li W, Yang J, Liu P (2014) Loss of LKB1 disrupts breast epithelial cell polarity and promotes breast cancer metastasis and invasion. J Exp Clin Cancer Res 33:70
68. Roy BC, Kohno T, Iwakawa R, Moriguchi T, Kiyono T, Morishita K, Sanchez-Cespedes M, Akiyama T, Yokota J (2010) Involvement of LKB1 in epithelial-mesenchymal transition (EMT) of human lung cancer cells. Lung Cancer 70:136–145
69. Hermeking H (2010) The miR-34 family in cancer and apoptosis. Cell Death Differ 17:193–199
70. Siegel R, Ma J, Zou Z, Jemal A (2014) Cancer statistics, 2014. CA Cancer J Clin 64:9–29
71. Galluzzi L, Vitale I, Michels J, Brenner C, Szabadkai G, Harel-Bellan A, Castedo M, Kroemer G (2014) Systems biology of cisplatin resistance: past, present and future. Cell Death Dis 5:e1257
72. Magee JA, Piskounova E, Morrison SJ (2012) Cancer stem cells: impact, heterogeneity, and uncertainty. Cancer Cell 21:283–296
73. Valent P, Bonnet D, De Maria R, Lapidot T, Copland M, Melo JV, Chomienne C, Ishikawa F, Schuringa JJ, Stassi G, Huntly B, Herrmann H, Soulier J, Roesch A, Schuurhuis GJ, Wohrer S, Arock M, Zuber J, Cerny-Reiterer S, Johnsen HE, Andreeff M, Eaves C (2012) Cancer stem cell definitions and terminology: the devil is in the details. Nat Rev Cancer 12:767–775
74. Varambally S, Dhanasekaran SM, Zhou M, Barrette TR, Sinha CK, Sanda MG, Ghosh D, Pienta KJ, Sewalt RG, Otte AP, Rubin MA, Chinnaiyan AM (2002) The polycomb group protein EZH2 is involved in progression of prostate cancer. Nature 419:624–629
75. Huqun Ishikawa R, Zhang J, Miyazawa H, Goto Y, Shimizu Y, Hagiwara K, Koyama N (2012) Enhancer of zeste homolog 2 is a novel prognostic biomarker in nonsmall cell lung cancer. Cancer 118:1599–1606
76. Raman JD, Mongan NP, Tickoo SK, Boorjian SA, Scherr DS, Gudas LJ (2005) Increased expression of the polycomb group gene, EZH2, in transitional cell carcinoma of the bladder. Clin Cancer Res 11:8570–8576
77. Zhang Q, Zhao W, Ye C, Zhuang J, Chang C, Li Y, Huang X, Shen L, Li Y, Cui Y, Song J, Shen B, Eliaz I, Huang R, Ying H, Guo H, Yan J (2015) Honokiol inhibits bladder tumor growth by suppressing EZH2/miR-143 axis. Oncotarget 6:37335–37348
78. Gupta GP, Massague J (2006) Cancer metastasis: building a framework. Cell 4:679–695
79. Chang KH, Yan MD, Yao CJ, Lin PC, Lai GM (2013) Honokiol-induced apoptosis and autophagy in glioblastoma multiforme cells. Oncol Lett 6:1435–1438
80. Kaushik G, Ramalingam S, Subramaniam D, Rangarajan P, Protti P, Rammamoorthy P, Anant S, Mammen JM (2012) Honokiol induces cytotoxic and cytostatic effects in malignant melanoma cancer cells. Am J Surg 204:868–873
81. De Craene B, Berx G (2013) Regulatory networks defining EMT during cancer initiation and progression. Nat Rev Cancer 13:97–110

82. Rosivatz E, Becker I, Specht K, Fricke E, Luber B, Busch R, Höfler H, Becker KF (2002) Differential expression of the epithelial-mesenchymal transition regulators snail, SIP1, and twist in gastric cancer. Am J Pathol 161:1881–1891
83. Liu WF, Ji SR, Sun JJ, Zhang Y, Liu ZY, Liang AB, Zeng HZ (2012) CD146 expression correlates with epithelial-mesenchymal transition markers and a poor prognosis in gastric cancer. Int J Mol Sci 13:6399–6406
84. Zhong XY, Zhang LH, Jia SQ, Shi T, Niu ZJ, Du H, Zhang GG, Hu Y, Lu AP, Li JY, Ji JF (2008) Positive association of up-regulated Cripto-1 and down-regulated E-cadherin with tumour progression and poor prognosis in gastric cancer. Histopathology 52:560–568
85. Vougioukalaki M, Kanellis DC, Gkouskou K, Eliopoulos AG (2011) Tpl2 kinase signal transduction in inflammation and cancer. Cancer Lett 304:80–89
86. Ohara R, Hirota S, Onoue H, Nomura S, Kitamura Y, Toyoshima K (1995) Identification of the cells expressing cot proto-oncogene mRNA. J Cell Sci 108:97–103
87. Pan HC, Lai DW, Lan KH, Shen CC, Wu SM, Chiu CS, Wang KB, Sheu ML (2013) Honokiol thwarts gastric tumor growth and peritoneal dissemination by inhibiting Tpl2 in an orthotopic model. Carcinogenesis 34:2568–2579
88. Li YL, Vergne J, Torchet C, Maurel MC (2009) In vitro selection of adenine-dependent ribozyme against Tpl2/Cot oncogene. FEBS J 276:303–314
89. Perfield JW 2nd, Lee Y, Shulman GI, Samuel VT, Jurczak MJ, Chang E, Xie C, Tsichlis PN, Obin MS, Greenberg AS (2011) Tumor progression locus 2 (TPL2) regulates obesity-associated inflammation and insulin resistance. Diabetes 60:1168–1176
90. Yunlan L, Juan Z (2014) Qingshan L (2014) Antitumor activity of di-n-butyl-(2,6-difluorobenzohydrox-amato)tin (IV) against human gastric carcino-ma SGC-7901 cells via G2/M cell cycle arrest and cell apoptosis. PLoS ONE 9:e90793
91. Su CC (2014) Tanshinone IIA inhibits gastric carcino-ma AGS cells through increasing p-p38, p-JNK and p53 but reducing p-ERK, CDC2 and cyclin B1 expression. Anticancer Res 34:7097–7110
92. Yan B, Peng ZY (2015) Honokiol induces cell cycle arrest and apoptosis in human gastric carcinoma MGC-803 cell line. Int J Clin Exp Med 8:5454–5461
93. Huang M, Stolina M, Sharma S, Mao JT, Zhu L, Miller PW, Wollman J, Herschman H, Dubinett SM (1998) Non-small cell lung cancer cyclooxygenase-2-dependent regulation of cytokine balance in lymphocytes and macrophages: up-regulation of interleukin 10 and down-regulation of interleukin 12 production. Cancer Res 58:1208–1216
94. Hida T, Yatabe Y, Achiwa H, Muramatsu H, Kozaki K, Nakamura S, Ogawa M, Mitsudomi T, Sugiura T, Takahashi T (1998) Increased expression of cyclooxygenase 2 occurs frequently in human lung cancers, specifically in adenocarcinomas. Cancer Res 58:3761–3764·
95. Wolff H, Saukkonen K, Anttila S, Karjalainen A, Vainio H, Ristimäki A (1998) Expression of cyclooxygenase-2 in human lung carcinoma. Cancer Res 58:4997–5001
96. Hosomi Y, Yokose T, Hirose Y, Nakajima R, Nagai K, Nishiwaki Y, Ochiai A (2000) Increased cyclooxygenase 2 (COX-2) expression occurs frequently in precursor lesions of human adenocarcinoma of the lung. Lung Cancer 30:73–81
97. Singh T, Katiyar SK (2013) Honokiol inhibits non-small cell lung cancer cell migration by targeting PGE_2-mediated activation of β-catenin signaling. PLoS ONE 8:e60749
98. Tuynman JB, Vermeulen L, Boon EM, Kemper K, Zwinderman AH, Peppelenbosch MP, Richel DJ (2008) Cyclooxygenase-2 inhibition inhibits c-Met kinase activity and Wnt activity in colon cancer. Cancer Res 68:1213–1220
99. Shlomo H, Simon JA (2008) A small-molecule inhibitor of Tcf/beta-catenin signaling down-regulates PPARgamma and PPARdelta activities. Mol Cancer Ther 7:521–529

100. Wharry CE, Haines KM, Carroll RG, May MJ (2009) Constitutive noncanonical NF-kappaB signaling in pancreatic cancer cells. Cancer Biol Ther 8:1567–1576
101. Arora S, Bhardwaj A, Srivastava SK, Singh S, McClellan S, Wang B, Singh AP (2011) Honokiol arrests cell cycle, induces apoptosis, and potentiates the cytotoxic effect of gemcitabine in human pancreatic cancer cells. PLoS ONE 6:e21573
102. Arora S, Singh S, Piazza GA, Contreras CM, Panyam J, Singh AP (2012) Honokiol: a novel natural agent for cancer prevention and therapy. Curr Mol Med 12:1244–1252

Chapter 12
Celastrol and Its Role in Controlling Chronic Diseases

Shivaprasad H. Venkatesha and Kamal D. Moudgil

Abstract Celastrol, a triterpenoid derived from traditional Chinese medicinal plants, has anti-inflammatory, antioxidant, and anticancer activities. Celastrol has shown preventive/therapeutic effects in experimental models of several chronic diseases. These include, chronic inflammatory and autoimmune diseases (e.g., rheumatoid arthritis, multiple sclerosis, systemic lupus erythematosus, inflammatory bowel disease, and psoriasis), neurodegenerative disorders (e.g., Alzheimer's disease, Parkinson's disease, and Amyotrophic lateral sclerosis), atherosclerosis, obesity, Type 2 diabetes, and cancer. Celastrol modulates intricate cellular pathways and networks associated with disease pathology, and it interrupts or redirects the aberrant cellular and molecular events so as to limit disease progression and facilitate recovery, where feasible. The major cell signaling pathways modulated by celastrol include the NF-kB pathway, MAPK pathway, JAK/STAT pathway, PI3K/Akt/mTOR pathway, and antioxidant defense mechanisms. Furthermore, celastrol modulates cell proliferation, apoptosis, proteasome activity, heat-shock protein response, innate and adaptive immune responses, angiogenesis, and bone remodeling. Current understanding of the mechanisms of action of celastrol and information about its disease-modulating activities in experimental models have set the stage for testing celastrol in clinical studies as a therapeutic agent for several chronic human diseases.

Keywords Celastrol · Inflammation · Autoimmune diseases · Neurodegenerative diseases · Metabolic disorders · Immune modulation · Natural products · Traditional Chinese medicine

S.H. Venkatesha · K.D. Moudgil (✉)
Department of Microbiology and Immunology, University of Maryland School of Medicine, 685 W. Baltimore Street, HSF-1, Suite-380, Baltimore, MD 21201, USA
e-mail: kmoudgil@som.umaryland.edu

K.D. Moudgil
Division of Rheumatology, Department of Medicine, University of Maryland School of Medicine, Baltimore, MD 21201, USA

S.C. Gupta et al. (eds.), *Anti-inflammatory Nutraceuticals and Chronic Diseases*,
Advances in Experimental Medicine and Biology 928,
DOI 10.1007/978-3-319-41334-1_12

12.1 Introduction

Celastrol is a bioactive component of several traditional Chinese medicinal plants including, *Tripterygium wilfordii* (Thunder God Vine), *Celastrus orbiculatus, Celastrus aculeatus, Celastrus reglii, Celastrus scandens,* and others that belong to the Celastraceae family [1–5]. The extracts of the root, bark, and stem of some of these plants have long been used in China and other Asian countries for the treatment of a wide range of chronic inflammatory disorders, including rheumatoid arthritis (RA), systemic lupus erythematosus (SLE), and allergies [1–5]. In this article, we describe the diverse molecular and cellular pathways modulated by celastrol, with emphasis on chronic inflammatory, autoimmune, neurodegenerative, and metabolic diseases [6–12]. Celastrol also possesses anticancer activity [5, 13–15]. A summary of the anticancer mechanisms employed by celastrol is presented at the end.

12.2 Physico-Chemical Properties of Celastrol

Celastrol is a pentacyclic triterpene (Fig. 12.1) that belong to a small class of organic compounds called quinone methides. It has a molecular weight of 450.6 and its molecular formula is $C_{29}H_{38}O_4$. It is a pale brown to orange red crystalline powder, and its melting point is between 219–230 °C. Celastrol has maximum UV/visible absorption spectra at 253 and 424 nm. It is sparingly soluble in water, but is soluble in nonpolar solvents such as dimethylsulfoxide (DMSO) and ethanol. Celastrol is an electrophilic compound and it can react with nucleophilic thiol groups of cysteine residues of a variety of proteins to form adducts or induce other

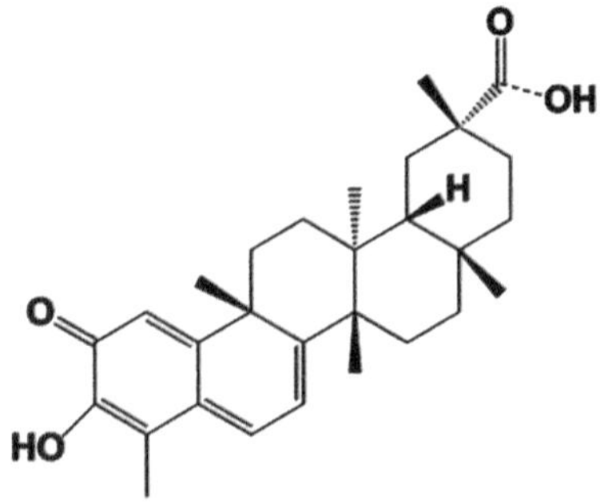

Fig. 12.1 Molecular structure of celastrol. Celastrol is a pentacyclic triterpenoid with a molecular weight 450.6 and molecular formula $C_{29}H_{38}O_4$. It belongs to a small class of organic compounds known as quinone methides. Celastrol has an acidic group at one end and a phenolic quinone at the other end

modifications within those proteins [6, 16–18]. Apparently, this is one of the mechanisms by which celastrol can affect biological functions of proteins. Celastrol is also known as tripterine/tripterin, but the name celastrol is commonly used.

12.3 Celastrol Controls Inflammation and Other Pathological Processes in Animal Models of Chronic Diseases

Celastrol has been shown to be beneficial in various chronic disease conditions in studies in animal models of immune-mediated diseases, neurodegenerative diseases, and others. The preventive/therapeutic potential of celastrol in various in vivo and in vitro models of these diseases is summarized in Table 12.1. Also mentioned therein are the cell signaling pathways as well as cellular and molecular targets of celastrol in various disease processes. The details of these and other mechanisms of action of celastrol are described below in separate sections. In addition, celastrol has potent anticancer activity. The mechanisms underlying the anticancer activity of celastrol are summarized at the end in a separate section.

12.3.1 Inflammatory, Autoimmune, and Allergic Diseases

For RA, using the rat adjuvant arthritis (AA) model, mouse collagen-induced arthritis (CIA) model and fibroblast-like synoviocytes from RA patients (RA-FLS) culture model, celastrol has been shown to reduce the severity of clinical and histopathological features of arthritis, as well as to modulate the production of pro-inflammatory cytokines and chemokines [8, 9, 19], to reset the T helper 17 (Th17)/T regulatory (Treg) cell balance to facilitate the suppression of arthritis [20], and to afford protection against bone damage [8, 9, 19] (Table 12.1A). Celastrol also inhibits RA-FLS invasion and protects against bone and cartilage damage [21]. For multiple sclerosis (MS), celastrol is shown to modulate Th17 responses, to shift Th1 responses toward Th2, and to increase the production of anti-inflammatory cytokines in the experimental autoimmune encephalomyelitis (EAE) model of MS [10, 22]. For SLE (also known as lupus), celastrol treatment decreases transforming growth factor (TGF)-β production, urine protein excretion, and serum autoantibody levels in BW F1 and BALB/c mouse models of SLE [23–25]. For ulcerative colitis, using the mouse dextran sulfate sodium (DSS)-induced colitis model, celastrol has been shown to modulate oxidative stress, inflammatory cytokines and intestinal homeostasis [11]. For asthma and other hypersensitivity reactions, celastrol inhibits histamine and eotaxin production and other mediators involved in hypersensitivity reactions [26–29]. The main mediators and pathways targeted by celastrol in above-mentioned diseases are described in Table 12.1A.

Table 12.1 Celastrol-induced prevention/treatment of chronic diseases of diverse etiology

Type of disease	Experimental model(s)	Targets/mechanisms of celastrol action	References
A. Inflammatory and autoimmune diseases			
Rheumatoid Arthritis (RA)	Rat AA, Rat/Mouse CIA, Human RA-FLS	Modulates pro-inflammatory cytokines, chemokines, and T helper 17 (Th17)/T regulatory (Treg) cell balance. Inhibits RA-FLS invasion and apoptosis. Decreases production of antibodies to the disease-related antigens and anti-cyclic citrullinated peptides (aCCP) antibodies. Also inhibits osteoclast differentiation, and reduces cartilage and bone damage	[8, 9, 19–21, 88, 118, 137–140]
Multiple sclerosis (MS)	Rat/mouse experimental autoimmune encephalomyelitis (EAE)	Modulates Th17 responses, shifts Th1 response towards Th2, decreases TNFα but increases IL-10. Inhibits NF-κB expression, nitrites levels, and expression of Toll-like receptor (TLR)2	[10, 22]
Systemic lupus erythematosus (SLE) (or Lupus)	BW F1 mice, BALB/c mice (chromatin injection)	Decreases transforming growth factor (TGF)-β, renal collagen type IV, urine protein excretion, and serum autoantibodies	[23–25]
Ulcerative colitis	DSS-induced colitis in mice	Modulates oxidative stress, inflammatory cytokines, and intestinal homeostasis	[11]
Psoriasis	HACaT keratinocytes	Inhibits NF-κB expression and induces apoptosis through caspase-3 activation	[141]
Hypersensitivity (e.g., Asthma and skin inflammation)	Ovalbumin/allergen-induced airway inflammation, phorbol myristate acetate-induced skin inflammation, and skin hypersensitivity to dinitrochlorobenzene in mice	Downregulates the expression of stem cell factor (SCF) in fibroblasts, and inhibits the production of histamine and eotaxin in mast cells. Inhibits antibody responses and immunoglobulin Fc epsilon receptor I signaling. Regulates the balance between isoforms of MMPs (MMP-2/9) and TIMPs (TIMP-1/2)	[26–29]

(continued)

Table 12.1 (continued)

Type of disease	Experimental model(s)	Targets/mechanisms of celastrol action	References
B. Neurodegenerative diseases			
Parkinson's disease (PD)	MPTP mouse model, SH-SY5Y cells	Modulates pro-inflammatory cytokines, prevents the generation of ROS, lipid peroxidation, and mitochondrial membrane potential. Protects against cellular injury and apoptotic cells death	[12, 31, 34]
Alzheimer's disease	Transgenic mouse model	Inhibits pro-inflammatory cytokines and expression of MHC-II molecules. Induces neuroprotective heat-shock proteins (Hsps). Lowers oxidative stress and regulates BACE-1 expression level via an NF-κB-dependent mechanism	[30, 32, 33, 36, 37]
Amyotrophic lateral sclerosis (ALS)	G93A SOD1 transgenic mouse model	Blocks neuronal cell death, reduces TNFα, iNOS, CD40, and GFAP immunoreactivity	[35]
Gaucher disease (GD)	GD fibroblasts	Modulates molecular chaperones and increases glucocerebrosidase activity	[38]
Age-related macular degeneration (AMD)	Human retinal pigment epithelial cells (ARPE-19 cells)	Reduces IL-6 and inhibits NF-κB	[39]
C. Atherosclerotic and metabolic diseases			
Atherosclerosis	ApoE-deficient mice, Rabbit carotid atherosclerosis model, and human platelets	Inhibits lectin-like oxidized low density lipoprotein receptor-1 (LOX-1) and generation of ROS. Reduces serum level of low density lipoproteins and VEGF expression. Inhibits platelet aggregation by reducing the expression of P-selectin and glycoprotein IIb/IIIa on platelets	[40, 41, 142]

(continued)

Table 12.1 (continued)

Type of disease	Experimental model(s)	Targets/mechanisms of celastrol action	References
Obesity	Hyperleptinemic diet-induced obese mice	Reduces food intake, increases energy expenditure, leading to weight loss by increasing leptin sensitivity	[42]
Type 2 diabetes	The db/db mouse	Acting on the liver, adipose tissue, and kidney, it Inhibits NF-kB, reduces insulin resistance, improves abnormal lipid metabolism and oxidative stress, reduces pro-inflammatory cytokines, and limits renal injury	[43]

AA adjuvant-induced arthritis, *CIA* collagen-induced arthritis, *DSS* dextran sulfate sodium, *FLS* fibroblasts-like synoviocytes, *Hsp* heat-shock proteins, *MMPs* matrix metalloproteases, *TIMPs* tissue inhibitor of matrix metalloproteases, *MPTP* 1-methyl-4-phenyl-1,2,3,6-tetrahydropyridin, *ROS* reactive oxygen species, *MHC-II* major histocompatibility complex class II, *BACE1* beta-site APP-cleaving enzyme 1, *iNOS* inducible nitric oxide synthase, *GFAP* glial fibrillary acidic protein, *p-JNK* phospho c-Jun N-terminal kinase, *NF-κB* nuclear factor kappa B, *ROS* reactive oxygen species, *VEGF* vascular endothelial growth factor

12.3.2 Neurodegenerative Disorders

The effects of celastrol on MS, a neurological disease of autoimmune origin, have been described above. For other neurological diseases such as Parkinson's disease, Alzheimer's disease and amyotrophic lateral sclerosis (ALS or Lou Gehrig's disease), celastrol has been shown to modulate pro-inflammatory cytokine production, to prevent the generation of reactive oxygen species (ROS), to limit oxidative damage, to protect against cell death, and to regulate heat-shock proteins (Hsps), as observed in mouse models and in vitro models of these diseases (Table 12.1B) [12, 30–37]. For Gaucher disease (GD), celastrol modulates molecular chaperones and increases glucocerebrosidase activity in the GD fibroblasts model [38]. Celastrol is also known to modulate age-related macular degeneration [39].

12.3.3 Other Diseases

Celastrol can inhibit platelet activation [40], prevent atherosclerotic plaque size in apo E-deficient mice [41], and decrease ratio of the plaque area and the arterial wall cross-section area in a rabbit model of carotid atherosclerosis [41], thus revealing the anti-atherosclerosis effect of this natural triterpene (Table 12.1C). Recently, celastrol has been reported to be a leptin sensitizer, whose effects are manifest as reduced intake of food, increased energy expenditure, and weight loss, and thereby it may potentially serve as an anti-obesity agent [42]. Celastrol is also effective in improving insulin resistance and limiting renal injury in a mouse model of type 2 diabetes (T2D) [43]. Furthermore, celastrol can modulate human immunodeficiency virus (HIV) 1-transactivator of transcription (Tat)-induced inflammatory responses in astrocytes in vitro by inhibiting the activation of various signaling pathways as well as the expression of pro-inflammatory chemokines and adhesion molecules such as intracellular adhesion molecule-1 (ICAM-1)/vascular cell adhesion molecule-1 (VCAM-1) [44]. Celastrol has also been reported to target defined functional components of pathogens such as the HIV-Tat [18] to inhibit the transcription and replication of that virus, and the enzyme enoyl-acyl carrier protein reductase of *Plasmodium falciparum* [45], which is a drug target for this malaria parasite. However, because of the limited scope of this article, we have not elaborated further on direct effects of celastrol on various pathogens.

12.4 Celastrol Modulates Cell Signaling Pathways

Inflammation involves interplays among a variety of cellular, molecular and biochemical mediators that are activated/induced in response to different pro-inflammatory stimuli. These mediators comprise diverse pathways (Fig. 12.2) that are described below. Inflammation is associated with multiple diseases, including chronic inflammatory diseases, autoimmune diseases, obesity, and cancer. Celastrol controls inflammation by targeting one or many of these pathways depending on the underlying disease process.

The nuclear factor kappa-light-chain-enhancer of activated B cells (NF-kB) pathway is a central regulator of inflammation. A broad range of pro-inflammatory stimuli including cytokines, growth factors, and microbial products activate the I-kappa B kinase (IKK) complex consisting of IKK1, IKK2 and NF-κB essential modulator (NEMO). Activated IKK complex phosphorylates I-kappa B (IκB), which leads to ubiquitination and proteasomal degradation of IκB. The degradation of IκB in turn activates NF-κB, which then translocates to the nucleus, where it binds to DNA and regulates the expression of several target genes. NF-kB activation enhances the production of pro-inflammatory cytokines (e.g., interleukin-1 β (IL-1β), IL-6 and tumor necrosis factor α (TNFα)) and other inflammatory mediators (e.g., matrix metalloproteinases (MMPs) and inducible nitric oxide synthase (iNOS)) [46, 47], without much effect on the induction of anti-inflammatory cytokines (e.g., IL-10 or IL-1 receptor antagonist (IL-1Ra)) [48]. Celastrol inhibits NF-κB activation and regulates NF-κB-regulated gene expression. It has been suggested that celastrol targets cysteine 179 in IKK [16] and blocks IKK activity as well as the degradation and phosphorylation of IκB [16, 21, 49]. This in turn blocks the activation of NF-κB and its nuclear translocation.

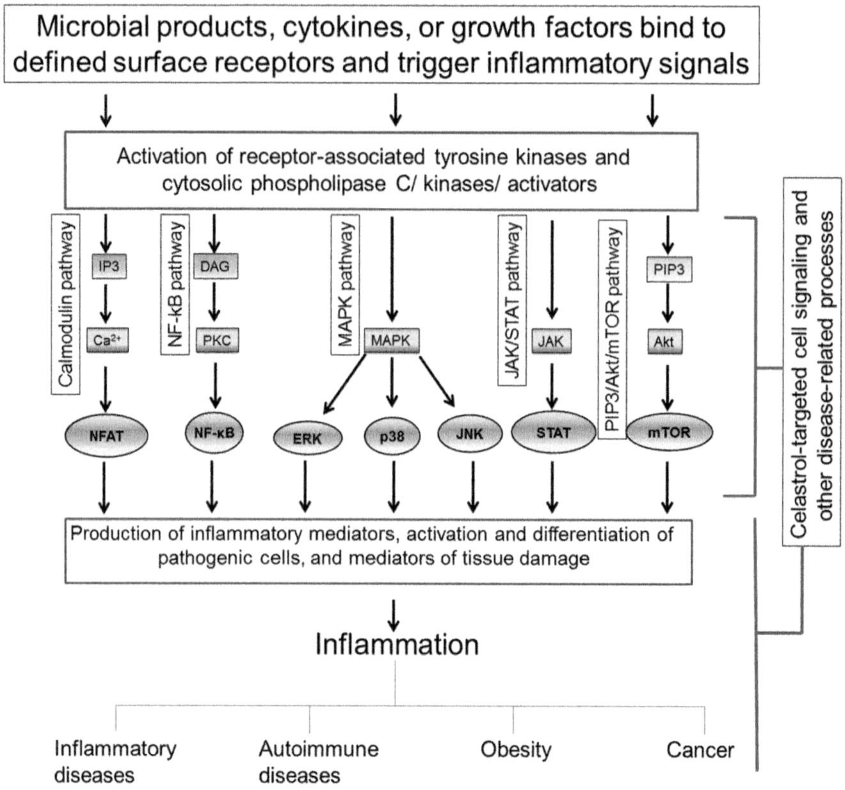

Fig. 12.2 Cell signaling pathways and other disease-related processes modulated by celastrol for the control of chronic diseases. A schematic representation of the cell signaling pathways that are regulated by celastrol is depicted here. These pathways are activated in response to diverse stimuli induced by specific ligand-cell surface receptor interaction. This interaction results in activation of receptor-associated tyrosine kinases, which subsequently activate other cytosolic targets, which then initiate various signaling pathways. The major pathways regulated by celastrol are described in the text and shown in the figure. Celastrol is known to target one or more of these pathways leading to the suppression of inflammation associated with various chronic diseases including, inflammatory diseases, autoimmune diseases, obesity, and cancer. There is no direct evidence for celastrol-induced modulation of calmodulin pathway. However, regulation of calcium release and AMPK activity by celastrol suggests the possibility of regulation of the calmodulin pathway by celsatrol. Besides cell signaling, celastrol modulates other disease-related processes (e.g., angiogenesis, heat-shock protein responses, and proteasome activity) to limit disease progression and to facilitate recovery, where feasible.

Mitogen activated protein kinase (MAPK) pathway is another important signal transduction pathway besides NF-κB pathway that is critical for immune-mediated inflammatory responses [50]. MAPKs are a family of serine/threonine protein kinases [51]. Three well-defined members of this family are the extracellular signal-regulated kinase (ERK), c-Jun N-terminal kinase (JNK), and p38 MAPK, and they are activated by pro-inflammatory stimuli, including cytokines [50]. ERK signal transduction pathway leads to the activation of transcription factors c-Jun, c-Fos, and activating transcription factor 2 (ATF-2), whereas JNK activation leads to the activation of c-Jun and ATF-2. Furthermore, the p38 MAPK-mediated processes involve the participation of transcription factors cAMP response element-binding protein (CREB) and ATF-2 [50, 52, 53]. Celastrol selectively regulates the MAPK pathway. It inhibits the phosphorylation of JNK and ERK in various models of inflammation and arthritis [8, 27, 54]. However, activation of JNK by celastrol has also been observed in another system [55]. For p38 MAPK, one report stated that phosphorylation of p38 MAPK is unaffected by celastrol [56], whereas another [57] indicated that celastrol can activate p38 MAPK; the latter effect has been associated with the anti-metastatic activity of celastrol against cancer.

The Janus kinase (JAK)-signal transducer and activator of transcription (STAT) pathway is a common signaling cascade for many cytokines [58, 59]. JAKs are known to associate with the cytoplasmic domain of cytokine receptors for interferon (IFN)-α/β, IFNγ, IL-2, IL-4, IL-6, IL-10, IL-12/23, and others [58]. In general, the binding of these cytokines to their respective receptors phosphorylates JAK, which then leads to the phosphorylation of STATs. Activated STATs dimerize and translocate to the nucleus, where they bind to promoter regions of cytokine-responsive genes and thereby activate gene transcription [58]. Different STATs are involved in the differentiation of naïve T cells into particular T cell subsets (Th1, Th2, Th17, and Treg). In our studies, we have shown that celastrol inhibits STAT3 activation and suppresses IL-17 expression as well as Th17 differentiation in the rat AA model [8, 20]. In models of cancer, such as multiple myeloma and hepatocellular carcinoma, constitutive STAT3 activation plays a role in cell proliferation, survival, and metabolism, and thereby to the disease process. Celastrol is shown to inhibit STAT3-mediated cell proliferation [60, 61]. It involves inhibition of activation of upstream JAK1 and JAK2. However, effects of celastrol on other JAKs and STATs remain to be determined.

Another signaling pathway affected by celastrol is phosphatidylinositol-3-kinase (PI3K)/Akt/mammalian target of rapamycin (mTOR) pathway, which is involved in immune-mediated diseases and cancer [62–67]. Altered activation of the PI3K/Akt/mTOR pathway is observed in many human tumors, and it regulates the proliferation, differentiation, metabolism and survival of cancer cells [68]. Furthermore, there is an association between the accumulation of hypoxia-inducible factor-1 (HIF-1) and amplified PI3K/Akt/mTOR pathway signaling [69]. HIF-1 is a transcription factor highly expressed under hypoxic conditions and regulates cell survival response to hypoxia and cancer [63, 70, 71]. Inhibitors of HIF-1 have been tried for cancer therapy [72]. Celastrol can inhibit both PI3K activity as well as HIF-1 [63, 66]. Celastrol inhibited HIF-1 activity in various cancer cell lines by decreasing the accumulation of HIF-1 and preventing the expression of HIF-1 target genes. Furthermore, the accumulation of HIF-1 by celastrol is correlated with inhibition of the phosphorylation of mTOR, ribosomal protein S6 kinase (p70S6K), eukaryotic initiation factor 4E (eIF4E), and ERK [63]. Contrary to the above, celastrol is also reported to induce HIF-1 accumulation through the induction of ROS and Akt/p70S6K signaling, and promote transcription of HIF target genes [70].

Therefore, additional studies are needed to clearly understand the role of celastrol in the regulation of mTOR and HIF-1.

Celastrol possesses antioxidant activity. Oxidative stress is one of the mediators of inflammation [73]. Oxidative stress builds up with the generation of high levels of reactive free radicals, such as reactive oxygen species (ROS; e.g., chemically reactive molecules derived from O_2 mainly O_2^- (superoxide anions), H_2O_2 (hydrogen peroxide) and $^{\bullet}OH$ (hydroxyl radicals)) and reactive nitrogen species (RNS; e.g., radicals derived from nitrogen and oxygen, particularly nitric oxide (NO)) in the cell [74, 75]. Celastrol is shown to inhibit lipid peroxidation in rat liver mitochondria by direct radical scavenging [76] as well as neutralizing oxygen radicals [77]. Celastrol also enhanced the antioxidant defense system and offered protection against bleomycin-induced pulmonary fibrosis in rats by restoring antioxidant enzymes such as hemoxygenase-1 (HO-1), glutathione-S-transferase (GSTs) and nicotinamide adenine dinucleotide phosphate (H) (NADP(H)): quinine oxidoreductase (NQO1) via the NF-E2-related factor-2 (Nrf2) pathway [78]. Similarly, celastrol decreased obesity-induced oxidative stress by increasing antioxidant enzymes and inhibiting NADH oxidase and ROS [79]. Defense against oxidant system by celastrol has also been attributed to decreased expression of iNOS and NO production [30, 34], and the blocking of reactive thiols [17]. In contrast to the above, celastrol has been reported to induce ROS accumulation and to initiate apoptosis through the downregulation on Hsp90 in tumor cells [80]. Similarly, in osteosarcoma, celastrol caused G2/M phase arrest, and induced apoptosis and autophagy via the ROS/JNK signaling pathway [81].

12.5 Celastrol has Anti-Angiogenic Activity and Protects Against Endothelial Barrier Dysfunction

Angiogenesis, the formation of new blood vessels, is a hallmark of cancer [82–84]. However, autoimmune diseases such as RA are also characterized by angiogenesis in the target organ, the inflamed joints [85, 86]. Accordingly, anti-angiogenic therapy has been considered for both these categories of disorders [86, 87]. As discussed above, celastrol treatment inhibits the progression of autoimmune arthritis in experimental models of AA and CIA [8, 9, 20, 88]. Similarly, celastrol suppresses tumor growth, for example, in mouse models and in vitro models of human prostate cancer [89, 90]. Interestingly, celastrol has been shown to inhibit angiogenesis, both in vitro and in vivo [83, 91], and to inhibit vascular endothelial growth factor (VEGF)-induced Akt/mTOR/p70S6 K signaling [83]. Furthermore, celastrol can inhibit hypoxia-mediated angiogenesis, which involves inhibition of HIF-1α and its downstream genes such as VEGF [92]. Celastrol's ability to inhibit Hsp90 was also implicated in reduced HIF-1α in this process. In another study, celastrol was shown to inhibit vasculogenesis by decreasing VEGF secretion, adhesion of endothelial cells to the extracellular matrix (ECM) and their subsequent migration, and tubule formation [93]. Inhibition of Akt/endothelial nitric oxide synthase (eNOS) signaling was implicated in this process. Celastrol has also been reported to inhibit lipopolysaccharide (LPS)-induced angiogenesis, which involved suppression of Toll-like receptor-4 (TLR-4)-mediated NF-kB activation [94], and to inhibit angiogenesis via suppression of VEGFR-1 and VEGFR-2 expression [95].

In RA, vascular endothelial cell physiology is relevant not only for angiogenesis but also for immune cell interaction and migration through blood vessels, as well as for maintaining a healthy endothelial barrier. In this regard, celastrol has been shown to inhibit the expression of cytokine-induced adhesion molecules such as ICAM-1 and VCAM-1 [96], and to prevent endothelial barrier dysfunction by inhibiting endogenous peroxynitrite formation in endothelial cells exposed to pro-inflammatory stimuli [97]. The latter effect involved inhibition of JAK-2-dependent iNOS and NADPH oxidase type 1 (Nox-1) induction.

12.6 Celastrol-Induced Modulation of Heat-Shock Response and Its Potential Therapeutic Applications in Chronic Diseases

Heat-shock proteins (Hsps), also known as "Stress proteins", can be induced by heat and other types of stimuli that cause cellular stress [98, 99]. These are highly conserved proteins evolutionarily. Hsps can be categorized into different families based on their molecular mass (kD), for example, Hsp110, Hsp90, Hsp70, Hsp60, Hsp40, and Small Hsps. One of the major functions of Hsps is to protect cells from damage under different types of stressful conditions [98, 99]. Acting as chaperones, Hsps bind to cellular proteins, ensure proper folding of cellular proteins, attempt to repair defective proteins, and protect them against denaturation and other types of damage. Hsps are also involved in signal transduction and apoptosis. Thus, heat-shock response is cytoprotective under situations that otherwise would promote apoptosis of cells. Stress-inducible heat-shock transcription factor-1 (HSF1) plays an important regulatory role in response to environmental stress and pathophysiological conditions.

Dysregulation of cellular stress pathways and protein folding can lead to intracellular accumulation of protein aggregates, which is turn can induce tissue pathology [100, 101]. Many pathophysiological conditions including, neurodegenerative disorders (e.g., Alzheimer's disease, Parkinson's disease), cardiovascular diseases, cancer, diabetes, and aging are associated with accumulation of misfolded and/or aggregated proteins within certain tissues, attributable in part to defective cellular stress response pathways [17, 32, 100–102]. In addition, inflammation and oxidant damage also contribute to the pathogenic processes in these disorders. Accordingly, pharmacological agents that possess anti-inflammatory and antioxidant activities, and can reset these defective pathways, are increasingly being sought [17, 32, 102].

Celastrol has been shown to have a cytoprotective effect in response to stress-induced cell death. Celastrol can induce the expression of various Hsps, for example, Hsp70, Hsp40, and Hsp27, by activation of HSF1 and these Hsps might contribute to its cytoprotective effect [103]. Celastrol's antioxidant attributes can also contribute to its cytoprotective effects. As described under cell signaling, the antioxidant response involves transcription factors Nrf-2 and Atf4, and celastrol has been shown to activate both these transcription factors [17]. In one study, celastrol's cytoprotective effect was shown to be mediated via induction of Hsp32 (also known as heme oxygenase-1; HO-1) [104]. This induction of Hsp32 was mediated via Nrf-2 instead of HSF-1, and Hsp32 in turn inhibited pro-apoptotic JNK. Besides the induction of Hsps mentioned above, inhibition of Hsp90 has been shown to have a therapeutic effect in certain neurodegenerative diseases; the latter effect is attributable to selective proteasomal degradation of Hsp90 client proteins [100]. Importantly, celastrol is an inhibitor of Hsp90 [105, 106], and it can modulate several nuclear transcription factors that are Hsp90 clients, including the aryl hydrocarbon receptor (AhR) [105, 106]. The involvement of celastrol-induced inhibition of Hsp90 and its anticancer effect is discussed below.

12.7 Anticancer Effects of Celastrol

Celastrol is known to have anticancer and anti-metastatic activities [15, 82, 83, 107, 108]. In addition, celastrol is shown to enhance the therapeutic efficacy of other anticancer drugs when used with them, and to potentiate the beneficial effects of radiotherapy [109, 110]. The major processes involved in these activities and affected by celastrol include, the inhibition of cellular proliferation, induction of apoptosis, prevention of malignant tissue invasion, and blockade of angiogenesis [7, 15, 82, 111]. Celastrol can inhibit cell proliferation and induce apoptosis via multiple actions. These include, potentiation of TNF-induced apoptosis via suppression of the NF-kB pathway [4]; downregulation of cytokines such as IL-6, which is an inducer of cell proliferation [112]; activation of caspases [113–115]; inhibition of the expression of anti-apoptotic proteins such as cellular inhibitor of apoptosis protein 1 and 2 (cIAP1 and cIAP2), cellular FLICE-inhibitory protein (FLIP), and B-cell lymphoma 2 (Bcl-2) [4, 114]; induction of cell cycle arrest [81, 116]; and downregulation of cell survival proteins coupled with upregulation of death receptors [117]. Furthermore, celastrol inhibits adhesion, migration and invasion of tumor cells via reduced expression of specific integrins, as well as reduced MMP activity [118–120]. In addition, as described above, celastrol can suppress angiogenesis [63, 83].

Two additional mechanisms contribute to the anticancer effects of celastrol, namely inhibition of Hsp90 and proteasome inhibition. In regard to Hsp90, celastrol directly binds to the C-terminal domain of Hsp90 inducing its oligomerization, and it interferes with specific biological functions through modulation of Hsp90-associated nuclear transcription factors [106, 121]. In addition, celastrol has been shown to inhibit Hsp90 in thiol-related reactions [116], and to downregulate Hsp90 client proteins via inhibition of enzymes of mitochondrial complexes and accumulation of ROS [80]. Furthermore, celastrol-induced inhibition of Hsp90 contributes to HIF-1α inhibition and cell cycle arrest [92]. As far as the proteasome is concerned, celastrol has been shown to inhibit proteasome function by targeting its chymotrypsin-like activity. This in turn results in the accumulation of ubiquitinated proteins and some of the known proteasomal substrates such as cell cycle-regulating proteins and others (IkBa, Bax and p27, etc.) leading to inhibition of cell proliferation coupled with induction of apoptosis [122, 123]. Accordingly, proteasomal inhibition has also been exploited in cancer therapy [123, 124]. Inhibition of NF-kB activation may contribute to the beneficial effect of proteasomal inhibition therapy. In addition, NF-kB inhibitors combined with standard chemotherapy drugs might be of benefit in the chronic inflammatory stage of tumor progression [125]. However, this aspect of cancer therapy needs further evaluation.

Another beneficial effect of celastrol in cancer relates to its ability to remodel bone by relatively reducing osteoclastic activity, while maintaining or increasing osteoblastic activity. Metastasis of cancer to the bone may cause osteolysis, which involves increased bone resorption. In regard to bone remodeling, the receptor activator of nuclear factor-κB ligand (RANKL) promotes the proliferation and differentiation of osteoclasts, whereas osteoprotegerin (OPG) secreted by the osteoblasts is a soluble decoy receptor for RANKL, and it serves as a natural inhibitor of osteoclast activation. In a study on an osteolytic bone metastasis model, celastrol suppressed trabecular bone loss; and reduced the number and size of osteolytic bone lesions, osteoclast number, and bone resorption [126]. In another study on human osteosarcoma cells, celastrol caused G2/M phase cell cycle arrest, and induced apoptosis and autophagy [81]. These observations in cancer studies are supported by the results of our study in the rat AA model [9]. Celastrol protected against bone and cartilage damage by regulating pro-inflammatory cytokines, inhibiting RANKL, increasing RANKL/OPG ratio, inhibiting the secretion of matrix-degrading enzymes such as MMPs, and reducing the number of osteoclasts without much effect on osteoblasts [9].

12.8 Use of Celastrol-Containing Natural Products for The Treatment of Chronic Inflammatory and Autoimmune Diseases in Humans

Celastrol is present in several plants belonging to the celastraceae family. Some of these plants have been used in traditional Chinese medicine (TCM) for several decades/centuries as medicinal herbs for the treatment of a wide range of chronic inflammatory disorders. For example, the extracts of the root, bark and stem of *Tripterygium wilfordii* (Thunder God Vine), *Celastrus orbiculatus*, *Celastrus aculeatus* and some other members of the Celastraceae family have been used for the treatment of RA, SLE, and other disorders [1–3, 5, 127]. However, a large part of this information is based on folklores as well as documented description of the use of these herbal products in old archived literature. Limited available information is derived from studies on small numbers of patients and/or scientifically controlled randomized clinical studies on the use of *T. wilfordii* in chronic inflammatory and autoimmune diseases such as RA, juvenile RA, ankylosing spondylitis, and SLE [5, 128–132]. Of these, the most reliable clinical studies have been performed using *T. wilfordii* in patients with RA. The efficacy of *T. wilfordii* extract against RA was compared with that of two of the mainstream anti-arthritic drugs, namely sulphasalazine and methotrexate. Interestingly, *T. wilfordii* extract reduced the severity of RA as assessed by well-established criteria, and the efficacy of *T. wilfordii* was comparable to, or better than, that of sulphasalazine/ methotrexate [128, 133–136]. Furthermore, the combination of *T. wilfordii* and methotrexate was better than methotrexate alone. However, the toxicity profile of this natural product needs further assessment before it can be approved for therapeutic purposes.

12.9 Conclusions

Celastrol, a natural triterpene, has anti-inflammatory, antioxidant, and anticancer activities. Besides targeting multiple cell signaling pathways, celastrol modulates several other pathophysiological processes involved in chronic inflammatory diseases, autoimmune diseases, and cancer [143]. Most of this information on celastrol is based on *in vitro* model systems in the laboratory and preclinical studies in animal models of human diseases. These studies have also offered mechanistic insights into the use of celastrol-containing herbal extracts from celastraceae family of plants for the treatment of some of these disorders in the traditional systems of medicine. This knowledge might encourage the clinical testing of herbal preparations as has been done for *T. wilfordii* in RA patients. It is hoped that in the near future, such natural products might be approved for use in mainstream therapy as adjuncts for, or in place of, conventional allopathic drugs for RA and some other chronic diseases. This would be a significant contribution to the therapeutic arsenal against several chronic debilitating human diseases.

Acknowledgments We thank Dr. Hua Yu, Dr. Brian Astry, Dr. Siddaraju Nanjundaiah, Dr. Rajesh Rajaiah, and Dr. Li Tong for their contribution to the original studies based on celastrol as well as for their helpful discussions.

Funding This work was supported by National Institutes of Health (NIH)/National Center for Complementary and Integrative Health (NCCIH) Grant Number AT004321.

References

1. Jin HZ, Hwang BY, Kim HS, Lee JH, Kim YH, Lee JJ (2002) Antiinflammatory constituents of Celastrus orbiculatus inhibit the NF-kappaB activation and NO production. J Nat Prod 65 (1):89–91
2. Luo DQ, Wang H, Tian X, Shao HJ, Liu JK (2005) Antifungal properties of pristimerin and celastrol isolated from Celastrus hypoleucus. Pest Manag Sci 61(1):85–90. doi:10.1002/ps.953
3. Tong L, Moudgil KD (2007) Celastrus aculeatus Merr. suppresses the induction and progression of autoimmune arthritis by modulating immune response to heat-shock protein 65. Arthritis Res Ther 9(4):R70. doi:10.1186/ar2268
4. Sethi G, Ahn KS, Pandey MK, Aggarwal BB (2007) Celastrol, a novel triterpene, potentiates TNF-induced apoptosis and suppresses invasion of tumor cells by inhibiting NF-kappaB-regulated gene products and TAK1-mediated NF-kappaB activation. Blood 109(7):2727–2735. doi:10.1182/blood-2006-10-050807
5. Wong KF, Yuan Y, Luk JM (2012) Tripterygium wilfordii bioactive compounds as anticancer and anti-inflammatory agents. Clin Exp Pharmacol Physiol 39(3):311–320. doi:10.1111/j.1440-1681.2011.05586.x
6. Salminen A, Lehtonen M, Paimela T, Kaarniranta K (2010) Celastrol: molecular targets of thunder god vine. Biochem Biophys Res Commun 394(3):439–442. doi:10.1016/j.bbrc.2010.03.050
7. Kannaiyan R, Shanmugam MK, Sethi G (2011) Molecular targets of celastrol derived from Thunder of God Vine: potential role in the treatment of inflammatory disorders and cancer. Cancer Lett 303(1):9–20. doi:10.1016/j.canlet.2010.10.025
8. Venkatesha SH, Yu H, Rajaiah R, Tong L, Moudgil KD (2011) Celastrus-derived celastrol suppresses autoimmune arthritis by modulating antigen-induced cellular and humoral effector responses. J Biol Chem 286(17):15138–15146. doi:10.1074/jbc.M111.226365
9. Nanjundaiah SM, Venkatesha SH, Yu H, Tong L, Stains JP, Moudgil KD (2012) Celastrus and its bioactive celastrol protect against bone damage in autoimmune arthritis by modulating osteoimmune cross-talk. J Biol Chem 287(26):22216–22226. doi:10.1074/jbc.M112.356816
10. Wang Y, Cao L, Xu LM, Cao FF, Peng B, Zhang X, Shen YF, Uzan G, Zhang DH (2015) Celastrol ameliorates EAE induction by suppressing pathogenic T cell responses in the peripheral and central nervous systems. J Neuroimmune Pharmacol 10(3):506–516. doi:10.1007/s11481-015-9598-9
11. Shaker ME, Ashamallah SA, Houssen ME (2014) Celastrol ameliorates murine colitis via modulating oxidative stress, inflammatory cytokines and intestinal homeostasis. Chem Biol Interact 210:26–33. doi:10.1016/j.cbi.2013.12.007
12. Faust K, Gehrke S, Yang Y, Yang L, Beal MF, Lu B (2009) Neuroprotective effects of compounds with antioxidant and anti-inflammatory properties in a Drosophila model of Parkinson's disease. BMC Neurosci 10:109. doi:10.1186/1471-2202-10-109
13. Liu Z, Ma L, Zhou GB (2011) The main anticancer bullets of the Chinese medicinal herb, thunder god vine. Molecules 16(6):5283–5297. doi:10.3390/molecules16065283
14. Abbas Bukhari SN, Jantan I, Seyed MA (2015) Effects of plants and isolates of celastraceae family on cancer pathways. Anticancer Agents Med Chem 15(6):681–693
15. Yadav VR, Prasad S, Sung B, Kannappan R, Aggarwal BB (2010) Targeting inflammatory pathways by triterpenoids for prevention and treatment of cancer. Toxins (Basel) 2 (10):2428–2466. doi:10.3390/toxins2102428
16. Lee JH, Koo TH, Yoon H, Jung HS, Jin HZ, Lee K, Hong YS, Lee JJ (2006) Inhibition of NF-kappa B activation through targeting I kappa B kinase by celastrol, a quinone methide triterpenoid. Biochem Pharmacol 72(10):1311–1321. doi:10.1016/j.bcp.2006.08.014
17. Trott A, West JD, Klaic L, Westerheide SD, Silverman RB, Morimoto RI, Morano KA (2008) Activation of heat shock and antioxidant responses by the natural product celastrol:

transcriptional signatures of a thiol-targeted molecule. Mol Biol Cell 19(3):1104–1112. doi:10.1091/mbc.E07-10-1004
18. Narayan V, Ravindra KC, Chiaro C, Cary D, Aggarwal BB, Henderson AJ, Prabhu KS (2011) Celastrol inhibits Tat-mediated human immunodeficiency virus (HIV) transcription and replication. J Mol Biol 410(5):972–983
19. Cascao R, Vidal B, Raquel H, Neves-Costa A, Figueiredo N, Gupta V, Fonseca JE, Moita LF (2012) Effective treatment of rat adjuvant-induced arthritis by celastrol. Autoimmun Rev 11 (12):856–862. doi:10.1016/j.autrev.2012.02.022
20. Astry B, Venkatesha SH, Laurence A, Christensen-Quick A, Garzino-Demo A, Frieman MB, O'Shea JJ, Moudgil KD (2015) Celastrol, a Chinese herbal compound, controls autoimmune inflammation by altering the balance of pathogenic and regulatory T cells in the target organ. Clin Immunol 157(2):228–238. doi:10.1016/j.clim.2015.01.011
21. Li G, Liu D, Zhang Y, Qian Y, Zhang H, Guo S, Sunagawa M, Hisamitsu T, Liu Y (2013) Celastrol inhibits lipopolysaccharide-stimulated rheumatoid fibroblast-like synoviocyte invasion through suppression of TLR4/NF-kappaB-mediated matrix metalloproteinase-9 expression. PLoS ONE 8(7):e68905. doi:10.1371/journal.pone.0068905
22. Abdin AA, Hasby EA (2014) Modulatory effect of celastrol on Th1/Th2 cytokines profile, TLR2 and CD3+ T-lymphocyte expression in a relapsing-remitting model of multiple sclerosis in rats. Eur J Pharmacol 742:102–112. doi:10.1016/j.ejphar.2014.09.001
23. Li H, Zhang YY, Huang XY, Sun YN, Jia YF, Li D (2005) Beneficial effect of tripterine on systemic lupus erythematosus induced by active chromatin in BALB/c mice. Eur J Pharmacol 512(2–3):231–237. doi:10.1016/j.ejphar.2005.02.030
24. Xu C, Wu Z (2002) The effect of tripterine in prevention of glomerulosclerosis in lupus nephritis mice. Zhonghua Nei Ke Za Zhi 41(5):317–321
25. Xu X, Zhong J, Wu Z, Fang Y, Xu C (2007) Effects of tripterine on mRNA expression of TGF-beta1 and collagen IV expression in BW F1 mice. Cell Biochem Funct 25(5):501–507. doi:10.1002/cbf.1338
26. Kim DY, Park JW, Jeoung D, Ro JY (2009) Celastrol suppresses allergen-induced airway inflammation in a mouse allergic asthma model. Eur J Pharmacol 612(1–3):98–105. doi:10.1016/j.ejphar.2009.03.078
27. Kim Y, Kim K, Lee H, Han S, Lee YS, Choe J, Kim YM, Hahn JH, Ro JY, Jeoung D (2009) Celastrol binds to ERK and inhibits FcepsilonRI signaling to exert an anti-allergic effect. Eur J Pharmacol 612(1–3):131–142. doi:10.1016/j.ejphar.2009.03.071
28. Liu RL, Liu ZL, Li Q, Qiu ZM, Lu HJ, Yang ZM, Hong GC (2004) The experimental study on the inhibitory effect of tripterine on airway inflammation in asthmatic mice. Zhonghua Jie He He Hu Xi Za Zhi 27(3):165–168
29. Zhang LX, Yu FK, Zheng QY, Fang Z, Pan DJ (1990) Immunosuppressive and antiinflammatory activities of tripterine. Yao Xue Xue Bao 25(8):573–577
30. Allison AC, Cacabelos R, Lombardi VR, Alvarez XA, Vigo C (2001) Celastrol, a potent antioxidant and anti-inflammatory drug, as a possible treatment for Alzheimer's disease. Prog Neuro-psychopharmacol Biol Psychiatry 25(7):1341–1357
31. Choi BS, Kim H, Lee HJ, Sapkota K, Park SE, Kim S, Kim SJ (2014) Celastrol from 'Thunder God Vine' protects SH-SY5Y cells through the preservation of mitochondrial function and inhibition of p38 MAPK in a rotenone model of Parkinson's disease. Neurochem Res 39(1):84–96. doi:10.1007/s11064-013-1193-y
32. Chow AM, Brown IR (2007) Induction of heat shock proteins in differentiated human and rodent neurons by celastrol. Cell Stress Chaperones 12(3):237–244
33. Chow AM, Tang DW, Hanif A, Brown IR (2014) Localization of heat shock proteins in cerebral cortical cultures following induction by celastrol. Cell Stress Chaperones 19(6):845–851. doi:10.1007/s12192-014-0508-5
34. Cleren C, Calingasan NY, Chen J, Beal MF (2005) Celastrol protects against MPTP- and 3-nitropropionic acid-induced neurotoxicity. J Neurochem 94(4):995–1004. doi:10.1111/j.1471-4159.2005.03253.x

35. Kiaei M, Kipiani K, Petri S, Chen J, Calingasan NY, Beal MF (2005) Celastrol blocks neuronal cell death and extends life in transgenic mouse model of amyotrophic lateral sclerosis. Neurodegener Dis 2(5):246–254. doi:10.1159/000090364
36. Paris D, Ganey NJ, Laporte V, Patel NS, Beaulieu-Abdelahad D, Bachmeier C, March A, Ait-Ghezala G, Mullan MJ (2010) Reduction of beta-amyloid pathology by celastrol in a transgenic mouse model of Alzheimer's disease. J Neuroinflammation 7:17. doi:10.1186/1742-2094-7-17
37. Tabuchi H, Konishi M, Saito N, Kato M, Mimura M (2014) Reverse Fox test for detecting visuospatial dysfunction corresponding to parietal hypoperfusion in mild Alzheimer's disease. Am J Alzheimers Dis Other Demen 29(2):177–182. doi:10.1177/1533317513511291
38. Yang C, Swallows CL, Zhang C, Lu J, Xiao H, Brady RO, Zhuang Z (2014) Celastrol increases glucocerebrosidase activity in Gaucher disease by modulating molecular chaperones. Proc Natl Acad Sci USA 111(1):249–254. doi:10.1073/pnas.1321341111
39. Paimela T, Hyttinen JM, Viiri J, Ryhanen T, Karjalainen RO, Salminen A, Kaarniranta K (2011) Celastrol regulates innate immunity response via NF-kappaB and Hsp70 in human retinal pigment epithelial cells. Pharmacol Res 64(5):501–508. doi:10.1016/j.phrs.2011.05.027
40. Hu H, Straub A, Tian Z, Bassler N, Cheng J, Peter K (2009) Celastrol, a triterpene extracted from Tripterygium wilfordii Hook F, inhibits platelet activation. J Cardiovasc Pharmacol 54 (3):240–245. doi:10.1097/FJC.0b013e3181b21472
41. Gu L, Bai W, Li S, Zhang Y, Han Y, Gu Y, Meng G, Xie L, Wang J, Xiao Y, Shan L, Zhou S, Wei L, Ferro A, Ji Y (2013) Celastrol prevents atherosclerosis via inhibiting LOX-1 and oxidative stress. PLoS ONE 8(6):e65477
42. Liu J, Lee J, Salazar Hernandez MA, Mazitschek R, Ozcan U (2015) Treatment of obesity with celastrol. Cell 161(5):999–1011. doi:10.1016/j.cell.2015.05.011
43. Kim JE, Lee MH, Nam DH, Song HK, Kang YS, Lee JE, Kim HW, Cha JJ, Hyun YY, Han SY, Han KH, Han JY, Cha DR (2013) Celastrol, an NF-kappaB inhibitor, improves insulin resistance and attenuates renal injury in db/db mice. PLoS ONE 8(4):e62068
44. Youn GS, Kwon DJ, Ju SM, Rhim H, Bae YS, Choi SY, Park J (2014) Celastrol ameliorates HIV-1 Tat-induced inflammatory responses via NF-kappaB and AP-1 inhibition and heme oxygenase-1 induction in astrocytes. Toxicol Appl Pharmacol 280(1):42–52. doi:10.1016/j.taap.2014.07.010
45. Tallorin L, Durrant JD, Nguyen QG, McCammon JA, Burkart MD (2014) Celastrol inhibits Plasmodium falciparum enoyl-acyl carrier protein reductase. Bioorganic Med Chem 22 (21):6053–6061
46. Simmonds RE, Foxwell BM (2008) Signalling, inflammation and arthritis: NF-kappaB and its relevance to arthritis and inflammation. Rheumatology (Oxford) 47(5):584–590. doi:10.1093/rheumatology/kem298
47. Tak PP, Firestein GS (2001) NF-kappaB: a key role in inflammatory diseases. J Clin Invest 107(1):7–11. doi:10.1172/JCI11830
48. Bondeson J, Foxwell B, Brennan F, Feldmann M (1999) Defining therapeutic targets by using adenovirus: blocking NF-kappaB inhibits both inflammatory and destructive mechanisms in rheumatoid synovium but spares anti-inflammatory mediators. Proc Natl Acad Sci USA 96(10):5668–5673
49. Ju SM, Youn GS, Cho YS, Choi SY, Park J (2015) Celastrol ameliorates cytokine toxicity and pro-inflammatory immune responses by suppressing NF-kappaB activation in RINm5F beta cells. BMB Rep 48(3):172–177
50. Hommes DW, Peppelenbosch MP, van Deventer SJ (2003) Mitogen activated protein (MAP) kinase signal transduction pathways and novel anti-inflammatory targets. Gut 52 (1):144–151
51. Kaminska B (2005) MAPK signalling pathways as molecular targets for anti-inflammatory therapy–from molecular mechanisms to therapeutic benefits. Biochim Biophys Acta 1754(1–2):253–262. doi:10.1016/j.bbapap.2005.08.017

52. Tan Y, Rouse J, Zhang A, Cariati S, Cohen P, Comb MJ (1996) FGF and stress regulate CREB and ATF-1 via a pathway involving p38 MAP kinase and MAPKAP kinase-2. EMBO J 15(17):4629–4642
53. Pierrat B, Correia JS, Mary JL, Tomas-Zuber M, Lesslauer W (1998) RSK-B, a novel ribosomal S6 kinase family member, is a CREB kinase under dominant control of p38alpha mitogen-activated protein kinase (p38alphaMAPK). J Biol Chem 273(45):29661–29671
54. Jung HW, Chung YS, Kim YS, Park YK (2007) Celastrol inhibits production of nitric oxide and proinflammatory cytokines through MAPK signal transduction and NF-kappaB in LPS-stimulated BV-2 microglial cells. Exp Mol Med 39(6):715–721. doi:10.1038/emm.2007.78
55. Kannaiyan R, Manu KA, Chen L, Li F, Rajendran P, Subramaniam A, Lam P, Kumar AP, Sethi G (2011) Celastrol inhibits tumor cell proliferation and promotes apoptosis through the activation of c-Jun N-terminal kinase and suppression of PI3 K/Akt signaling pathways. Apoptosis 16(10):1028–1041
56. Kim DH, Shin EK, Kim YH, Lee BW, Jun JG, Park JH, Kim JK (2009) Suppression of inflammatory responses by celastrol, a quinone methide triterpenoid isolated from Celastrus regelii. Eur J Clin Investig 39(9):819–827. doi:10.1111/j.1365-2362.2009.02186.x
57. Zhu H, Liu XW, Cai TY, Cao J, Tu CX, Lu W, He QJ, Yang B (2010) Celastrol acts as a potent antimetastatic agent targeting beta1 integrin and inhibiting cell-extracellular matrix adhesion, in part via the p38 mitogen-activated protein kinase pathway. J Pharmacol Exp Ther 334(2):489–499. doi:10.1124/jpet.110.165654
58. Shuai K, Liu B (2003) Regulation of JAK-STAT signalling in the immune system. Nat Rev Immunol 3(11):900–911. doi:10.1038/nri1226
59. Darnell JE Jr (1997) STATs and gene regulation. Science 277(5332):1630–1635
60. Kannaiyan R, Hay HS, Rajendran P, Li F, Shanmugam MK, Vali S, Abbasi T, Kapoor S, Sharma A, Kumar AP, Chng WJ, Sethi G (2011) Celastrol inhibits proliferation and induces chemosensitization through down-regulation of NF-kappaB and STAT3 regulated gene products in multiple myeloma cells. Br J Pharmacol 164(5):1506–1521. doi:10.1111/j.1476-5381.2011.01449.x
61. Rajendran P, Li F, Shanmugam MK, Kannaiyan R, Goh JN, Wong KF, Wang W, Khin E, Tergaonkar V, Kumar AP, Luk JM, Sethi G (2012) Celastrol suppresses growth and induces apoptosis of human hepatocellular carcinoma through the modulation of STAT3/JAK2 signaling cascade in vitro and in vivo. Cancer Prev Res (Phila) 5(4):631–643. doi:10.1158/1940-6207.CAPR-11-0420
62. Chen S, Gu C, Xu C, Zhang J, Xu Y, Ren Q, Guo M, Huang S, Chen L (2014) Celastrol prevents cadmium-induced neuronal cell death via targeting JNK and PTEN-Akt/mTOR network. J Neurochem 128(2):256–266. doi:10.1111/jnc.12474
63. Ma J, Han LZ, Liang H, Mi C, Shi H, Lee JJ, Jin X (2014) Celastrol inhibits the HIF-1alpha pathway by inhibition of mTOR/p70S6 K/eIF4E and ERK1/2 phosphorylation in human hepatoma cells. Oncol Rep 32(1):235–242. doi:10.3892/or.2014.3211
64. Mabuchi S, Kuroda H, Takahashi R, Sasano T (2015) The PI3 K/AKT/mTOR pathway as a therapeutic target in ovarian cancer. Gynecol Oncol 137(1):173–179. doi:10.1016/j.ygyno.2015.02.003
65. Sha M, Ye J, Zhang LX, Luan ZY, Chen YB, Huang JX (2014) Celastrol induces apoptosis of gastric cancer cells by miR-21 inhibiting PI3 K/Akt-NF-kappaB signaling pathway. Pharmacology 93(1–2):39–46. doi:10.1159/000357683
66. Shrivastava S, Jeengar MK, Reddy VS, Reddy GB, Naidu VG (2015) Anticancer effect of celastrol on human triple negative breast cancer: possible involvement of oxidative stress, mitochondrial dysfunction, apoptosis and PI3 K/Akt pathways. Exp Mol Pathol 98(3):313–327. doi:10.1016/j.yexmp.2015.03.031
67. Zhao J, Sun Y, Shi P, Dong JN, Zuo LG, Wang HG, Gong JF, Li Y, Gu LL, Li N, Li JS, Zhu WM (2015) Celastrol ameliorates experimental colitis in IL-10 deficient mice via the up-regulation of autophagy. Int Immunopharmacol 26(1):221–228. doi:10.1016/j.intimp.2015.03.033

68. Polivka J Jr, Janku F (2014) Molecular targets for cancer therapy in the PI3 K/AKT/mTOR pathway. Pharmacol Ther 142(2):164–175. doi:10.1016/j.pharmthera.2013.12.004
69. Hudson CC, Liu M, Chiang GG, Otterness DM, Loomis DC, Kaper F, Giaccia AJ, Abraham RT (2002) Regulation of hypoxia-inducible factor 1alpha expression and function by the mammalian target of rapamycin. Mol Cell Biol 22(20):7004–7014
70. Han X, Sun S, Zhao M, Cheng X, Chen G, Lin S, Guan Y, Yu X (2014) Celastrol stimulates hypoxia-inducible factor-1 activity in tumor cells by initiating the ROS/Akt/p70S6 K signaling pathway and enhancing hypoxia-inducible factor-1alpha protein synthesis. PLoS ONE 9(11):e112470. doi:10.1371/journal.pone.0112470
71. Bellot G, Garcia-Medina R, Gounon P, Chiche J, Roux D, Pouyssegur J, Mazure NM (2009) Hypoxia-induced autophagy is mediated through hypoxia-inducible factor induction of BNIP3 and BNIP3L via their BH3 domains. Mol Cell Biol 29(10):2570–2581. doi:10.1128/MCB.00166-09
72. Onnis B, Rapisarda A, Melillo G (2009) Development of HIF-1 inhibitors for cancer therapy. J Cell Mol Med 13(9A):2780–2786. doi:10.1111/j.1582-4934.2009.00876.x
73. Holmstrom KM, Finkel T (2014) Cellular mechanisms and physiological consequences of redox-dependent signalling. Nat Rev Mol Cell Biol 15(6):411–421. doi:10.1038/nrm3801
74. Ye ZW, Zhang J, Townsend DM, Tew KD (2015) Oxidative stress, redox regulation and diseases of cellular differentiation. Biochim Biophys Acta 1850(8):1607–1621. doi:10.1016/j.bbagen.2014.11.010
75. Halliwell B (1987) Free radicals and metal ions in health and disease. Proc Nutr Soc 46 (1):13–26
76. Sassa H, Takaishi Y, Terada H (1990) The triterpene celastrol as a very potent inhibitor of lipid peroxidation in mitochondria. Biochem Biophys Res Commun 172(2):890–897
77. Sassa H, Kogure K, Takaishi Y, Terada H (1994) Structural basis of potent antiperoxidation activity of the triterpene celastrol in mitochondria: effect of negative membrane surface charge on lipid peroxidation. Free Radic Biol Med 17(3):201–207
78. Divya T, Dineshbabu V, Soumyakrisnan S, Sureshkumar S, Sudandiran G (2016) Celastrol enhances Nrf2 mediated antioxidant enzymes and exhibits anti-fibrotic effect through regulation of collagen production against bleomycin-induced pulmonary fibrosis. Chem Biol Interact 246:52–62
79. Wang C, Shi C, Yang X, Yang M, Sun H, Wang C (2014) Celastrol suppresses obesity process via increasing antioxidant capacity and improving lipid metabolism. Eur J Pharmacol 744:52–58. doi:10.1016/j.ejphar.2014.09.043
80. Chen G, Zhang X, Zhao M, Wang Y, Cheng X, Wang D, Xu Y, Du Z, Yu X (2011) Celastrol targets mitochondrial respiratory chain complex I to induce reactive oxygen species-dependent cytotoxicity in tumor cells. BMC Cancer 11:170. doi:10.1186/1471-2407-11-170
81. Li HY, Zhang J, Sun LL, Li BH, Gao HL, Xie T, Zhang N, Ye ZM (2015) Celastrol induces apoptosis and autophagy via the ROS/JNK signaling pathway in human osteosarcoma cells: an in vitro and in vivo study. Cell Death Dis 6:e1604. doi:10.1038/cddis.2014.543
82. Gupta SC, Kim JH, Prasad S, Aggarwal BB (2010) Regulation of survival, proliferation, invasion, angiogenesis, and metastasis of tumor cells through modulation of inflammatory pathways by nutraceuticals. Cancer Metastas Rev 29(3):405–434. doi:10.1007/s10555-010-9235-2
83. Pang X, Yi Z, Zhang J, Lu B, Sung B, Qu W, Aggarwal BB, Liu M (2010) Celastrol suppresses angiogenesis-mediated tumor growth through inhibition of AKT/mammalian target of rapamycin pathway. Cancer Res 70(5):1951–1959
84. Khan KA, Bicknell R (2015) Anti-angiogenic alternatives to VEGF blockade. Clin Exp Metastas 33(2):197–210
85. Szekanecz Z, Besenyei T, Paragh G, Koch AE (2009) Angiogenesis in rheumatoid arthritis. Autoimmunity 42(7):563–573
86. Koch AE (2000) The role of angiogenesis in rheumatoid arthritis: recent developments. Ann Rheum Dis 59(Suppl 1):i65–i71

87. Al-Husein B, Abdalla M, Trepte M, Deremer DL, Somanath PR (2012) Antiangiogenic therapy for cancer: an update. Pharmacotherapy 32(12):1095–1111. doi:10.1002/phar.1147
88. Gan K, Xu L, Feng X, Zhang Q, Wang F, Zhang M, Tan W (2015) Celastrol attenuates bone erosion in collagen-induced arthritis mice and inhibits osteoclast differentiation and function in RANKL-induced RAW264.7. Int Immunopharmacol 24(2):239–246. doi:10.1016/j.intimp.2014.12.012
89. Dai Y, Desano J, Tang W, Meng X, Meng Y, Burstein E, Lawrence TS, Xu L (2010) Natural proteasome inhibitor celastrol suppresses androgen-independent prostate cancer progression by modulating apoptotic proteins and NF-kappaB. PLoS ONE 5(12):e14153. doi:10.1371/journal.pone.0014153
90. Ji N, Li J, Wei Z, Kong F, Jin H, Chen X, Li Y, Deng Y (2015) Effect of celastrol on growth inhibition of prostate cancer cells through the regulation of hERG channel in vitro. Biomed Res Int 2015:308475. doi:10.1155/2015/308475
91. Zhou YX, Huang YL (2009) Antiangiogenic effect of celastrol on the growth of human glioma: an in vitro and in vivo study. Chin Med J (Engl) 122(14):1666–1673
92. Huang L, Zhang Z, Zhang S, Ren J, Zhang R, Zeng H, Li Q, Wu G (2011) Inhibitory action of Celastrol on hypoxia-mediated angiogenesis and metastasis via the HIF-1alpha pathway. Int J Mol Med 27(3):407–415
93. Huang S, Tang Y, Cai X, Peng X, Liu X, Zhang L, Xiang Y, Wang D, Wang X, Pan T (2012) Celastrol inhibits vasculogenesis by suppressing the VEGF-induced functional activity of bone marrow-derived endothelial progenitor cells. Biochem Biophys Res Commun 423(3):467–472
94. Ni H, Zhao W, Kong X, Li H, Ouyang J (2013) Celastrol inhibits lipopolysaccharide-induced angiogenesis by suppressing TLR4-triggered nuclear factor-kappa B activation. Acta Haematol 131(2):102–111
95. Huang Y, Zhou Y, Fan Y, Zhou D (2008) Celastrol inhibits the growth of human glioma xenografts in nude mice through suppressing VEGFR expression. Cancer Lett 264(1):101–106. doi:10.1016/j.canlet.2008.01.043
96. Zhang DH, Marconi A, Xu LM, Yang CX, Sun GW, Feng XL, Ling CQ, Qin WZ, Uzan G, d'Alessio P (2006) Tripterine inhibits the expression of adhesion molecules in activated endothelial cells. J Leukoc Biol 80(2):309–319. doi:10.1189/jlb.1005611
97. Wu F, Han M, Wilson JX (2009) Tripterine prevents endothelial barrier dysfunction by inhibiting endogenous peroxynitrite formation. Br J Pharmacol 157(6):1014–1023
98. Lindquist S, Craig EA (1988) The heat-shock proteins. Annu Rev Genet 22:631–677
99. Rajaiah R, Moudgil KD (2009) Heat-shock proteins can promote as well as regulate autoimmunity. Autoimmun Rev 8(5):388–393
100. Adachi H, Katsuno M, Waza M, Minamiyama M, Tanaka F, Sobue G (2009) Heat shock proteins in neurodegenerative diseases: pathogenic roles and therapeutic implications. Int J Hyperth 25(8):647–654
101. Arawaka S, Machiya Y, Kato T (2010) Heat shock proteins as suppressors of accumulation of toxic prefibrillar intermediates and misfolded proteins in neurodegenerative diseases. Curr Pharm Biotechnol 11(2):158–166
102. Muchowski PJ, Wacker JL (2005) Modulation of neurodegeneration by molecular chaperones. Nat Rev Neurosci 6(1):11–22
103. Westerheide SD, Bosman JD, Mbadugha BN, Kawahara TL, Matsumoto G, Kim S, Gu W, Devlin JP, Silverman RB, Morimoto RI (2004) Celastrols as inducers of the heat shock response and cytoprotection. J Biol Chem 279(53):56053–56060
104. Francis SP, Kramarenko II, Brandon CS, Lee FS, Baker TG, Cunningham LL (2011) Celastrol inhibits aminoglycoside-induced ototoxicity via heat shock protein 32. Cell Death Dis 2:e195
105. Hughes D, Guttenplan JB, Marcus CB, Subbaramaiah K, Dannenberg AJ (2008) Heat shock protein 90 inhibitors suppress aryl hydrocarbon receptor-mediated activation of CYP1A1 and CYP1B1 transcription and DNA adduct formation. Cancer Prev Res (Phila) 1(6):485–493

106. Zhang D, Xu L, Cao F, Wei T, Yang C, Uzan G, Peng B (2010) Celastrol regulates multiple nuclear transcription factors belonging to HSP90's clients in a dose- and cell type-dependent way. Cell Stress Chaperones 15(6):939–946
107. Petronelli A, Pannitteri G, Testa U (2009) Triterpenoids as new promising anticancer drugs. Anticancer Drugs 20(10):880–892. doi:10.1097/CAD.0b013e328330fd90
108. Yadav VR, Sung B, Prasad S, Kannappan R, Cho SG, Liu M, Chaturvedi MM, Aggarwal BB (2010) Celastrol suppresses invasion of colon and pancreatic cancer cells through the downregulation of expression of CXCR4 chemokine receptor. J Mol Med 88(12):1243–1253
109. Zheng L, Fu Y, Zhuang L, Gai R, Ma J, Lou J, Zhu H, He Q, Yang B (2014) Simultaneous NF-kappaB inhibition and E-cadherin upregulation mediate mutually synergistic anticancer activity of celastrol and SAHA in vitro and in vivo. Int J Cancer 135(7):1721–1732. doi:10.1002/ijc.28810
110. Dai Y, DeSano JT, Meng Y, Ji Q, Ljungman M, Lawrence TS, Xu L (2009) Celastrol potentiates radiotherapy by impairment of DNA damage processing in human prostate cancer. Int J Radiat Oncol Biol Phys 74(4):1217–1225. doi:10.1016/j.ijrobp.2009.03.057
111. Li-Weber M (2013) Targeting apoptosis pathways in cancer by Chinese medicine. Cancer Lett 332(2):304–312. doi:10.1016/j.canlet.2010.07.015
112. Chiang KC, Tsui KH, Chung LC, Yeh CN, Chen WT, Chang PL, Juang HH (2014) Celastrol blocks interleukin-6 gene expression via downregulation of NF-kappaB in prostate carcinoma cells. PLoS ONE 9(3):e93151. doi:10.1371/journal.pone.0093151
113. Lu L, Shi W, Deshmukh RR, Long J, Cheng X, Ji W, Zeng G, Chen X, Zhang Y, Dou QP (2014) Tumor necrosis factor-alpha sensitizes breast cancer cells to natural products with proteasome-inhibitory activity leading to apoptosis. PLoS ONE 9(11):e113783. doi:10.1371/journal.pone.0113783
114. Mi C, Shi H, Ma J, Han LZ, Lee JJ, Jin X (2014) Celastrol induces the apoptosis of breast cancer cells and inhibits their invasion via downregulation of MMP-9. Oncol Rep 32(6):2527–2532. doi:10.3892/or.2014.3535
115. Yang HS, Kim JY, Lee JH, Lee BW, Park KH, Shim KH, Lee MK, Seo KI (2011) Celastrol isolated from Tripterygium regelii induces apoptosis through both caspase-dependent and -independent pathways in human breast cancer cells. Food Chem Toxicol 49(2):527–532. doi:10.1016/j.fct.2010.11.044
116. Peng B, Xu L, Cao F, Wei T, Yang C, Uzan G, Zhang D (2010) HSP90 inhibitor, celastrol, arrests human monocytic leukemia cell U937 at G0/G1 in thiol-containing agents reversible way. Mol Cancer 9:79. doi:10.1186/1476-4598-9-79
117. Sung B, Park B, Yadav VR, Aggarwal BB (2010) Celastrol, a triterpene, enhances TRAIL-induced apoptosis through the down-regulation of cell survival proteins and up-regulation of death receptors. J Biol Chem 285(15):11498–11507
118. Li GQ, Liu D, Zhang Y, Qian YY, Zhu YD, Guo SY, Sunagawa M, Hisamitsu T, Liu YQ (2013) Anti-invasive effects of celastrol in hypoxia-induced fibroblast-like synoviocyte through suppressing of HIF-1alpha/CXCR4 signaling pathway. Int Immunopharmacol 17(4):1028–1036. doi:10.1016/j.intimp.2013.10.006
119. Xu J, Wu CL, Huang J (2015) Effect of celastrol in inhibiting metastasis of lung cancer cells by influencing Akt signaling pathway and expressing integrins. Zhongguo Zhong Yao Za Zhi 40(6):1129–1133
120. Xu J, Wu CL (2015) Anti-metastasis of celastrol on esophageal cancer cells and its mechanism. Sheng Li Xue Bao 67(3):341–347
121. Zanphorlin LM, Alves FR, Ramos CH (2014) The effect of celastrol, a triterpene with antitumorigenic activity, on conformational and functional aspects of the human 90 kDa heat shock protein Hsp90alpha, a chaperone implicated in the stabilization of the tumor phenotype. Biochim Biophys Acta 10:3145–3152. doi:10.1016/j.bbagen.2014.06.008
122. Wang WB, Feng LX, Yue QX, Wu WY, Guan SH, Jiang BH, Yang M, Liu X, Guo DA (2012) Paraptosis accompanied by autophagy and apoptosis was induced by celastrol, a natural compound with influence on proteasome, ER stress and Hsp90. J Cell Physiol 227(5):2196–2206

123. Yang H, Landis-Piwowar KR, Chen D, Milacic V, Dou QP (2008) Natural compounds with proteasome inhibitory activity for cancer prevention and treatment. Curr Protein Pept Sci 9 (3):227–239
124. Dou QP, Zonder JA (2014) Overview of proteasome inhibitor-based anticancer therapies: perspective on bortezomib and second generation proteasome inhibitors versus future generation inhibitors of ubiquitin-proteasome system. Curr Cancer Drug Targets 14(6):517–536
125. Hoesel B, Schmid JA (2013) The complexity of NF-kappaB signaling in inflammation and cancer. Mol Cancer 12:86
126. Idris AI, Libouban H, Nyangoga H, Landao-Bassonga E, Chappard D, Ralston SH (2009) Pharmacologic inhibitors of IkappaB kinase suppress growth and migration of mammary carcinosarcoma cells in vitro and prevent osteolytic bone metastasis in vivo. Mol Cancer Ther 8(8):2339–2347. doi:10.1158/1535-7163.MCT-09-0133
127. Wang KW, Mao JS, Tai YP, Pan YJ (2006) Novel skeleton terpenes from Celastrus hypoleucus with anti-tumor activities. Bioorg Med Chem Lett 16(8):2274–2277. doi:10.1016/j.bmcl.2006.01.021
128. Tao X, Cush JJ, Garret M, Lipsky PE (2001) A phase I study of ethyl acetate extract of the chinese antirheumatic herb Tripterygium wilfordii hook F in rheumatoid arthritis. J Rheumatol 28(10):2160–2167
129. Zhang W, Shi Q, Zhao LD, Li Y, Tang FL, Zhang FC, Zhang X (2010) The safety and effectiveness of a chloroform/methanol extract of Tripterygium wilfordii Hook F (T2) plus methotrexate in treating rheumatoid arthritis. J Clin Rheumatol 16(8):375–378. doi:10.1097/RHU.0b013e3181fe8ad1
130. Ji W, Li J, Lin Y, Song YN, Zhang M, Ke Y, Ren Y, Deng X, Zhang J, Huang F, Yu D (2010) Report of 12 cases of ankylosing spondylitis patients treated with Tripterygium wilfordii. Clin Rheumatol 29(9):1067–1072. doi:10.1007/s10067-010-1497-0
131. Gao ZG, Zang AC, Bai RX (1986) Radix Tripterygium Wilfordii Hook F in rheumatoid arthritis, ankylosing spondylitis and juvenile rheumatoid arthritis. Chin Med J (Engl) 99 (4):317–320
132. Patavino T, Brady DM (2001) Natural medicine and nutritional therapy as an alternative treatment in systemic lupus erythematosus. Altern Med Rev 6(5):460–471
133. Tao X, Younger J, Fan FZ, Wang B, Lipsky PE (2002) Benefit of an extract of Tripterygium Wilfordii Hook F in patients with rheumatoid arthritis: a double-blind, placebo-controlled study. Arthritis Rheum 46(7):1735–1743
134. Goldbach-Mansky R, Wilson M, Fleischmann R, Olsen N, Silverfield J, Kempf P, Kivitz A, Sherrer Y, Pucino F, Csako G, Costello R, Pham TH, Snyder C, van der Heijde D, Tao X, Wesley R, Lipsky PE (2009) Comparison of Tripterygium wilfordii Hook F versus sulfasalazine in the treatment of rheumatoid arthritis: a randomized trial. Ann Intern Med 151 (4):229–240
135. Lv QW, Zhang W, Shi Q, Zheng WJ, Li X, Chen H, Wu QJ, Jiang WL, Li HB, Gong L, Wei W, Liu H, Liu AJ, Jin HT, Wang JX, Liu XM, Li ZB, Liu B, Shen M, Wang Q, Wu XN, Liang D, Yin YF, Fei YY, Su JM, Zhao LD, Jiang Y, Li J, Tang FL, Zhang FC, Lipsky PE, Zhang X (2014) Comparison of Tripterygium wilfordii Hook F with methotrexate in the treatment of active rheumatoid arthritis (TRIFRA): a randomised, controlled clinical trial. Ann Rheum Dis. doi:10.1136/annrheumdis-2013-204807
136. Moudgil KD, Berman BM (2014) Traditional Chinese medicine: potential for clinical treatment of rheumatoid arthritis. Expert Rev Clin Immunol 10(7):819–822
137. Li H, Zhang YY, Tan HW, Jia YF, Li D (2008) Therapeutic effect of tripterine on adjuvant arthritis in rats. J Ethnopharmacol 118(3):479–484. doi:10.1016/j.jep.2008.05.028
138. Li H, Jia YF, Pan Y, Pan DJ, Li D, Zhang LX (1997) Effect of tripterine on collagen-induced arthritis in rats. Zhongguo Yao Li Xue Bao 18(3):270–273
139. Xu Z, Wu G, Wei X, Chen X, Wang Y, Chen L (2013) Celastrol induced DNA damage, cell cycle arrest, and apoptosis in human rheumatoid fibroblast-like synovial cells. Am J Chin Med 41(3):615–628. doi:10.1142/S0192415X13500432

140. Li GQ, Zhang Y, Liu D, Qian YY, Zhang H, Guo SY, Sunagawa M, Hisamitsu T, Liu YQ (2012) Celastrol inhibits interleukin-17A-stimulated rheumatoid fibroblast-like synoviocyte migration and invasion through suppression of NF-kappaB-mediated matrix metalloproteinase-9 expression. Int Immunopharmacol 14(4):422–431. doi:10.1016/j.intimp.2012.08.016
141. Zhou LL, Lin ZX, Fung KP, Cheng CH, Che CT, Zhao M, Wu SH, Zuo Z (2011) Celastrol-induced apoptosis in human HaCaT keratinocytes involves the inhibition of NF-kappaB activity. Eur J Pharmacol 670(2–3):399–408. doi:10.1016/j.ejphar.2011.09.014
142. Zhu F, Li C, Jin XP, Weng SX, Fan LL, Zheng Z, Li WL, Wang F, Wang WF, Hu XF, Lv CL, Liu P (2014) Celastrol may have an anti-atherosclerosis effect in a rabbit experimental carotid atherosclerosis model. Int J Clin Exp Med 7(7):1684–1691
143. Venkatesha SH, Dudics S, Astry B, Moudgil KD (2016) Control of autoimmune inflammation by celastrol, a natural triterpenoid. Pathog Dis 74(6). pii:ftw059. doi: 10.1093/femspd/ftw059

Chapter 13
Boswellic Acids and Their Role in Chronic Inflammatory Diseases

H.P.T. Ammon

Abstract Boswellic acids, which are pentacyclic triterpenes belong to the active pharmacological compounds of the oleogum resin of different Boswellia species. In the resin, more than 12 different boswellic acids have been identified but only KBA and AKBA received significant pharmacological interest. *Biological Activity:* In an extract of the resin of Boswellia species multiple factors are responsible for the final outcome of a therapeutic effect, be it synergistic or antagonistic. Moreover, the anti-inflammatory actions of BAs are caused by different mechanisms of action. They include inhibition of leukotriene synthesis and to a less extend prostaglandin synthesis. Furthermore inhibition of the complement system at the level of conversion of C3 into $C3_a$ and $C3_b$. A major target of BAs is the immune system. Here, BEs as well as BAs including KBA and AKBA, have been shown to decrease production of proinflammatory cytokines including IL-1, IL-2, IL-6, IFN-γ and TNF-α which finally are directed to destroy tissues such as cartilage, insulin producing cells, bronchial, intestinal and other tissues. NFκB is considered to be the target of AKBA. The complex actions of BEs and BAs in inflamed areas may be completed by some effects that are localized behind the inflammatory process as such tissue destruction. In this case, in vitro- and animal studies have shown that BAs and BEs suppress proteolytic activity of cathepsin G, human leucocyte elastase, formation of oxygen radicals and lysosomal enzymes. *Pharmacokinetics:* Whereas KBA is absorbed reaching blood levels being close to in vitro $IC_{50,}$ AKBA which is more active in in vitro studies than KBA, but undergoes much less absorption than KBA. However, absorption of both is increased more than twice when taken together with a high-fat meal.*Clinical Studies* There are a variety of chronic inflammatory diseases which respond to treatment with extracts from the resin of Boswellia species. Though, the number of cases is small in related clinical studies, their results are convincing and supported by the preclinical data. These

H.P.T. Ammon (✉)
Department of Pharmacology and Toxicology, Institute of Pharmaceutical Sciences, University of Tuebingen, Auf der Morgenstelle 8, 72076 Tuebingen, Germany
e-mail: info@hptammon.de; sekretariat.ammon@uni-tuebingen.de

H.P.T. Ammon
Im Kleeacker 30, 72072 Tuebingen, Germany

S.C. Gupta et al. (eds.), *Anti-inflammatory Nutraceuticals and Chronic Diseases*, Advances in Experimental Medicine and Biology 928,
DOI 10.1007/978-3-319-41334-1_13

studies include rheumatoid arthritis, osteoarthritis, chronic colitis, ulcerative colitis, collagenous colitis, Crohn's disease and bronchial asthma. It can not be expected that there is cure from these diseases but at least improvement of symptoms in about 60–70 % of the cases. *Side Effects* The number and severity of side effects is extremely low. The most reported complaints are gastrointestinal symptoms. Allergic reactions are rare. And most authors report, that treatment with BEs is well tolerated and the registered side effects in BE- and placebo groups are similar.

Keywords Boswellic acids · Boswellic extracts · Leukotrienes · Prostaglandins · Proteolytic enzymes · Cytokines · Pharmacokinetics · Rheumatoid arthritis · Inflammatory bowel diseases · Bronchial asthma · Diabetes · Side effects

Abbreviations

AA	Arachidonic Acid
ABA	Acetyl-boswellic acid
Ac-OH-LA	3α-Acetoxy-28-hydroxylup-20 (29)
AKBA	Acetyl-11-keto-β-Boswellic acid
α-BA	α-Boswellic acid
β-BA	β-Boswellic acid
BA	Boswellic acid
BE	Boswellic extract
BS	*Boswellia serrata*
BSA	Bovine serum albumin
CD4	CD4 lymphocytes
CD8	CD8 lymphocytes
CIA	Collagen-induced arthritis
COX	Cyclooxygenase
CRP	C-reactive protein
CDAI	Crohn's Disease Activity Index
ConA	Concavalin A
ESR	Erythrocyte Sedimentation Rate
FCV	Forced vital capacity
FEV_1	Forced expiratory volume
GSH	Reduced glutathione
Hb	Hemoglobin
HETE	Hydroxyeicosatetraenoic acid
12-HHT	12-Hydroxyheptadecatrienoic acid
HLE	Human Leucozyte Elastase
IA_2-A	Tyrosinephosphatase antibody
IFN-γ	Interferon-γ
IgG	Immunoglobulin G
IgM	Immunoglobulin M
IL	Interleukin
IMG	Immune globulin

KBA	11-Keto-β-Boswellic acid
LA	Lupenoic acid
LADA	Late onset autoimmune diabetes of the adult
5-LO	5-Lipoxigenase
12-LO	12-Lipoxigenase
LPO	Lipid peroxidase
LPS	Lipopolysaccharide
LTB_4	Leukotriene B
LTC_4	Leukotriene C_4
LTD_4	Leukotriene D_4
LTE_4	Leukotriene E_4
MIC	Minimal inhibitory concentration
f-MLP	n-formylmethionyl-leucyl-phenylalanine
MLD-STZ	Multiple low-dose streptozotocin
NADPH	Nicotinamide adenine dinucleotide phosphate hydrate
$NF_{\kappa}B$	Nuclear transcription factor $_{\kappa}B$
NK cells	Natural killer cells
NO	Nitrogen monoxide
NSAID	Nonsteroidal anti-inflammatory drugs
OA	Osteoarthritis
PEFR	Peak expiratory flow rate
PGE_2	Prostaglandin E_2
PBMC	Peripheral blood mononuclear cells
PEFR	Peak expiratory flow rate
PGE_1	Prostaglandin E_1
PHA	Phytohemagglutinin
PMA	Phorbol 12-myristate 13-acetate
PMN	Polymorph mononuclear neutrophil leucocyte
RA	Rheumatoid arthritis
SG	Salai guggal
SOD	Superoxid dismutase
STZ	Streptozotocin
TA	Tirucallic acid
Th_1	Th_1 lymphocytes
Th_2	Th_2 lymphocytes
TNF-α	Tumor necrosis factor alpha
t1/2	Half-life

13.1 Introductory Remarks

Boswellic acids (BAs) belong to the active pharmacological principles of the oleo gum resin from the trees of different Boswellia species. These trees are plants typically found in the deserts, where the aborigines since thousands of years, scratch the bark and collect fluid, during dry periods. Burning the resin, the fumes are used for disinfection, improvement of the scent of the air, as well as for ceremonial and medical purposes. The resins are known as salai guggal (India), frankincense (pure incense), incense and olibanum.

This chapter summarizes the present knowledge about medical history, pharmacological active ingredients and therapeutical uses of the resin with special impact on the anti-inflammatory mechanisms of boswellic acids.

13.2 Medical History

The oldest written document, which mentions frankincense as a drug is the Papyrus Ebers. In 1873, Moritz Fritz Ebers, professor of Egyptology, received a more than 20 m long papyrus from an Arab businessman [40] describing the medical use of frankinsence in Egypt. In India, the therapeutic applications of the oleogum resin of *Boswellia serrata*, called Salai guggal (SG), are already described in early Ayurvedic textbooks (Charaka Samhita, 1st–2nd century AD and in Astangahrdaya Samhita, seventh century AD).

Remedies containing preparations from frankincense (here *Boswellia carterii*) were also prescribed by the famous physicians Hippocrates, Celsus, Galenus, Dioskurides and others for the treatment of tumours, carcinomas, edemas, inflammatory diseases including diarrhoea, and diseases of the respiratory tract [40].

Olibanum, the resin of various Boswellia species (Table 13.1), was also known as a remedy in Europe from ancient times till the beginning of the twentieth century. Then it disappeared from the list of doctoral prescriptions since *scientific* evidence for therapeutical efficacy was missing. Only when Singh and Atal [69] and Ammon et al. [3] showed that an extract from resin of *Boswellia serrata* inhibited inflammation in an animal model resp. formations of leukotrienes in an in vitro model, the scientific community became interested and the first human pilot studies were initiated. By now, preparations of the resin are widely used to treat a variety of chronic inflammatory disorders.

Table 13.1 Some species of *Boswellia* trees producing incense and the respective areas of growth [40]

Species	Growing	Product
B. carteri Birdw.	Somalia	Olibanum
B. sacra Flueck	Nubia Saudi Arabia	Olibanum
B. frereana Birdw.	Somalia	Olibanum
B. bhau-dajiana Birdw.	North Somalia	Olibanum
B. papyrifera Hochst.	Ethiopia	Olibanum
B. neglecta S. Moore	Somalia	Olibanum
B. odOrata Hutch.	Tropical Africa	Olibanum
B. dalzielli Hutch.	Tropical Africa	Olibanum
B. serrata Roxb.	India	Salai Gugal

13.3 Composition of the Resin

The resin of Boswelli species consists of mucus, volatile oil and resin acids (Table 13.2). However, the quantitative composition of these constituents varies from species to species.

The *resin* acids contain pentacyclic and tetracyclic triterpenes. Among the pentacyclic triterpenes, only some boswellic acids are responsible for many of the pharmacological effects; but also tirucallic acids (TAs), from the tetracyclic triterpenic acids, have been shown to be biologically active .

Pentacyclic Triterpenes: Büchele et al. [9] identified 12 different pentacyclic triterpenes in the samples of Boswellia extracts (BEs) (Table 13.3). From these 12, the chemical structures of the two most active boswellic acids (BAs) are shown in Fig. 13.2.

The authors reported significant quantitative differences of pentacyclic triterpenes between various species: A striking difference was observed in the content of the boswellic acids, i.e. KBA and AKBA (Table 13.3). Recently Beisner et al. [5] identified a new pentacyclic triterpene from *Boswellia serrata*, it was just one, 3α-acetyl-20(29)-lupene-24-oic acid and Verhoff et al. [80] observed biological activity of a novel C(28)-hydroxylated lupeolic acid. Though BAs received most attention through the group of pentacyclic triterpenes, some other, including lupeol, exhibit pharmacological activity as well, which are also considered boswellic acids [49].

Tetracyclic Triterpenes: Among the tetracyclic triterpenes, three TAs have been identified: 3-oxotirucallic acid, 3-hydroxytirucallic acid and 3-acetoxytirucallic acid. Other resin compounds with pharmacological activities are: betulinic acid, epi-lupeol, lupenoic acid, 1-ursene-2-diketone-incensole acetate, isoincensole and isoincensole acetate and as well as terpenes that can be found in the volatile oil.

13.4 Preclinical Studies

13.4.1 Anti-inflammatory Actions

The first scientific publication with the title "Analgesic effect of the oleogum resin of *Boswellia serrata* Roxb". by Karr and Mennon appeared 1969 [31]. Singh and

Table 13.2 Composition of oleogum resin of two different *Boswellia* species [9]

	Boswellia carteri Birdw. (%)	*Boswellia serrata* Roxb. (%)
Volatile oil	5–9	7.5–9 to 15
Pure resin	ca. 66	55–57
Mucus	~12–20	~23

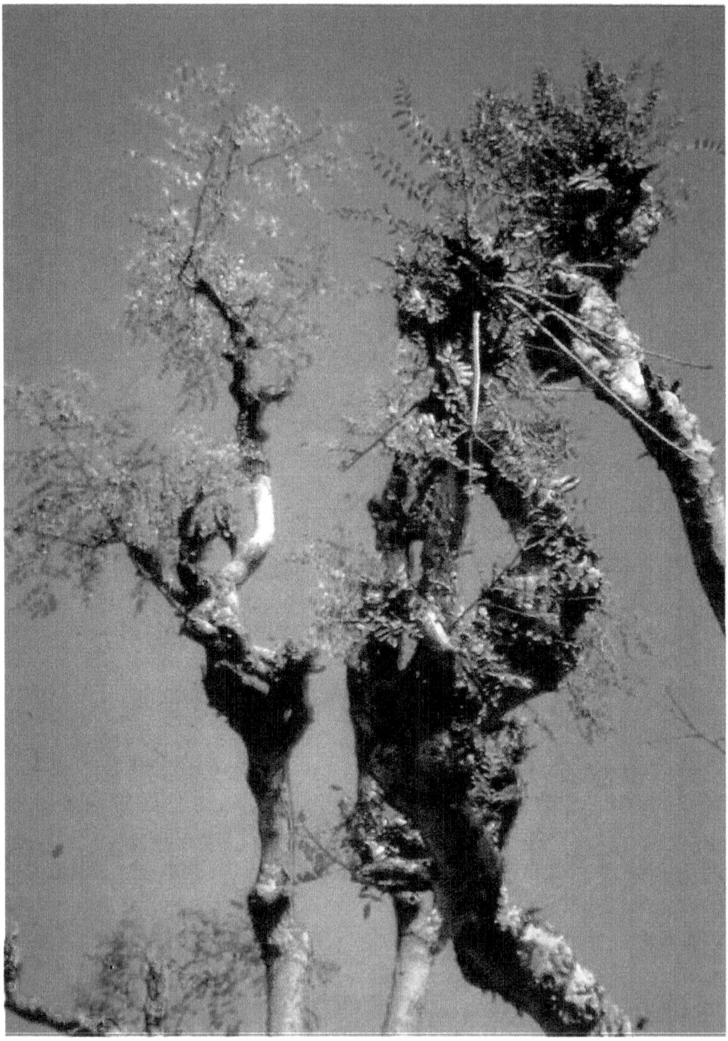

Fig. 13.1 *Boswellia serrata* Roxb. Desert of Radschastan, India, taken by the author

Table 13.3 Contents of different pentacyclic triterpenic acids in a frankincense extract determined by Büchele and Simmet [8]

α-Boswellic acid	13.78 %	β-Boswellic acid	19.20 %
Acetyl-α-boswellic acid	3.37 %	Acetyl-β-boswellic acid	10.04 %
Lupeoloc acid	2.61 %	11-Keto-β-boswellic acid	6.66 %
Acetyl-lupeoloc acid	1.10 %	Aetyl-11-keto-β-boswellic acid	3.81 %
11-Dehydro-α-boswellic acid	0.18 %	9,11-Dehydro-β-boswellic acid	0.83 %
Acetyl-9-11-dehydro-α-boswellic acid	0.06 %	Acetyl-9-11-dehydro-β-boswellic acid	0.52 %

Fig. 13.2 Structures of 11-keto-β-boswellic acid and acetyl-11-keto-β-boswellic acid

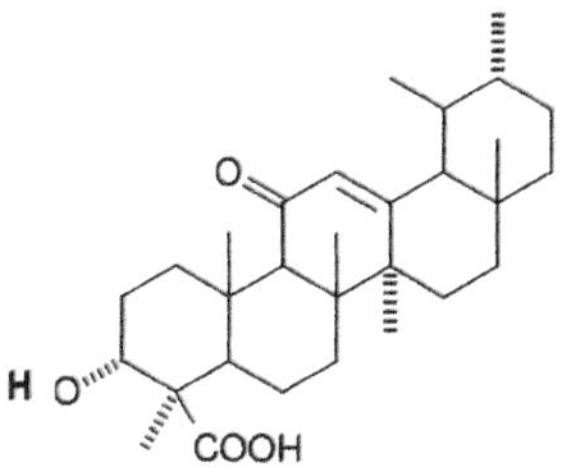

11-Keto-β-boswellic acid

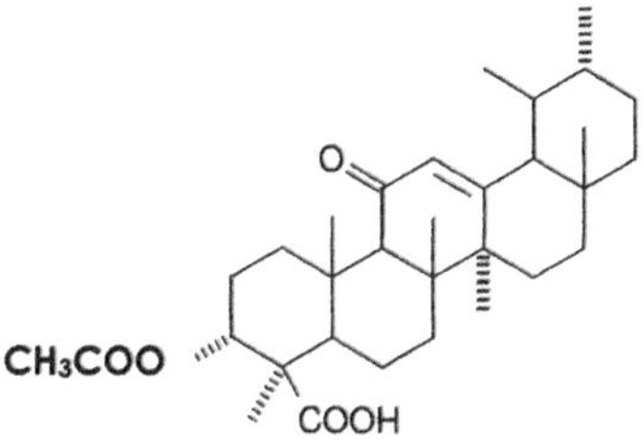

Acetyl-11-Keto-β-boswellic acid

Atal [69] published a paper entitled: "Pharmacology of an extract of salai guggal ex-*Boswellia serrata*, a new non steroidal anti-inflammatory agent". In this study, Singh and Atal [69] observed that the oral administration of an *alcoholic* extract of the oleogum resin of *Boswellia serrata* caused inhibition of the carrageenan- and dextran-induced edema in the paws of rats and mice, suggesting anti-phlogistic action of a BE. Since such an effect could also be observed in adrenalectomized rats, the authors concluded that the anti-inflammatory effect of the BE was not due to the liberation of glucocorticoids. Significant anti-arthritic activity of an acetone extract from *Boswellia carterii* in lewis rats was reported by Fan et al. [19]. Moreover, anti-inflammatory, anti-noceptive and antioxidant activities have been described using extracts from other Boswellia species; in this case, *Boswellia longata* [44]. Boswellia extracts were also effective in the treatment of skin inflammations [71].

A reduction of the carrageenan-induced edema in the paws of mice after oral or intraperitoneal application of 1 mg/kg β-BA was recently reported by Siemoneit et al. [68].

Introducing a new model, i.e. papaya latex also causing rat paw inflammation, Gupta et al. [21] tested a variety of anti-rheumatic agents and BAs and compared their effects with the actions of carrageenan in relation to rat paw inflammation. It turned out that in the carrageenan model the inhibitory effects of indomethacin, piroxicam, ibuprofen and acetylsalicylic acid were more pronounced than those of BAs, whereas BAs were much more effective in the papaya latex model. The action of prednisolone was almost similar in both models. This suggests that the

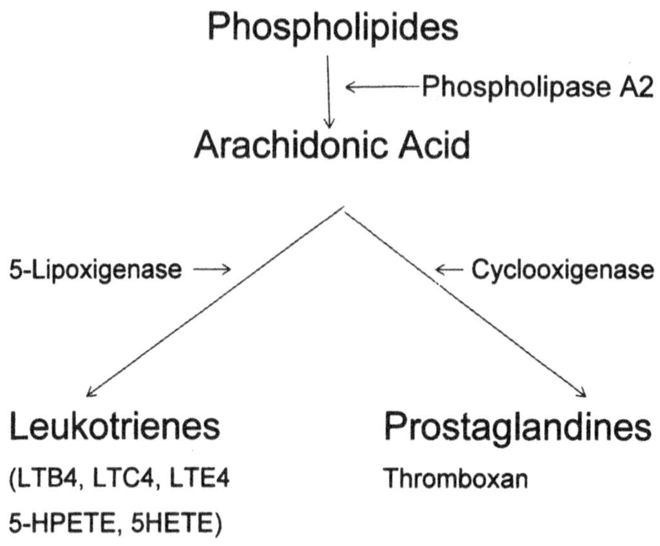

Fig. 13.3 Arachidonic acid cascade

anti-inflammatory mechanism of BAs is different from the so-called "aspirin-like" drugs and prednisolone (Fig. 13.3).

13.4.1.1 The Arachidonic Acid Cascade: Cyclooxygenase and Cyclooxygenase Products

Activation of the arachidonic acid cascade by the membrane bound enzyme phospholipase A_2 (PLA_2) is the initial step to start production of mediators of inflammation. In this cascade (Fig. 13.3) cyclooxygenases and 5-lipoxigenase produce prostaglandines and leukotrienes, which eventually lead to the typical inflammatory symptoms. The mechanism of anti-inflammatory action of BEs and BAs on members of the arachidonic acid cascade has been studied by several scientists.

Boswellic Extracts: Based on the observations of Singh and Atal [69], Ammon et al. [3] studied whether or not an alcoholic extract of the BS resin, could affect prostaglandin synthesis in vitro. For this study, human platelets which contain cyclooxygenase-1 (COX-1) were used. After in vitro stimulation with the Ca ionophore A 23187, the extract inhibited 6-keto-PKF-1α synthesis, a product of COX-1, up to 50 % at a concentration of *100* µg/ml (Fig. 13.4).

In another in vitro model extracts from *Boswellia frereana* suppressed cytokine IL-1A-induced prostaglandin E_2 synthesis and COX-2. In this case, epi-lupeol was identified as a principal constituent [6].

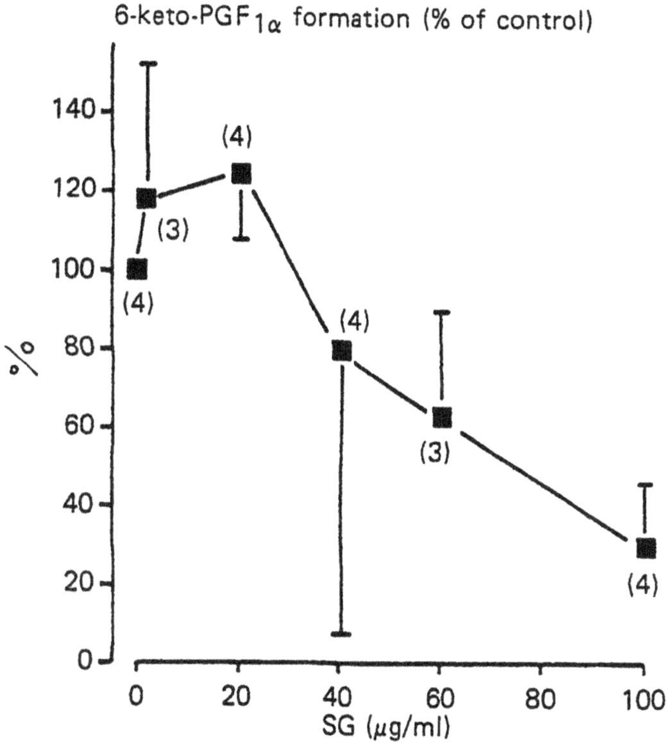

Fig. 13.4 Inhibition of 6-keto-$PGF_{1\alpha}$ formation in human platelets by an alcoholic extract of salai guggal (SG). 100 % = 277 pg 6-keto-$PGF_{1\alpha}/10^7$ cells. Number of experiments are given in parentheses [3]

Boswellic Acids: As discussed above, the resins contain a variety of compounds which could be responsible for their anti-inflammatory actions. These boswellic acids are listed in Fig. 13.2.

Among these in a variety of studies most evidence has been gained from acetyl-11-keto-β-boswellic acid (AKBA) and 11-keto-β-boswellic acid (KBA). Thus, it was near at hand to study their effect on the production of the arachidonic acid cascade intermediates. In the assay that used human platelets, AKBA produced 50 % inhibition of 12-hydroxyheptadecatrienoic acid (12-HHT) at a concentration of 10 μM. Acetyl-boswellic acid (ABA) on the contrary showed no such effect. Inhibition of COX products by AKBA was also observed by Siemoneit et al. [66, 68], using the human platelets model. BAs, preferably AKBA, inhibited COX-1 product formation with an $IC_{50} \sim 6$ μM. The authors also reported that COX-1 is more sensitive to inhibition by AKBA than COX-2. In this sense, Siemoneit et al. [68] described the inhibition of prostaglandin E 2 synthase-1 as the molecular basis for the anti-inflammatory actions of boswellic acids. This means that BAs, in particular AKBA, directly interfere with COX-1 and may mediate their anti-inflammatory actions not only by suppression of lipoxygenases, as discussed later, but also by inhibiting cyclooxygenases, preferentially COX-1 [66]. On the other hand, β-boswellic acid (β-BA) and AKBA stimulated arachidonic acid release and 12-lipoxigenase activity in human platelets, where AKBA was less potent than β-BA [47].

Cao et al. [12] observed, that, in addition to AKBA, β-BA, acetyl-α-BA, acetyl-β-BA and betulinic acid are also inhibitors of COX-1. The IC_{50} was estimated to be 10 μM.

Other compounds: Verhoff et al. [80] reported that a novel, yet unknown C(28)-hydroxylated lupenoic acid (LA), that is 3α-acetoxy-28-hydroxylup-20(29)-en-4β-oic acid (Ac-OH-LA) inhibits the biosynthesis of COX-, 5-LO- and 12-Lipoxigenase (12-LO)-derived eicosanoids from endogenous arachidonic acid (AA) in activated platelets, neutrophils and monocytes from human blood with consistent IC_{50} values of 2.3–6.9 μM. Thus, the data discussed suggests that cyclooxygenases are targets of a variety of compounds in the resins of Boswellia species.

13.4.1.2 The Arachidonic Acid Cascade: 5-Lipoxigenase and 5-Lipoxigenase Products

Until 1991, there was no drug known which could predominantly inhibit the synthesis of leukotrienes despite the need for such compounds to treat diseases where leukotrienes have a major impact. It was the publication of Ammon et al. [3] that showed that BEs not only affected formation of COX products, but to a much larger extend also inhibited LTB_4 synthesis. This publication and a later paper [50], indicating that certain BAs are responsible for this effect, received large attention by the scientific community.

Boswellic Extracts: After the stimulation of leukotriene synthesis with the calcium ionophore A 231876 in polymorphmononuclear neutrophils (PMN)—which contained 5-LO but no COX the same extract that was used for the studies on prostaglandin synthesis [3] in a concentration-dependent manner inhibited synthesis of leukotriene B4 (LTB4) and 5-hydroxyeicosatetraenoic acid (5-HETE) (a metabolite of the 5-LO cascade) formation at concentrations between 10 and 80 μg/ml (Fig. 13.5). In this case, 50 % inhibition occurred at a concentration of 30 μg/ml, indicating that the inhibitory action of the extract was significantly more pronounced than its effect on COX-1 [3].

Boswellic Acids: Concerning the actions of BAs, Safayhi et al. reported in 1992 BAs to be specific, non-redox inhibitors of 5-LO. In this study, isomers of (α- and β-) of BAs and their acetyl derivatives were isolated from the oleogum resin of BS. It was observed that BAs partly decreased the formation of LTB4 in calcium-ionophore-stimulated PMN in a concentration-dependent manner. AKBA was most effective with an IC_{50} value of 1.5 μM.

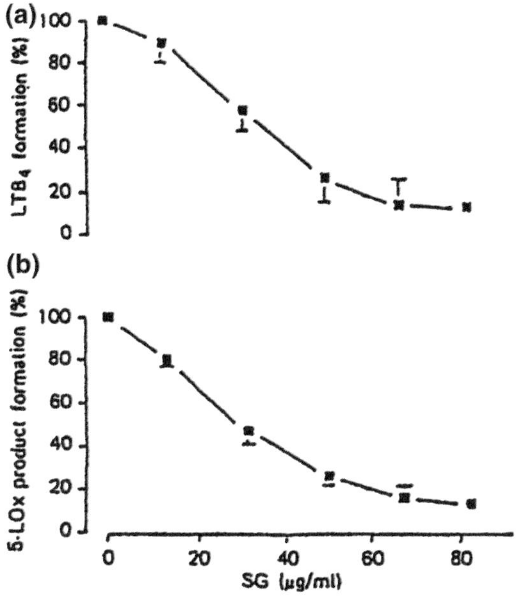

Fig. 13.5 Concentration-dependent inhibition of LTB_4-formation by salai guggal (SG) ethanolic extract in stimulated rat peritoneal PMNL (**a**), and the decrease in the inhibition of the sum of 5-LOx products (**b**) [3]. *x*-axis represents a and b

Structure–Action Relationships: This observation posed the question whether or not certain chemical motif in the *molecular structure* of BAs are required for the inhibition of leukotriene production. In this sense, Sailer et al. [53] studied the effect of a variety of derivatives of BAs on leukotriene synthesis in Ca ionophore-stimulated PMN. From the IC_{50} values, it was obvious that not all tested compounds inhibited synthesis of leukotrienes and that some of them exhibited only a partial effect. Taking into account the different chemical structures of the tested BAs, the data revealed that a hydrophilic function at C-4 position in combination with an 11-keto group appears to be essential for the inhibition of leukotriene synthesis by BAs (Table 13.4).

5-L*O as target*: *In intact PMN, signal transduction cascade of events that starts with* the external stimulation of leukocytes, where the participation of calcium ions

Table 13.4 Inhibitory effect of different boswellic acids on leukotriene formation/5-lipoxygenase activity

	R^1	R^2	IC_{50} (µM)
AKBA	AcO	O	2.7 (1.5)
3-Acetyl-11-OH-BA	AcO	OH/H	Not tested
3-Acetyl-11-MeO-BA	AcO	MeO/H	Partial inhibition
KBA	OH	O	3.0
β-BA	OH	2H	Partial inhibition
3-Acetyl-β-BA	AcO	2H	Partial inhibition
Acetyl-9,11-dehydro-BA	AcO	–	0.75
9.11-Dehydro-BA	OH	–	Partial inhibition

is necessary, results in the production of leukotrienes by intracellular 5-LO. In order to study whether or not BAs might directly interfere with 5-LO, in a cell-free system from PMN, where this cascade is interrupted, the effect of various derivatives of BAs on 5-LO activity was tested after addition of exogenous arachidonic acid. It was found that the effects of different BAs were qualitatively similar to those in intact PMN. However, the IC_{50} was higher than in intact cells which may be due to the different environment of 5-LO in a cell-free system. [54].

Mechanism of 5-LO Inhibition: Further studies addressing the mechanism of direct 5-LO inhibition used the supernatant of PMN. In this study, pentacyclic triterpenes lacking the 11-keto function and/or carboxyl function on ring A (e.g. amyrin and ursolic acid) did not or only partially inhibit 5-LO (Table 13.4). These compounds even caused a concentration-dependent reversal of 5-LO inhibition by AKBA, whereas the inhibitory actions of 5-LO inhibitors from different chemical classes were not modified. Thus, it was concluded that AKBA acts directly on the 5-LO enzyme at a site selective for pentacyclic triterpenes which is different from the arachidonate substrate binding site [51]. Using photoaffinity labelling, it was studied whether or not 4-azido-5-125 iodo-salicyl-β-alanyl-11-keto-β-boswellic acid, a photoaffinity analogue inhibiting 5-LO activity as efficiently as a lead compound, could be displaced from its binding site by AKBA. This was in fact the case. On the other hand, AA had no such effect. This data also suggests that AKBA in the presence of calcium binds to a site distinct from the substrate (AA) binding site of 5-LO [54].

13.4.2 Proteolytic Enzymes: Human Leucocyte Elastase (HLE)

Another factor in the inflammatory process is the release of proteolytic enzymes from PMN which are involved in the destruction of cartilage. Tausch et al. [78] observed that BAs suppressed the proteolytic activity of cathepsin G in a competitive reversible manner with an estimated IC_{50} value of 0.6 μM. The same effect was observed in humans after oral administration of a BE.

HLE is a serine protease produced and released by PMN. Using pure HLE, Safayhi et al. [52] screened several pentacyclic triterpenes for inhibitory actions on HLE. In this study AKBA decreased the activity of HLE with an IC_{50} value of roughly 15 μM. Among the pentacyclic triterpenes, tested in concentrations up to 20 μM, substantial inhibition by β-BA, amyrin and ursolic acid was observed.

13.4.3 Oxygen Radicals

Oxygen radicals which are formed in PMN through the action of leukotrienes are also involved *in* cartilage destruction *in* rheumatoid arthritis. Heil et al. [27] studied the effects of AKBA and of BEs on SOD-quenchable O_2-radical formation in intact PMNs and in a cell-free system. AKBA (IC_{50} ~ 10 μM) and extracts (IC_{50} ~ 13 μg/ml) consistently inhibited phorbol-12-myristate-13-acetate (PMA)-stimulated NADPH oxidase activity in rat peritoneal PMNs and reduced *n*-formyl-methionyl-leucyl-phenylazanin (f-MLP) and PMA-induced oxidative burst in stimulator-sensitive human blood PMN preparations.

13.4.4 The Complement System

The complement system is part of the non-specific humoral defence. It is an important link between immuno- and inflammatory reactions.

Boswellic Acids: As early as 1987, inhibition of the guinea pig complement system by α-BA and β-BA in concentration range between 5 and 100 μM has been reported by Wagner et al. Anticomplementary activities of a mixture of BAs were also described by Kapil and Moza [30]. They observed that BAs inhibited the in vitro immunohemolysis of antibody-coated sheep erythrocytes by pooled guinea pig serum. The reduced immunohemolysis was found to be due to an inhibition of C3 convertase of the classical complement pathway.

The threshold concentration for inhibition was 100 μg per 0.1 ml diluted buffer added to the assay. Thus, at least in vitro, BAs can suppress the conversion of C3 into C3a and C3b and therefore its proinflammatory actions of this system.

Summarizing the anti-inflammatory actions of BEs and BAs:

The resin of Boswellia species contains a variety of compounds with anti-inflammatory properties. Among these are BAs but also some other constituents have been described. Members of the arachidonic acid cascade are targets of BEs and BAs as well as proteolytic enzymes, oxygen radicals, and the complement system.

Most information is available from AKBA and KBA. Among the cyclooxygenases, COX-1 seems to be most sensible to inhibition by BAs. Of special interest is the inhibitory action of BAs on 5-LO. 5-LO produces leukotrienes, which are responsible for plasma exudation, edema production, chemotaxis and activation of white blood cells which release proteolytic enzymes and oxygen radicals. 5-LO is more sensitive to BAs than cyclooxygenases. In addition, BAs directly inhibit proteolytic enzymes and oxygen radical formation in PMN, and last but not least also the complement system, which is an important link between immune and inflammatory reaction. Thus, especially BEs—a multicomponent product as well as BAs—in contrast to the widely used NSAID drugs—exhibit their anti-inflammatory action simultaneously affecting a variety of parameters that are involved in inflammatory processes.

13.4.5 The Immunosystem

White blood cells play an important role in the defence system of the body. Granulocytes, monocytes, macrophages and lymphocytes cover the non-specific as well as the humoral and cellular defence. However, under certain conditions, they are also closely related to inflammatory autoimmune disorders. Humoral and cellular defence have also been the subject of studies with BEs and BAs.

13.4.5.1 Humoral Defence

Humoral defence is one of the important measures of the body against infectious diseases. It is related to the activation of B lymphocytes. After contact with antigens, B cells differentiate to plasma cells, which then produce antibodies belonging to the family of immunoglobulins.

Antibody Titres

Boswellic Acids: Humoral antibody synthesis in mice treated with sheep erythrocytes was studied by Sharma et al. [62] by determining the hemagglutinating antibody titers in the serum. Here, *primary* antibody production (after a first antigen injection) and *secondary* antibody production (after a second injection) were tested.

It was found that a single dose of a mixture of BAs (*50–200* mg/kg)—as isolated by Singh et al. [70] on the day of sensitization produced a dose related reduction (10.4–32.8 %) in *primary* hemagglutinating antibody titers on day 4. Significant reduction in antibody production was obtained with 100 and 200 mg/kg doses. On the other hand the *secondary* antibody titers were significantly enhanced at *lower* doses, the effect being more prominent at 50 mg/kg. Azathioprine was administered as a reference compound (200 mg/kg p.o.) following the same schedule and resulted in only 10.4 % inhibition of *primary* antibody synthesis and had no effect on the *secondary* antibody production.

Usually, the second injection of antigens causes earlier antibody production with higher affinity and is mainly due to immunoglobulin G (IgG).

Using the technique of complement fixing, a method for analysing antigen and antibody titers, oral administration of a mixture containing BAs for 5 days around the time of immunization resulted in a significant decrease in *primary* and *secondary* complement fixing antibody titers at 100 mg/kg [62]. On the contrary, when a BA mixture (25–100 mg/kg) was given orally for 5 days *around* immunization a marked increase (15.38–26.92 %) in antibody production on day +7 was observed. The effect was more pronounced at a dose of 25 mg/kg than at 50 or 100 mg/kg. The *secondary* antibody titers were only marginally increased. Azathioprine treatment (100 mg/kg) had no significant effects on *primary* as well as on *secondary* antibody titers.

In mice, in which treatment with BAs was initiated 7 days prior to immunization, BAs (25–100 mg/kg) elicited a dose related increase (37.93–63.79 %) in the *primary* humoral response without significantly affecting the expression of the *secondary* response. Levamisole (2.5 mg/kg, p.o.), an immunopotentiating agent, displayed only a 25 % increase in *primary* and a 6.66 % increase in *secondary* antibody titers.

Immunoglobulins

Boswellic Extract As far as low doses of BEs are concerned, the data received with antibody titers finds their equivalent when immunoglobulins were determined in the blood of sensitized mice. Previously, it was shown by Khajuria et al. [33] that oral administration of a biopolymeric fraction (BOS 2000) from *B. serrata* (1–10 mg/kg) elicited a dose related increase in the delayed hypersensitivity reaction (early 24 h and delayed 48 h) in mice. It also stimulated the immunoglobulin M (IgM) and IgG titers expressed in the form of plaques (PFC) and the complement fixing antibody titre.

Gupta et al. [26] studied a possible immunological adjuvant effect of BOS 2000 on specific antibody and the cellular response to ovalbumin in mice. Mice were immunized s. c. with ovalbumin 100 μg and received BOS 2000, 80 μg on days 1 and 15. Two weeks later, BOS 2000, 80 μg corresponding to about 3.5 mg/kg bw significantly increased IgG, IgG_1 and IgG_{2a} antibody levels in the serum compared to the ovalbumin group.

At a dose of 80 μg BOS 2000, there was also a significant increase of lymphocytes CD4/CD8 and CD80/CD 86 analyzed in spleen cells and with cytokines (IL-2 and IFN-γ) profiles in the spleen cell culture supernatant. From their data, the authors conclude, that BOS 2000 seems to be a promising balanced Th1- and Th2 lymphocytes directing immunological adjuvant which can enhance the immunogenicity of vaccines.

Thus, regarding the humoral defence in the in vivo experiments, it appears that BAs have a dual effect on antibody titers: at lower doses, there is an increased formation, whereas at higher doses, BAs may even have inhibitory effects. Whether or not this data is of relevance for humans remains to be established. And the question remains: what is a high and what is a low-dose regarding humans.

13.4.5.2 Cellular Defence: Effect on Leucocytes

Cellular defence against infectious microorganisms is mediated by the actions of white blood cells. This includes proliferation, transformation, and activation of lymphocytes, as well as induction of infiltration and phagocytosis by macrophages and neutrophil granulocytes.

Their functions are organized through the crosstalking among related cells via cytokines produced and released from various leucocytes. Numerous authors have dealt with the question whether or not extracts from the Boswellia resin, its volatile oil, and/or boswellic acids would affect the activity of white blood cells and whether or not such effects could be attributed to an interaction with the system of cross talking between white blood cells by cytokines.

Boswellic Extracts and Essential Oils: In their studies on lymphocyte transformation, Badria et al. [4] used an assay with lymphocytes isolated from venous human blood. In this study, a methylene chloride extract from the oleogum resin of Boswellia carterii in the presence of phytohemaglutinin (PHA) or concanavalin A (CON A) at 1 mg/ml *stimulated lymphocyte transformation* by 90 % (EC_{50} = 0.55 mg/ml). Several compounds from the essential oil were also biologically active. The different BAs and TAs tested, including acetyl-β-BA, acetyl-α-BA, 3-oxo-TA, AKBA, β-BA, 3-hydroxy-TA and KBA, showed a similar activity with EC_{50} values from 0.001 to 0.005 μM.

Mikhaeil et al. [41], who studied the chemical composition of frankincense oil, also reported that the oil exhibited strong immunostimulant activity (90 %) of *lymphocyte transformation*, when assessed in a lymphocyte proliferation assay. From these studies, it may be concluded, that a variety of components of an extract from *Boswellia* resins are effective in stimulating *lymphocyte transformation* and thus can contribute to cellular defence.

Boswellic Acids: Sharma et al. [62] reported that, if spleen cells from non-immunized mice were used, a mixture of various BAs in the range of 1.95–125.0 μg/ml showed no spontaneous mitogenic activity and the cell viability was comparable to controls. However, when, the test, was performed in the presence of mitogen stimulating lipopolysaccharides (LPS, PHA, CON A and alloantigen), a concentration-dependent *inhibition* of *lymphocyte proliferation* by BAs was observed.

The effect of a mixture of BAs on *phagocytosis* was also studied by Sharma et al. [62]. Preincubation of peritoneal macrophages with different concentrations of BAs (1.95–125 μg/ml) resulted in an enhanced *phagocytotic* function of adherent macrophages with a maximal effect occurring at 62.25 μg/ml.

The studies discussed so far have been performed *in vitro*. They showed stimulating and inhibitory effects of BA_s and BE_s, respectively, employing different concentrations. At present, the data is difficult to interpret and transferred to the human situation.

In an in vivo experiment studying the anti-arthritic activity of boswellic acids employing bovine serum albumin (BSA) induced arthritis, Sharma et al. [61] observed that oral administration of a mixture of BAs (25, 50 and 100 mg/kg/day) reduced *the population of leucocytes* when BSA was injected into the knee, and changed the electrophoretic pattern of the synovial fluid proteins. The local injection of BAs (5, 10 and 20 mg) into the knee 15 min prior to BSA challenge also reduced *infiltration of leucocytes* into the knee joint and inhibited the migration properties of PMN in vitro. As discussed above some BAs are inhibitors of 5-Lo. So, the mechanism of action of BAs on leucocyte infiltration could be the inhibition of LTB_4—synthesis, i.e. reducing their chemotactic action.

13.4.5.3 The Cross Talk in Cellular Defence

NFκB plays a key role for the function of cytokines in their crosstalk between immune competent cells. NFκB, which is usually present in the cytosol, is produced by neutrophil granulocytes. This compound regulates the release of cytokines from various white blood cells being responsible for proliferation, activation and function of these cells.

Nuclear Transcription Factor κB (NFκB)

As far as possible effects of BEs are concerned, AKBA, as one of their pharmacological active compounds, has turned out to be a natural inhibitor of NFκB [16]. Thus, AKBA applied in vivo in mice (100 μmol/kg) for 1 week inhibited the NFκB activation. Suppression of NFκB and NFκB-regulated gene expression by AKBA is also reported by Takada et al. [77].

When AKBA was given systemically or locally in a mouse model with psoriasis, the signalling action of NFκB and subsequent NFκB-dependent cytokine production by macrophages was significantly suppressed. This was associated with profound improvement of the psoriasis disease activity score [82]. As far as the mechanism of action on NFκB is concerned, Syrovets et al. [76] reported that acetyl-boswellic acids inhibit constitutively activated NFκB signalling by intercepting the IκB-kinase activity in an in vitro model of PC-3 prostate cancer cells. However, inhibition of NFκB is not only due to an action of BAs in extracts from Boswellia species. Previously, Moussaieff et al. [45] reported that incensole acetate, a compound isolated from *Boswellia* resins, also inhibits NFκB activation. This action was combined with an anti-inflammatory effect in the inflamed mouse paw model.

Cytokines

Crosstalk between leucocytes is organized by a group of compounds released from monocytes, macrophages and T cells, called cytokines. These include interleukines (IL), interferone-γ (IFN-γ) and tumornekrosisfactor-α (TNF-α), which regulate different functions of white blood cells. Since on the one hand cytokines are under regulation of NFκB but on the other hand NFκB is a target of AKBA a compound of the resin of Boswellia species it was just logical to study whether or not BEs and BAs would affect production/serum levels of various cytokines.

Interleukines/IFN-γ

Interleukins belong to the group of cytokines. There are pro- and anti-inflammatory interleukins produced by macrophages and T cells following the recognition of a pathogen.

Chervier et al. [13] studied the effect of an extract from *Boswellic carterii* on the production of T_H-1 and T_H-2 cytokines by murine splenocytes. The use of an extract with sesame oil as solvent resulted in a dose-dependent inhibition of IL-2 and IFN-γ and a dose-dependent potentiation of IL-4 and IL-10. Gayathri et al. [19] observed that a crude methanolic extract from BS and 12-ursine-2-diketone, a pure compounds of BS, inhibited TNF-α, IL-1 B and IL-6 in cultured Peripheral Blood Mononuclear Cells (PBMC). Observations on T_{H1}/T_{H2} cytokines also revealed marked down regulation of IFN-γ and IL-12, whereas IL-4 and IL-10—which are anti-inflammatory interleukins—was upregulated upon treatment with a crude extract and the pure compound 1-ursene-2-diketone. This indicates that both are capable of carrying out anti-inflammatory activities at sites where chronic inflammation is present by switching off the proinflammatory cytokines.

Employing an acetone extract from *Boswellia carterii* Birdw. Fan et al. [18], in an adjuvant arthritis model in lewis rats *900 mg/kg* for 10 consecutive days, observed significant decrease of arthritic scores. This was associated with suppression of local tissue IL-1B and TNF-α. On the other hand, in a study of Khajuria et al. [33], the authors demonstrated that oral administration of *1–10 mg/kg* of a polymeric fraction from BS (BOS 2000) increased levels of IL-4, IFN-γ and TNF-α in the serum.

Tumor Necrosis Factor-alpha (TNF-α)

TNF-α ***is*** also an important cytokine which activates local restriction of infections.

TNF-α released from macrophages, natural killer (NK) cells, and T cells activates vascular endothel, increases permeability of vessels for proteins and cells and entry of IgG and complement into tissues. TNF-α induces fever. Massive liberation of TNF-α from macrophages can even cause shock.

Inhibition of TNF-α and its signalling has been recognized as a highly successful strategy for the treatment of chronic inflammatory diseases such as rheumatoid arthritis. Previously it has been shown by Syrovets et al. [76] that acetyl-α-BA and AKBA inhibited the generation of TNF-α in concentrations between 1 and 10 μM in LPS-stimulated human monocytes. AKBA was found to be the most active compound. The effect was mediated by an indirect inhibition of NFκB and subsequent downregulation of TNF-α expression in human monocytes. In these cells, Borsches and Grim (personal communication 2000) observed a concentration-dependent decrease of TNF-α and IL-1B production in a concentration range of 5–20 μM.

The data from this chapter, covering cytokines, suggest that low doses of Boswellia preparations increase production of proinflammatory cytokines, whereas high doses are even suppressive. In other words, low doses of BEs may stimulate cellular defence f.i. in case of infections and high doses may be useful in defeating the proinflammatory actions of cytokines in autoimmune inflammatory disorders.

Cytokines in Autoimmune Diabetes

Type 1 diabetes is an autoimmune disease, where a chronic inflammatory process finally causes death of insulin producing β-cells of pancreatic islets and insulin deficiency. Autoimmune diseases are—as discussed—associated with overexpression of proinflammatory cytokines. Among these, in patients with type 1 diabetes NFκB, TNF-α, IFN-γ, IL-1B and IL-2 have been found to be increased in splenocytes and PBMC [15].

Application of multiple low doses of streptozotocin (MLD-STZ) is a method to induce autoimmune diabetes in animals similar to type 1 diabetes in humans.

Shehata et al. [64] studied whether or not a BE could prevent hyperglycemia, inflammation of pancreatic islets and increase of proinflammatory cytokines in the blood in MLD-STZ treated mice. In this study, treatment with streptozotocin (STZ) (40 mg/kg i.p. for 5 days) after 10 days produced a permanent increase of blood glucose, infiltration of lymphocytes into pancreatic islets, apoptosis of periinsular cells and after 35 days shrinking of islet tissue. This was associated with

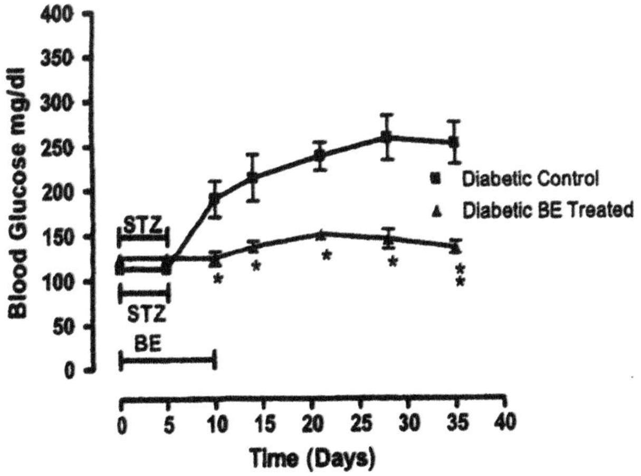

Fig. 13.6 Effect of boswellic extract (150 mg/kg i.p. for 10 days) on blood glucose levels of MLD-STZ-treated mice (mean ± SE; $n = 4$) [64]

an increase of proinflammatory cytokines (IL-1A, IL-1B, IL-2, IL-6, IFN-γ, TNF-α) in the blood. In STZ treated mice, simultaneous i.p. injection of 150 mg/kg of BE over a period of 10 days prevented animals from increase of blood glucose levels (Fig. 13.6). Histochemical studies showed, that BE avoided lymphocyte infiltration into pancreatic islets, apoptosis of peri-insular cells and shrinking of islet size.

As far as the cytokines tested are concerned, there was a significant inhibition of the increase of IL-1A, IL-1B, IL-2, IL-6, IFN-γ and TNF-α in the blood. It was concluded that extracts from the gum resin of *Boswellia serrata* prevent islet destruction and consequent hyperglycemia in an animal model of type 1 diabetes,

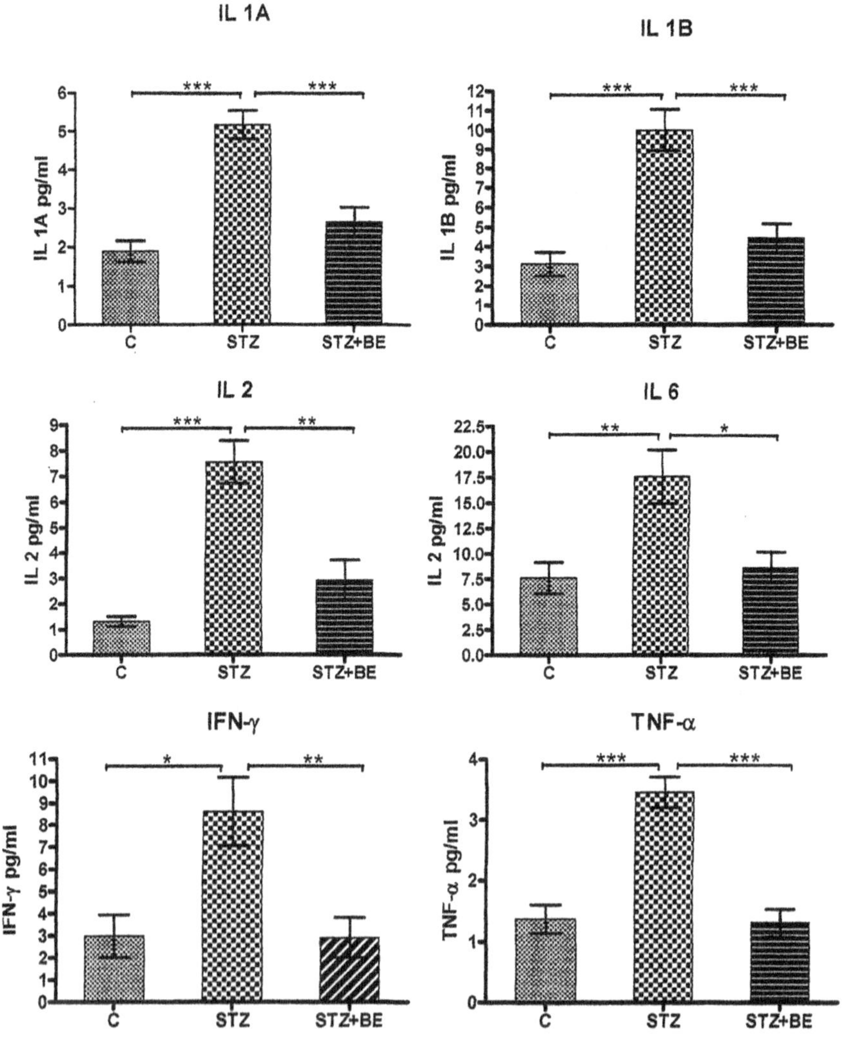

Fig. 13.7 Effect of Boswellic extract (150 mg/kg i.p. for 10 days) on proinflammatory cytokines in the serum of MLD-STZ-treated mice. *C* control (mean ± SE; *n* = 4) [64]

probably by inhibition of the production/action of cytokines related to induction of islet inflammation in an autoimmune process (Fig. 13.7).

When these experiments were repeated with KBA or AKBA the same results were achieved [65]. So far, however, no clinical data *is* available to support these animal experiments.

13.5 Antimicrobial and Antiparasitical Effects

Resins in general protect the stems of trees from any microbial attack.

Raja et al. [48] studied the antimicrobial activities of various Boswellic acids against 112 pathogenic bacterial isolates including ATCC strains. Here, AKBA exhibited the most potent antibacterial activity showing a Minimal Inhibitory Concentration (MIC) range of 2–8 μg/ml against the entire Gram-positive bacterial pathogens tested. It exhibited a concentration-dependent toxicity of Staphylococcus aureus ATCC 29213 up to 8 × MIC. The antibacterial mode of action of AKBA probably occurred via disruption of the microbial membrane structure.

In another study, methanolic and aqueous extracts from *Boswellia dalziellia* also showed a broad spectrum of inhibitory activity against bacteria, both Gram positive, Gram negative and fungi [2].

Serratol, a diterpene isolated from the gum resin of *Boswellia serrata*, was previously tested by Schmidt et al. [57] for its antiprotozoal activity. It was found to be active against *Tripanosoma brucie*, *Rhode siense* (sleeping sickness) and *Plasmodium falciparum* (Tropical Malaria).

Essential oils of the gum resin from different Boswellia species including *Boswellia carterii* (Somalia), *Boswellia papyrifera* (Ethiopia), *Boswellia serrata* (India) and *Boswellia rivae* (Ethiopia) were tested by Camardes et al. [11] and showed antimicrobial activity.

13.6 Clinical Studies

So far, only extracts from the gum resin of *Boswellia serrata* have been used for clinical trials. Studies with isolated compounds are still missing. The studies focus on chronic inflammatory diseases.

13.6.1 Pharmacokinetics of Boswellic Acids

In modern pharmacology, the therapeutic effects of drugs are closely related to their pharmacokinetic properties. However, as far as extracts from herbal medicine are concerned, it is impossible to establish pharmacokinetic data since they contain a

Table 13.5 Antimicrobial and antiparasitical effects of extracts, essential oils, and chemical constituents from different Boswellia species

Extracts		
Methanolic extract (stem bark) *B. dalzielli*	Broad spectrum of gram positive and gram negative bacteria and fungi	[2]
Methanolic extract *B. ameero* *B. elongata*	Gram positive multiresistent Staphylococcus strains	[42]
Boswellic extract *B. ameero* *B. elongata*	Influenza virus A	[43]
Methanolic extract *B. carterii*	Hepatitis virus C	[29]
Methanolic extract from stem bark	Musceocideal	[23]
Essential oils		
Essential oil different B. species	Gram positive bacteria, gram negative bacteria, antifungal	[11]
Essential oil *B. riva*	*Candida albicans*	[56]
Chemical constituents		
Serratol (diterpene from *B. serrata*)	*Tripanosoma brucei rhodesiense* (sleeping sicknes) *Plasmodium falsiparum* (tropical Malaria)	[57]
AKBA	*Staphylococcus aureus,* gram positive bacterial pathogens	[48]

variety of compounds which are involved in the final therapeutic actions. Moreover, their contents vary from species to species. Thus, the only possibility for a rough standardization is to determine one or more components of an extract where significant pharmacological effects can be expected. At present, in case of BEs, these are KBA and AKBA. Studies with isolated KBA and AKBA in humans do not exist yet. (Table 13.5)

13.6.1.1 Blood Levels of AKBA and KBA

In an open uncontrolled trial with 12 healthy male volunteers [63], a single oral dose of a commercial product of an extract out of gum resin from *Boswellia serrata* (WokVel™) containing 333 mg was given after standard breakfast. The extract contained 6.44 % KBA, 2 % AKBA, 18.51 % β-BA, 8.58 % 3-*O*-acetyl-β-BA, 6.93 % α-BA and 1.85 % 3-*O*-acetyl-αBA. In this study, only the concentration of KBA in the plasma was measured (Fig. 13.8). As shown in Table 13.6 maximum concentration of KBA was found after 4.5 h 2.72 μM. This concentration is in the range of the IC_{50} of KBA for the inhibition of leukotriene synthesis in vitro. In this study, the elimination half life (t1/2b) was 5.97 h. This suggests that when the above treatment is given every 6 h, the steady state plasma concentration of KBA ***is reached*** after approximately 30 h.

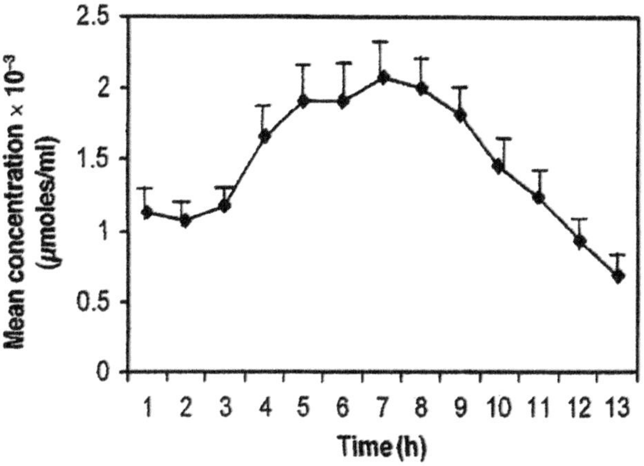

Fig. 13.8 Mean plasma concentration of 11-keto-β-boswellic acid versus time after oral administration of 333 mg *Boswellia serrata* extract WokVel™ containing 6.44 % KBA [63]

Table 13.6 Pharmacokinetic parameters of KBA after oral administration of 333 mg *Boswellia serrata* extract Wok Vel™ containing 6.44 % KBA [63

Pharmacokinetic parameters	Mean	SEM
C_{max} (μmol/ml)	2.72×10^{-3}	0.18
t_{max} (h)	4.5	0.55
Kel (per h)	0.17	0.04
$t½\ b$ (h)	5.97	0.94
$AUC_{0-\infty}$ (μmol/ml h)	27.33×10^{-3}	1.99
Ka (per h)	0.62	0.17
$t^1/_2\ a$ (h)	2.35	0.63
Vd (1)	142.87	22.78
Cl (ml/min)	296.10	24.09

As discussed in Sect. 3, Büchele and Simmet [8] identified 12 different pentacyclic triterpenic acids in an extract of *Boswellia serrata*. Their structures and contents are shown in Fig. 13.2 and Table 13.3. Using high-performance liquid chromatography and photodiode array detection, after 10 days of treatment with an oleogum resin extract of *Boswellia serrata* (4 × 786 mg per day), the authors could most of them (Table 13.3) identify in the plasma of a patient with brain tumor.

After intake of BEs by humans AKBA in the blood is below its IC_{50} in vitro, but at least KBA is near to its in vitro value of about 2.4 μM. As far as β-BA is concerned, which represents the highest percentage in a BE (around 19 % s. Table 13.3) its concentration in the blood after oral injection of a BE was found to be there in effective concentrations [68].

Effect of Food Intake: It is very well known that absorption of drugs may be related to food intake and to the kind of food. In this sense, Sterk et al. [74] studied the effect of food intake on the bioavailability of BAs from a herbal preparation of

Boswellia. Twelve healthy subjects fasted 10 h before and 4 h after drug administration (group A). A second group (B) received a *high-fat* meal together with the drug. The volunteers swallowed a single dose of 3 capsules with 282 mg (total of 786 mg) extract, containing 143.4 mg β-BA, 103.71 mg α-BA, 82.71 mg acetyl-β-BA, 48.12 mg KBA, 28.71 mg AKBA and 26.25 mg acetyl-α-BA. The time course of the plasma concentrations of the most active boswellic acids, i.e. KBA and AKBA, was dramatically different between fasted and high-fat meal volunteers. The calculated pharmacokinetic parameters are shown in Table 13.7.

It is obvious that in the high-fat meal group C_{max} of KBA is about 2.7 times and AKBA 4.8 times higher than in the fasting group. This can be explained by the lipophilic character of KBA and AKBA. Consequently, BEs should be taken together with food.

Table 13.7 Pharmacokinetics parameters of 11-keto-β-boswellic acid (KBA) and acetyl-11-keto-β-bosellic acid (AKBA) after administration of three capsules BSE–018 (786 mg dry extract of the oleogum resin from *Boswellia serrata*) as a single oral dose under fasted conditions (treatment A) and under fed conditions (treatment B) [74]

Parameters	Values (geometric mean + range) Treatment A (fasted conditions) n = 12	Treatment B (fed conditions) n = 12
11-Keto-β-boswellic acid		
$AUC_{(0-\infty)inf}$ (ng h ml^{-1})	1.660.72(940.3–3778.1)	3037.15(1481.9–6583.1)
$AUC_{(0-tz)}$ (ng h ml^{-1})	658.4(137.0–2747.3)	2451.8(1085.0–6125.4)
C_{max} (ng ml^{-1})	83.8 (24.9–243.8)	227.1 (101.0–418.1)
T_{max} (h)[a]	3.5(2.0–4.0)	4.0 (3.0–8.0)
K(h^{-1})	0.017	0.027
$T_{½}$ (h)	40.8	25.7
Acetyl-11-keto-β-boswellic acid		
$AUC_{(0-\infty)}$ (ng h ml^{-1})	153.6 (59.2–647.9)	748.9(271.4–5316.8)
$AUC_{(0-tz)}$ (ng h ml^{-1})	47.4 (8.0–232.0)	243.7(53.0–3528.0)
C_{max} (ng ml^{-1})	6.0 (0.9–45.7)	28.8 (13.0–264.5)
T_{max} (h)[a]	2.0 (0.0–24.0)	3.0 (0.5–60.0)
K (h^{-1})	0.066	0.046
$T_{½}$ (h)	10.5	15.0

$AUC(_{O-oo})$ = area under the concentration time curve, extrapolated to infinity
$AUC_{(0-tz)}$ = area under the concentration time curve
O = last quantifiable sample
C_{max}: = maximum plasma concentration
K = overall elimination rate constant by log linear regression
T_{max} = time to C_{max}
$T_{½}$ = terminal elimination half-life from K
[a]Median (and range)

13.6.1.2 Absorption

Extract preparations from the resin of Boswellia species, in most cases, are administered by oral route. Compared to the concentrations of BAs, in extract preparations their concentrations in the blood after oral application are very low. This holds true, especially for the most active BA, i.e. AKBA. Krüger et al. [37] explain this phenomenon to be due to poor permeability of AKBA and also moderate absorption of KBA.

13.6.1.3 Distribution

According to Siemoneit et al. [67] 11-keto-boswellic acids show > 95 % plasma protein binding. However, due to their lipophilic properties it is possible, that BAs may accumulate in lipophilic tissues.

13.6.1.4 Metabolism

In rat liver microsomes, human liver microsomes and hepatocytes, Krüger et al. [36] found that KBA but not AKBA undergoes extensive phase I metabolism. Oxidation to hydroxylated metabolites is the principal metabolic route. In vitro, KBA yielded metabolic profiles similar to those obtained in vivo in rat plasma and liver, whereas no metabolites of AKBA could be identified in vivo. Unexpectedly, AKBA is not deacetylated to KBA.

13.6.1.5 Topical Administration

Extracts from the gum resin of BS are frequently used topically in ointment preparations for skin diseases. Singh et al. [71] reported anti-inflammatory activity of BAs through this route in different acute and chronic models of inflammation such as arachidonic acid- and croton-oil-induced mouse ear edema, carrageenan-induced rats paw edema and adjuvant-induced arthritis in rats. The results of the study revealed that the antiphlogistic effect observed through this route is in accordance with the study conducted with the systemic application.

13.6.2 Chronic Inflammatory Diseases

From the preclinical studies it is reasonable to conclude that BEs and their active constituents will be effective in inflammatory disorders, since they inhibit the responsible related factors, i.e. products of the arachidonic acid cascade, especially leukotrienes, members of the complement system—and especially factors of the immune system which are related to the inflammatory autoimmune system. However, their actions will not be as immediate as it is the case with nonsteroidal anti-inflammatory drugs (NSAIDs) or glucocorticoids since it is evident, from pharmacokinetc studies, that the concentration of the most active compounds, i.e. KBA and AKBA in the blood does not reach effective levels after a single administration. This is in accordance with the experience of patients who report that the therapeutic effect of BEs occurs with a certain delay of 1 or 2 weeks.

13.6.2.1 Rheumatoid Diseases

As early as 1986, Singh and Atal [69] reported that in an arthritic model in rats a mixture of boswellic acids showed anti-inflammatory activity and Sharma et al. [61] observed that in another arthritis model a mixture of BAs reduced infiltration of leucocytes into an arthritic knee. Very recently, Umar [79] studied the effect of an extract from *Boswellia serrata* in the collagen-induced arthritis model in rats on most of the inflammatory parameters discussed. BE was administered at doses of 100 and 200 mg/kg body weight once daily for 21 days. The effects of the treatment in rats were assessed by biochemical parameters (articular elastase, LPO, GSH, catalase, SOD and NO), inflammatory mediators (IL-1B, IL-6, TNF-α, IL-10, IFN-γ and PGE_2), and histopathology in joints. In this study, BE was effective bringing significant changes to all the tested parameters (articular elastase, LPO, GSH, catalase, SOD and NO). Oral administration of BE resulted in significantly reduced levels of inflammatory mediators (IL-1B, IL-6, TNF-α, IFN-γ and PGE_2), and increased levels of IL-10. The protective effects of BE against RA were also evident from the decrease in arthritis scores and bone histology. On the basis of these studies and traditional experiences, a variety of clinical studies have been initiated including subjects suffering from rheumatoid arthritis and osteoarthritis.

Rheumatoid Arthritis

Rheumatoid arthritis belongs to the class of autoimmune diseases. The rheumatoid lesion, which is located in the synovial membrane, includes invasion of macrophages and lymphocytes that release cytokines such as interleukines and TNF-α. Neutrophils which are present in the synovial fluid of the inflamed joints produce leukotrienes, oxygen radicals and elastase activity, which finally cause synovialitis and destruction of cartilage.

Boswellic Extracts: Etzel [17] summarized the results of 11 mostly unpublished studies using extracts from the oleogum resin of *Boswellia serrata* in patients with chronic polyarthritis. The criteria were pain, swelling, sensitivity and tolerance. In five studies, patients were treated intraindividually in 2 placebo-controlled studies. In a meta-analysis of the above studies, about 50–60 % of the patients responded to this treatment. Pain and swelling of joints were improved by the commercial product H15™ (produced by Gufic Ltd. Mumbai, India), when compared to the placebo group ($p < 0.05$). Unfortunately, not all of these studies could be re-examined by the author of this chapter as they were not published. As a consequence, the quality and the outcome of these studies were critiqued by the German Society of Rheumatology in 1998. The arguments are mainly based on a study of Sander et al. [55]. In this multicentre controlled trial, the authors studied the effect of H 15™ versus placebo over a period of 12 weeks in 37 outpatients with rheumatoid arthritis and chronic polyarthritis being under constant therapy with steroids and disease-modifying antirheumatic drugs. The patients received 9 tablets of H 15™ (3600 mg) or placebo daily *in addition* to their previous therapy. Doses of NSAIDs could be adjusted on demand. Efficacy parameters were the index for swelling and pain, ESR and CRP. Pain and NSAID doses were documented at the beginning and at 6 and 12 weeks after initiation. In this study, treatment with H15™ resulted in no measurable effect. However, this study suffers from the drawback that the effect of the BE alone in comparison to standard therapy was not tested. It can be assumed that administration of H15™ to patients who are being already treated with steroids and patients with basic therapy will not experience an additional effect.

Osteoarthritis

Osteoarthritis is a common chronic, progressive, skeletal degenerative disorder, which often affects the knee joint and the shoulder.

Gupta et al. [22] investigated the effect of S-Compound™ (Rahul Pharma, Jammu Tawi, India), a mixture of various boswellic acids in patients suffering from chronic osteoarthritis (OA) of the primary type. A total of 50 patients were treated with either S-Compound™ (30 patients) or with Ibuprofen (20 patients) for 12–24 weeks. In this study, 60 % of the patients treated with S-Compound™ showed relief of symptoms in 12 weeks. 33.3 % out of the remaining 40 % recovered in 24 weeks but 2 patients had no relief. Only 30 % of the patients improved with Ibuprofen.

In a randomized, double-blind, placebo-controlled cross-over study, Kimmatkar et al. [34] studied efficacy, safety and tolerability of a BE preparation (trade name WokVel™ capsules) in 30 patients with osteoarthritis in the knee, 15 of them receiving the drug or placebo for 8 weeks. Each capsule of WokVel™ contained a standardized extract of *Boswellia serrata* oleogum resin with a minimum of 65 % organic acids or a minimum of 40 % total boswellic acids. The patients received one capsule with 333 mg of the extract three times a day and after a washout phase the alternative treatment. All patients reported decreased knee pain, increased knee flexion, an increase in the walking distance and in the ability to climb stairs. The symptoms returned after withdrawal of the treatment.

In a different double-blind, randomized, placebo-controlled study, Sengupta et al. [59] evaluated the efficacy and safety of 5-Loxin™ (Laila Natura, New Dehli,

India) for treatment of OA of the knee. 5-Loxin™ is a novel *Boswellia serrata* extract enriched with 30 % AKBA.

Seventy-five OA patients were included in the study. The patients received either 100 mg ($n = 25$) or 250 mg ($n = 25$) of 5-Loxin™ daily or a placebo ($n = 25$) for 90 days. Each patient was evaluated for pain and physical functions using the standard tools (visual analogue scale, Lequesne's Functional Index, and Western Ontario and McMaster Universities Osteoarthritis Index) at the baseline (day 0), and at days 7, 30, 60 and 90. Additionally, the cartilage degrading enzyme matrix metalloproteinase-3 was evaluated in the synovial fluid from OA patients. Measurement of a battery of biochemical parameters in the serum, haematological parameters and urine analysis were performed to evaluate the safety of 5-Loxin™. At the end of the study, both doses of 5-Loxin™ conferred clinically and statistically significant improvements in pain scores and physical function scores. Interestingly, improvements in pain score and functional ability were recorded not immediately but first 7 days after the start of treatment. Corroborating the improvements in pain scores in the treatment groups, the authors also noted significant reduction in synovial fluid matrix metalloproteinase-3. In a further study with 40 patients (20 with the same product and 20 with placebo), Sengupta et al. [60] reported similar results. Moreover, in an open randomized controlled study, Sontakke et al. [72] compared the effect of the Boswellia extract preparation WokVel™ capsules three times daily with a selective COX-2-inhibitor Valdecoxib (10 mg once daily) over a period of 6 months. Both groups showed comparable improvement as far as pains, stiffness and physical movement are concerned.

13.6.2.2 Chronic Inflammatory Bowel Diseases

Treatment of the symptoms of bowel disease with preparations containing olibanum/frankincense has a long tradition (see Chap. 2). Modern science has attributed these symptoms to different acute and chronic disorders. The latter include ulcerative colitis, chronic colitis, collagenous colitis and Crohn's disease. Moreover, it has been recognized that certain mediators of inflammation and immunological parameters, i.e. cytokines, play an important role in these disorders.

Thus, it is known that the mucosa of patients with chronic inflammatory bowel diseases is synthesizing considerable amounts of leukotrienes LTB_4, LTD_4 and LTE_4, which increase the production of mucus and stimulate contraction of the smooth muscle of the gastrointestinal tract. As far as the immune system is concerned, autoimmune antibodies have been detected in patients with ulcerative colitis and Crohn's disease. In addition, IL-1 and TNF-α have also been shown to be of importance in intestinal inflammations [73]. Based on these findings, the effect of oleogum resin *preparations* from *Boswellia serrata* were tested in patients with different chronic inflammatory bowel diseases.

Ulcerative Colitis

Ulcerative colitis is a chronic inflammatory disease with remissions and exacerbations affecting primarily the rectal mucosa, the left colon, but in many instances also the entire colon. It is characterized by rectal bleeding and diarrhoea affecting mainly, but not exclusively, the youth and early middle age.

Boswellic Extract: In 34 patients, suffering from ulcerative colitis grades II and III, the effect of an alcoholic extract of *Boswellia serrata* oleogum resin was studied according to Singh et al. [70] 350 mg thrice daily for 6 weeks, analyzing stool properties, histopathology, rectal biopsies via scan microscopy, and blood parameters including Hb, serum iron, calcium phosphorus, proteins, total leucocytes, and eosinophils [23]. Eight patients received sulfasalazine (1 g thrice daily) serving as controls. All parameters tested improved after treatment with the extract. 82 % out of treated patients went into remission while the remission rate for sulfasalazine was 75 %.

Chronic Colitis

This disease was characterized by the authors [25] as vague lower abdominal pain, bleeding per rectum with diarrhoea and palpable tender descending and sigmoid colon. Its pathophysiology seems to be different from that of ulcerative colitis.

Boswellic Extract: In this study, 30 patients, 17 males and 13 females age 18–48 years, were included. Twenty patients were given a preparation of the oleogum resin of *Boswellia serrata* (S-Compound™) containing KBA 0.63 %, AKBA 0.7 %, acetyl-β-BA and β-BA 1.5 % (900 mg daily divided in three doses for 6 weeks) and ten patients receiving sulfasalazine (3 mg daily divided in three doses for 6 weeks) served as controls. Out of the 20 patients treated with *Boswellia* oleogum resin, 18 patients showed an improvement in one or more of the following parameters: stool properties, histopathology as well as scanning electron microscopy, Hb, serum iron, calcium, phosphorus, proteins, total leukocytes, and eosinophils.

Collagenous Colitis

A rarer chronic inflammatory bowel disease is collagenous colitis. It is characterized by aqueous diarrhoea, histological thickness of the mucosa and a subepithelial collagen band.

Boswellic Extract: In a randomized, placebo-controlled, double-blind multicenter study, quality of life and histology were studied in 25 patients receiving either 400 mg BE (H15™) three times a day or a placebo. After 6 weeks of treatment, significant improvements were reported for 58.3 % of the *Boswellia* group and for 30.8 % in the placebo group [38].

Crohn's Disease

Crohn's disease (Ileitis terminalis) is a chronic inflammatory disease of the entire gastrointestinal tract from the oral cavitity up to the anal area. Most common locations are the terminal ileum, colon and rectum. Typical symptoms are abdominal pain, diarrhoea with mucus, purulency and aqueous stools. The anti-inflammatory treatment at present consists of the use of mesalazine and sulfasalazine.

Boswellic Extracts: Gerhardt et al. [20] studied the effect of a BE (H15™) on symptoms in an active state of Crohn's disease. In a double-blind, verum-controlled parallel group comparison, 102 patients were randomized. The protocol population included 44 patients treated with BE H15™ and 39 patients treated with mesalazine. As primary parameter, the change of the Crohn's Disease Activity Index (CDAI) from the beginning to the end of the therapy was chosen. H15™ was tested for non-inferiority compared to the standard treatment with mesalazine. In this study, the CDAI after treatment with H15™ was reduced by 90 and after therapy with mesalazine by 53 score points in the mean. A difference between both treatments could not be proven to be statistically significant. Thus, the data suggest that in treatment of Crohn's disease in an *active* state the extract from the oleogum resin of *Boswellia serrata* is at least as effective as a standard medication under the conditions of this study.

In a previous study [28] it was investigated whether or not, in a period of 2 years, permanent treatment with Boswellan™ (special BE extract from Pharmasan Company—Freiburg, Germany) would increase the time of remission. This was, however, not the case. Obviously, the Boswellia preparations are only effective in an *acute* phase of the disease, improving factors related to the CDAI.

13.6.2.3 Respiratory Diseases: Bronchial Asthma

Since ancient times (see Chap. 2) respiratory symptoms are treated with preparations of olibanum/frankincense. This still holds for bronchitis including cough and expectoration. A special case is bronchial asthma.

Bronchial asthma is a chronic inflammatory condition characterized by bronchial hyper-responsiveness and reversible airways obstruction.

Increased production of leukotrienes both during episodes of asthma and in patients with stable asthma was shown by Chanarin and Johnston [14]. Bronchial asthma is also a case of autoimmune diseases.

Boswellia Extracts: In a double-blind, placebo-controlled trial with asthma patients Gupta et al. [24] tested forty patients with a mean duration of bronchial asthma of 9.58 ± 6.07 years. They received a preparation of oleogum resin of *Boswellia serrata* (S-Compound™) of 300 mg three times daily over a period of 6 weeks. In this study, 70 % of the patients showed improvement of the disease measured by the disappearance of physical symptoms and by signs such as dyspnoea, rhonchi, the number of obstructive attacks, increase in respiratory parameters, including FEV_1, FVC and PEFR as well as by a decrease in eosinophilic count and ESR. In the control group of 40 patients only 27 % of these patients showed improvements.

13.6.2.4 Autoimmune Diabetes: Tyrosinephosphatase Antibody

Autoimmune Diabetes is associated with an increase of specific markers in the blood including tyrosinephosphatase antibody (IA_2-A), which indicate presence of insulitis. So far there exists no clinical study whether or not a BE or BA are effective in human autoimmune diabetes.

Recently in a case report it was shown that a BE decreased blood levels of IA_2-A in a patient with "Late onset Autoimmune Diabetes of the Adult" (LADA). A female patient 50 years old with a body weight of 72 kg where diabetes was first diagnosed in November 2012 and who was under insulin therapy (Humalog™, Humaninsulin basal™) received a BE "Indian Boswellia the Original™, a new product from Indian Boswellia Laboratory, Agra India, containing 3.6 % KBA and 1.4 % AKBA. The patient received 3 times daily 2 tablets (400 mg BE each) per oral route over a period of 8.5 weeks.

During this time IA_2-A levels in the blood dropped from 25 to 10 K/U/L indicating improvement of insulitis [58].

The authors are aware, that this is only one case with all its restrictions. But it may stimulate other attempts to strengthen the hypothesis that BEs or BAs including KBA and AKBA may be an option for prevention/treatment of autoimmune diabetes.

What do the clinical studies teach:

In the clinical studies, that have been performed so far between 6 and 13 weeks and with a limited number of patients, improvement of symptoms in patients suffering from rheumatoid arthritis, osteoarthritis, chronic inflammatory bowel diseases and bronchial asthma were reported. This is in line with preclinical in vitro and in vivo studies showing pharmacological activity of BEs and some BAs on mediators of inflammation as well as on factors related to autoimmune disorders. It should, however, be taken into consideration that the effects of BEs are more likely to be an overall action of several components of the extract than of single compounds. Nevertheless, for future clinical studies, extracts should be standardized according to regional pharmacopoeias, for instance European Pharmacopoea, using KBA and or AKBA as leading compounds.

13.6.3 Side Effects

Taking into account the wide use of oleogum resin from different *Boswellia* species in ancient times and nowadays, side effects do not appear to be a critical point. This is also the outcome of the published material. Most of the side effects, if at all, are related to the gastrointestinal tract. In detail:

Gastrointestinal Tract: In the study using S-Compound™ [22], dyspeptic symptoms in form of pain in abdomen, distension of abdomen, sour eructation and loss of appetite were reported in 8 % while 60 % of patients treated with Ibuprofen had dyspeptic symptoms.

In a further trial with S-Compound™, two from 40 patients complained about epigastric pain, hyperacidity, and nausea [24]. In a study dealing with ulcerative colitis [23], 6 out of 34 patients reported retrosternal burning, nausea, fullness of abdomen, epigastric pain and anorexia.

Böker and Winking [7], studying the effect of H15™, reported that some patients developed nausea and vomiting. The side effects were reversible after omission of the treatment. Comparing the effect of H15™ (44 patients) with mesalazine (39 patients) suffering from Crohn's disease), Gerhardt et al. [20] reported no drug related side effects in the H15™ group but 4 patients treated with mesalazine suffered from headache and gastrointestinal symptoms. In the study of Gupta et al. [25], out of 20 patients treated with Boswellia gum resin, only 2 patients complained of heartburn and Streffer et al. [75] reported that the preparation H15™ was well tolerated, only some gastrointestinal complains were observed. BE (15 patients) was also well tolerated in the study of Kimmatkar et al. [34] exept for minor gastrointestinal reactions. In the study of Sontakke et al. [72], one patient out of 33 receiving BE complained about diarrhoea and abdominal cramps.

Boswellic extracts in higher doses are used in treatment of cerebral edemas caused by brain tumours. In a prospective, randomized, placebo-controlled double-blind pilot study [35], where 22 patients with brain tumours received 4200 mg of a BE (H15™) or placebo, diarrhoea grade 1–2 occurred in 6 patients of the BE group. Other side effects were the same as in the placebo group.

Respiratory Tract: There is a case report from a patient who complained about asthma symptoms after exposure to fume of incense in the church [46].

Skin: In an other case report Acebo et al. [1] describe a patient suffering from allergic contact dermatitis using an extract from *Boswellia serrata* in a naturopathic cream.

In two patients being treated with H15™ for brain edema, Böker and Winking [7] described skin irritations. The side effects were reversible after omission of the treatment.

General Tolerability: No adverse reactions were observed in a double-blind placebo-controlled study in 20 volunteers receiving topical formulation cream containing boswellic acids [39]. No side effects were also observed in the pharmacokinetic study of Sharma et al. [63] and in the study on OA by Sengupta et al. [59]. And the study of Holtmeier et al. [28] confirmed good tolerance of the preparation Boswellan™ over a period of 52 weeks.

When Aflapin™ (Laila Impex R & D Center, New Dehli, India) and 5-Loxin™ were used to treat osteoarthritis in comparison to a placebo [59, 60], the safety parameters were almost unchanged in the treatment group. In a retrospective analysis in 2000, the laboratory parameters before and after the treatment of patients suffering from rheumatoid arthritis, ulcerative colitis, Crohn's disease, neurodermitis, lupus erythematosus, multiple sclerosis, astrocytoma, glioblastoma, bronchial asthma and psoriasis were tested receiving the Boswellia preparation H15™ over a period of 6 years.

No significant changes related to the therapy were observed [10].

All together, it appears that extracts from the oleogum resin of Boswellia species are relatively safe as far as side effects are concerned. This is one of the big advantages compared to all anti-inflammatory remedies being in use presently.

References

1. Acebo E, Raton JA, Saulua S, Eizaguirre X, Trébol J, Perez JLD (2004) Allergic contact dermatitis from *Boswellia serrata* extract in a naturopathic cream. Contact Dermat 51:91
2. Adelakun EA, Finbar EA, Agina SE, Makinde AA (2001) Antimicrobial activity of *Boswellia dalzielii* stem bark. Fitoterapia 72:822–824
3. Ammon HP, Mack T, Singh GB, Safayhi H (1991) Inhibition of leukotriene B4 formation in rat peritoneal neutrophils by an ethanolic extract of the gum resin exudates of *Boswellia serrata*. Planta Med 57:203–207
4. Badria FA, Mikhaeil BR, Maatooq GT, Amer MM (2003) Immunmodulatory terpenoids from the oleogum resin of *Boswellia carterii* Bordwood. Z Naturforsch 58:506–516
5. Beisner K, Büchele B, Werz U, Simmet T (2003) Structural analysis of 3-α-acetyl-20(29)-lupene-24-oic acid, a novel pentacyclic triterpene isolated from the gum resin of *Boswellia serrata*, by NMR spectroscopy. Magn Reson Chem 41:629–632
6. Blain EJ, Ali AY, Duance VC (2010) *Boswellia frereana* (frankincense) suppresses cytokine-induced matrix metalloproteinase expression and production of proinflammatory molecules in articular cartilage. Phytother Res 24:905–912
7. Böker DK, Winking M (1997) Die Rolle von *Boswellia*-Säuren in der Therapie maligner Gliome. Dtsch Ärztebl 94:B-958–B-960
8. Büchele B, Simmet T (2003) Analysis of 12 different pentacyclic triterpenic acids from frankincense in human plasma by high performance liquid chromatography and photodiode array detection. J Chromatogr B 795:355–362
9. Büchele B, Zugmaier W, Simmet T (2003) Analysis of pentacyclic triterpenic acids from frankincense gum resins and related phytopharmaceuticals by high-performance liquid chromatography. Identification of lupeolic acid, a novel pentacyclic triterpene. J Chromatogr B 791:21–30
10. Buvari PG (2001) Wirksamkeit und Unbedenklichkeit der H15 Ayurmedica-Therapie bei chronisch entzündlichen Erkrankungen. Dissertation, University of Mannheim-Heidelberg

11. Camardes L, Dayton T, Di Stefano V, Pitonzo R, Schillaci D (2007) Chemical composition and antimicrobial activity of some oleogum resin essential oils from Boswellia spp. (Burseraceae). Ann Chim 97:837–844
12. Cao H, Yu R, Choi Y, Ma ZZ, Zhang H, Xiang W, Lee DY et al (2010) Discovery of cyclooxygenase inhibitors from medicinal plants used to treat inflammation. Pharmacol Res 61:519–524
13. Chervier MR, Ryan AE, Lee DY, Zhongze M, Wu-Yan Z, Via CS (2005) *Boswellia carterii* extract inhibits TH1 cytokines and promotes TH2 cytokines *in vitro*. Clin Diagn Lab Immunol 1:575–580
14. Chanarin N, Johnston SL (1994) Leukotrienes as a target in asthma therapy. Drugs 47:12–24
15. Cnop M, Welsh N, Jonas JC et al (2005) Mechanisms of pancreatic beta-cell death in type 1 and type 2 diabetes: many differences, few similarities. Diabetes 54(Suppl. 2):97–107
16. Cuaz-Pérolin C, Billiel L, Baugé E, Copin C, Scott-Algaria D, Genze F, Rouis M et al (2008) Antiinflammatory and antiatherogenic effects of NF-Kappa B inhibitor acetyl-11-beta-boswellic acid in LPS-challenged ApoE-/- mice. Arterioscler Thromb Vasc Biol 28:272–277
17. Etzel R (1996) Special extract of *Boswellia serrata* (H15) in the treatment of rheumatoid arthritis. Phytomedicine 3:91–94
18. Fan AY, Lao L, Zhang RX, Wang LB, Lee DY, Ma ZZ et al (2005) Effects of an acetone extract of *Boswellia carterii* Birdw. (Burseraceae) gum resin on rats with persistent inflammation. J Altern Complement Med 11:323–331
19. Gayathri B, Manjula N, Vinaykumar KS, Lakshmi BS, Balakrishnan A (2007) Pure compound from *Boswellia serrata* extract exhibits anti-inflammatory property in human PBMCs and mouse macrophages through inhibiton of TNF alpha, IL-1beta, NO and MAP kinases. Int Immunopharmacol 7:472–482
20. Gerhardt H, Seifert F, Buvari P, Vogelsang H, Repges RZ (2001) Therapie des aktiven Morbus Crohn mit *Boswellia serrata* Extract H 15. Z Gastroenterol 39:11–17
21. Gupta OP, Sharma N, Chand DA (1992) Sensitive and relevant model for evaluating anti-inflammatory activity-papaya latex-induced rat paw inflammation. J Pharmacol Toxicol Methods 28:15–19
22. Gupta J, Gupta S (1993) Parihar A. S-compound-A traditional drug for osteoarthritis patients. The Indian Practitioner 46:69–72
23. Gupta I, Parihar A, Malhotra P, Singh GB, Lüdtke R, Safayhi H, Ammon HP (1997) Effects of *Boswellia serrata* gum resin in patients with ulcerative colitis. Eur J Med Res 2:37–43
24. Gupta I, Gupta V, Parihar A, Gupta S, Lüdtke R, Safayhi H, Ammon HP (1998) Effects of *Boswellia serrata* gum resin in patients with bronchial asthma: results of a double-blind, placebo-controlled, 6-week clinical study. Eur J Med Res 3:511–514
25. Gupta I, Parihar A, Malhorta P, Gupta S, Ludtke R, Safayhi H et al (2001) Effects of gum resin of *Boswellia serrata* in patients with chronic colitis. Planta Med 67:391–395
26. Gupta A, Khajuria A, Singh J, Singh S, Suri KA, Qazi GN (2011) Immunological adjuvant effect of *Boswellia serrata* (BOS 2000) on specific antibody and cellular response to ovalbumin in mice. Int Immunopharmacol 11:968–975
27. Heil K, Ammon HP, Safayhi H (2001) Inhibiton of NADPH-oxidase by AKBA in intact PMNs. Naunyn Schmiedebergs Arch Pharmacol 3635:R14
28. Holtmeier WH, Zeuzem S, Preiß J, Kruis W, Böhm S, Maaser Ch et al (2010) Randomized, placebo-controlled, double-blind trial of *Boswellia serrata* in maintaining remission of Crohn's Disease: good safety profile but lack of efficacy. Inflamm Bowel Dis 17(2):573–582
29. Hussein G, Miyashiro H, Nakamura N, Hattori M, Kakiuchi N, Shimotohno K (2000) Inhibitory effects of sudanese medicinal plant extracts on hepatitis C virus (HCV) protease. Phytother Res 14:510–516
30. Kapil A, Moza N (1991) Anticomplementary activity of *Boswellia* acids—an inhibitor of C3-convertase of the classical complement pathway. Int J Immunopharmacol 14:1139–1143
31. Karr A, Menon MK (1969) Analgesic effect of the gum resin of *Boswellia serrata* Roxb. Life Sci 8:1023–1028

32. Kela SL, Ogunsusi RA, Ogbogu VC, Nwude N (1989) Screening of some Nigeria plants for molluscicidal activity. Rev Elev Med Vet Pays Trop 42:195–202
33. Khajuria A, Gupta A, Suden P, Singh S, Malik F, Singh J et al (2008) Immunmodulatory activity of biopolymeric fraction BOS 2000 from *Boswellia serrata*. Phytother Res 22:340–348
34. Kimmatkar N, Thawani V, Hingorani L, Khiyani R (2003) Efficacy and tolerability of *Boswellia serrata* extract in treatment of osteoarthritis of knee—a randomized double blind placebo controlled trial. Phytomedicine 10:3–7
35. Kirsten S, Treier M, Wehrle SJ, Becker G, Abdel-Tawab M, Gerbeth K et al (2011) *Boswellia serrata* acts on cerebral edema in patients irradiated for brain tumors. Cancer 117:3788–3795
36. Krüger P, Daneshfar R, Eckert GP, Klein J, Volmer DA et al (2008) Metabolism of boswellic acids in vitro and in vivo. Drug Metabol Distpos 36:1135–1142
37. Krüger P, Kanzer J, Hummel J, Fricker G, Schubert-Zsilavecz M, Abdel-Tawab M (2009) Permeation of Boswellia extract in the Caco-2 model and possible interactions of its constituents KBA and AKBA with OATP1B3 and MRP2. Eur J Pharm Sci 36:275–284
38. Madisch A, Miehlke S, Eichele O, Bethke B, Mrwa J, Kuhlisch E et al (2005) *Boswellia serrata* Extrakt bei kollagener Kolitis – eine randomisierte, placebo-kontrollierte, doppelblinde Multicenterstudie. Dtsch Ges Verdau Stoffw Erkr. Gastroenterol 43(Suppl. Z):P061
39. Martelli L, Berardesca E, Martelli M (2000) Topical formulation of a new plant extract complex with refirming properties. Clinical and non-invasive evaluation in a double-blind trial. Int J Cosmet Sci 22:201–206
40. Martinez D, Lohs K, Janzen J (1989) Weihrauch und Myrrhe. Kulturgeschichte und wirtschaftliche Bedeutung. Botanik, Chemie, Medizin. Wissenschaftliche Verlagsgesellschaft, Stuttgart
41. Mikhaeil BR, Maatooq GT, Badria FA, Amer MM (2003) Chemistry and immunomodulatory activity of frankincense oil. Z Naturforsch C 58:230–238
42. Mothana RA, Lindequist U (2005) Antimicrobial activity of some medicinal plants of the island Sogotra. J Ethnopharmacol 96:177–181
43. Mothana RA, Mentel R, Reiss C, Lindequist U (2006) Phytochemical screening and antiviral activity of some medicinal plants from the island Sogotra. Phytother Res 20:298–302
44. Mothana RA (2011) Anti-inflammatory, antinociceptive and antioxidant activities of the endemic Sogotraen *Boswellia elongata* Balf. F. and *Jatropha unicostata* Balf. F. in different experimental models. Food Chem Toxicol 49:2594–2599
45. Moussaieff A, Shohami E, Kashman Y, Fride E, Schmitz ML, Renner F et al (2007) Incensolate acetate, a novel anti-inflammatory compound isolated from *Boswellia* resin, inhibits nuclear factor-kappa B activation. Mol Pharmacol 72:1657–1664
46. O'Connor TM, Cusack R, Lauders S, Bredin CP (2014) Holy Saturday asthma. BMJ Case Rep doi:10.1136/bcr-2014-203861
47. Poeckel D, Tausch L, Kather N, Jauch J, Werz O (2006) Boswellic acids stimulate arachidonic acid release and 12-lipoxygenase activity in human platelets independent of Ca^{2+} and differentially interact with platelet-type 12-lipoxygenase. Mol Pharmacol 70:1071–1078
48. Raja AF, Ali F, Khan IA, Shawl AS, Arora DS (2011) Acetyl-11-keto-β-boswellic acid (AKBA); targeting oral cavity pathogens. BMC Res Notes 4:406
49. Reddy KP, Singh AB, Puri A, Srivastava K, Narender T (2009) Synthesis of novel triterpenoid (lupeol) derivatives and their in vivo antihyperglycemic and antidyslipidemic activity. Bioorg Med Chem Lett 19:4463–4466
50. Safayhi H, Mack T, Sabieraj J, Anazodo MI, Subramanian LR, Ammon HP (1992) Boswellic acids: novel, specific, nonredox inhibitors of 5-lipoxygenase. J Pharmacol Exp Ther 261:1143–1146
51. Safayhi H, Sailer ER, Ammon HP (1995) Mechanism of 5-lipoxygenase inhibition by acetyl-11-keto-beta-boswellic acid. Mol Pharmacol 47:1212–1216
52. Safayhi H, Rall B, Sailer ER, Ammon HP (1997) Inhibition by Boswellic acids of human leukocyte elastase. J Pharmacol Exp Ther 281:460–463

53. Sailer ER, Subramanian LR, Rall B, Hoernlein RF, Ammon HP, Safayhi H (1996) Acetyl-11-keto-beta-boswellic acid (AKBA): structure requirements for binding and 5-lipoxygenase inhibitory activity. Br J Pharmacol 117:615–618
54. Sailer ER, Schweizer S, Boden SE, Ammon HP, Safayhi H (1998) Characterization of an acetyl-11-keto-beta-boswellic acid and arachidonate-binding regulatory site of 5-lipoxygenase using photoaffinity labeling. Eur J Biochem 256:364–368
55. Sander O, Herborn G, Rau R (1998) Is H15 (extract of *Boswellia serrata* "incense") an efficient supplementation to established drug therapy of rheumatoid arthritis? Results of a double-blind pilot trial. Z Rheumatol 57:11–16
56. Schillaci D, Arizza V, Dayton T, Camarda L, Di SV (2008) In vitro anti-biofilm activity of Boswellia spp. Oleogum resin essential oils. Lett Appl Microbiol 47:433–438
57. Schmidt TJ, Kaiser M, Brun R (2011) Complete structural assignment of serratol, a cembrane-type diterpene from *Boswellia serrata* and evaluation of its antiprotozoal activity. Planta Med 77:849–850
58. Schrott E, Laufer S, Lämmerhofer M, Ammon HPT (2014) Extract from gum resin of *Boswellia serrata* decreases IA_2-antibody in a patient with "Late onset Autoimmune Diabetes of the Adult" (LADA). Phytomedicine 21:786
59. Sengupta K, Alluri KV, Satish AR, Mishra S, Golakoti T, Sarma KV et al (2008) A double blind, randomised, placebo controlled study of the efficacy and safety of 5-Loxin for treatment of osteoarthritis of the knee. Arthritis Res Ther 10:R85
60. Sengupta K, Krishnaraju AV, Vishal AA, Mishra A, Trimurtulu G, Sarma KV et al (2010) Comperative efficacy and tolerability of 5-Loxin and Aflapin. Against osteoarthritis of the knee: a double blind, randomized, placebo controlled clinical study. Int J Med Sci 7:366–379
61 Sharma ML, Bani S, Singh CB (1989) Antiarthritic activity of boswellic acids in bovine serum albumin (BSA)-induced arthritis. Int J Immunopharmacol 11:647-652
62. Sharma ML, Kaul A, Khajuria A, Singh S, Singh GB (1996) Immunomodulatory activity of boswellic acids (pentacyclic triterpene acids) from *Boswellia serrata*. Phytother Res 10: 107–112
63. Sharma S, Thawani V, Hingorani L, Shrivastava M, Bhate VR, Khiyani R (2004) Pharmacokinetic study of 11-keto-beta-boswellic acid. Phytomedicine 11:255–260
64. Shehata AM, Quintanilla-Fend L, Bettio S, Singh CB, Ammon HP (2011) Prevention of multiple low-dose streptozotocin (MLD-STZ) diabetes in mice by an extract from gum resin of *Boswellia serrata* (BE). Phytomedicine 18:1037–1044
65. Shehata AM, Quintanilla-Fend L, Bettio S, Jauch J, Scior T, Scherbaum WA, Ammon HPT (2015) 11-Keto-β-Boswellic acids prevent development of autoimmune reactions, insulitis and reduce hyperglycemia during induction of multiple low dose streptozotocin (MLD-STZ) diabetes in mice. Horm Metab Res 47:463–469
66. Siemoneit U, Hofmann B, Kather N, Lamkemeyer T, Madlung J, Franke L et al (2008) Identification and functional analysis of cyclooxygenase-1 as a molecular target of Boswellic acids. Biochem Pharmacol 75:503–513
67. Siemoneit U, Pergola C, Jazzar B, Northoff H, Skarke C, Jauch J, Werz O (2009) On the interference of Boswellic acids with 5-lipoxygenase: mechanistic studies in vitro and pharmacological relevance. Eur J Pharmacol 606:246–254
68. Siemoneit U, Koeberle A, Rossi A, Dehm F, Verhoff M, Reckel S et al (2011) Inhibition of microsomal prostaglandin E2 synthase-1 as a molecular basis for the anti-inflammatory actions of Boswellic acids from frankincense. Br J Pharmacol 162:147–162
69. Singh GB, Atal CH (1986) Pharmacology of an extract of salai guggal ex *Boswellia serrata*, a new non-steroidal anti-inflammatory agent. Agents Actions 18:407–412
70. Singh GB, Singh S, Bani S (1996) Alcoholic extract of salai-guggal ex *Boswellia serrata*, a new natural source NSAID. Drugs Today 32:109–112
71. Singh S, Khajuria A, Taneja SC, Khajuria RK, Singh J, Johri RK, Qazi GN (2008) Boswellic acids: a leukotriene inhibitor also effective through topical application in inflammatory disorders. Phytomedicine 15:400–407

72. Sontakke S, Thawani V, Pimpalkhute S, Kabra P, Bubhulkar S, Hingorani L (2007) Open, randomized controlled clinical trial of *Boswellia serrata* extract as compared to valdecocib in osteoarthritis of knee. Indian J Pharmacol 39:27–29
73. Stange EF, Schreiber S, Raedler A et al (1997) Therapie des Morbus Crohn. Z Gastroenterol 35:541–554
74. Sterk V, Büchele B, Simmet T (2004) Effect of food intake on the bioavailability of boswellic acids from a herbal preparation in healthy volunteers. Planta Med 70:1155–1160
75. Streffer JR, Bitzer M, Schabet M, Dichganz J, Weller M (2001) Response of radiochemotherapy-associated cerebral edema a phytotherapeutic agent, H15. Neurology 56:1219–1221
76. Syrovets T, Büchele B, Krauss C, Laumonnier Y, Simmet T (2005) Acetylboswellic acids inhibit lipopolysaccharide-mediated TNF-alpha induction in monocytes by direct interaction with IkappaB kinase. J Immunol 174:498–506
77. Takada Y, Ichikawa H, Badmaev V, Aggarwal BB (2006) Acetyl-11-keto-beta-boswellic acid potentiates apoptosis, inhibits invasion and abolishes osteoclastogenesis by suppressing NF-kappa B and NF-kappa B-regulated gene expression. J Immunol 176:3127–3140
78. Tausch L, Henkel A, Siemoneit U, Poeckel D, Kather N, Franke L et al (2009) Identification of human cathepsin G as a functional target of boswellic acids from the anti-inflammatory remedy frankincense. J Immunol 183:3433–3442
79. Umar S, Umar K, Saarwar AH, Khan A, Ahmad N (2014) *Boswellia serrata* extract attenuates inflammatory mediators and oxidative stress in collagen induced arthritis. Phytomedicine 21:847–856
80. Verhoff M, Seitz S, Northoff H, Jauch J, Schaible AM, Werz O (2012) A novel C(28)-hydroxylated lupeolic acid suppresses the biosynthesis of eicosanoids through inhibition of cytosolic phospholipase A(2). Biochem Pharmacol 84:681–691
81. Wagner H, Knaus W, Jordan E (1987) Pflanzeninhaltsstoffe mit Wirkung auf das Komplementsystem. Z Phytother 8:148–149
82. Wang H, Syrovets T, Kess D, Büchele B, Hainzl H, Lunov O et al (2009) Targeting NF-kappa B with a natural triterpenoid alleviates skin inflammation in a mouse model of psoriasis. J Immunol 1:4755–4763

Chapter 14
Natural Withanolides in the Treatment of Chronic Diseases

Peter T. White, Chitra Subramanian, Hashim F. Motiwala and Mark S. Cohen

Abstract Withanolides, and in particular extracts from *Withania somnifera*, have been used for over 3,000 years in traditional Ayurvedic and Unani Indian medical systems as well as within several other Asian countries. Traditionally, the extracts were ascribed a wide range of pharmacologic properties with corresponding medical uses, including adaptogenic, diuretic, anti-inflammatory, sedative/anxiolytic, cytotoxic, antitussive, and immunomodulatory. Since the discovery of the archetype withaferin A in 1965, approximately 900 of these naturally occurring, polyoxygenated steroidal lactones with 28-carbon ergostane skeletons have been discovered across 24 diverse structural types. Subsequently, extensive pharmacologic research has identified multiple mechanisms of action across key inflammatory pathways. In this chapter we identify and describe the major withanolides with anti-inflammatory properties, illustrate their role within essential and supportive inflammatory pathways (including NF-κB, JAK/STAT, AP-1, PPARγ, Hsp90 Nrf2, and HIF-1), and then discuss the clinical application of these withanolides in inflammation-mediated chronic diseases (including arthritis, autoimmune, cancer, neurodegenerative, and neurobehavioral). These naturally derived compounds exhibit remarkable biologic activity across these complex disease processes, while showing minimal adverse effects. As novel compounds and analogs continue to be discovered, characterized, and clinically evaluated, the interest in withanolides as a novel therapeutic only continues to grow.

Keywords Autoimmune · Cancer · Inflammation · Neurodegenerative · NF-κB · Withaferin A · Withanolide

These authors contributed equally

P.T. White · C. Subramanian · H.F. Motiwala · M.S. Cohen (✉)
Department of Surgery, University of Michigan Hospital and Health Systems, 2920K Taubman Center, SPC 5331, 1500 East Medical Center Drive, Ann Arbor, MI 48109-5331, USA
e-mail: cohenmar@med.umich.edu

S.C. Gupta et al. (eds.), *Anti-inflammatory Nutraceuticals and Chronic Diseases*, Advances in Experimental Medicine and Biology 928,
DOI 10.1007/978-3-319-41334-1_14

Abbreviations

5XFAD	5 FAD mutations carried on APP and PS1 transgenes
AChE	Acetylcholinesterase
AD	Alzheimer's disease
ADAM10	Adisintegrin and metalloproteinase domain-containing protein 10, or α-secretase
AP-1	Activator protein 1
APP	Amyloid precursor protein
BACE	APP cleaving enzyme 1 or β-secretase
BChE	Butyrylcholinesterase
Bfl-1/A1	Bcl-2-related protein A1
C/EBPα	CCAAT/enhancer-binding proteinα
CCR7	Chemokine (C–C motif) receptor 7
cFLIP	C-FADD-like IL-1β-converting enzyme–inhibitory proteins
CNS	Central nervous system
COX	Cyclooxygenase
CSC	Cancer stem cell
EGF	Epidermal growth factor
EGFR	EGF receptor
ERK	Extracellular signal-regulated kinase
FDA	Food and Drug Administration
GABA	Gamma-aminobutyric acid
GMP	Good manufacturing process
HD	Huntington's disease
HIF-1	Hypoxia inducible factor-1
HMGB1	High mobility group box 1
hnRNP-K	Heterogeneous nuclear ribonucleoprotein
KHPA	Hypothalamic–pituitary–adrenal
Hsp	Heat shock protein
HTT	Mutant Huntingtin
IAP1	Inhibitor of apoptosis protein-1
IBD	Inflammatory bowel disease
ICAM	Intercellular adhesion molecule
IFN	Interferon
IKK	I kappa B kinase
IL	Interleukin
iNOS	Inducible nitric oxide synthase
JAK	Janus kinase
JNK1	c-Jun N-terminal protein kinase
Keap1	Kelch like ECH-associated protein-1
LPS	Lipopolysaccharide

LTB_4	Leukotriene B4
MAPK	Mitogen-activated protein kinase
MCE	Mitotic clonal expansion,
MCP-1	Monocyte chemoattractant protein-1
MMPs	Matrix metalloproteinases
MMTV-neu	Mouse mammary tumor virus-neu
MPTP	1-Methyl-4-phenyl-1,2,3,6-tetrahydropyridine
MS	Mass spectrometry
mTOR	Mechanistic target of rapamycin
MUC-1	Mucin 1
NF-κB	Nuclear factor kappa B
NO	Nitric oxide
Nrf2	Nuclear factor erythroid 2-related factor 2
OCD	Obsessive-compulsive disorder
PBMC	Peripheral blood mononuclear cells
PD	Parkinson's disease
PDGF	Platelet-derived growth factor
PGE_2	Prostaglandin E2
PI3K	Phosphatidylinositol-3-kinase
PPARs	Peroxisome proliferator-activated receptors
QR	Quinone reductase
RA	Rheumatoid arthritis
ROS	Reactive oxygen species
RTKs	Receptor tyrosine kinases
SAR	Structural–activity relationship
SFMC	Synovial fluid mononuclear cells
SOD	Super oxide dismutase
STAT	Signal transducer and activator of transcription
TAK1	Transforming growth factor-β-activating kinase
TGF-β	Transforming growth factor beta
Th	T-helper
TLRs	Toll-like receptors
TNBS	Trinitrobenzyl sulfonic acid
TNF	Tumor necrosis factor
TRAIL	Tumor necrosis factor-related apoptosis-inducing ligand
TWIST	T*wist* family BHLH transcription factor
UPLC	Ultra-performance liquid chromatography
VEGF	Vascular endothelial growth factor
WA	Withaferin A
WS	*Withania somnifera*

14.1 Introduction

Withanolides are a group of naturally occurring polyoxygenated steroidal lactones assembled on a C_{28} ergostane skeleton. The structural skeleton of withanolides usually varies in the nature and number of oxygenated substituents and the degree of unsaturation of the rings. Structurally diverse withanolides are typically classified based on the arrangement of the C-17 side chain into a major C-22/C-26 δ-lactone/lactol group and a minor C-23/C-26 γ-lactone/lactol group with few exceptions and about 90 % of these compounds possess ketone functionality at C-1 (Figs. 14.1, 14.2) [1–4]. Additionally, withanolides with a C-17 δ-lactone side chain, as shown in Fig. 14.1, can be further categorized into withanolides with an unmodified skeleton (e.g., withaferin A and withaperuvin B) and into those with a

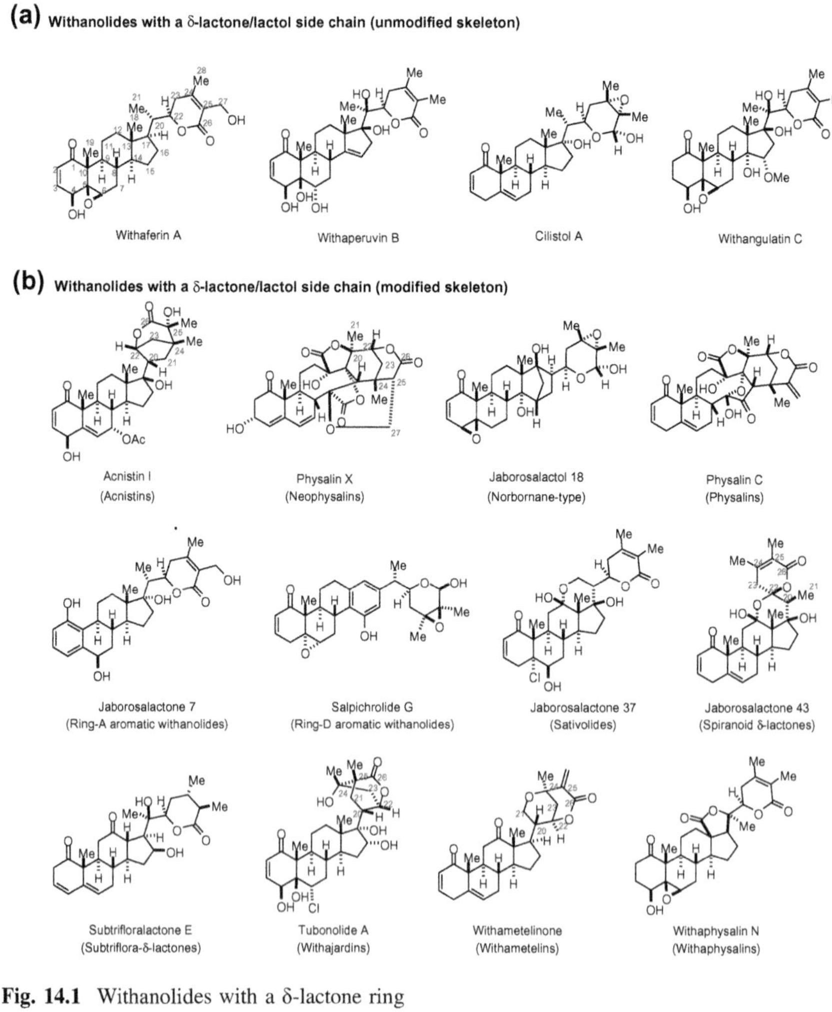

Fig. 14.1 Withanolides with a δ-lactone ring

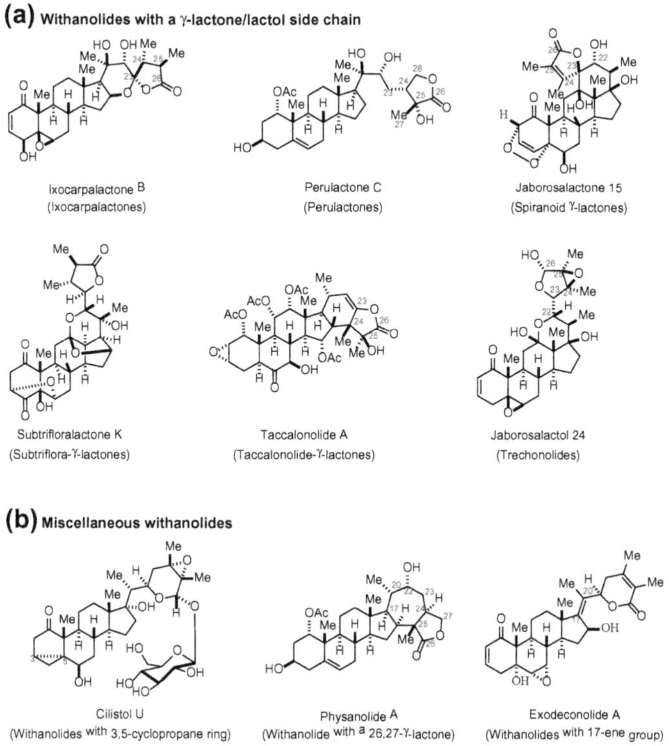

Fig. 14.2 Withanolides with a γ-lactone ring and unclassified structural type

modified skeleton (e.g., physalin C and withametelinone) [1, 2, 4]. The occurrence of unmodified withanolides is more common in nature with approximately 580 of these naturally occurring withanolides reported in the family Solanaceae alone [1–3]. Structurally more complex withanolides with a modified skeleton both in the steroid nucleus and the side chain could possibly result from the biogenetic transformations of unmodified withanolides [3, 5].

Withaferin A (WA), an archetype of this class was discovered from *Withania somnifera* (WS) or Ashwagandha in 1965 [6]. In the past 50 years, approximately 900 withanolides falling into 24 diverse structural types have been discovered [1, 3]. Withanolides are mainly distributed in various genera of Solanaceae, which includes Acnistus, Aureliana, Brachistus, Browallia, Datura, Deprea, Discopodium, Dunalia, Exodeconus, Hyoscyamus, Iochroma, Jaborosa, Larnax, Lycium, Mandragora, Nicandra, Physalis, Salpichroa, Saracha, Solanum, Trechonaetes, Tubocapsicum, Vassobia, Withania, and Witheringia [1–3, 7–9]. A minor population of withanolides has been isolated from other plant sources such as Dioscoreaceae, Fabaceae, Labiatae, Lamiaceae, Leguminosae, Myrtaceae, and Taccaceae [1–3] and interestingly from marine sources of Alcyoniidae family [10–12].

Structurally varied withanolides have received significant attention due to their versatile biological activities demonstrated in vitro and/or in vivo. These activities have been described as antitumor [7, 13–15], cytotoxic [16–20], apoptotic [21–23], anti-inflammatory [9, 10, 24–31], immunomodulating [32–34], antimicrobial [35–37], antistress [34], antioxidant [38], anti-neurodegenerative [39–41], radiosensitizing [42, 43], and insect antifeedant [44, 45]. Withaferin A, the most studied withanolide, possesses a wide array of the pharmacological activities described above and thus carries a great clinical potential for drug development [1, 4, 46–51]. Most notably, the antitumor and associated anti-inflammatory activities of WA and other withanolides results from targeting multiple signaling pathways simultaneously, particularly the nuclear factor kappa B (NF-κB), signal transducer and activator of transcription (STAT), and ubiquitin proteasome pathways (see Tables 14.1, 14.2) [52–57]. The potent biological activities of withanolides such as WA and tubocapsenolide A, especially the antitumor and anti-inflammatory properties have been attributed to the presence of key structural features such as an α,β-unsaturated ketone in ring A, a 5β,6β-epoxide in ring B, and a lactone side chain [1, 4, 7, 13, 30, 58–62]. Cysteine residues in the proteins are often implicated to react with these key electrophilic sites on the withanolide molecule [59, 60, 63, 64]. While other withanolides may possess α,β-unsaturated ketone and/or epoxide in some respect (e.g., paraminabeolides, capsisteroids, and chantriolides) and are bioactive, they are generally less potent than those withanolides possessing all three crucial functional groups.

14.2 Modulation of Inflammatory Cell Signaling Pathways by Withanolides

Inflammation is a complex immunological process by which our body fights against infection, cancer, or injury. The initial, acute stage of inflammation is mediated through the activation of immune cells, the resultant inflammatory cytokines and intracellular pathways. The initial immune mediators are $CD4^+$ T-cells or T-helper (Th) cells and are classified as Th-1, Th-2, and Th-17. They play a crucial role in regulating the cellular and humoral immune responses through recognition of antigens presented on antigen presenting cells via the major histocompatibility complex II. Th-1 cells promote the cellular immune response (macrophages) and primarily produce interferon (IFN)-γ, tumor necrosis factor (TNF)-β, and interleukin (IL)-2, whereas Th-2 cells promote the humoral immune system (antibodies) and primarily produce IL-4 and IL-10, and Th-17 cells help recruit neutrophils early in the adaptive response, produce IL-17 cytokine, and are involved in many autoimmune diseases [82]. The alteration of normal homeostasis of any of the Th cells through aberrant recognition of self or dysregulated production of cytokines plays a major role in the formation of chronic inflammatory or autoimmune/immunomodulatory diseases. Excess cytokine production leads to the over activation of multiple downstream inflammatory pathways, including Janus kinase

Table 14.1 Natural and semi-synthetic anti-inflammatory withanolides

Active compounds	Structures	Plant source	Targets inhibited/Inflammation models	Diseases involved	Ref.
Chantriolide A	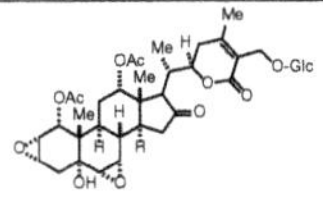 Chantriolide A Glc = β-D-Glucopyranosyl	*Tacca plantaginea* (Dioscoreaceae)*	TNFα-induced NF-κB	Inflammation	(29)
Cilistol G, Capsisteroids A and E	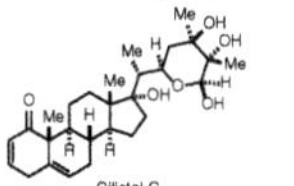 Cilistol G 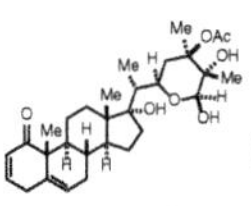 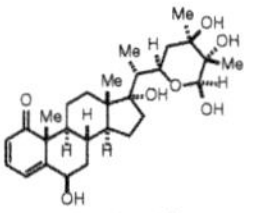 Capsisteroid A Capsisteroid E	*Solanum capsicoides* (Solanaceae)	superoxide anion and elastase release by human neutrophils	Inflammation and cancer	(9)
Coagulin L	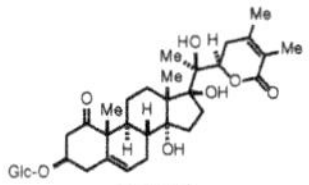 Coagulin L Glc = β-D-Glucopyranosyl	*Withania coagulans* (Solanaceae)	PPARγ, C/EBPα, and MCE	Obesity and metabolic syndrome	(65)
Daturafolisides A and B, Baimantuoluoside B, and 12-Deoxywithastramonolide	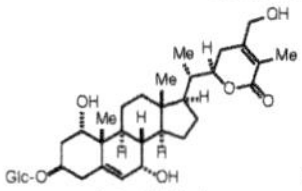 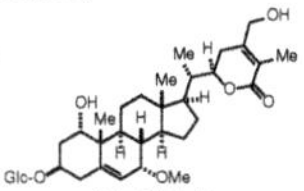 Daturafoliside A Daturafoliside B 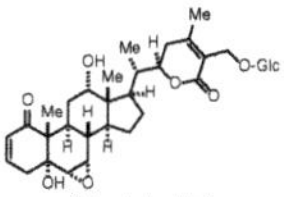 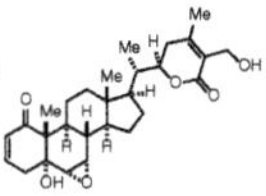 Baimantuoluoside B 12-Deoxywithastramonolide Glc = β-D-Glucopyranosyl	*Datura metel*(Solanaceae)	LPS-induced NO production in macrophages	Inflammation	(27)
Denosomin	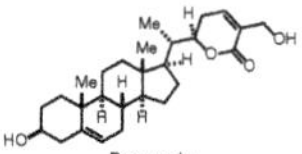 Denosomin	Synthetic	Increases vimentin, neuroprotective	Spinal cord injury	(66)
2,3-Dihydrowithaferin A and 4-(2,2-Dimethyl-3-oxocyclopropoxy)-2,3-dihydrowithaferin A	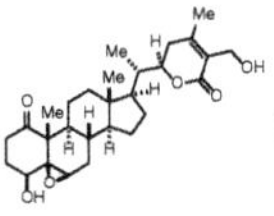 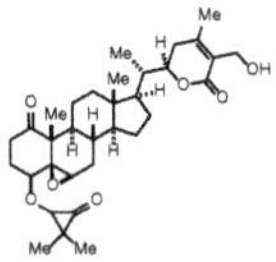 2,3-Dihydrowithaferin A 4-(2,2-Dimethyl-3-oxocyclopropoxy)-2,3-dihydrowithaferin A	*Withania somnifera*(Solanaceae)	COX-2	Inflammation and cancer	(30)
6α,7α-Epoxy-1-oxo-5α,12α,17α-trihydroxywitha-2,24-dienolide	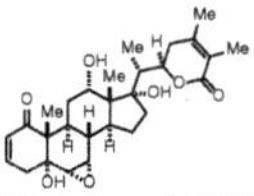 6α,7α-Epoxy-1-oxo-5α,12α,17α-trihydroxywitha-2,24-dienolide	*Discopodium penninervium*(Solanaceae)	LTB_4 and COX-2	Inflammation and cancer	(26)
4β-Hydroxywithanolide E	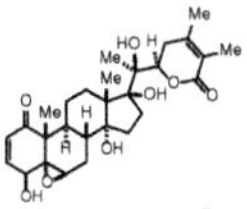 4β-Hydroxywithanolide E	*Physalis pruinosa* (Solanaceae)	NF-κB and MCP-1	Diabetes and obesity	(67)

3β-Hydroxy-2,3-dihydrowithanolide F	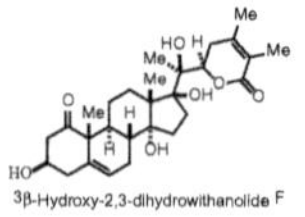	*Withania coagulans* (Solanaceae)	Formalin-induced arthritis model and cotton pellet granuloma method for sub-acute inflammation	Inflammation	(68)
Minabeolides-1, -2, -4, and -5	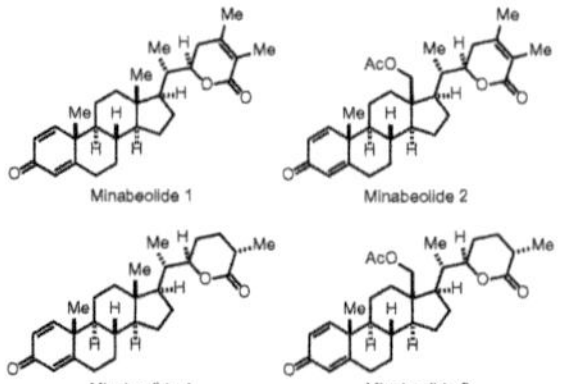	*Paraminabea acronocephala*(Alcyoniidae)	LPS-induced iNOS and COX-2 proteins in macrophages	Inflammation and cancer	(10)
Paraminabeolides A–D	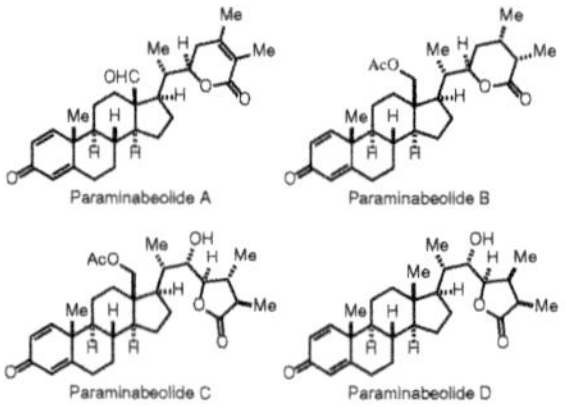	*Paraminabea acronocephala*(Alcyoniidae)	LPS-induced iNOS protein in macrophages	Inflammation and cancer	(10)
Physalins A and O, and Isophysalin A	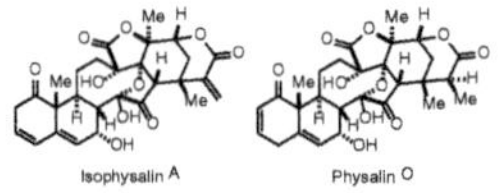	*Physalis alkekengi* (Solanaceae)	IKKβ, NF-κB, and LPS-induced NO production in macrophages	Inflammation	(64)
Physalins C, B, A, N, F and Withanolides E, F, G	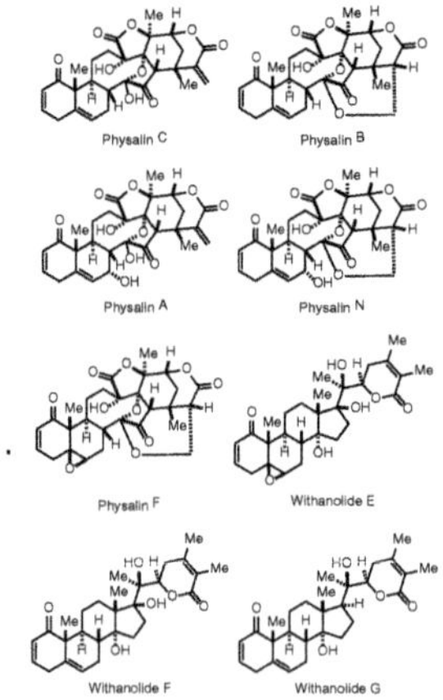	*Physalis alkekengi and Physalis peruviana* (Solanaceae)	TNFα-induced NF-κB	Inflammation and cancer	(59)

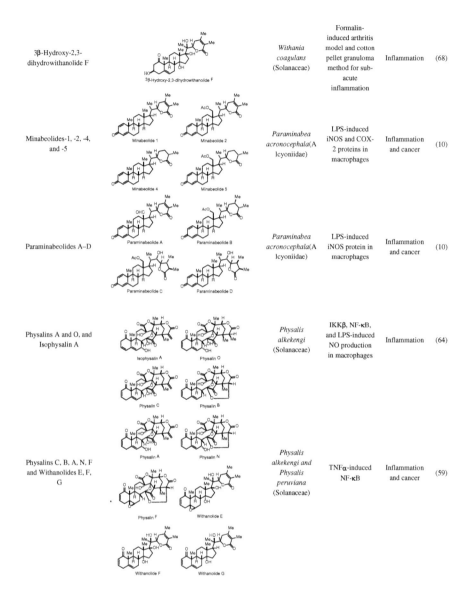

Plantagiolide I	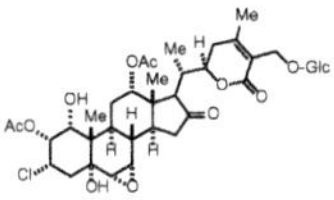 Plantagiolide I Glc = β-D-Glucopyranosyl	*Tacca plantaginea* (Dioscoreaceae)*	PPARs	Inflammation and metabolic disorders such as diabetes and obesity	(29)
Sominone and Withanoside IV	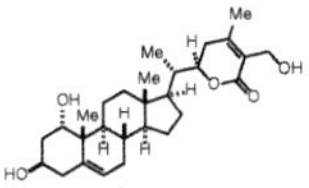 Sominone 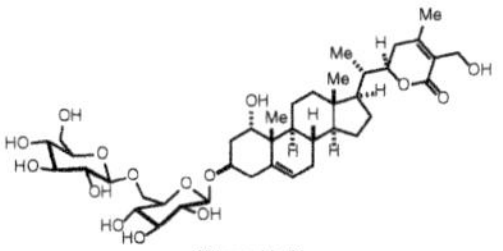 Withanoside IV	*Withania somnifera*(Solanaceae)	Induces neurite outgrowth	Dementia and Alzheimer's disease	(39, 40)
Tubocapsanolide A	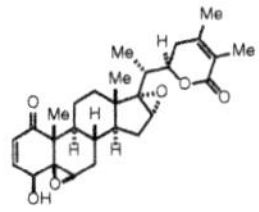 TubocapsanolideA	*Tubocapsicum anomalum* (Solanaceae)	CCR7 expression, IKK, and NF-κB	Cancer	(69)
Tubocapsenolide A	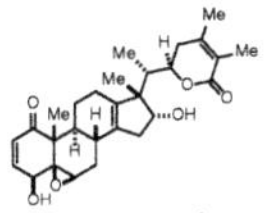 Tubocapsenolide A	*Tubocapsicum anomalum* (Solanaceae)	Hsp90-Hsp70 chaperone complex	Cancer	(62, 70)
Virginols A–C	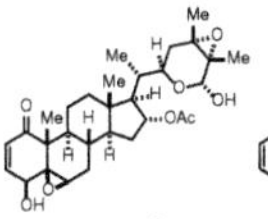 Virginol A 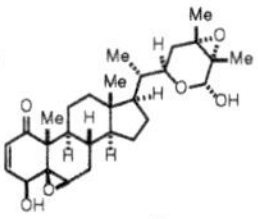 Virginol B 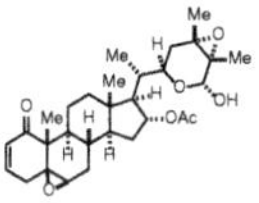 Virginol C	*Physalis virginiana*(Solanaceae)	TPA-induced ear edema assay	Inflammation	(28)
Viscosalactone B	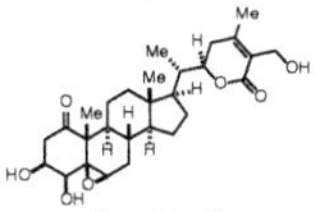 Viscosalactone B	*Withania somnifera*(Solanaceae)	TNFα-induced NF-κB	Inflammation and cancer	(54)
			COX-2	Inflammation and cancer	(30)
Withacnistin	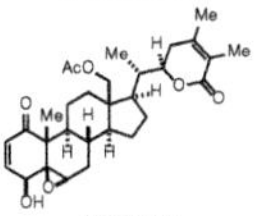 Withacnistin	–†	STAT3 and STAT5	Inflammation and cancer	(71)
			TNFα-induced NF-κB and Ubiquitin proteasome pathway NF-κB and	Angio-inflammatory diseases and cancer	(55)

Withaferin A	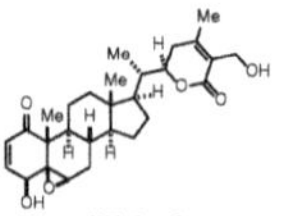 Withaferin A	*Withania somnifera*(Solanaceae)	zymosan-induced inflammed paw model	Inflammation and cancer	(24)
			NF-κB, AP-1, Nrf2, and IL-6	Inflammation and cancer	(72)
			COX-2	Inflammation and cancer	(30)
			STAT3	Inflammation and cancer	(53, 57)
			COX-2, PGE_2, STAT1, and STAT3	Microglial activation	(73)
			LPS-mediated HMGB1 release, ICAMs, and NF-κB	Vascular inflammatory diseases such as atherosclerosis	(51)
			NF-κB and AP-1	Inflammation and cancer	(56)
Withaferin A 4,27-diacetate	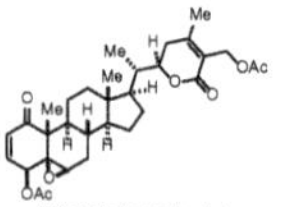 Withaferin A 4,27-diacetate	Semisynthetic	TNFα-induced IKK and NF-κB	Inflammation and cancer	(54)
Withanolide D	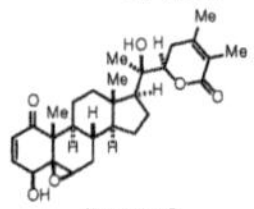 Withanolide D	*Withania somnifera*(Solanaceae)	Ubiquitin proteasome pathway and NF-κB network	Age-related macular degeneration	(52)
Withanolide sulfoxide	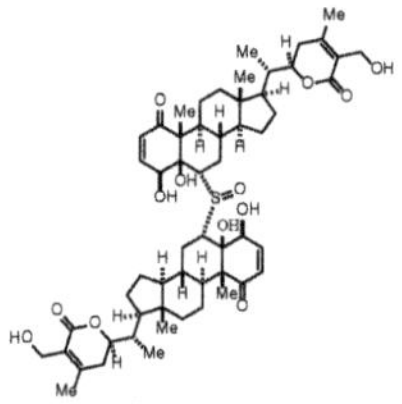 Withanolide sulfoxide	*Withania somnifera* (Solanaceae)	COX-2 and TNFα-induced NF-κB	Inflammation and cancer	(74)

* Reference 28 had the genus Tacca assigned to family Taccaceae, which has been found in older texts but the APG II system has incorporated this genus into the family Dioscoreaceae. † Obtained from National Cancer Institute Developmental Therapeutics Program

(JAK)/STAT, NF-κB, phosphatidylinositol-3-kinase (PI3K)/Akt, and mitogen-activated protein kinase (MAPK). A number of withanolides have demonstrated significant immunomodulatory effects, including WS extract (primarily aqueous extract), withanolide A, physalins and coagulins; however, both immunostimulatory and inhibitory actions have been attributed to different withanolides. WS extract (primarily withanolide A and 2,3 dihydro-3-sulphonile withanone components) is able to shift the immune response toward Th-1 polarization, activate cytotoxic natural killer cells [83, 84], and recover depleted T-cells and increase expression of Th-1 cytokines IL-2 and IFN-γ in models of stress [32, 34, 85, 86]. Conversely, coagulins isolated from *Withania coagulans* and primarily coagulin-H have demonstrated immunosuppressive effects similar to prednisolone, inhibiting stimulated T and B-cell lymphocyte proliferation, and Th-1 cytokine production

Table 14.2 Anti-inflammatory activity of withanolides in plant extracts

Plant extract	Plant part	Active components	Effects	Therapeutic uses	References
Physalis peruviana (Solanaceae)	Fruits	Withanolides, polyphenols, and phytosterols	Antioxidant, anti-inflammatory, and renoprotective	Acute renal injury	[75]
	Calyces	–	Anti-inflammatory and immunosuppressive effect on macrophages apoptopic (downregulates IL-6, TNF, and MCP-1)	Inflammation	[76]
Withania somnifera (Solanaceae)	Roots	Withanolides such as withanolide A and alkaloids	Neuroprotective	Alzheimer's disease	[77]
	Roots	Withanolides, alkaloids, and flavanoids	Immunomodulatory, anti-inflammatory, and proapoptopic (downregulates IL-6, IL-1β, IL-8, Hsp70, and STAT-2)	Cancer	[78]
	Roots	–	Antioxidant, anti-inflammatory, and cytoprotective	Inflammatory bowel disease	[79]
	Leaves	–	Neuroprotective against glutamate neurotoxicity	Stroke and neurodegenerative disorders	[80]
Withania coagulans (Solanaceae)	Fruits	–	Antioxidant, anti-inflammatory, antihyperglycemic, immunomodulatory, and renoprotective (downregulates IL-1β, IL-6, TNFα, IL-4, and IFN-γ)	Diabetes and associated renal complications	[81]

possibly through IL-2 receptor binding [87, 88]. Similar to coagulins, physalins B, F, G, and H isolated from *Physalis angulata* have demonstrated immunosuppressive properties. Physalins B, F, and G showed inhibition of lipopolysaccharide (LPS)-activated macrophages along with their cytokine (TNF-α, IL-6 and IL-12) and nitric oxide (NO) production, whereas concanavalin A-induced T-cell proliferation and cytokine production in a mechanism distinct from dexamethasone [89, 90]. Physalin H has demonstrated polarization to Th-2 cells with inhibition of Th-1 cytokines IL-2 and IFN-γ, increased Th-2 cytokines IL-4 and IL-10, and induction of the heme oxygenase-1 [91].

There are strong preclinical and clinical studies that demonstrate that inflammation initially started by immune cell mediators may persist chronically, resulting in ongoing stimulation of inflammatory mediators and regulatory pathways that contribute to the pathogenesis of chronic diseases including cardiovascular, neurologic, and pulmonary diseases, as well as cancer, diabetes, and obesity [92–94]. As with acute inflammation, chronic inflammation is mediated through various signaling factors, which include proinflammatory cytokines such as TNFα, IL-1, IL-6, IL-8, IL-12, NO, adhesion molecules, and chemokines [95]. Additionally, transcription factors that regulate the expression of inflammatory mediators such as NF-κB, activator protein 1 (AP-1), peroxisome proliferator-activated receptor (PPAR)-γ, STAT3, hypoxia inducible factor-1 (HIF-1), β-catenin/Wnt, hedgehog, and nuclear factor erythroid 2-related factor 2 (Nrf2) have been linked to chronic diseases. The DNA-binding capacity of these transcription factors is modified by several signaling cascades such as JAK/STAT, MAPKs, PI3K/Akt/mechanistic target of rapamycin (mTOR), and ubiquitin proteasome system [96]. These signaling pathways have a wide range of functions and show complex crosstalk depending on the cell type and the chronic disease involved. Withanolides have emerged recently as potential therapeutics for chronic diseases due to their unique ability to modulate multiple signaling pathways. In this chapter, we will discuss several different withanolides and their seemingly broad mechanism of action in modulating key molecular pathways that connect inflammation and chronic diseases.

14.2.1 Withanolides Modulate the NF-κB Pathway

The NF-κB family of transcription factors plays a prominent role in the immune system and inflammation. In response to ligation by Toll-like receptors (TLRs) and IL-1 receptor family members (B-cell and T-cell receptors), NF-κB regulates the expression of several factors such as inhibitor of apoptosis protein-1 (IAP1), inducible nitric oxide synthase (iNOS), cytokines, cyclooxygenase (COX)-2, prostaglandins, growth factors, and effector enzymes [97–99]. NF-κB is activated by inflammatory cytokines, stress, free radicals, radiation, growth receptors, and TNFα leading to transcriptional regulation of several genes that are involved in proliferation, inflammation, cellular survival, apoptosis, angiogenesis, and differentiation [100–103]. The mammalian transcription NF-κB family of proteins includes RelA (p65), RelB, NF-κB2 (p52), c-Rel, and NF-κB1 (p50). In the absence of stimuli, inactive forms of NF-κB proteins are present in the cytoplasm due to their interaction with several inhibitors of kappaB (IκB) proteins. Upon exposure to stimuli, NF-κB is activated either through canonical or noncanonical pathways by regulatory IκB kinases (IKK) such as IKKα, IKKβ, and IKKγ. In the most common classical pathway, IKK phosphorylation leads to IκBα phosphorylation at serine 32 and serine 36, followed by phosphorylation, nuclear localization, DNA binding of p65–p50 complex, and transcriptional activation of NF-κB responsive genes [104].

Activation of NF-κB is essential for the survival and expression of inflammatory mediators. Hence, constitutively active NF-κB is associated with several inflammation-mediated chronic diseases such as cancer, neurological, and metabolic disorders [98].

A number of naturally occuring withanolides such as chantriolide A, physalins A, B, C, and O, viscosalactone B, WA, withanolides D, E, F and withaferin A 4,27-diacetate, a diacetyl derivative of WA have been reported to modulate the regulation of NF-κB [24, 29, 34, 52, 54, 59, 64]. Several studies have examined the beneficial effect of inhibiting transcriptional activity of NF-κB in chronic inflammatory diseases including cancer [24, 55, 56, 72]. In a study led by Aggarwal et al., various withanolides isolated from the leaf extract of WS along with their semi-synthetic acetylated derivatives were tested for their inhibitory effects on NF-κB activation induced by activators such as cigarette smoke condensate, TNF, doxorubicin, and IL-1β [54]. Withaferin A and viscosalactone B along with their 4,27-diacetyl derivative inhibited TNF-induced NF-κB activation in human myeloid leukemia KBM-5 cells, whereas physagulin D and related glycosidic withanolides were inactive. The mechanism through which the above withanolides blocked NF-κB was through the inhibitory effects of activated IκBα, with subsequent phosphorylation of IκBα and p65, followed by prevention of IκBα degradation. Blocking the degradation of IκBα in turn prevents nuclear localization of p65, and activation of NF-κB-dependent gene products such as Bcl-2-related protein A1 (Bfl-1/A1), IAP-1, c-FADD-like cFLIP, ICAM1, and COX-2 [54]. To further understand the SAR, the authors examined TNF-induced NF-κB activity after treatment of human myeloid leukemia KBM-5 cells with various withanolides isolated from the leaf extract of WS along with their synthetically modified acetylated derivatives by electrophoretic mobility shift assay (EMSA). This analysis pointed toward the importance of the α,β-unsaturated ketone in ring A as a required structure for the potent inhibition of NF-κB activity [54].

Physalins A, L, G and O, and isophysalin A isolated from *Physalis alkekengi* were evaluated for their anti-inflammatory properties and Physalins A, O and isophysalin A showed significant inhibition of LPS-induced NO production in macrophages [64]. Based on their structural features characterized by the presence of either an α,β-unsaturated ketone in ring A (physalin O) or an α,β-unsaturated ester in lactone side chain featuring an exomethylene group (physalin A and isophysalin A), these physalins were able to conjugate with glutathione as identified by ultra-performance liquid chromatography tandem mass-spectrometry (UPLC-MS/MS) analysis. Furthermore, peptide mapping and sequencing of alkylated IKKβ using micrOTOF-MS revealed alkylation of six cysteine residues on IKKβ by physalin A indicating IKKβ as a potential target for its anti-inflammatory mechanism of action. In another related and complementary study, SARs were performed on a library of withanolides including the physalins. This study revealed the importance of the oxygenated right-side partial structure (including the lactone side chain) and the 5β,6β-epoxide, or C5–C6 olefin in the B-ring for the inhibition of NF-κB activation [59]. Withanolides and physalins with 5β,6β-epoxide inhibited NF-κB signaling through prevention of IκBα degradation and p65 nuclear localization, whereas those with C5–C6 olefin inhibited NF-κB function by blocking p65/p50 dimer binding to DNA [59].

Chantriolide A, one of the eight compounds isolated from *Taccaplantaginea* exhibited potent inhibition of TNFα-induced NF-κB transcriptional activity in human hepatocellular carcinoma (HepG2) cells in an NF-κB-luciferase assay [29]. In another study, withanolide D and WA from WS inhibited angiogenesis through blocking of NF-κB activity by suppressing proteasome-mediated ubiquitin degradation of IκBα in human umbilical vein endothelial cells [52]. Additionally, 4β-hydroxywithanolide E was shown to inhibit inflammatory response in adipocytes via inhibition of NF-κB transcriptional activity [67]. Inhibition of IKKβ activation by 4β-hydroxy withanolide E through suppression of IKKβ phosphorylation was mechanistically distinct from the NF-κB inhibition observed for WA, where the induction of IKKβ over-phosphorylation was shown to inhibit IKKβ activation [24]. Moreover in vivo, 4β-hydroxy withanolide E demonstrated an improvement of impaired glucose tolerance suggesting its potential role for the treatment/prevention of metabolic disorders including type 2 diabetes [67]. Overexpression of CCR7 in metastatic breast cancer cells has been associated with lymph node metastasis [69]. In breast cancer cells MDA-MB-231, tubocapsanolide A inhibited TAK1 to suppress NF-κB-mediated CCR7 expression leading to the inhibition of lymphatic invasion of breast cancer in vitro and in vivo.

In addition to the inhibition of NF-κB activation, WA and several other withanolides have been shown to directly block the expression of LPS- or TNFα-induced NF-κB-regulated inflammatory genes such as iNOS, COX-1, COX-2, and NO [10, 13, 14, 25, 26, 64, 74]. Nitric oxide is a small molecule that regulates MMPs and joints extracellular matrix, and is modulated through iNOS. COX-1 and COX-2 convert arachidonic acid to prostaglandins, which in turn cause a significant inflammatory response. COX-1 is constitutively expressed in most cell types, and is responsible for maintenance of normal physiologic function, whereas COX-2 is inducible in response to proinflammatory cytokines [26]. Nair and co-workers were the first to demonstrate the role of withanolides in inhibiting COX enzymes and provide insight into their anti-inflammatory mechanism [30]. Withaferin A, viscosalactone B, 2,3-dihydrowithaferin A, and 4-(2,2-dimethyl-3-oxocyclopropoxy)-2,3-dihydrowithaferin A were shown to inhibit COX-2 enzyme but not COX-1. Interestingly, during this study it was observed that the presence of a double bond between C-24 and C-25 in the lactone ring was essential for COX inhibitory activities and a withanolide lacking this unsaturation in the lactone ring was found to be inactive against both COX-1 and COX-2 enzymes [30].6α,7α-Epoxy-1-oxo-5α,12α,17α-trihydroxywitha-2,24-dienolide from *Discopodiumpenninervium* was found to inhibit COX-2 and leukotriene B_4 (LTB_4) but was inactive against the COX-1 enzyme [26]. Like other withanolides, withanolide sulfoxide, a sulfoxide dimer of WA was highly selective in inhibiting COX-2 compared to COX-1[74].

Daturafolisides A and B along with other known withanolides from *Datura metel* were shown to exhibit significant reduction in NO production in LPS-induced RAW 264.7 macrophage cells [27]. Of note, both of these compounds lack the α,β-unsaturated ketone in ring A and the 5β,6β-epoxide in ring B, however, they do possess a δ-lactone side chain. Additionally, withanolides such as paraminabeolides and minabeolides obtained from a marine source were found to inhibit LPS-induced iNOS expression in RAW 264.7 macrophages, with minabeolides also effectively inhibiting COX-2 expression [10].

14.2.2 Withanolide Modulation of the JAK/STAT Pathway

The JAK/STAT pathway is a key-signaling mediator of cytokines and growth factors such as platelet-derived growth factor (PDGF), epidermal growth factor (EGF), IL6, as well as oncogenic proteins [105]. Activation of STAT proteins depends on their binding to cytokines and growth factor receptors on the plasma membrane followed by tyrosine phosphorylation either directly by receptor tyrosine kinases (RTKs) or by non RTKs such as JAK or Src [106, 107]. Upon phosphorylation, cytoplasmic STAT proteins undergo dimerization via reciprocal SH2-domain/phosphotyrosine interactions followed by translocation to the nucleus for DNA binding to STAT-specific response elements leading to transcriptional activation. There are eight known STAT proteins (STATs 1A, 1B, 2, 3, 4, 5A, 5B, and 6) that play diverse biochemical roles in several important processes such as survival, proliferation, apoptosis, invasion, immune response, inflammation, and angiogenesis [105, 108, 109]. Among the eight isoforms STAT3 and STAT5 are constitutively activated in several solid tumors, including lung, bladder, breast, colon, as well as in hematological malignancies [108]. Additionally, STAT3 is also interconnected with the NF-κB pathway and plays a central role in inflammation [107].

Several chronic diseases including cancer have been shown to induce aberrant regulation of STAT3. This transcription factor promotes oncogenic processes such as invasion, metastasis, and angiogenesis as several genes involved in these mechanisms such as cyclin D1, c-Myc, vascular endothelial growth factor (VEGF), mucin 1 (MUC-1), twist family BHLH transcription factor (TWIST) are all regulated by STAT3 [110–114]. Studies have investigated the role of WA from WS in regulating STAT proteins in different cancer models including colon cancer, breast cancer, multiple myeloma, and neuroblastoma [53, 57, 115, 116]. In breast cancer, WA treatment of triple negative MDA-MB-231 and hormonally active MCF-7 cells effectively decreased the constitutive as well as the IL-6 inducible phosphorylation of JAK 2 and its downstream target STAT3 thereby inhibiting the transcriptional activity of STAT3 [115]. In renal carcinoma Caki cells, WA had a similar effect and also downregulated the expression levels of anti-apoptotic proteins that are regulated by STAT3 like Bcl-2, cyclin D1, survivin, and Bcl-xL, thereby inducing apoptosis [116]. Docking studies showed that WA not only downregulates the phosphorylation of STAT3 at the tyrosine Y705, but also prevents dimerization of STAT3 [57]. In addition to cancer cells, WA also is able to suppress the phosphorylation of STAT1/3 in murine BV2 microglial cells, leading to a reduction in LPS-induced COX-2 downregulation and PGE_2 production [73]. Withacnistin, an unmodified withanolide blocked both IL-6 as well as EGF-stimulated binding of STAT3 and STAT5 to gp130 and EGF-receptor (EGFR) in MDA-MB-468 breast cancer cells. This resulted in subsequent downregulation of STAT3 tyrosine phosphorylation and decreased nuclear translocation. Further evaluation of STAT3-DNA binding and transcriptional activity after Withacnistin treatment revealed blocking of both DNA binding as well as STAT3 reporter activity. This in turn caused downregulation of STAT3 target genes Bcl-xL and MCL-1 resulting in apoptosis [71].

14.2.3 Modulation of the AP-1 Pathway by Withanolides

The transcription factor AP-1, which plays a key role in the inflammatory response is implicated in several diseases such as cancer, psoriasis, inflammatory bowel disease (IBD), rheumatoid arthritis (RA) and fibrosis [117]. The AP-1 complex consists of homo and hetero dimers of Jun (JunD, C-Jun, and JunB) and the Fos (FosB, C-Fos, Fra-1 and Fra-2) family of proteins [118, 119]. Cytokines, chemokines, hormones, and growth factors as well as external stress factors are known to activate AP-1 signaling. The AP-1 complex translocates to the nucleus in response to stress signaling cascades, such MAPKs and c-Jun terminal kinases [120]. This in turn leads to activation of AP-1 and regulates multiple functions such as differentiation, transformation, proliferation, and survival [121]. The crude ethanol extract of WS has been shown to inhibit the nuclear localization of both AP-1 and NF-κB in LPS-activated peripheral blood mononuclear cells (PBMC) of both normal and RA patients, as well as synovial fluid mononuclear cells (SFMC) of RA patients. This in turn led to decreased downstream transcription target genes such as MMPs, COX-2, and iNOS, all of which are known mediators of RA [122].

14.2.4 Withanolides Can Modulate the PPARγ Pathway

PPARγ was first discovered in adipocyte differentiation and lipid metabolism and is one of three members in this nuclear receptor family of transcription factors [123]. The other members of the PPARs in mammals are PPARα and PPARβ/δ. The PPARs activate several genes involved in inflammation, adipogenesis, lipid metabolism, glucose metabolism, cellular differentiation, development, and tumorigenesis via binding of the PPAR/retinoid X receptor heterodimer to PPAR-responsive regulatory elements [124, 125]. PPARγ plays a key role in inflammation through modulation of proinflammatory transcription factors such as NF-κB and AP-1 [113]. Treatment of 3T3-L1 adipocytes with WA resulted in phosphorylation of extracellular signal-regulated kinase (ERK), followed by decreased expressions of PPARγ leading to altered levels of Bcl_2 and Bax expression, induction of apoptosis, and inhibition of adipogenesis [126]. In addition to WA, other withanolides such as plantagiolide J and I isolated from *Taccaplantaginea* [29] and coagulin-L isolated from *Withania coagulans* [65] also modulate PPARγ transcriptional activity.

14.2.5 Modulation of the Hsp90 Pathway by Withanolides

Heat shock proteins (Hsp) are ATP-dependent ubiquitously expressed molecular chaperones that are involved in the folding, assembly, maintenance, and transport of key regulatory proteins involved in numerous signaling pathways in the cell. Several environmental and physiological stimuli such as hypoxia, oxidative damage, inflammation, infection, and elevated temperature induce the expression of these highly conserved molecular chaperone family of proteins as a protein homeostasis and survival response [70, 114]. The Hsp90 family of proteins (Hsp90α, Hsp90β, GRP94, and TRAP1) form a large complex with other co-chaperones such as cdc37, HSP70-HSP90 organizing protein, p27, Hsp32, and Hsp70. This complex then stabilizes and maintains functional activity of proteins/kinases in many key signaling pathways, such as PI3K/Akt/mTOR, p38/MAPK, and NF-κB, all of which play critical roles in inflammation, chronic inflammatory diseases, and oncogenesis. Through inhibition of Hsp90, and therefore inhibition of its oncogenic chaperone clients, cancer cells undergo apoptosis [124, 125].

Several studies have shown that withanolides such as WA, withalongolides A and B, tubocapsenolide A, and some of their synthetically modified analoges such as withalongolide A triacetate and withalongolide B diacetateare are able to target multiple cancers such as colon, prostate, brain, breast, head and neck, skin, adrenal, and thyroid both in vitro and in vivo [17, 20, 21, 53, 63, 70, 127–137]. Withanolides such as WA and withalongolide A are known to block Hsp90 chaperone function through blocking the Hsp90/cdc37 complex, and induction of thiol-mediated oxidative stress [63, 138, 139]. The Hsp90/cdc37 complex facilitates active conformation of client kinases in particular, such as Akt, cyclin-D1, raf-1, and cdk4. Blocking this complex leads to dysfunctional or proteasome mediated degradation of these kinases within multiple oncogenic, pro-survival, and proliferative kinase cascades (p38/MAPK, PI3K/Akt/mToR, NF-κB pathways), which ultimately leads to cancer cell apoptosis [136, 138]. In addition to targeting the bulk cancer cell population, WA and withalongolide A triacetate may also target the cancer stem cell (CSC) population. These CSCs comprise a small fraction of cancer cells, and are characterized by their tumor initiating and self-renewal capacity. WA and withalongolide A triacetate block several developmental pathways such as Wnt/β-catenin, notch, and NF-κB, as well as vimentin and VEGF, all of which are important in inflammation, self-renewal, and CSC epithelial-to-mesenchymal transition [115, 140–145].

14.2.6 Withanolide Modulation of Nrf2 Pathway

Nuclear factor erythroid 2 related factor 2(Nrf2) is a transcription factor that regulates genes involved in redox homeostasis, inflammation, energy metabolism and cellular growth [146]. Under normal homeostatic conditions, Nrf2 is anchored in the cytoplasm as a complex with Kelch like ECH-associated protein-1 (Keap1), which facilitates ubiquitin mediated proteasome degradation of Nrf2 and decreased expression of Nrf2 target genes. However, in response to stimulation by growth factors, electrophilic stressors, and changes in redox signal, Nrf2 ubiquitination is disrupted and levels increase rapidly. Nrf2 translocates to the nucleus and upregulates expression of proteins involved in glutathione and thioredoxin-based antioxidant defense, drug metabolism and efflux, and proteins associated with heme and iron metabolism [147]. Nrf2 is engaged in crosstalk with several signaling pathways that play a critical role in the pathogenesis and progression of chronic diseases, including NF-κB, PI3K, MAPK, glycogen synthase kinase-3β, and notch [146, 147]. Molecular docking studies have shown that both WA and withanone interact with the amino acids Ala 69, Gln 75, and Phe 71 of Nrf2 [148]. In another study, WA induced reactive oxygen species (ROS) that activated JNK and stabilized Nrf2 that resulted in activation of NADPH quinone oxidoreductase and Tap73 transcriptional function leading to apoptosis of cancer cells [149]. WA was also shown to inhibit NFκB, AP-1, and Nrf2 in adriamycin-resistant human myelogenous erythroleukemic K562/Adr cells in a dose-dependent manner [72]. Moreover, compared to other tested natural products such as quercetin, only WA overcomes attenuated caspase activation and blocking of apoptosis in K562/Adr cells [72].

14.2.7 Modulation of the HIF-1 Pathway by Withanolides

Under normal oxygen conditions, the HIF-1 α protein is synthesized at a high rate and rendered transcriptionally inactive due to immediate hydroxylation-dependent proteasome/ubiquitin degradation by the VHL E3 ligase. However, when hypoxia is induced through impaired cellular oxygen balance, hydroxylase activity is downregulated, HIF-α protein is stabilized, and HIF-1 is activated [150]. Transcriptional activation of HIF-1 upregulates several genes that control glycolytic metabolism, angiogenesis, invasion, metastasis, and cell survival, such as VEGF, MMPs, stromal cell-derived factor-1, e-cadherin, chemokine receptor 4, EGF, and transforming growth factor beta (TGF-β) 3 [151–155]. Crosstalk between NF-κB and HIF pathways has been shown to be associated with several chronic inflammatory diseases such as cancer, RA, asthma, and chronic obstructive pulmonary diseases [156]. In solid tumors, the availability of oxygen within the tumor decreases as distance from blood vessels increases resulting in the creation of hypoxic regions [157]. This is known to be responsible in part for therapy resistance and metastatic spread [158]. Although, no study thus far directly demonstrates inhibition of HIF-1 transcriptional activation by withanolides, a few note down-regulation of migration-promoting HIF-mediated genes such as VEGF, heterogeneous nuclear ribonucleoprotein K (hnRNP-K) and MMPs, which lead to restriction of angiogenesis and metastasis [159].

14.3 Withanolides for Clinical Development

As discussed above, studies show the ability of withanolides to target multiple interconnected signaling pathways such as PI3K/Akt/mTOR, JAK/STAT, AP-1, NF-κB, PPARγ, Nrf2 and MAPK. Withanolides target these pathways through multiple mechanism, such as blocking Hsp90-Cdc37 co-chaperone interaction, targeting Akt and its downstream pathways, and induction of thiol-mediated oxidative stress (summarized in Fig. 14.3). Each of these mechanisms and pathway interactions play important roles in the development of chronic inflammatory diseases. Building on the studies identifying mechanisms of action of withanolides, we will discuss the clinical importance of withanolides on inflammatory mediated diseases including chronic inflammatory/autoimmune, cancer, and neurologic.

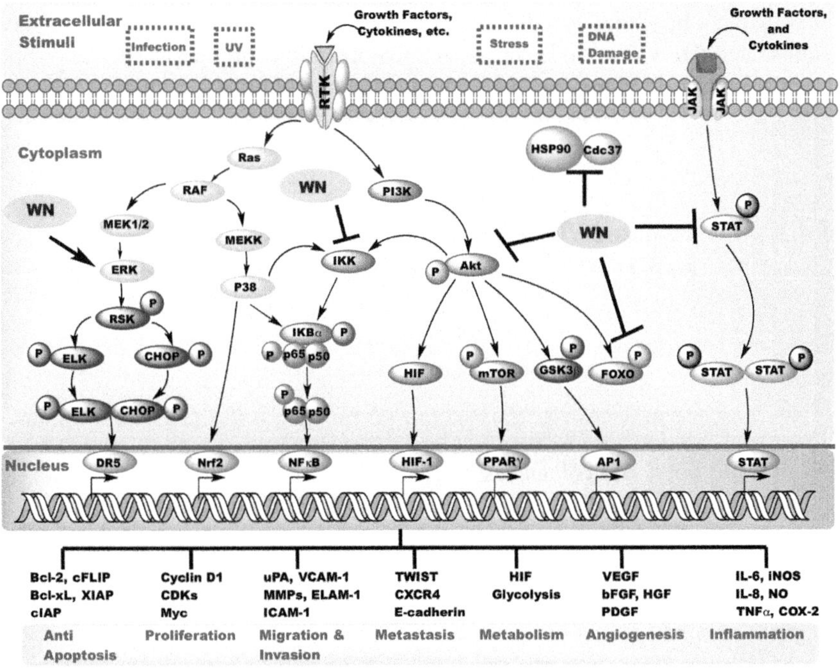

Fig. 14.3 Schematic diagram representing modulation of various inflammatory pathways by withanolides

14.4 Application of Withanolides in Inflammatory/Autoimmune Diseases

14.4.1 Osteoarthritis and Rheumatoid Arthritis

In Ayurvedic medicine, withanolides are frequently used to treat both osteoarthritis (OA) and RA and there are several anti-inflammatory pathways affected by withanolides that contribute to chondro protection and treatment. The previously described NF-κB pathway plays a key role in arthritic inflammation, as do the downstream effectors NO via iNOS, COX-1, and COX-2 enzymes [160]. NO has been implicated in chondrocyte apoptosis in RA [161] and WS extracts have demonstrated reductions in NO in murine macrophage cell lines [122] and human chondrocytes [162]. Nonsteroidal anti-inflammatory drugs nondiscriminately inhibit COX enzymes, which with chronic use increases the risk of upper GI ulcers. Withanolides have been demonstrated to exhibit significant selective COX-2 inhibition while sparing COX-1 [13, 26, 163]. Additionally, along a parallel proinflammatory pathway with arachidonic acid, withanolides inhibited the production of LTB_4 [26].

Another important mediator of arthritis is the formation of ROS leading to oxidative stress, and the protective role of Nrf2 pathway in glutathione and thioredoxin-based antioxidant defense [164]. However, the exact mechanism by which withanolides act within this pathway is still unclear as studies have demonstrated that withanolides are both ROS protective through inhibition of lipid peroxidation [13, 163] and can induce oxidative stress in rabbit chondrocytes [165, 166].

14.4.2 Therapeutic Benefits of Withanolides for Osteoarthritis and Rheumatoid Arthritis In Vivo

There have been several studies indicating that withanolides have a chrondroprotective aspect. WS extract has been shown in animal models to significantly reduce the effects of collagenase on bovine Achilles tendons with even a suggestion of collagen stabilization [167]. This has also been demonstrated with inhibition of the gelatinase activity of collagenase type 2 enzyme in vitro [168]. Several collagen-induced arthritic rat models have noted significant amelioration of paw and ankle arthritis, oxidative stress, degradation of cartilage, and improvements in functional recovery and radiological score [24, 169–171]. Aqueous extracts of WS have demonstrated a significant dose-dependent reduction in adjuvant-induced hind foot pad thickness, reductions in immune complement activity [172], as well as reduced arthritic index, autoantibodies, and CRP levels with results comparable to methotrexate treatment. These rats similarly demonstrate reductions in oxidative stress through decreased lipid peroxidation, glutathione-S-transferase activity, and an increase in glutathione content and ferric-reducing ability [170]. In a monosodium urate crystal-induced rat model of gout, WS extract demonstrated a significant reduction in paw pad volume down to that of normal controls as well as analgesic and antipyretic effects without any evidence of gastric injury [173]. Despite the conflicting reports of WA increasing oxidative stress and reducing type II collagen through induction of COX-2 by microRNA-25 [166], the majority of evidence continues to support the chondroprotective and analgesic properties of withanolides in arthritis.

14.4.3 Clinical Activity of Withanolides for Osteoarthritis and Rheumatoid Arthritis

On the basis of the long-standing use of WS extract in the treatment of arthritis in Ayurvedic medicine and the support from animal models, there have been several human tissue and blood studies performed in recent years. WS root powder extracts were given to patients with chronic OA and mild to moderate (Grade 1–2) articular cartilage and a portion of the cartilage was explanted for analysis. Half of the cartilage samples had a significant short-term chondroprotective response as demonstrated by significant decreases in proteoglycan release [168]. Further research on the explanted cartilage also demonstrated a significant reduction in NO production as an inflammatory regulator molecule in 50 % of the patient samples [162].

In RA, WS crude ethanol extract significantly inhibited LPS-induced expression of multiple proinflammatory cytokines from PBMCs and SFMCs taken from RA and normal patients, including TNF-α, IL-1β, and IL-12 p40. The reduction in inflammatory cytokines may have resulted from suppression of LPS-activated NF-κB and AP-1, in addition to inhibition of AP-1 nuclear translocation and LPS-induced phosphorylation of IκBα [122].

Although there have been several human trials for OA and RA, they were developed using combinations of Ayurvedic drugs. Combination therapy RA-11 (that includes WS, *Boswelliaserrata*, *Zingiberofficinale*, and *Curcumalonga*) was given to patients in a randomized, placebo-controlled OA trial. Results demonstrated a mean reduction in pain (using visual analog scale) and in the modified WOMAC index (Western Ontario McMaster University OA Index) at 16 and 32 weeks compared to placebo without any significant in adverse events [174]. A pilot prospective study of the combination Ashwagandha and SidhMakardhwaj in RA demonstrated a significant ACR20 (20 % improvement in tender joint/swollen join counts and 20 % reduction in 3 of 5 areas, physician global assessment score, patient global assessment score, pain assessment score, patient self-assessed disability index score, and ESR) response in 56 % of patients, and a moderate response in 40 % of patients by EULAR criteria (European League Against Rheumatism) [175]. Although only part of a combination therapy and the effects of WS alone cannot be determined, these trials suggest that withanolides may have chondroprotective, anti-inflammatory, and analgesic characteristics in human joints without significant adverse events.

14.4.4 Applications in Systemic Lupus Erythematous and Inflammatory Bowel Disease

The pathogenesis of systemic lupus erythematous (SLE) and IBD is rooted in chronic, aberrant activation of the immune system and inflammatory pathways. SLE is a complex B-cell mediated autoimmune disease characterized by the generation of autoantibodies against nuclear antigens (antinuclear antibody) and a type III hypersensitivity reaction (antibody–antigen complexes) leading to chronic inflammation and deposition of the antibody–antigen complexes within small vessels of end organs, such as the kidneys, skin, and brain [176]. In IBD, although chronic, intermittent inflammation is a cornerstone of disease progression, the pathogenesis is more complex, involving genetic susceptibilities, perturbation of mucosal physiology/epithelial barrier, and homeostasis of intestinal innate immune system [177]. For both SLE and IBD, current therapies are based upon anti-inflammatory, immunosuppressive, or immune/biologic therapies. Ongoing therapeutic research is focused on identifying additional immune targets including modulation of the Th-1, Th-2 and Th-17 responses, inflammatory cytokines, and downstream inflammatory pathways [178, 179]. As discussed previously, withanolides including *Withania coagulin,* and *Physalis angulata* have demonstrated significant immunomodulatory effects on Th cells and inflammatory cytokines making these compounds an exciting new area of therapeutic development for inflammatory and autoimmune diseases.

14.4.5 Therapeutic Benefits of Withanolides for SLE and IBD In Vivo

The recent characterization of the effects of withanolides on immunomodulation has given rise to several in vivo animal models of SLE and IBD. Aqueous WS extracts were used to treat a nonautoimmune pristane-induced model of SLE in mice, which develop SLE-like symptoms, including autoantibody production, proteinuria, and nephritis. The prophylactic effects of WS extract were characterized by orally administering WS for one month prior and six months following pristane injections. WS treatment resulted in significant reductions in ROS formation within intraperitoneal macrophages, as well as reductions in inflammatory cytokines (IL-6 and TNF-α), and decreased inflammation within the kidneys, liver, and lung, however, no reduction in the humoral response autoantibodies or immune complex deposition [180, 181].

Using trinitrobenzylsulfonic acid (TNBS)-induced IBD model in rats, a rectal gel formulation from aqueous WS extract was administered from the fourth to fourteenth day, and demonstrated a dose-dependent inhibition of lipid peroxidation up to 96 %, hydrogen peroxide scavenging up to 82 %, and NO scavenging ability similar to curcumin. Histopathology demonstrated a significant decrease in colonic injury with WS treatment along with improvement in macroscopic damage when compared to untreated controls. WS-treated rats also retained their weight with improved recovery following induction of the TNBS model [79].

While the animal data for these inflammatory and autoimmune diseases remains relatively sparse, there has yet to be any major human studies using withanolides in these diseases. In the meantime, the immunomodulatory effects of withanolides continue to be characterized and hold therapeutic potential for the treatment of a number of autoimmune and immune-modulating diseases.

14.5 Application of Withanolides in Cancer Therapy

The discovery that most withanolides have cytotoxic capabilities against a wide range of cancers has initiated a large breadth of research into the cytotoxic mechanisms and potential therapeutic benefits of withanolides for cancer treatment and prevention. As previously described and depicted in Fig. 14.3, withanolides inhibit multiple aspects of inflammatory pathways. While these inflammatory pathways have complex interactions between one another, they also interact with proliferative and oncogenic pathways. Several key mechanisms of cytotoxicity from withanolides have been described and these include: (a) induction of oxidative stress, (b) inhibition of proteasome mediated ubiquitin degradation of IκBα (leading to inhibition of NF-κB and its downstream effectors AP-1 and Nrf-2), (c) inhibition of transcription factor STAT3, (d) inhibition of Hsp90 (by blocking interaction of the Cdc37 co-chaperone with Hsp90) with resultant Hsp90 client inhibition in the PI3K/Akt and MAPK pathways, (e) dysregulation of cytoskeletal and structural proteins, and (f) angiogenesis inhibition though HIF-1 [1, 137, 182, 183]. Withanolides with significant activity and identified mechanisms are depicted in Table 14.1, and their cytotoxic characteristics have been demonstrated in multiple cancer types, including breast, ovarian, colon, head and neck, renal, prostate, pancreatic, thyroid, glioblastoma, and hematologic cancers such as lymphoma, leukemia, and multiple myeloma [1, 70, 136, 182–186].

14.5.1 Anticancer Benefits of Withanolides in Animal Models

The groundwork done in vitro to establish the cytotoxic effect of withanolides against cancer cell lines and characterize their multiple mechanisms of therapeutic potential led to the translational evaluation of these compounds in several cancer animal models. Since cancer is a heterogeneous complex disease process, different cancers utilize different key oncogenic pathways for survival. Because different aspects of the inflammatory pathways are important in various cancer models, withanolides demonstrate cytotoxic effects on tumor growth, rate of metastatic spread, and even prevention. Looking at the STAT3 pathway in a colorectal cancer in vivo model, WS extract treatment attenuated IL-6 activation of STAT3 and demonstrated a 1.44 fold decrease in average tumor volume [53].

Following the initial characterization of a novel withanolide tubocapsenolide A to inhibit Hsp90–Hsp70 complex function in breast cancer through direct thiol oxidation [70], WA was shown to bind to the C-terminal of Hsp90, disrupt the Hsp90–Cdc37 complex, and inhibit chaperone activity in pancreatic cancer. Pancreatic cancer xenografts treated daily with withanolides demonstrated a 58 % reduction in average tumor volume compared to controls [63]. In medullary thyroid cancer, RET, a known Hsp90 client, is a key proto-oncogene that encodes for a transmembrane RTK. WA treatment of medullary thyroid xenografts not only inhibited RET phosphorylation and activation, but also inhibited phospho-Akt and phospho-ERK protein expression ex vivo. The xenograft tumors also demonstrated significant, 2-week delayed growth kinetics with 80 % of mice responding to WA treatment, as well as improved survival when compared to controls [187]. Withanolide E has also been shown to sensitize renal carcinoma cells to tumor necrosis factor-related apoptosis-inducing ligand (TRAIL)-mediated apoptosis through cFLIP degradation as a result of inhibited Hsp90 chaperone function. Combination treatment of mouse renal carcinoma xenografts with withanolide E and a TRAIL death receptor agonist demonstrated complete and sustained tumor responses in 55 % of treated mice compared to control or either treatment alone [188].

Cytoskeletal and structural protein inhibition by withanolides has been shown to lead to cell cycle arrest, decreased epithelial-to-mesenchymal transition (EMT), and decreased metastasis. In breast cancer, WA binds to and inhibits β-tubulin, decreasing β-tubulin protein levels in G_0–G_1 phase cells and severely disrupting normal spindle morphology, both of which lead to cell cycle arrest [14]. Withaferin A also induces perinuclear vimentin (a mesenchymal protein) accumulation leading to rapid vimentin depolymerization and disrupted morphology. In both murine mammary carcinoma and human xenograft breast cancer models in mice, WA and WS treatment showed a dose-dependent inhibition of tumor growth kinetics, a decrease in number of metastatic lung nodules, and an increase in ser56 phosphorylated vimentin that is indicative of disassembly [189, 190]. Subsequent studies also showed that WA treatment attenuated TNF-α and TGF-β induced EMT, increased the epithelial phenotype protein E-cadherin, and inhibited vimentin expression in addition to inhibited tumor grown kinetics and cell proliferation [23, 143]. Together, these studies characterize the ability of WA to inhibit EMT both in vitro and in vivo, which may inhibit the metastatic potential of these tumors.

Another area of research in cancer therapy is the inhibition of angiogenesis which limits the oxygen and nutrient supply to growing tumors as well as their metastatic capabilities. Withanolides demonstrate significant angiogenesis inhibition [55] and as previously described, mechanisms include blocking NF-κB activity along with inhibition of cyclin D1 expression through suppressing proteasome-mediated ubiquitin degradation of IκBα [52, 55], and the interplay between NF-κB, JAK/STAT, HIF-1 and downstream targets VEGF, hnRNP-K, and MMPs [52, 140, 159]. Using both a subcutaneous flank xenograft and lung metastasis murine model with fibrosarcoma cells, withanone and WA demonstrated significant suppression of both subcutaneous and lung metastasis tumor growth compared to controls. The ex vivo tumors then demonstrated decreased expression of hnRNP-K and downstream effectors VEGF, Erk p44/42, and MMP2 [159]. In an in vivo assay of neovascularization using subcutaneously injected Matrigel that contained VEGF and bFGF, mice treated with 3-azido withaferin A (3-azidoWA) demonstrated a marked reduction in neovascularization with both preventative and treatment dosing when compared to untreated controls [50].

Not only have withanolides demonstrated significant cytotoxicity in multiple cancer models, but they have also demonstrated the capability to prevent cancer growth and implantation [137]. The induction of the phase II enzyme quinone reductase (QR) in mouse hepatoma cells has been used as a biological screen for chemopreventive compounds, and multiple withanolides have demonstrated robust induction of QR with minimal toxicity [191]. Subsequently in rodent models, pretreatment with the WS root isolate 1-oxo-5beta, 6beta-epoxy-witha-2-enolide prevented the formation of cutaneous malignancy and were absent p53 + foci that were noted in untreated rats that had been exposed to ultraviolet B radiation and benzoyl peroxide [192]. Additionally, WS root extract inhibited benzo(a) pyrene-induced forestomach papillomagenesis by 60 % and 7,12-dimethylbenzanthracene-induced skin papillomagenesis by 45 % [193]. It has been proposed that one mechanism of cutaneous chemoprevention is through inhibition of carcinogen-induced upregulation of acetyl-CoA carboxylase by suppressing AP-1 activation [194]. In a mouse mammary tumor virus-neu (MMTV-neu) transgenic model that forms spontaneous tumors, preventative WA treatment led to a significant 50 % reduction in average mammary tumor weight, a 95 % reduction in average area of invasive carcinoma, and a 73 % reduction in incidence of lung metastasis [195]. Another important antitumor effect of these withanolides is that they can also target breast cancer stem cells. Treatment of breast cancer cells with WA resulted in decreased ability to form mammospheres as well as significantly decreased aldehyde dehydrogenase activity within the mammary tumor cells [196]. WS root extract has also been shown to reduce the formation of spontaneous estrogen receptor negative mammary tumors in the MMTV-neu mice when mice were fed a diet containing the extract [197].

Overall these in vivo studies also noted that withanolides were well tolerated without significant reductions in animal weight, necrosis, or fibrosis when compared to placebo [23, 143, 159, 189, 190, 192, 193, 195]. The promising results of withanolides observed thus far in cancer models have led to ongoing research by many centers to both identify new withanolides and evaluate existing withanolides in multiple cancer models. In the last few years, withanolides have also been shown to demonstrate tumor cytotoxicity using animal xenografts in gliomas [198], B-cell lymphomas [199], ovarian cancer [200, 201], prostate cancer [202, 203], soft tissue sarcoma [204], cervical carcinoma [205], melanoma, and mesothelioma [206]. These exciting results all point toward the incredible potential of these natural products for future clinical treatment regimens.

14.5.2 Clinical Applications of Withanolides for Cancer

Despite having improvements in our understanding of the multiple mechanisms of cytotoxicity with withanolide treatment across an expanding range of cancers, there has yet to be a significant human clinical placebo-controlled trial brought to completion and published that evaluates the efficacy of withanolides for the treatment of cancer. Withanolides are generally regarded as safe and have been used in human clinical trials for inflammatory and neurologic diseases, and have been evaluated for the treatment of fatigue for breast cancer patients undergoing chemotherapy [207]. Additional in vivo research on withanolides is ongoing and has overall been quite promising to identify withanolides as an important cancer therapy, however, further supporting research is needed to initiate the human clinical trials required to obtain a better understanding of the clinical treatment effects of withanolides on cancer. To date, there is no Food and Drug Administration (FDA)-approved good manufacturing process (GMP) facility currently purifying and producing purified withanolide compounds for use in clinical trials, although several facilities in other countries produce capsules of withanolide plant products and extracts that are not regulated by the FDA.

14.6 Application of Withanolides in Neurologic Diseases

14.6.1 Neurodegenerative Diseases

Neurodegenerative diseases are characterized by the progressive dysfunction and loss of neurons in the central nervous system (CNS) and are a major cause of dementia, cognitive and motor dysfunction. As the pathophysiology of neurodegenerative diseases such as Alzheimer's disease (AD), Parkinson's disease (PD), and Huntington's disease (HD) are better understood, the major role of the immune system and neuroinflammation has become readily apparent [208]. Although the blood–brain barrier maintains some degree of separation of the CNS from the systemic immune system to aid in the immune privileged state of the CNS (its relative inability of nonself antigens to illicit an immune response), the role of the innate and adaptive immune responses has become a major focus of both study and intervention [209]. In addition to the formation and deposition of amyloid β plaques in AD, activation of microglia (macrophage-like CNS cell) and astrocytes, increased complement components, cytokines, and TLR pathways, and alterations in peripheral Th cell responses have also been described [210, 211]. In PD, mitochondrial dysfunction, oxidative stress, and altered protein handling with Lewy body deposition as well as inflammation through microglial activation, increased IL-1β, IL-6, TNF-α, and TLRs, formation of antibodies to neuronal antigens, and Th cell modulation are important. Finally in HD, mutant Huntingtin (HTT) expression in neurons and glia leading to microglia proliferation/activation, increased complement 3, 9 and neuroinflammation are keys to the pathogenesis of the disease [208, 209].

As previously discussed, withanolides inhibit multiple inflammatory pathways, and within the CNS astrocytes, Withaferin A has been shown to attenuate LPS-induced NF-κB, TNF-α, COX-2 and iNOS [212]. In addition to neuroinflammatory modulation, several withanolides including WS extract, withanosides (particularly withanoside IV and its active metabolite sominone), the synthetic withanolidedenosomin, withanolide A and coagulin Q have all demonstrated important effects on stimulating neurite outgrowth and regeneration [66, 210, 211]. In AD, additional key findings demonstrated that withanolide A significantly downregulates beta-site amyloid precursor protein (APP) cleaving enzyme 1 (BACE1; known as *β*-secretase, enzyme involved in production of Aβ) while it upregulates a disintegrin and metalloproteinase domain-containing protein 10 (ADAM10; *α*-secretase, non-amyloidogenic enzymatic processing of APP). Additionally, withanolide A increases expression of insulin-degrading enzyme, which is important in the proteolytic degradation of Aβ [213]. Multiple withanolides (WS, WA, and bracteosins) have also demonstrated significant acetylcholinesterase (AChE) or butyrylcholinesterase (BChE) inhibition [214, 215] with computational docking analysis supporting withanolide A high-affinity binding for active sites on AChE [216]. These results, combined with the known antioxidant and anti-inflammatory effects of withanolides have propelled their research forward in neurodegenerative disorders to further elucidate their mechanism of action.

14.6.2 In Vivo Activities of Withanolides in the Treatment of Neurodegenerative Diseases

In a systematic review and meta-analysis, Durg et al. identified and analyzed 28 studies evaluating the use of WS in neurobehavioral disorders (including AD, PD, HD and anxiety/stress) induced by brain oxidation in rodent models [217]. Overall, WS treatment had a protective effect on brain oxidative stress that corrected abnormal activity levels of super oxide dismutase (SOD), catalase, glutathione peroxidase and glutathione, lipid peroxidation, and levels of nitrite and AChE [217]. In several types of AD mouse models, including Aβ-[25–35] induced memory deficit and 5XFAD mice (5 FAD mutations carried on APP and PS1 transgenes), withanolides (withanolide A, withanoside IV and its main active metabolite, sominone, and WS extract) significantly ameliorated the impairment of spatial memory and behavioral deficits [39, 40, 210, 217], while ex vivo brains showed increased axonal and dendritic protein markers back to control levels [39, 211], increased axonal densities [40], and reduced Aβ levels and plaque depositions through upregulation of low-density lipoprotein receptor-related protein within the liver [218].

Parkinson's disease is characterized by an age-related neurodegenerative progression that leads to resting tremor, rigidity, and akinesia though loss of dopaminergic nigro-striatal neurons, particularly within the substantia nigra [219]. The rodent models of Parkinsonism are created through brain injection of 6-Hydroxydopamine [220] or systemic administration of 1-methyl-4-phenyl-1,2,3,6-tetrahydropyridine (MPTP) [221] or the combination of manganese ethylene-bis-dithiocarbamate (maneb) and *N,N′*-dimethyl-4,4′-bipyridinium dichloride (paraquat) [222]. They cause specific degeneration and toxicity to catecholaminergic and dopaminergic neurons though oxidative stress and formation of hydrogen peroxide, hydroxyl, and superoxide radicals [220–222]. Using these models, treatment with WS extract resulted in significant improvements in locomotor control (including rotation, locomotion, muscular coordination and rearing), amelioration of oxidative parameters (including LPO, glutathione and associated enzymes, SOD and catalase), correction of ex vivo rodent brain alterations to catecholamine, dopamine, and dopamine metabolites (DOPAC/HVA) in ex vivo rat brains [222–226]. Some of these effects may be due to mediation of the otherwise proapototic state through reductions of Bax and Bcl-2 expression and neuroinflammatory astrocyte activation [227].

Huntington's disease has autosomal dominant transmission of the mutated HTT gene that leads to neuron destruction within the basal ganglia, leading to dementia and the characteristic involuntary writhing movements characteristic of Huntington's chorea. Mutant HTT aggregates have been implicated in oxidative stress through the formation of free radicals, which creates imbalance and plays a role in subsequent neuroinflammation [228]. Huntington's disease-like neurobehavioral and biochemical changes are induced in rodent models using neurotoxin 3-Nitropropionic acid. Treatment with WS root extract demonstrated significant dose-dependent attenuation of AChE levels, significantly improved oxidative stress markers, and improvement in general locomotor, performance and behavioral changes tested by Rotarod and Morris water [229, 230].

Although the involvement of the immune response and neuroinflammation plays a significant role in the pathogenesis of neurodegenerative diseases, the specific connections between these inflammatory pathways and the effects of withanolide treatment have not been well defined. The role of WS on reducing the oxidative stress within neurons has been demonstrated in multiple animal models of different disease processes, as well as the neuro-regenerative role of several withanolides on axonal and dendritic outgrowths and functional locomotor improvements. Connecting these effects to neuroinflammation and immunomodulation identifies an important area of future research.

14.6.3 Clinical Activity of Withanolides in Neurodegenerative Diseases

There is an overall paucity of research on the effects of withanolides in patients with neurodegenerative diseases. WS was a component of one study that evaluated the efficacy of a traditional Ayurveda treatment in clinically diagnosed PD patients. Treatment with a combination of eliminative cleansing and a concoction of cow's milk with powdered *Mucunapruriens*, *Hyoscyamusreticulatus* seeds, WS and *Sidacordifolia* roots (analyzed to contain 200 mg L-DOPA per dose) showed significant improvements in tremor/bradykinesia, stiffness and cramp-like pain resulting in improved activities of daily living, however, no changes in other symptoms like dysphonia, dysarthria, wasting, cogwheel rigidity, shuffling gait, or other locomotor symptoms [231]. However, conclusions regarding the role of WS cannot be reached due to the mixed nature of the L-DOPA containing herbal treatment. However, the growing in vitro and animal data continue to support the use of withanolides in neurodegenerative diseases, and illustrates the potential for its use in a more controlled clinical trial.

14.6.4 Withanolides in Neurobehavioral/Psychiatric Diseases

There is a broad range of neurological diseases in which inflammation and particularly cytokines and microglial activation have been shown to play a pathophysiological role. These include chronic stress [232], anxiety [233], depression [234], schizophrenia [235, 236], bipolar disorder [237, 238], and obsessive–compulsive disorder (OCD) [239]. Although the study of how the immune system and inflammation contribute to these diseases is relatively recent, major inflammatory pathways and cytokines have been identified. One proposed mechanism is through the stress response, whether through external stimuli or psychological imbalances, which leads to activation of the hypothalamic-pituitary-adrenal (HPA) axis and short-term elevations in glucocorticoids (mainly cortisol) and a subsequent anti-inflammatory response. However, prolonged stress and sustained HPA activation causes cortisol resistance and initiation of pro-inflammatory pathways, such Th cell release of IL-1α and β, IL-2, IL-6, IL-10, TNF-α cytokines, activation of NF-κB pathway, and microglial activation [232–238]. In addition to the known anti-inflammatory effects of withanolides previously discussed, they have also been described as adaptogens that assist with balance and regulation of the body's physiologic response to stressors [240]. The adaptogen mechanism of effect has been proposed to occur through modulation of the HPA axis, inducing stress-activated c-Jun N-terminal protein kinase (JNK1), inhibiting iNOS expression, and modulation of Hsp70 chaperone function [241]. Additionally, the inhibitory neurotransmitter gamma-aminobutyric acid (GABA), which plays an important inhibitory role in neurological disorders, has more recently been shown to have key anti-inflammatory interactions within the immune system through suppression of T-cells and macrophages, and inhibition of NF-κB on lymphocytes [242]. The GABA-mimetic activity of WS root extract has been shown for several decades [243] with a recent study identifying a 27 times greater affinity of WS for the highly sensitive GABAρ1 receptors compared to $GABA_A$ receptors, though WA and withanolide A were not the active GABA-mimetics [244]. These GABA-mimetic and adaptogenic effects likely play a significant role in the long-standing history of using Ashwagandha for the treatment of anxiety and neurobehavioral disorders, though the vast majority of animal and human studies have been performed in the last several decades.

14.6.5 In Vivo Activity of Withanolides for Neurobehavioral/Psychiatric Diseases

Most animal studies evaluating neurologic disorders have focused on the effects of WS extract using models of either chronic stress or withdrawal to induce anxiety and depression. Using a chronic, unpredictable, mild footshock to create a chronic stress model in rats, treatment with aqueous ethanol WS root extract significantly attenuated chronic, stress-induced abnormalities with improvements in biochemical imbalances (elevated blood glucose and corticosteroid levels), reduced number and severity of gastric ulcers, improved behavioral depression and sexual responses, improved cognitive memory function, and rescued immunosuppression in macrophage activity and immunologic pedal edema [245]. In depression and anxiety rodent models using chronic stress, isolation, sleep deprivation, WS extract treatment demonstrated significant antidepressant effects, and potentiated conventional antidepressants (tricyclic antidepressant imipramine and selective serotonin-reuptake inhibitor fluoxetine) measured by reduced immobility time in the forced open swim test ("behavioral despair/learned helplessness"), and an anxiolytic effect similar to benzodiazepines (lorazepam and diazepam) in the elevated plus maze, the social interaction test, and the feeding latency test [246–250].

In an OCD rodent model of marble-burying behavior, intraperitoneal injections of both methanolic and aqueous WS root extracts 30 min prior to evaluation resulted in significant dose-dependent reductions in marble-burying behavior similar to standard fluoxetine alone, and a synergistic effect in combination with fluoxetine [251]. These in vivo studies demonstrate a consistent amelioration of stress, anxiety, depressant, and OCD behaviors with corresponding corrections in biochemical abnormalities, however, the modulation of inflammatory pathways in these diseases requires further characterization.

14.6.6 Clinical Activities of Withanolides in Neurobehavioral/Psychiatric Diseases

Recent clinical trials using WS extract as a neurological treatment have evaluated effects on psychomotor function in patients with anxiety, bipolar disorder, and schizophrenia and provide clinical support for centuries of WS use in Ayurvedic medicine. There have been several randomized controlled trials that demonstrate significant improvement in anxiety and stress relief [252–257]. Studying ICD-10 anxiety disorders (generalized anxiety disorder, mixed anxiety and depression, panic disorder, and adjustment disorder with anxiety) assessed by Hamilton Anxiety Scale, patients were treated with 500 mg WS extract or placebo twice daily with subsequent clinically guided dose titrations. At 6 weeks, the WS extract treatment response of 88 % was significantly improved compared to the 50 % placebo response with no significant difference in overall adverse outcomes or with abrupt cessation of WS treatment [253]. Subsequent randomized controlled studies have corroborated their results and demonstrated either significantly decreased anxiety or improved stress relief using multiple anxiety scales (Hamilton Anxiety Scale, Beck Anxiety Inventory, Perceived Stress Scale), a range of WS dosing primarily between 125 and 600 mg/day for extract (one study 12,000 mg/day whole dried root powder) over the course of 60–84 days [252, 254–257]. None of the studies reported significant adverse events with WS treatment, with all described as mild or comparable to the placebo groups. However, significant limitations existed in each of the studies that included high rates of patient withdrawal from study [253], low sample size leading to bias risk and under powering, inconsistent dosing or lack of withanolide standardization, lack of comparison to standard of care anti-anxiolytics, and possible methodological flaws [252–257]. The limitations impair making definitive conclusions regarding the effectiveness of WS in anxiety disorders, but the body of study identifies WS as a relatively safe therapeutic and supports the role for conducting additional clinical studies.

In both bipolar disease and schizophrenia, cognitive impairments are consistently associated with poorer functional outcomes. As discussed previously, WS improves memory and cognitive function when treating neurodegenerative rodent models, and in healthy adults significantly improves psychomotor function as demonstrated by simple reaction times, choice discrimination, digit symbol substitution, digit vigilance, and card sorting tests compared to placebo [258]. In well maintained bipolar disease patients, a randomized controlled, trial of WS in adjunct to maintenance bipolar treatment resulted specific improvement in several cognitive function tests including the digit span backward, Flanker neutral response time, and social cognition response rating from the Penn Emotional Acuity Test, though no global cognitive improvement [259]. In schizophrenia, there is currently an ongoing randomized controlled clinical trial in the United States evaluating the effect of WS extract on symptom severity and associated stress that also aims to characterize alterations in inflammatory cytokines [260]. The results from this study will help provide valuable insight into the effect of WS on neuroinflammation and schizophrenia symptoms.

14.7 Conclusions

Withanolides are an incredibly bio-diverse group of naturally occurring steroidal lactones. These plant-derived compounds have ongoing use within Ayurvedic medical practices and are important plant-derived medicinal compounds for a variety of human diseases and conditions. With WA as the archetype of this novel class drugs, there are now approximately 900 withanolides identified from a natural source or synthetically modified. Significant strides have been made in recent years to advance our understanding of the biochemical, immunomodulatory, and anti-inflammatory mechanisms of these compounds and plant extracts. Added to this is emerging in vivo and clinical evidence of safe, efficacious treatment effects across multiple disease processes ranging from autoimmune/inflammatory disorders, cancer, neurodegenerative diseases, and neurobehavioral/psychiatric diseases. Ongoing research on withanolides continues to identify new compounds and analogs, both plant derived and synthetically altered, that are more potent or specific for use in particular diseases. Given their impressive biologic activity in a number of challenging and complex disease processes and their unique ability to synergize with many standard drug treatments, these naturally derived drug compounds undoubtedly will have an important role clinically in well-designed combination strategies once disease-specific mechanisms of action and synergy are further validated and characterized. As such, they remain a very hot area of research as a novel group of medicinal therapeutics.

References

1. Chen L-X, He H, Qiu F (2011) Natural withanolides: an overview. Nat Prod Rep 28(4):705–740
2. Misico R, Nicotra V, Oberti J, Barboza G, Gil R, Burton G (2011) Withanolides and related steroids. In: Kinghorn AD, Falk H, Kobayashi J (eds) Progress in the chemistry of organic natural products. Fortschritte der Chemie organischer Naturstoffe/Progress in the chemistry of organic natural products, vol 94. Springer, Vienna, pp 127–229
3. Zhang H, Cao C-M, Gallagher RJ, Timmermann BN (2014) Antiproliferative withanolides from several solanaceous species. Nat Prod Res 28(22):1941–1951
4. Glotter E (1991) Withanolides and related ergostane-type steroids. Nat Prod Rep 8(4):415–440
5. Misico RI, Song LL, Veleiro AS, Cirigliano AM, Tettamanzi MC, Burton G et al (2002) Induction of quinone reductase by withanolides. J Nat Prod 65(5):677–680
6. Lavie D, Glotter E, Shvo Y (1965) Constituents of *Withania somnifera* Dun. Part IV. The structure of withaferin A. J Chem Soc (1): 7517–7531

7. Zhang H, Samadi AK, Cohen MS, Timmermann BN (2012) Antiproliferative withanolides from the Solanaceae: a structure–activity study. Pure Appl Chem 84(6):1353–1367
8. Cao C-M, Wu X, Kindscher K, Xu L, Timmermann BN (2015) Withanolides and Sucrose Esters from Physalis neomexicana. J Nat Prod 78(10):2488–2493
9. Chen B-W, Chen Y-Y, Lin Y-C, Huang C-Y, Uvarani C, Hwang T-L et al (2015) Capsisteroids A–F, withanolides from the leaves of Solanum capsicoides. RSC Adv 5 (108):88841–88847
10. Chao C-H, Chou K-J, Wen Z-H, Wang G-H, Wu Y-C, Dai C-F et al (2011) Paraminabeolides A-F, cytotoxic and anti-inflammatory marine withanolides from the soft coral *Paraminabea acronocephala*. J Nat Prod 74(5):1132–1141
11. Ksebati MB, Schmitz FJ (1988) Minabeolides: a group of withanolides from a soft coral, *Minabea* sp. J Organ Chem 53(17):3926–3929
12. Huang C-Y, Liaw C-C, Chen B-W, Chen P-C, Su J-H, Sung P-J et al (2013) Withanolide-based steroids from the cultured soft coral *Sinularia brassica*. J Nat Prod 76 (10):1902–1908
13. Jayaprakasam B, Zhang Y, Seeram NP, Nair MG (2003) Growth inhibition of human tumor cell lines by withanolides from *Withania somnifera* leaves. Life Sci 74(1):125–132
14. Antony ML, Lee J, Hahm E-R, Kim S-H, Marcus AI, Kumari V et al (2014) Growth arrest by the antitumor steroidal lactone withaferin A in human breast cancer cells is associated with down-regulation and covalent binding at cysteine 303 of β-tubulin. J Biol Chem 289 (3):1852–1865
15. Shohat B, Joshua H (1971) Effect of withaferin a on Ehrlich ascites tumor cells. II. Target tumor cell destruction in vivo by immune activation. Int J Cancer 8(3):487–496
16. Zhang H, Bazzill J, Gallagher RJ, Subramanian C, Grogan PT, Day VW et al (2012) Antiproliferative Withanolides from *Datura wrightii*. J Nat Prod 76(3):445–449
17. Zhang H, Samadi AK, Gallagher RJ, Araya JJ, Tong X, Day VW et al (2011) Cytotoxic withanolide constituents of *Physalis longifolia*. J Nat Prod 74(12):2532–2544
18. Minguzzi S, Barata LES, Shin YG, Jonas PF, Chai H-B, Park EJ et al (2002) Cytotoxic withanolides from *Acnistus arborescens*. Phytochemistry 59(6):635–641
19. He Q-P, Ma L, Luo J-Y, He F-Y, Lou L-G, Hu L-H (2007) Cytotoxic withanolides from *Physalis angulata* L. Chem Biodivers 4(3):443–449
20. Grogan PT, Sleder KD, Samadi AK, Zhang H, Timmermann BN, Cohen MS (2013) Cytotoxicity of withaferin A in glioblastomas involves induction of an oxidative stress-mediated heat shock response while altering Akt/mTOR and MAPK signaling pathways. Invest New Drugs 31(3):545–557
21. Samadi AK, Tong X, Mukerji R, Zhang H, Timmermann BN, Cohen MS (2010) Withaferin A, a cytotoxic steroid from *Vassobia breviflora*, induces apoptosis in human head and neck squamous cell carcinoma. J Nat Prod 73(9):1476–1481
22. Choi JK, Murillo G, Su B-N, Pezzuto JM, Kinghorn AD, Mehta RG (2006) Ixocarpalactone A isolated from the Mexican tomatillo shows potent antiproliferative and apoptotic activity in colon cancer cells. FEBS J 273(24):5714–5723
23. Stan SD, Hahm E-R, Warin R, Singh SV (2008) Withaferin A causes FOXO3a- and Bim-dependent apoptosis and inhibits growth of human breast cancer cells in vivo. Cancer Res 68(18):7661–7669
24. Kaileh M, Vanden Berghe W, Heyerick A, Horion J, Piette J, Libert C et al (2007) Withaferin A strongly elicits IκB Kinase β hyperphosphorylation concomitant with potent inhibition of its kinase activity. J Biol Chem 282(7):4253–4264
25. Oh JH, Lee T-J, Park J-W, Kwon TK (2008) Withaferin A inhibits iNOS expression and nitric oxide production by Akt inactivation and down-regulating LPS-induced activity of NF-κB in RAW 264.7 cells. Eur J Pharmacol 599(1–3):11–17
26. Wube AA, Wenzig E-M, Gibbons S, Asres K, Bauer R, Bucar F (2008) Constituents of the stem bark of *Discopodium penninervium* and their LTB4 and COX-1 and -2 inhibitory activities. Phytochemistry 69(4):982–987

27. Yang B-Y, Guo R, Li T, Wu J-J, Zhang J, Liu Y et al (2014) New anti-inflammatory withanolides from the leaves of *Datura metel* L. Steroids 87:26–34
28. Maldonado E, Amador S, Martínez M, Pérez-Castorena AL (2010) Virginols A–C, three new withanolides from *Physalis virginiana*. Steroids 75(4–5):346–349
29. Quang TH, Ngan NTT, Minh CV, Kiem PV, Yen PH, Tai BH et al (2012) Plantagiolides I and J, two new withanolide glucosides from *Tacca plantaginea* with nuclear factor-kappaB inhibitory and peroxisome proliferator-activated receptor transactivational activities. Chem Pharm Bull 60(12):1494–1501
30. Jayaprakasam B, Nair MG (2003) Cyclooxygenase-2 enzyme inhibitory withanolides from *Withania somnifera* leaves. Tetrahedron 59(6):841–849
31. Qiu L, Zhao F, Jiang Z-H, Chen L-X, Zhao Q, Liu H-X et al (2008) Steroids and flavonoids from *Physalis alkekengi* var. franchetii and their inhibitory effects on nitric oxide production. J Nat Prod 71(4):642–646
32. Malik F, Singh J, Khajuria A, Suri KA, Satti NK, Singh S et al (2007) A standardized root extract of *Withania somnifera* and its major constituent withanolide-A elicit humoral and cell-mediated immune responses by up regulation of Th1-dominant polarization in BALB/c mice. Life Sci 80(16):1525–1538
33. Habtemariam S (1997) Cytotoxicity and immunosuppressive activity of withanolides from *Discopodium penninervium*. Planta Med 63(01):15–17
34. Kour K, Pandey A, Suri KA, Satti NK, Gupta KK, Bani S (2009) Restoration of stress-induced altered T cell function and corresponding cytokines patterns by Withanolide A. Int Immunopharmacol 9(10):1137–1144
35. Abou-Douh AM (2002) New withanolides and other constituents from the fruit of *Withania somnifera*. Arch Pharm 335(6):267–276
36. Bravo BJA, Sauvain M, Gimenez TA, Balanza E, Serani L, Laprévote O et al (2001) Trypanocidal withanolides and withanolide glycosides from *Dunalia brachyacantha*. J Nat Prod 64(6):720–725
37. Choudhary MI, Yousuf S, Samreen AS, Atta UR (2007) New leishmanicidal physalins from *Physalis minima*. Nat Prod Res 21(10):877–883
38. Bhattacharya SK, Satyan KS, Ghosal S (1997) Antioxidant activity of glycowithanolides from *Withania somnifera*. Indian J Exp Biol 35(3):236–239
39. Kuboyama T, Tohda C, Komatsu K (2006) Withanoside IV and its active metabolite, sominone, attenuate Aβ(25–35)-induced neurodegeneration. Eur J Neurosci 23(6):1417–1426
40. Joyashiki E, Matsuya Y, Tohda C (2011) Sominone Improves Memory Impairments and Increases axonal density in Alzheimer's Disease Model Mice, 5XFAD. Int J Neurosci 121 (4):181–190
41. Baitharu I, Jain V, Deep SN, Shroff S, Sahu JK, Naik PK et al (2014) Withanolide A prevents neurodegeneration by modulating hippocampal glutathione biosynthesis during hypoxia. PLoS ONE 9(10):e105311
42. Devi PU (1996) Withaferin A: a new radiosensitizer from the Indian medicinal plant *Withania somnifera*. Int J Radiat Biol 69(2):193–197
43. Devi PU, Kamath R (2003) Radiosensitizing effect of withaferin A combined with hyperthermia on mouse fibrosarcoma and melanoma. J Radiat Res 44(1):1–6
44. Budhiraja RD, Krishan P, Sudhir S (2000) Biological activity of withanolides. J Sci Ind Res 59(11):904–911
45. Mareggiani G, Picollo MI, Zerba E, Burton G, Tettamanzi MC, Benedetti-Doctorovich MOV et al (2000) Antifeedant Activity of Withanolides from *Salpichroa origanifolia* on Musca domestica. J Nat Prod 63(8):1113–1116
46. Mandal C, Dutta A, Mallick A, Chandra S, Misra L, Sangwan R et al (2008) Withaferin A induces apoptosis by activating p38 mitogen-activated protein kinase signaling cascade in leukemic cells of lymphoid and myeloid origin through mitochondrial death cascade. Apoptosis 13(12):1450–1464

47. Khan ZA, Ghosh AR (2010) Possible nitric oxide modulation in protective effects of withaferin A against stress induced neurobehavioural changes. J Med Plants Res 4(6):490–495
48. Machin RP, Veleiro AS, Nicotra VE, Oberti JC, Padrón JM (2010) Antiproliferative activity of withanolides against human breast cancer cell lines. J Nat Prod 73(5):966–968
49. Koduru S, Kumar R, Srinivasan S, Evers MB, Damodaran C (2010) Notch-1 inhibition by Withaferin-A: a therapeutic target against colon carcinogenesis. Mol Cancer Ther 9(1):202–210
50. Rah B, Amin H, Yousuf K, Khan S, Jamwal G, Mukherjee D et al (2012) A novel MMP-2 inhibitor 3-azidowithaferin A (3-azidoWA) abrogates cancer cell invasion and angiogenesis by modulating extracellular par-4. PLoS ONE 7(9):e44039
51. Lee W, Kim TH, Ku S-K, K-j Min, Lee H-S, Kwon TK et al (2012) Barrier protective effects of withaferin A in HMGB1-induced inflammatory responses in both cellular and animal models. Toxicol Appl Pharmacol 262(1):91–98
52. Bargagna-Mohan P, Ravindranath PP, Mohan R (2006) Small molecule anti-angiogenic probes of the ubiquitin proteasome pathway: Potential application to choroidal neovascularization. Invest Ophthalmol Vis Sci 47(9):4138–4145
53. Choi BY, Kim B-W (2015) Withaferin-A inhibits colon cancer cell growth by blocking STAT3 transcriptional activity. J Cancer Prevent 20(3):185–192
54. Ichikawa H, Takada Y, Shishodia S, Jayaprakasam B, Nair MG, Aggarwal BB (2006) Withanolides potentiate apoptosis, inhibit invasion, and abolish osteoclastogenesis through suppression of nuclear factor-κB (NF-κB) activation and NF-κB-regulated gene expression. Mol Cancer Ther 5(6):1434–1445
55. Mohan R, Hammers H, Bargagna-Mohan P, Zhan X, Herbstritt C, Ruiz A et al (2004) Withaferin A is a potent inhibitor of angiogenesis. Angiogenesis 7(2):115–122
56. Ndlovu MN, Van Lint C, Van Wesemael K, Callebert P, Chalbos D, Haegeman G et al (2009) Hyperactivated NF-κB and AP-1 transcription factors promote highly accessible chromatin and constitutive transcription across the interleukin-6 gene promoter in metastatic breast cancer cells. Mol Cell Biol 29(20):5488–5504
57. Yco LP, Mocz G, Opoku-Ansah J, Bachmann AS (2014) Withaferin A Inhibits STAT3 and induces tumor cell death in neuroblastoma and multiple myeloma. Biochem Insights 7:1–13
58. Ishiguro M, Kajikawa A, Haruyama T, Morisaki M, Ikekawa N (1974) Synthetic studies of withanolide I synthesis of AB ring moiety of withaferin A. Tetrahedron Lett 15(15):1421–1424
59. Ozawa M, Morita M, Hirai G, Tamura S, Kawai M, Tsuchiya A et al (2013) Contribution of cage-shaped structure of physalins to their mode of action in inhibition of NF-κB activation. ACS Med Chem Lett 4(8):730–735
60. Wijeratne EMK, Xu Y-M, Scherz-Shouval R, Marron MT, Rocha DD, Liu MX et al (2014) Structure–activity relationships for withanolides as inducers of the cellular heat-shock response. J Med Chem 57(7):2851–2863
61. Damu AG, Kuo P-C, Su C-R, Kuo T-H, Chen T-H, Bastow KF et al (2007) Isolation, structures, and structure-cytotoxic activity relationships of withanolides and physalins from *Physalis angulata*. J Nat Prod 70(7):1146–1152
62. Wang H-C, Tsai Y-L, Wu Y-C, Chang F-R, Liu M-H, Chen W-Y et al (2012) Withanolides-induced breast cancer cell death is correlated with their ability to inhibit heat protein 90. PLoS ONE 7(5):e37764
63. Yu Y, Hamza A, Zhang T, Gu M, Zou P, Newman B et al (2010) Withaferin A targets heat shock protein 90 in pancreatic cancer cells. Biochem Pharmacol 79(4):542–551
64. Ji L, Yuan Y, Luo L, Chen Z, Ma X, Ma Z et al (2012) Physalins with anti-inflammatory activity are present in *Physalis alkekengi* var. franchetii and can function as Michael reaction acceptors. Steroids 77(5):441–447
65. Beg M, Chauhan P, Varshney S, Shankar K, Rajan S, Saini D et al (2014) A withanolide coagulin-L inhibits adipogenesis modulating Wnt/β-catenin pathway and cell cycle in mitotic clonal expansion. Phytomedicine 21(4):406–414

66. Teshigawara K, Kuboyama T, Shigyo M, Nagata A, Sugimoto K, Matsuya Y et al (2013) A novel compound, denosomin, ameliorates spinal cord injury via axonal growth associated with astrocyte-secreted vimentin. Br J Pharmacol 168(4):903–919
67. Takimoto T, Kanbayashi Y, Toyoda T, Adachi Y, Furuta C, Suzuki K et al (2014) 4β-Hydroxywithanolide E isolated from *Physalis pruinosa* calyx decreases inflammatory responses by inhibiting the NF-κB signaling in diabetic mouse adipose tissue. Int J Obes 38 (11):1432–1439
68. Budhiraja RD, Sudhir S, Garg KN (1984) Antiinflammatory activity of 3 β-hydroxy-2,3-dihydro-withanolide F. Planta Med 50(02):134–136
69. Pan M-R, Chang H-C, Wu Y-C, Huang C-C, Hung W-C (2009) Tubocapsanolide A inhibits transforming growth factor-β-activating kinase 1 to suppress NF-κB-induced CCR7. J Biol Chem 284(5):2746–2754
70. Chen W-Y, Chang F-R, Huang Z-Y, Chen J-H, Wu Y-C, Wu C-C (2008) Tubocapsenolide A, a novel withanolide, inhibits proliferation and induces apoptosis in MDA-MB-231 cells by thiol oxidation of heat shock proteins. J Biol Chem 283(25):17184–17193
71. Zhang X, Blaskovich MA, Forinash KD, Sebti SM (2014) Withacnistin inhibits recruitment of STAT3 and STAT5 to growth factor and cytokine receptors and induces regression of breast tumours. Br J Cancer 111(5):894–902
72. Suttana W, Mankhetkorn S, Poompimon W, Palagani A, Zhokhov S, Gerlo S et al (2010) Differential chemosensitization of P-glycoprotein overexpressing K562/Adr cells by withaferin A and Siamois polyphenols. Mol Cancer 9(1):1–22
73. Min K-J, Choi K, Kwon TK (2011) Withaferin A down-regulates lipopolysaccharide-induced cyclooxygenase-2 expression and PGE2 production through the inhibition of STAT1/3 activation in microglial cells. Int Immunopharmacol 11(8):1137–1142
74. Mulabagal V, Subbaraju GV, Rao CV, Sivaramakrishna C, DeWitt DL, Holmes D et al (2009) Withanolide sulfoxide from Aswagandha roots inhibits nuclear transcription factor-kappa-B, cyclooxygenase and tumor cell proliferation. Phytother Res 23(7):987–992
75. Ahmed LA (2014) Renoprotective effect of egyptian cape gooseberry fruit (*Physalis peruviana* L.) against acute renal injury in rats. Sci World J 2014:273870 (273871–273877)
76. Martínez W, Ospina LF, Granados D, Delgado G (2010) In vitro studies on the relationship between the anti-inflammatory activity of *Physalis peruviana* extracts and the phagocytic process. Immunopharmacol Immunotoxicol 32(1):63–73
77. Kurapati KRV, Atluri VSR, Samikkannu T, Nair MPN (2013) Ashwagandha (*Withania somnifera*) reverses β-Amyloid$_{1\text{-}42}$ induced toxicity in human neuronal cells: implications in HIV-associated neurocognitive disorders (HAND). PLoS ONE 8(10):e77624 (77621–77615)
78. Aalinkeel R, Hu Z, Nair BB, Sykes DE, Reynolds JL, Mahajan SD et al (2010) Genomic analysis highlights the role of the JAK-STAT signaling in the anti-proliferative effects of dietary flavonoid—'Ashwagandha' in prostate cancer cells. Evid Based Complement Altern Med 7(2):177–187
79. Pawar P, Gilda S, Sharma S, Jagtap S, Paradkar A, Mahadik K et al (2011) Rectal gel application of *Withania somnifera* root extract expounds anti-inflammatory and muco-restorative activity in TNBS-induced Inflammatory Bowel Disease. BMC Complement Altern Med 11(1):1–9
80. Kataria H, Wadhwa R, Kaul SC, Kaur G (2012) Water extract from the leaves of *Withania somnifera* protect RA differentiated C6 and IMR-32 cells against glutamate-induced excitotoxicity. PLoS ONE 7(5):e37080
81. Ojha S, Alkaabi J, Amir N, Sheikh A, Agil A, Fahim MA et al (2014) Withania coagulans fruit extract reduces oxidative stress and inflammation in kidneys of streptozotocin-induced diabetic rats. Oxid Med Cell Longev 2014:201436 (201431–201439)
82. Chaplin DD (2010) Overview of the immune response. J Allergy Clin Immunol 125(2 Suppl 2):S3–S23
83. Mikolai J, Erlandsen A, Murison A, Brown KA, Gregory WL, Raman-Caplan P et al (2009) In vivo effects of Ashwagandha (*Withania somnifera*) extract on the activation of lymphocytes. J Altern Complement Med 15(4):423–430

84. Davis L, Kuttan G (2002) Effect of *Withania somnifera* on cell mediated immune responses in mice. J Exp Clin Cancer Res. 21(4):585–590
85. Khan B, Ahmad SF, Bani S, Kaul A, Suri KA, Satti NK et al (2006) Augmentation and proliferation of T lymphocytes and Th-1 cytokines by *Withania somnifera* in stressed mice. Int Immunopharmacol 6(9):1394–1403
86. Bani S, Gautam M, Sheikh FA, Khan B, Satti NK, Suri KA et al (2006) Selective Th1 up-regulating activity of *Withania somnifera* aqueous extract in an experimental system using flow cytometry. J Ethnopharmacol 107(1):107–115
87. Mesaik MA, Zaheer Ul H, Murad S, Ismail Z, Abdullah NR, Gill HK et al (2006) Biological and molecular docking studies on coagulin-H: Human IL-2 novel natural inhibitor. Mol Immunol 43(11):1855–1863
88. Huang C-F, Ma L, Sun L-J, Ali M, Arfan M, Liu J-W et al (2009) Immunosuppressive withanolides from withania coagulans. Chem Biodivers 6(9):1415–1426
89. Soares MB, Bellintani MC, Ribeiro IM, Tomassini TC, dos Santos RR (2003) Inhibition of macrophage activation and lipopolysaccaride-induced death by seco-steroids purified from *Physalis angulata* L. Eur J Pharmacol 459(1):107–112
90. Soares MBP, Brustolim D, Santos LA, Bellintani MC, Paiva FP, Ribeiro YM et al (2006) Physalins B, F and G, seco-steroids purified from *Physalis angulata* L., inhibit lymphocyte function and allogeneic transplant rejection. Int Immunopharmacol 6(3):408–414
91. Yu Y, Sun L, Ma L, Li J, Hu L, Liu J (2010) Investigation of the immunosuppressive activity of Physalin H on T lymphocytes. Int Immunopharmacol 10(3):290–297
92. Aggarwal BB, Vijayalekshmi RV, Sung B (2009) Targeting inflammatory pathways for prevention and therapy of cancer: short-term friend, long-term foe. Clin Cancer Res 15 (2):425–430
93. Costa G, Francisco V, Lopes MC, Cruz MT, Batista MT (2012) intracellular signaling pathways modulated by phenolic compounds: application for new anti-inflammatory drugs discovery. Curr Med Chem 19(18):2876–2900
94. Libby P (2007) Inflammatory mechanisms: the molecular basis of inflammation and disease. Nutr Rev 65(12 Pt 2):S140–S146
95. Santangelo C, Vari R, Scazzocchio B, Di Benedetto R, Filesi C, Masella R (2007) Polyphenols, intracellular signalling and inflammation. Ann Ist Super Sanita 43(4):394–405
96. O'Neill LA (2006) Targeting signal transduction as a strategy to treat inflammatory diseases. Nat Rev Drug Discov 5(7):549–563
97. Ghosh DM, George BS, Bhatia A, Sidhu OP (2014) Characterization of *Withania somnifera* leaf transcriptome and expression analysis of pathogenesis-related genes during salicylic acid signaling. PLoS ONE 9(4):e94803
98. Li Q, Verma IM (2002) NF-kappaB regulation in the immune system. Nat Rev Immunol 2 (10):725–734
99. Bonizzi G, Karin M (2004) The two NF-kappaB activation pathways and their role in innate and adaptive immunity. Trends Immunol 25(6):280–288
100. Brasier AR (2006) The NF-kappaB regulatory network. Cardiovasc Toxicol 6(2):111–130
101. Gilmore TD (2006) Introduction to NF-kappaB: players, pathways, perspectives. Oncogene 25(51):6680–6684
102. Perkins ND (2007) Integrating cell-signalling pathways with NF-kappaB and IKK function. Nat Rev Mol Cell Biol 8(1):49–62
103. Tian B, Brasier AR (2003) Identification of a nuclear factor kappa B-dependent gene network. Recent Prog Horm Res 58:95–130
104. Karin M (2009) NF-kappaB as a critical link between inflammation and cancer. Cold Spring Harb Perspect Biol 1(5):a000141
105. Darnell JE Jr (1997) STATs and gene regulation. Science 277(5332):1630–1635
106. Darnell JE Jr (2002) Transcription factors as targets for cancer therapy. Nat Rev Cancer 2 (10):740–749
107. Yu H, Pardoll D, Jove R (2009) STATs in cancer inflammation and immunity: a leading role for STAT3. Nat Rev Cancer 9(11):798–809

108. Yu H, Jove R (2004) The STATs of cancer—new molecular targets come of age. Nat Rev Cancer 4(2):97–105
109. Takeda K, Noguchi K, Shi W, Tanaka T, Matsumoto M, Yoshida N et al (1997) Targeted disruption of the mouse Stat3 gene leads to early embryonic lethality. Proc Natl Acad Sci USA 94(8):3801–3804
110. Cheng GZ, Zhang WZ, Sun M, Wang Q, Coppola D, Mansour M et al (2008) Twist is transcriptionally induced by activation of STAT3 and mediates STAT3 oncogenic function. J Biol Chem 283(21):14665–14673
111. Niu G, Wright KL, Huang M, Song L, Haura E, Turkson J et al (2002) Constitutive Stat3 activity up-regulates VEGF expression and tumor angiogenesis. Oncogene 21(13):2000–2008
112. Ahmad R, Rajabi H, Kosugi M, Joshi MD, Alam M, Vasir B et al (2011) MUC1-C oncoprotein promotes STAT3 activation in an autoinductive regulatory loop. Sci Signal 4 (160):ra9
113. Kiuchi N, Nakajima K, Ichiba M, Fukada T, Narimatsu M, Mizuno K et al (1999) STAT3 is required for the gp130-mediated full activation of the c-myc gene. J Exp Med 189(1):63–73
114. Masuda M, Suzui M, Yasumatu R, Nakashima T, Kuratomi Y, Azuma K et al (2002) Constitutive activation of signal transducers and activators of transcription 3 correlates with cyclin D1 overexpression and may provide a novel prognostic marker in head and neck squamous cell carcinoma. Cancer Res 62(12):3351–3355
115. Lee J, Hahm ER, Singh SV (2010) Withaferin A inhibits activation of signal transducer and activator of transcription 3 in human breast cancer cells. Carcinogenesis 31(11):1991–1998
116. Um HJ, Min K-J, Kim DE, Kwon TK (2012) Withaferin A inhibits JAK/STAT3 signaling and induces apoptosis of human renal carcinoma Caki cells. Biochem Biophys Res Commun 427(1):24–29
117. Schonthaler HB, Guinea-Viniegra J, Wagner EF (2011) Targeting inflammation by modulating the Jun/AP-1 pathway. Ann Rheum Dis 70(Suppl 1):i109–i112
118. Zenz R, Wagner EF (2006) Jun signalling in the epidermis: From developmental defects to psoriasis and skin tumors. Int J Biochem Cell Biol 38(7):1043–1049
119. Hess J, Angel P, Schorpp-Kistner M (2004) AP-1 subunits: quarrel and harmony among siblings. J Cell Sci 117(Pt 25):5965–5973
120. Wagner EF, Nebreda AR (2009) Signal integration by JNK and p38 MAPK pathways in cancer development. Nat Rev Cancer 9(8):537–549
121. Eferl R, Wagner EF (2003) AP-1: a double-edged sword in tumorigenesis. Nat Rev Cancer 3 (11):859–868
122. Singh D, Aggarwal A, Maurya R, Naik S (2007) *Withania somnifera* inhibits NF-kappaB and AP-1 transcription factors in human peripheral blood and synovial fluid mononuclear cells. Phytother Res 21(10):905–913
123. Pratt WB, Toft DO (2003) Regulation of signaling protein function and trafficking by the hsp90/hsp70-based chaperone machinery. Exp Biol Med (Maywood) 228(2):111–133
124. Sawai A, Chandarlapaty S, Greulich H, Gonen M, Ye Q, Arteaga CL et al (2008) Inhibition of Hsp90 down-regulates mutant epidermal growth factor receptor (EGFR) expression and sensitizes EGFR mutant tumors to paclitaxel. Cancer Res 68(2):589–596
125. Stebbins CE, Russo AA, Schneider C, Rosen N, Hartl FU, Pavletich NP (1997) Crystal structure of an Hsp90-geldanamycin complex: targeting of a protein chaperone by an antitumor agent. Cell 89(2):239–250
126. Park HJ, Rayalam S, Della-Fera MA, Ambati S, Yang JY, Baile CA (2008) Withaferin A induces apoptosis and inhibits adipogenesis in 3T3-L1 adipocytes. Biofactors 33(2):137–148
127. Subramanian C, Zhang H, Gallagher R, Hammer G, Timmermann B, Cohen M (2014) Withanolides are potent novel targeted therapeutic agents against adrenocortical carcinomas. World J Surg 38(6):1343–1352
128. Samadi AK, Bazzill J, Zhang X, Gallagher R, Zhang H, Gollapudi R et al (2012) Novel withanolides target medullary thyroid cancer through inhibition of both RET phosphorylation and the mammalian target of rapamycin pathway. Surgery 152(6):1238–1247

129. Yadav VR, Prasad S, Sung B, Kannappan R, Aggarwal BB (2010) Targeting inflammatory pathways by triterpenoids for prevention and treatment of cancer. Toxins 2:2428–2466
130. Zhang X, Mukerji R, Samadi AK, Cohen MS (2011) Down-regulation of estrogen receptor-alpha and Rearranged during Transfection tyrosine kinase is associated with Withaferin A-induced apoptosis in MCF-7 breast cancer cells. BMC Complement Altern Med 11:84
131. Zhang X, Samadi AK, Roby KF, Timmermann B, Cohen MS (2012) Inhibition of cell growth and induction of apoptosis in ovarian carcinoma cell lines CaOV3 and SKOV3 by natural withanolide Withaferin A. Gynecol Oncol 124(3):606–612
132. Zhang X, Timmermann B, Samadi AK, Cohen MS (2012) Withaferin a induces proteasome-dependent degradation of breast cancer susceptibility gene 1 and heat shock factor 1 proteins in breast cancer cells. ISRN Biochem 2012:707586
133. Samadi AK, Cohen SM, Mukerji R, Chaguturu V, Zhang X, Timmermann BN et al (2012) Natural withanolide withaferin A induces apoptosis in uveal melanoma cells by suppression of Akt and c-MET activation. Tumor Biol 33(4):1179–1189
134. Cohen SM, Mukerji R, Timmermann BN, Samadi AK, Cohen MS (2012) A novel combination of withaferin A and sorafenib shows synergistic efficacy against both papillary and anaplastic thyroid cancers. Am J Surg 204(6):895–900; (discussion 900–891)
135. Motiwala HF, Bazzill J, Samadi A, Zhang H, Timmermann BN, Cohen MS et al (2013) Synthesis and cytotoxicity of semisynthetic withalongolide A analogues. ACS Med Chem Lett 4(11):1069–1073
136. Grogan PT, Sarkaria JN, Timmermann BN, Cohen MS (2014) Oxidative cytotoxic agent withaferin A resensitizes temozolomide-resistant glioblastomas via MGMT depletion and induces apoptosis through Akt/mTOR pathway inhibitory modulation. Invest New Drugs 32 (4):604–617
137. Vyas AR, Singh SV (2014) Molecular targets and mechanisms of cancer prevention and treatment by withaferin A, a naturally occurring steroidal lactone. AAPS J 16(1):1–10
138. Grover A, Shandilya A, Agrawal V, Pratik P, Bhasme D, Bisaria VS et al (2011) Hsp90/Cdc37 chaperone/co-chaperone complex, a novel junction anticancer target elucidated by the mode of action of herbal drug withaferin A. BMC Bioinform 12(Suppl 1):S30
139. Gambhir L, Checker R, Sharma D, Thoh M, Patil A, Degani M et al (2015) Thiol dependent NF-kappaB suppression and inhibition of T-cell mediated adaptive immune responses by a naturally occurring steroidal lactone withaferin A. Toxicol Appl Pharmacol 289(2):297–312
140. Saha S, Islam MK, Shilpi JA, Hasan S (2013) Inhibition of VEGF: a novel mechanism to control angiogenesis by *Withania somnifera*'s key metabolite withaferin A. In Silico Pharmacol 1:11
141. White PT, Subramanian C, Zhu Q, Zhang H, Zhao H, Gallagher R et al (2016) Novel HSP90 inhibitors effectively target functions of thyroid cancer stem cell preventing migration and invasion. Surgery 159(1):142–151
142. Lee DH, Lim I-H, Sung E-G, Kim J-Y, Song I-H, Park YK et al (2013) Withaferin A inhibits matrix metalloproteinase-9 activity by suppressing the Akt signaling pathway. Oncol Rep 30 (2):933–938
143. Lee J, Hahm ER, Marcus AI, Singh SV (2015) Withaferin A inhibits experimental epithelial-mesenchymal transition in MCF-10A cells and suppresses vimentin protein level in vivo in breast tumors. Mol Carcinog 54(6):417–429
144. Lee J, Sehrawat A, Singh SV (2012) Withaferin A causes activation of Notch2 and Notch4 in human breast cancer cells. Breast Cancer Res Treat 136(1):45–56
145. Amin H, Nayak D, Ur Rasool R, Chakraborty S, Kumar A, Yousuf K et al (2016) Par-4 dependent modulation of cellular beta-catenin by medicinal plant natural product derivative 3-azido withaferin A. Mol Carcinog 55(5):864–881
146. O'Connell MA, Hayes JD (2015) The Keap1/Nrf2 pathway in health and disease: from the bench to the clinic. Biochem Soc Trans 43(4):687–689

147. Hayes JD, Chowdhry S, Dinkova-Kostova AT, Sutherland C (2015) Dual regulation of transcription factor Nrf2 by Keap1 and by the combined actions of beta-TrCP and GSK-3. Biochem Soc Trans 43(4):611–620
148. Vaishnavi K, Saxena N, Shah N, Singh R, Manjunath K, Uthayakumar M et al (2012) Differential activities of the two closely related withanolides, Withaferin A and Withanone: bioinformatics and experimental evidences. PLoS ONE 7(9):e44419
149. Kostecka A, Sznarkowska A, Meller K, Acedo P, Shi Y, Mohammad Sakil HA et al (2014) JNK-NQO1 axis drives TAp73-mediated tumor suppression upon oxidative and proteasomal stress. Cell Death Dis 5:e1484
150. Scholz CC, Taylor CT (2013) Targeting the HIF pathway in inflammation and immunity. Curr Opin Pharmacol 13(4):646–653
151. Arya M, Ahmed H, Silhi N, Williamson M, Patel HR (2007) Clinical importance and therapeutic implications of the pivotal CXCL12-CXCR4 (chemokine ligand-receptor) interaction in cancer cell migration. Tumour Biol 28(3):123–131
152. Hanahan D, Weinberg RA (2000) The hallmarks of cancer. Cell 100(1):57–70
153. Conway EM, Collen D, Carmeliet P (2001) Molecular mechanisms of blood vessel growth. Cardiovasc Res 49(3):507–521
154. Laderoute KR, Calaoagan JM, Gustafson-Brown C, Knapp AM, Li GC, Mendonca HL et al (2002) The response of c-jun/AP-1 to chronic hypoxia is hypoxia-inducible factor 1 alpha dependent. Mol Cell Biol 22(8):2515–2523
155. Masoud GN, Li W (2015) HIF-1 pathway: role, regulation and intervention for cancer therapy. Acta Pharm Sin B. 5(5):378–389
156. D'Ignazio L, Bandarra D, Rocha S (2016) NF-kappaB and HIF crosstalk in immune responses. FEBS J 283(3):413–424
157. Semenza GL (2010) Defining the role of hypoxia-inducible factor 1 in cancer biology and therapeutics. Oncogene 29(5):625–634
158. Vaupel P (2009) Prognostic potential of the pre-therapeutic tumor oxygenation status. Adv Exp Med Biol 645:241–246
159. Gao R, Shah N, Lee JS, Katiyar SP, Li L, Oh E et al (2014) Withanone-rich combination of Ashwagandha withanolides restricts metastasis and angiogenesis through hnRNP-K. Mol Cancer Ther 13(12):2930–2940
160. Hitchon CA, El-Gabalawy HS (2004) Oxidation in rheumatoid arthritis. Arthritis Res Ther 6 (6):265–278
161. van't Hof RJ, Hocking L, Wright PK, Ralston SH (2000) Nitric oxide is a mediator of apoptosis in the rheumatoid joint. Rheumatology (Oxford) 39(9):1004–1008
162. Sumantran VN, Chandwaskar R, Joshi AK, Boddul S, Patwardhan B, Chopra A et al (2008) The relationship between chondroprotective and antiinflammatory effects of *Withania somnifera* root and glucosamine sulphate on human osteoarthritic cartilage in vitro. Phytother Res 22(10):1342–1348
163. Subbaraju GV, Vanisree M, Rao CV, Sivaramakrishna C, Sridhar P, Jayaprakasam B et al (2006) Ashwagandhanolide, a bioactive dimeric thiowithanolide isolated from the roots of *Withania somnifera*. J Nat Prod 69(12):1790–1792
164. Wruck CJ, Fragoulis A, Gurzynski A, Brandenburg LO, Kan YW, Chan K et al (2011) Role of oxidative stress in rheumatoid arthritis: insights from the Nrf2-knockout mice. Ann Rheum Dis 70(5):844–850
165. Yu SM, Kim SJ (2013) Production of reactive oxygen species by withaferin A causes loss of type collagen expression and COX-2 expression through the PI3K/Akt, p38, and JNK pathways in rabbit articular chondrocytes. Exp Cell Res 319(18):2822–2834
166. Kim JH, Kim SJ (2014) Overexpression of microRNA-25 by withaferin A induces cyclooxygenase-2 expression in rabbit articular chondrocytes. J Pharmacol Sci 125(1):83–90
167. Ganesan K, Sehgal PK, Mandal AB, Sayeed S (2011) Protective effect of *Withania somnifera* and *Cardiospermum halicacabum* extracts against collagenolytic degradation of collagen. Appl Biochem Biotechnol 165(3–4):1075–1091

168. Sumantran VN, Kulkarni A, Boddul S, Chinchwade T, Koppikar SJ, Harsulkar A et al (2007) Chondroprotective potential of root extracts of *Withania somnifera* in osteoarthritis. J Biosci 32(2):299–307
169. Rasool M, Varalakshmi P (2007) Protective effect of *Withania somnifera* root powder in relation to lipid peroxidation, antioxidant status, glycoproteins and bone collagen on adjuvant-induced arthritis in rats. Fundam Clin Pharmacol 21(2):157–164
170. Khan MA, Subramaneyaan M, Arora VK, Banerjee BD, Ahmed RS (2015) Effect of *Withania somnifera* (Ashwagandha) root extract on amelioration of oxidative stress and autoantibodies production in collagen-induced arthritic rats. J Complement Integr Med 12 (2):117–125
171. Gupta A, Singh S (2014) Evaluation of anti-inflammatory effect of *Withania somnifera* root on collagen-induced arthritis in rats. Pharm Biol 52(3):308–320
172. Rasool M, Varalakshmi P (2006) Immunomodulatory role of *Withania somnifera* root powder on experimental induced inflammation: an in vivo and in vitro study. Vascul Pharmacol 44(6):406–410
173. Rasool M, Varalakshmi P (2006) Suppressive effect of *Withania somnifera* root powder on experimental gouty arthritis: an in vivo and in vitro study. Chem Biol Interact 164(3):174–180
174. Chopra A, Lavin P, Patwardhan B, Chitre D (2004) A 32-week randomized, placebo-controlled clinical evaluation of RA-11, an Ayurvedic drug, on osteoarthritis of the knees. J Clin Rheumatol 10(5):236–245
175. Kumar G, Srivastava A, Sharma SK, Rao TD, Gupta YK (2015) Efficacy & safety evaluation of Ayurvedic treatment (Ashwagandha powder & Sidh Makardhwaj) in rheumatoid arthritis patients: a pilot prospective study. Indian J Med Res 141(1):100–106
176. Gottschalk TA, Tsantikos E, Hibbs ML (2015) Pathogenic inflammation and its therapeutic targeting in systemic lupus erythematosus. Front Immunol 6:550
177. Khor B, Gardet A, Xavier RJ (2011) Genetics and pathogenesis of inflammatory bowel disease. Nature 474(7351):307–317
178. Yildirim-Toruner C, Diamond B (2011) Current and novel therapeutics in the treatment of systemic lupus erythematosus. J Allergy Clin Immunol 127(2):303–312; (quiz 313–304)
179. Triantafillidis JK, Merikas E, Georgopoulos F (2011) Current and emerging drugs for the treatment of inflammatory bowel disease. Drug Des Dev Ther 5:185–210
180. Minhas U, Minz R, Bhatnagar A (2011) Prophylactic effect of *Withania somnifera* on inflammation in a non-autoimmune prone murine model of lupus. Drug Discov Ther 5 (4):195–201
181. Minhas U, Minz R, Das P, Bhatnagar A (2012) Therapeutic effect of *Withania somnifera* on pristane-induced model of SLE. Inflammopharmacology 20(4):195–205
182. Samadi AK (2015) Potential anticancer properties and mechanisms of action of withanolides. Enzymes 37:73–94
183. Dar NJ, Hamid A, Ahmad M (2015) Pharmacologic overview of *Withania somnifera*, the Indian Ginseng. Cell Mol Life Sci 72(23):4445–4460
184. Widodo N, Priyandoko D, Shah N, Wadhwa R, Kaul SC (2010) Selective killing of cancer cells by Ashwagandha leaf extract and its component withanone involves ROS signaling. PLoS ONE 5(10):e13536
185. Nishikawa Y, Okuzaki D, Fukushima K, Mukai S, Ohno S, Ozaki Y et al (2015) Withaferin A induces cell death selectively in androgen-independent prostate cancer cells but not in normal fibroblast cells. PLoS ONE 10(7):e0134137
186. Park JW, Min KJ, Kim DE, Kwon TK (2015) Withaferin A induces apoptosis through the generation of thiol oxidation in human head and neck cancer cells. Int J Mol Med 35(1):247–252
187. Samadi AK, Mukerji R, Shah A, Timmermann BN, Cohen MS (2010) A novel RET inhibitor with potent efficacy against medullary thyroid cancer in vivo. Surgery 148(6):1228–1236
188. Henrich CJ, Brooks AD, Erickson KL, Thomas CL, Bokesch HR, Tewary P et al (2015) Withanolide E sensitizes renal carcinoma cells to TRAIL-induced apoptosis by increasing cFLIP degradation. Cell Death Dis 6:e1666

189. Thaiparambil JT, Bender L, Ganesh T, Kline E, Patel P, Liu Y et al (2011) Withaferin A inhibits breast cancer invasion and metastasis at sub-cytotoxic doses by inducing vimentin disassembly and serine 56 phosphorylation. Int J Cancer 129(11):2744–2755
190. Yang Z, Garcia A, Xu S, Powell DR, Vertino PM, Singh S et al (2013) *Withania somnifera* root extract inhibits mammary cancer metastasis and epithelial to mesenchymal transition. PLoS ONE 8(9):e75069
191. Su B-N, Gu J-Q, Kang Y-H, Park E-J, Pezzuto JM, Kinghorn AD (2004) Induction of the phase II enzyme, quinone reductase, by withanolides and norwithanolides from solanaceous species. Mini Rev Org Chem 1(1):115–123
192. Mathur S, Kaur P, Sharma M, Katyal A, Singh B, Tiwari M et al (2004) The treatment of skin carcinoma, induced by UV B radiation, using 1-oxo-5beta, 6beta-epoxy-witha-2-enolide, isolated from the roots of *Withania somnifera*, in a rat model. Phytomedicine 11(5):452–460
193. Padmavathi B, Rath PC, Rao AR, Singh RP (2005) Roots of *Withania somnifera* inhibit forestomach and skin carcinogenesis in mice. Evid Based Complement Altern Med 2 (1):99–105
194. Li W, Zhang C, Du H, Huang V, Sun B, Harris JP et al (October 2015) Withaferin A suppresses the up-regulation of acetyl-coA carboxylase 1 and skin tumor formation in a skin carcinogenesis mouse model. Mol Carcinog 1–8. doi: 10.1002/mc.22423. (Epub ahead of print)
195. Hahm ER, Lee J, Kim SH, Sehrawat A, Arlotti JA, Shiva SS et al (2013) Metabolic alterations in mammary cancer prevention by withaferin A in a clinically relevant mouse model. J Natl Cancer Inst 105(15):1111–1122
196. Kim SH, Singh SV (2014) Mammary cancer chemoprevention by withaferin A is accompanied by in vivo suppression of self-renewal of cancer stem cells. Cancer Prev Res (Phila) 7(7):738–747
197. Khazal KF, Hill DL, Grubbs CJ (2014) Effect of *Withania somnifera* root extract on spontaneous estrogen receptor-negative mammary cancer in MMTV/Neu mice. Anticancer Res 34(11):6327–6332
198. Kataria H, Kumar S, Chaudhary H, Kaur G (2016) *Withania somnifera* suppresses tumor growth of intracranial allograft of glioma cells. Mol Neurobiol 53(6):4143–4158
199. McKenna MK, Gachuki BW, Alhakeem SS, Oben KN, Rangnekar VM, Gupta RC et al (2015) Anti-cancer activity of withaferin A in B-cell lymphoma. Cancer Biol Ther 16 (7):1088–1098
200. Kakar SS, Ratajczak MZ, Powell KS, Moghadamfalahi M, Miller DM, Batra SK et al (2014) Withaferin a alone and in combination with cisplatin suppresses growth and metastasis of ovarian cancer by targeting putative cancer stem cells. PLoS ONE 9(9):e107596
201. Fong MY, Jin S, Rane M, Singh RK, Gupta R, Kakar SS (2012) Withaferin A synergizes the therapeutic effect of doxorubicin through ROS-mediated autophagy in ovarian cancer. PLoS ONE 7(7):e42265
202. Yang H, Shi G, Dou QP (2007) The tumor proteasome is a primary target for the natural anticancer compound Withaferin A isolated from "Indian winter cherry". Mol Pharmacol 71 (2):426–437
203. Srinivasan S, Ranga RS, Burikhanov R, Han SS, Chendil D (2007) Par-4-dependent apoptosis by the dietary compound withaferin A in prostate cancer cells. Cancer Res 67 (1):246–253
204. Lahat G, Zhu QS, Huang KL, Wang S, Bolshakov S, Liu J et al (2010) Vimentin is a novel anti-cancer therapeutic target; insights from in vitro and in vivo mice xenograft studies. PLoS ONE 5(4):e10105
205. Munagala R, Kausar H, Munjal C, Gupta RC (2011) Withaferin A induces p53-dependent apoptosis by repression of HPV oncogenes and upregulation of tumor suppressor proteins in human cervical cancer cells. Carcinogenesis 32(11):1697–1705
206. Yang H, Wang Y, Cheryan VT, Wu W, Cui CQ, Polin LA et al (2012) Withaferin A inhibits the proteasome activity in mesothelioma in vitro and in vivo. PLoS ONE 7(8):e41214

207. Biswal BM, Sulaiman SA, Ismail HC, Zakaria H, Musa KI (2013) Effect of *Withania somnifera* (Ashwagandha) on the development of chemotherapy-induced fatigue and quality of life in breast cancer patients. Integr Cancer Ther 12(4):312–322
208. Amor S, Peferoen LA, Vogel DY, Breur M, van der Valk P, Baker D et al (2014) Inflammation in neurodegenerative diseases–an update. Immunology 142(2):151–166
209. Amor S, Woodroofe MN (2014) Innate and adaptive immune responses in neurodegeneration and repair. Immunology 141(3):287–291
210. Zhao J, Nakamura N, Hattori M, Kuboyama T, Tohda C, Komatsu K (2002) Withanolide derivatives from the roots of *Withania somnifera* and their neurite outgrowth activities. Chem Pharm Bull (Tokyo) 50(6):760–765
211. Kuboyama T, Tohda C, Komatsu K (2005) Neuritic regeneration and synaptic reconstruction induced by withanolide A. Br J Pharmacol 144(7):961–971
212. Martorana F, Guidotti G, Brambilla L, Rossi D (2015) Withaferin A inhibits nuclear factor-kappaB-dependent pro-inflammatory and stress response pathways in the astrocytes. Neural Plast 2015:381964
213. Patil SP, Maki S, Khedkar SA, Rigby AC, Chan C (2010) Withanolide A and asiatic acid modulate multiple targets associated with amyloid-beta precursor protein processing and amyloid-beta protein clearance. J Nat Prod 73(7):1196–1202
214. Choudhary MI, Yousuf S, Nawaz SA, Ahmed S, Atta ur R (2004) Cholinesterase inhibiting withanolides from *Withania somnifera*. Chem Pharm Bull (Tokyo) 52(11):1358–1361
215. Riaz N, Malik A, Nawaz SA, Muhammad P, Choudhary MI (2004) Cholinesterase-inhibiting withanolides from Ajuga bracteosa. Chem Biodivers 1(9):1289–1295
216. Grover A, Shandilya A, Agrawal V, Bisaria VS, Sundar D (2012) Computational evidence to inhibition of human acetyl cholinesterase by withanolide a for Alzheimer treatment. J Biomol Struct Dyn 29(4):651–662
217. Durg S, Dhadde SB, Vandal R, Shivakumar BS, Charan CS (2015) *Withania somnifera* (Ashwagandha) in neurobehavioural disorders induced by brain oxidative stress in rodents: a systematic review and meta-analysis. J Pharm Pharmacol 67(7):879–899
218. Sehgal N, Gupta A, Valli RK, Joshi SD, Mills JT, Hamel E et al (2012) *Withania somnifera* reverses Alzheimer's disease pathology by enhancing low-density lipoprotein receptor-related protein in liver. Proc Natl Acad Sci 109(9):3510–3515
219. Galvan A, Wichmann T (2008) Pathophysiology of parkinsonism. Clin Neurophysiol 119 (7):1459–1474
220. Przedborski S, Levivier M, Jiang H, Ferreira M, Jackson-Lewis V, Donaldson D et al (1995) Dose-dependent lesions of the dopaminergic nigrostriatal pathway induced by intrastriatal injection of 6-hydroxydopamine. Neuroscience 67(3):631–647
221. Przedborski S, Vila M (2003) The 1-methyl-4-phenyl-1,2,3,6-tetrahydropyridine mouse model: a tool to explore the pathogenesis of Parkinson's disease. Ann N Y Acad Sci 991:189–198
222. Prakash J, Yadav SK, Chouhan S, Singh SP (2013) Neuroprotective role of *Withania somnifera* root extract in maneb-paraquat induced mouse model of parkinsonism. Neurochem Res 38(5):972–980
223. RajaSankar S, Manivasagam T, Sankar V, Prakash S, Muthusamy R, Krishnamurti A et al (2009) *Withania somnifera* root extract improves catecholamines and physiological abnormalities seen in a Parkinson's disease model mouse. J Ethnopharmacol 125(3):369–373
224. Ahmad M, Saleem S, Ahmad AS, Ansari MA, Yousuf S, Hoda MN et al (2005) Neuroprotective effects of *Withania somnifera* on 6-hydroxydopamine induced Parkinsonism in rats. Hum Exp Toxicol 24(3):137–147
225. RajaSankar S, Manivasagam T, Surendran S (2009) Ashwagandha leaf extract: a potential agent in treating oxidative damage and physiological abnormalities seen in a mouse model of Parkinson's disease. Neurosci Lett 454(1):11–15
226. Sankar SR, Manivasagam T, Krishnamurti A, Ramanathan M (2007) The neuroprotective effect of *Withania somnifera* root extract in MPTP-intoxicated mice: an analysis of behavioral and biochemical variables. Cell Mol Biol Lett 12(4):473–481

227. Prakash J, Chouhan S, Yadav SK, Westfall S, Rai SN, Singh SP (2014) *Withania somnifera* alleviates parkinsonian phenotypes by inhibiting apoptotic pathways in dopaminergic neurons. Neurochem Res 39(12):2527–2536
228. Crotti A, Glass CK (2015) The choreography of neuroinflammation in Huntington's disease. Trends Immunol 36(6):364–373
229. Kumar P, Kumar A (2008) Effects of root extract of *Withania somnifera* in 3-nitropropionic acid-induced cognitive dysfunction and oxidative damage in rats. Int J Health Res 1(3):139–149
230. Kumar P, Kumar A (2009) Possible neuroprotective effect of *Withania somnifera* root extract against 3-nitropropionic acid-induced behavioral, biochemical, and mitochondrial dysfunction in an animal model of Huntington's disease. J Med Food 12(3):591–600
231. Nagashayana N, Sankarankutty P, Nampoothiri MR, Mohan PK, Mohanakumar KP (2000) Association of L-DOPA with recovery following Ayurveda medication in Parkinson's disease. J Neurol Sci 176(2):124–127
232. Tian R, Hou G, Li D, Yuan TF (2014) A possible change process of inflammatory cytokines in the prolonged chronic stress and its ultimate implications for health. Sci World J 2014:780616
233. Furtado M, Katzman MA (2015) Neuroinflammatory pathways in anxiety, posttraumatic stress, and obsessive compulsive disorders. Psychiatry Res 229(1–2):37–48
234. Raison CL, Capuron L, Miller AH (2006) Cytokines sing the blues: inflammation and the pathogenesis of depression. Trends Immunol 27(1):24–31
235. Tohmi M, Tsuda N, Watanabe Y, Kakita A, Nawa H (2004) Perinatal inflammatory cytokine challenge results in distinct neurobehavioral alterations in rats: implication in psychiatric disorders of developmental origin. Neurosci Res 50(1):67–75
236. Potvin S, Stip E, Sepehry AA, Gendron A, Bah R, Kouassi E (2008) Inflammatory cytokine alterations in schizophrenia: a systematic quantitative review. Biol Psychiatry 63(8):801–808
237. Goldstein BI, Kemp DE, Soczynska JK, McIntyre RS (2009) Inflammation and the phenomenology, pathophysiology, comorbidity, and treatment of bipolar disorder: a systematic review of the literature. J Clin Psychiatry 70(8):1078–1090
238. Berk M, Kapczinski F, Andreazza AC, Dean OM, Giorlando F, Maes M et al (2011) Pathways underlying neuroprogression in bipolar disorder: focus on inflammation, oxidative stress and neurotrophic factors. Neurosci Biobehav Rev 35(3):804–817
239. Gray SM, Bloch MH (2012) Systematic review of proinflammatory cytokines in obsessive–compulsive disorder. Curr Psychiatry Rep 14(3):220–228
240. Rege NN, Thatte UM, Dahanukar SA (1999) Adaptogenic properties of six rasayana herbs used in Ayurvedic medicine. Phytother Res 13(4):275–291
241. Panossian A, Wikman G (2009) Evidence-based efficacy of adaptogens in fatigue, and molecular mechanisms related to their stress-protective activity. Curr Clin Pharmacol 4 (3):198–219
242. Prud'homme GJ, Glinka Y, Wang Q (2015) Immunological GABAergic interactions and therapeutic applications in autoimmune diseases. Autoimmun Rev 14(11):1048–1056
243. Mehta AK, Binkley P, Gandhi SS, Ticku MK (1991) Pharmacological effects of *Withania somnifera* root extract on GABAA receptor complex. Indian J Med Res 94:312–315
244. Candelario M, Cuellar E, Reyes-Ruiz JM, Darabedian N, Feimeng Z, Miledi R et al (2015) Direct evidence for GABAergic activity of *Withania somnifera* on mammalian ionotropic GABAA and GABArho receptors. J Ethnopharmacol 171:264–272
245. Bhattacharya SK, Muruganandam AV (2003) Adaptogenic activity of *Withania somnifera*: an experimental study using a rat model of chronic stress. Pharmacol Biochem Behav 75 (3):547–555
246. Gupta GL, Rana AC (2007) Protective effect of *Withania somnifera* dunal root extract against protracted social isolation induced behavior in rats. Indian J Physiol Pharmacol 51(4):345–353
247. Gupta GL, Rana AC (2008) Effect of *Withania somnifera* Dunal in ethanol-induced anxiolysis and withdrawal anxiety in rats. Indian J Exp Biol 46(6):470–475

248. Bhattacharya SK, Bhattacharya A, Sairam K, Ghosal S (2000) Anxiolytic-antidepressant activity of *Withania somnifera* glycowithanolides: an experimental study. Phytomedicine 7 (6):463–469
249. Kumar A, Kalonia H (2007) Protective effect of *Withania somnifera* Dunal on the behavioral and biochemical alterations in sleep-disturbed mice (Grid over water suspended method). Indian J Exp Biol 45(6):524–528
250. Shah PC, Trivedi NA, Bhatt JD, Hemavathi KG (2006) Effect of *Withania somnifera* on forced swimming test induced immobility in mice and its interaction with various drugs. Indian J Physiol Pharmacol 50(4):409–415
251. Kaurav BP, Wanjari MM, Chandekar A, Chauhan NS, Upmanyu N (2012) Influence of *Withania somnifera* on obsessive compulsive disorder in mice. Asian Pac J Trop Med 5 (5):380–384
252. Cooley K, Szczurko O, Perri D, Mills EJ, Bernhardt B, Zhou Q et al (2009) Naturopathic care for anxiety: a randomized controlled trial ISRCTN78958974. PLoS ONE 4(8):e6628
253. Andrade C, Aswath A, Chaturvedi SK, Srinivasa M, Raguram R (2000) A double-blind, placebo-controlled evaluation of the anxiolytic efficacy of an ethanolic extract of *withania somnifera*. Indian J Psychiatry 42(3):295–301
254. Chandrasekhar K, Kapoor J, Anishetty S (2012) A prospective, randomized double-blind, placebo-controlled study of safety and efficacy of a high-concentration full-spectrum extract of ashwagandha root in reducing stress and anxiety in adults. Indian J Psychol Med 34 (3):255–262
255. Auddy B, Hazra J, Mitra A, Abedon B, Ghosal S (2008) A standardized *Withania somnifera* extract significantly reduces stress-related parameters in chronically stressed humans: a double-blind, randomized, placebo-controlled study. J Am Neutraceut Assoc 11:50–56
256. Khyati S, Anup T (2013) A randomized double blind placebo controlled study of ashwagandha on generalized anxiety disorder. Int Ayurvedic Med J 1:1–7
257. Pratte MA, Nanavati KB, Young V, Morley CP (2014) An alternative treatment for anxiety: a systematic review of human trial results reported for the Ayurvedic herb ashwagandha (*Withania somnifera*). J Altern Complement Med 20(12):901–908
258. Pingali U, Pilli R, Fatima N (2014) Effect of standardized aqueous extract of *Withania somnifera* on tests of cognitive and psychomotor performance in healthy human participants. Pharmacogn Res 6(1):12–18
259. Chengappa KN, Bowie CR, Schlicht PJ, Fleet D, Brar JS, Jindal R (2013) Randomized placebo-controlled adjunctive study of an extract of *withania somnifera* for cognitive dysfunction in bipolar disorder. J Clin Psychiatry 74(11):1076–1083
260. Chengappa KN (2014) *Withania Somnifera*: an immunomodulator and anti-inflammatory agent for schizophrenia. In: ClinicalTrials.gov. National Library of Medicine (US), Bethesda (MD). [cited 2015 Dec 10]. https://clinicaltrials.gov/show/NCT01793935. p NLM identifier: NCT01793935

Chapter 15
Gambogic Acid and Its Role in Chronic Diseases

Manoj K. Pandey, Deepkamal Karelia and Shantu G. Amin

Abstract Kokum, a spice derived from the fruit of the *Garcinia hanburyi* tree, is traditionally used in Ayurvedic medicines to facilitate digestion and to treat sores, dermatitis, diarrhoea, dysentery, and ear infection. One of the major active components of kokum is gambogic acid, also known as guttic acid, guttatic acid, beta-guttilactone, and beta-guttiferin. Gambogic acid's anti-proliferative, anti-bacterial; antioxidant and anti-inflammatory effects result from its modulation of numerous cell-signaling intermediates. This chapter discusses the sources, chemical components, mechanism of action, and disease targets of the kokum spice.

Keywords Neutraceuticals · Dietary agents · Gambogic acid · Kokum · Cancer · Signal transduction pathways

15.1 Introduction

Mother Nature has gifted us a variety of natural agents, including nutraceuticals. One of the well-known nutraceuticals is Gambogic acid (GA), which is a xanthonoid derived from the brownish or orange resin from *Garcinia hanburyi* (Fig. 15.1). *Garcinia hanburyi* is a small to medium-sized evergreen tree with smooth gray bark, and it is native to Cambodia, southern Vietnam, and Thailand. *Garcinia indica*, primarily of Indian origin, is known by many names: bindin, biran, bhirand, bhinda, kokum, katambi, panarpuli, ratamba, amsol, and tamal. In English language, it is commonly known as mangosteen, wild mangosteen, red mango, Hanbury's Garcinia, gambojia, gamboge, and Indian gamboge tree. Germans called this gummi-gutti.

The *Garcinia indica* seed contains 23–26 % oil, which is used in confectionery, medicines, and cosmetics. It is used in curries and other dishes as a slightly bitter spice, a souring agent, and as a substitute for tamarind.

M.K. Pandey (✉) · D. Karelia · S.G. Amin
Department of Pharmacology, College of Medicine, Pennsylvania State University, 500 University Dr., Hershey, PA 17033, USA
e-mail: mkp13@psu.edu

S.C. Gupta et al. (eds.), *Anti-inflammatory Nutraceuticals and Chronic Diseases*, Advances in Experimental Medicine and Biology 928,
DOI 10.1007/978-3-319-41334-1_15

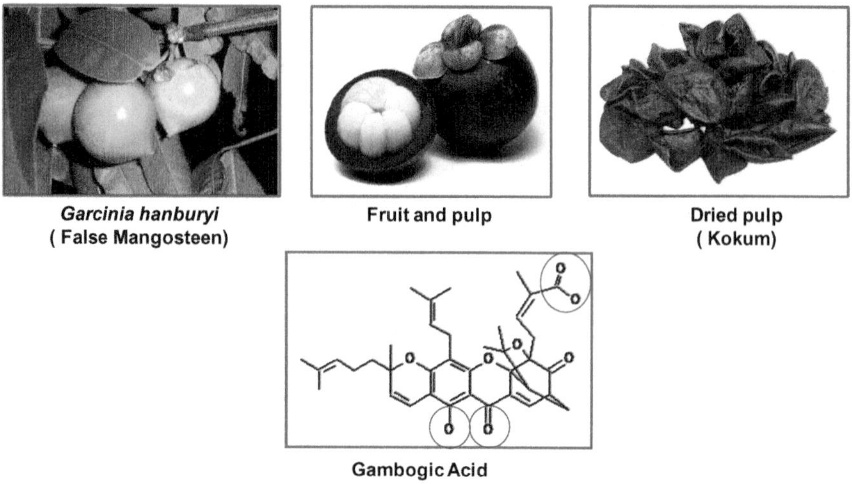

Fig. 15.1 Plant species and fruits by which gambogic acid is derived. *Highlighted circles* on GA structure indicate the most common sites for novel derivative generation

In traditional medicine, such as ayurveda, kokum is prescribed for edema, rheumatism, delayed menstruation, constipation and other bowel complaints, and intestinal parasites. The extract of *Garcinia cambogia* is used as an herbal appetite suppressant and weight-loss supplement.

In last decades, worldwide extensive studies have been performed on Gambogic acid to understand its full potential as therapeutic agents against variety of diseases including chronic diseases such as cancers which is summarized in following sections.

15.2 Physciochemical Properties of GA

GA is also chemically called as Guttic acid, Guttatic acid, beta-Guttilactone, and beta-Guttiferin. The molecular formula and weight of GA is $C_{38}H_{44}O_8$ and 628.76, respectively. The appearance of this xanthone is amorphous orange solid. The core of GA is known as xanthone core and contains a unique 4-oxatricyclo [4.3.1.03,7] decan-2-one scaffold [1, 2]. Earlier studies regarding its structural activity relationships (SAR) revealed that the C¼C bond of the α,β-unsaturated ketone in GA is critical for its antitumor activity, while the HOC(6), C(8)¼O, and C(30)OOH groups could tolerate a variety of modifications Fig. 15.1 [3, 4]. Along these lines various modifications have been performed to make GA as a better antitumor agent [5, 6].

15.3 Modulation of Cell Signaling Pathways by GA

Enthusiasm shown by researchers from around the globe clearly suggests that GA has been one of the "hot" nutraceuticals. GA has shown to be effective on different chronic diseases (Sect. 4.1 covers different chronic diseases), but its effect on cancer has been studied the most. Almost a decade ago our group showed that the anti-inflammatory and anticancer response of GA is associated with its inhibitory response on Nuclear Factor-Kappa B (NF-κB) [7], since then plethora of studies suggest that GA regulates several key signaling pathways. GA exhibits anti-proliferative, antioxidant, and anti-inflammatory effects by modulating cell signaling pathways, enzymes, and molecular targets, such as epigenetic regulators, protein kinases, transcription factors, inflammatory biomarkers, and growth regulators. Through microarray analysis, GA modulates many gene products [8, 9] (Table 15.1).

15.3.1 GA Inhibits Signaling of Nuclear Factor-Kappa B (NF-κB)

The transcription factor NF-κB is one of the major mediators of inflammation and is linked with many diseases including cancer, diabetes, arthritis, and neurological disorders. Therefore, an agent that can suppress NF-κB activation has potential for clinical use against various chronic illnesses. GA suppression of NF-κB activation induced by TNF-α, LPS, and various agents [7, 10] leads to the suppression of NF-κB regulated products, such as cyclooxygenase type 2 (COX-2), inducible nitric oxide synthase (iNOS), and survival proteins [7, 10, 11]. These actions give it great potential as a broad-spectrum clinical agent.

15.3.2 GA Inhibits Phosphatidylinositol 3′-Kinase/Protein Kinase B (PI3K/Akt)

Serine/threonine-specific protein kinase B, commonly designated Akt, is a central regulator of widely divergent cellular processes, including proliferation, differentiation, migration, survival, and metabolism [12, 13]. Akt is activated by a variety of stimuli, through growth factor receptors, in a PI3K-dependent manner [12, 13]. Frequently in human cancer, normal signaling along the Akt/PKB/phosphatase, and tensin homolog (PTEN) pathway is disrupted [14]. Akt plays important roles in development, progression, and resistance to chemotherapy in cells [12, 13]. Blocking Akt signaling can mediate apoptosis and inhibit the growth of tumor cells in vitro [14]. GA inhibits Akt activation, which leads to inhibition of tumor cell proliferation and survival [15–19].

Table 15.1 A list of molecular targets of Gambogic acid

Transcription factor
Nuclear factor—kappa B ↓
STAT-3 - ↓
STAT-5 ↓
Inflammatory cytokines
IL-6 ↓
Tumor necrosis factor alpha↓
Enzymes
Cyclooxygenase-2 ↓
Inducible nitric oxide synthase↓
Matrix metalloproteinase↓
Src homology 2 domain-containing typrosine phosphate 2↓
Kinases
Focal adhesion kinase↓
Janus kinase ↓
Mitogen-activated protein kinase ↓
Protein kinase A↓
Protein kinase B↓
Protein kinase C↓
Growth factors
Vascular endothelial growth factor ↓
Receptors
Chemokine (C-X-C motif) receptor 4 ↓
Transferrin receptor ↓
Adhesion molecules
Endothelial leukocyte adhesion molecule-1
Intracellular adhesion molecule-1 ↓
Anti-apoptotic proteins
B-cell lymphoma protein-2 ↓
Bcl-xL ↓
Inhibitory apoptosis protein-1 ↓
Mcl-1 ↓
Survivin ↓
Others
Cyclin D1 ↓
Heat shock protein 90 ↓
Heat shock protein 70 ↑

15.3.3 GA Inhibits Mitogen-Activated Protein Kinase (MAPK)

MAPKs are evolutionarily conserved enzymes that play a key role in the inflammatory stimuli and environmental stresses that lead to the activation of three independent pathways: p44/42 MAPK extracellular signal-regulated kinases 1 and 2 (ERK1/ERK2), c-Jun N-terminal kinase, and p38 MAPK [20]. In vitro studies of several cancer cells showed that GA inhibits MAPK pathways [21]. Moreover, this phytochemical also inhibited ERK in HT-29, HepG2, KBM5, and NCI-H460 cancer cells [22–24].

15.3.4 GA Inhibits Src

The Src family of proteins consists of eight non-receptor tyrosine kinases characterized by a common structure [25]. Src kinases are involved in signal transduction pathways that are triggered by a variety of surface receptors, including receptors for tyrosine kinases, integrin, and antigens, as well as receptors coupled with the G-protein [25, 26]. As a consequence of changes observed in protein expression and kinase activity in cancer cells, the Src family has been implicated in the development of cancer [25, 26]. This prompted the design of specific inhibitors, the most common of which are adenine mimetics, to treat solid tumors and leukemia clinically [25, 26]. In addition, some of the Src kinases expressed in hematopoietic cells play pivotal roles in lymphocyte maturation and activation [25]. This finding encouraged the development of safe and effective Src-specific inhibitors that are currently in clinical trials as immune-suppressants for the treatment of immunological disorders [15, 27]. Separate research showing that GA inhibits Src in PC3, and K562 cells suggests that GA may also have clinical potential against cancers and immunological disorders in which Src plays a pivotal role [15, 16].

15.3.5 GA Inhibits Signal Transducer and Activator of Transcription-3 (STAT-3) Pathways

Proteins in the STAT family are among the best studied of the latent cytoplasmic signal-dependent transcription factors [28–30]. In vitro studies of the MCF-7, MCF-10A, U266, and MM1.s cell lines suggest that GA modulates the nuclear translocation and DNA binding of STAT3 and inhibits genes modulated by this transcription factor [28, 31].

15.3.6 GA Inhibits Chemokine X-Receptor 4 (CXCR4) and Downstream Signaling Pathways

Chemokine receptors belong to class A seven transmembrane G-protein-coupled receptors and consist of 350 amino acids on average. Primary receptors are defined as CXCR, CCR, CR, or CX3CR [32]. The function of atypical chemokine receptors is to modulate immune responses by scavenging, sequestration, buffering as well as intracellular transport of chemokines from inflammatory sites [33–35]. The receptor CXCR4 is expressed on almost all of the hematopoietic cells, embryonic pluripotent, and tissue-committed stem cells, allowing them to migrate and invade along CXCL12 gradients. In malignant cells the chemokine receptor that is most commonly found is the receptor CXCR4 [34, 36]. At least 23 different types of tumor cells from human cancers of epithelial, mesenchymal and hematopoietic origin express CXCR4 [37]. In cancer, CXCL12 plays a role in the mobilization and recruitment of these cells to the inflammatory tumor microenvironment, neo-angiogenic niches, supporting revascularization, tumor growth, and metastasis [32, 38]. Thus an inhibitor of CXCR4/CXCL12 axis will inhibit tumor metastasis, GA is one of those inhibitors. Recently, we showed that GA directly interacts with CXCR4 and inhibits the migration of multiple myeloma cells [17]. We further demonstrate that GA inhibits CXCR4 regulated pathways and suppresses the bone loss [17]. Overall, GA has a tremendous potential to be used a therapeutic agent.

15.3.7 GA Inhibits CBP/p300 Histone Aceyltransferase (HAT) and Histone Deacetylase (HDAC)

The process of histone acetylation and deacetylation in eukaryotic cells alters chromatin structure and thereby modulates gene expression [39]. HATs and HDACs are classes of enzymes that effect histone acetylation [40]. These enzymes can also acetylate and deacetylate several nonhistone substrates, which can have functional consequences. Altered HAT and HDAC activities can lead to several diseases, ranging from cancer to neurodegenerative disorders. Therefore, HAT and HDAC inhibitors are being developed as therapeutic agents. GA inhibits HAT and HDAC activity in A549 lung cancer cells [41]. These activities of GA demonstrate its great potential as a therapeutic candidate.

15.3.8 GA Inhibits the Activation of Focal Adhesion Kinase (FAK)

FAK is a 119- to 121-kDa non-receptor protein kinase widely expressed in various tissues and cell types [42]. Several studies showed that FAK plays an important role in integrin signaling [43–45]. Once activated, whether by integrin or non-integrin stimuli, FAK binds to and activates several other molecules, such as Src, Src adaptor protein p130Cas, the growth factor receptor-bound protein 2 (Grb2), PI3K, and paxillin, and thus promotes signaling transduction [44, 46–50]. In a recent study, FAK was held responsible for uninhibited proliferation, protection from apoptosis, invasion, migration, adhesion, and spread, as well as tumor angiogenesis [46, 47]. Our group showed that GA modulates the tyrosine phosphorylation of FAK and subsequently induce apoptosis by downregulating Src, ERK, and Akt signaling in prostate cancer PC3 cells [16].

15.3.9 GA Inhibits iNOS

iNOS is expressed in a variety of cell types, particularly inflammatory cells, in response to diverse pro-inflammatory stimuli [51–53]. iNOS, which may be induced by bacterial LPS or its derivative lipid A, is expressed by a variety of solid tumors and generates high levels of nitric oxide inside tumor cells [10]. In vitro studies showed that GA inhibits LPS- and interferon-gamma-induced iNOS in RAW246.6 cells [10].

15.3.10 GA Induces the Production of Reactive Oxygen Species (ROS)

ROS have been linked with various cell signaling pathways [54, 55]. GA, induces the production of ROS [56].

15.3.11 GA Inhibits COX-2

Overexpression of COX-2 is associated with many cancers and is linked with tumor cell proliferation and suppression of apoptosis [57, 58]. Therefore, COX-2 inhibitors have great potential in the treatment of cancers and inflammatory conditions, as evidenced by the U. S. Food and Drug Administration's approval of celecoxib, a known COX-2 inhibitor, for the treatment of various inflammatory conditions [59]. GA, too, has been shown to inhibit COX-2 activation induced by TNF-α in KBM5 leukemic cells [7].

15.3.12 GA Inhibits Matrix Metalloproteinase 7 & 9 (MMP-7 & 9)

Also known as matrilysin, MMP-7 is a “minimal domain” MMP that exhibits proteolytic activity against components of the extracellular matrix [60–62]. MMP-7 is frequently overexpressed in human cancer tissues and is associated with cancer progression [63]. Therefore, MMP-7 inhibitors have great potential in the treatment of cancer [64]. The studies showed that GA inhibits the expression of MMP-7 in breast cancer cells like MDA-MB-231 and MDA-MB-435 [65, 66], further supporting the idea that GA may be effective against breast cancer in humans.

15.3.13 GA Inhibits Tubulin

Microtubules are a major component of the cytoskeleton. They are important in many cellular events and play a crucial role in cell division [67]. As such, microtubules are a highly attractive target for anticancer-drug design. Tubulin-binding agents, also called anti-microtubule or microtubule-targeted agents, are widely used chemotherapeutic drugs with a proven clinical efficacy against breast, lung, ovarian, prostate, and hematologic malignancies, as well as childhood cancers [68, 69]. Research has shown that GA belongs to this class of agents because it inhibits microtubule assembly and prevents cell division [20].

15.3.14 GA Inhibits Expression of Cyclin D1

The sequential transcriptional activation of cyclins, the regulatory subunits of cell cycle-specific kinases, is thought to regulate progress through the cell cycle [70]. Thus, cyclins are potential oncogenes, and overexpression of cyclin D1 or amplification at its genomic locus, 11q13, is commonly seen in breast cancer, head, and neck cancer, non-small-cell lung cancer, and mantle cell lymphoma [71, 72]. GA has been shown to inhibit Cyclin D1 in several cancers including leukemia and multiple myeloma [7, 31].

15.3.15 GA Induces Cleavage of Poly(ADP-Ribose) Polymerases (PARPs)

PARPs are cell signaling enzymes present in eukaryotes and are involved in poly (ADP ribosylation) of DNA-binding proteins [73]. Pharmacological degradation of PARP-1 may enhance the activity of antitumor drugs by inhibiting necrosis and activating apoptosis [74]. In vitro studies have shown that GA induces PARP degradation and enhances apoptosis in T98 glioma, HeLa, non-small lung cancer A549 and NCI-H460, breast cancer, and multiple myeloma cells [7, 11, 17, 22, 24, 31, 66, 75–77].

15.3.16 GA Inhibits Tumor Necrosis Factor-α (TNF-α)

TNF-α is a vital member of the multifunctional superfamily of TNFs and plays important roles in immunity and cellular remodeling, as well as apoptosis and cell survival [78]. Because TNF-α is a key player in inflammation and cancer, several efforts are underway to develop therapeutic TNF-α antagonists. Two such antagonists are from the *Garcinia* species. At a dose of 5 μM, both GA and cambogin inhibited the release of TNF-α by LPS-activated macrophages [79, 80], suggesting another mechanism for their antitumor activity.

15.3.17 GA Inhibits the Expression of Bcl-2 Family Proteins

The bcl-2 gene family consists of at least 25 genes that are proapoptotic or anti-apoptotic and share at least one of the four characteristic BH domains [81]. The anti-apoptotic protein bcl-2, which displays sequence homology in all four domains (i.e., BH1–BH4), promotes cell survival [82]. Increased expression of the bcl-2 protein commonly occurs in human malignancies and is associated with disease maintenance and progression, resistance to chemotherapy, and poor clinical outcome. Antisense oligonucleotides targeting bcl-2 have been shown to facilitate apoptosis in various tumor types [83]. Therefore, bcl-2 inhibitors have great potential in the treatment of cancer. In vitro and in vivo studies showed that GA inhibits bcl-2 expression in MGC-803, HL-60, MCF-7, A375M, SMMC-7721, BGC-823, Jeko-1, and K562 [15, 84–88].

15.3.18 GA Induces BID

Pro-apoptotic BID activates the multi-domain bcl-2 family members bcl-2–associated X protein (BAX) and bcl-2 homologous antagonist killer (BAK) [89]. Activation of either BAX or BAK produces an allosteric conformational change and releases cytochrome *c* [90]. This means that compounds that can induce BID could be very useful in the treatment of cancer. GA and its derivative GA3 are such inducers because these agents activate BID and induces apoptosis in cancer cells [91].

15.3.19 GA Induces BAD

BAD is proapoptotic and proliferative, suggesting that the cell cycle functions of the multi-domain bcl-2 family members [89]. BAD antagonizes both the cell cycle and anti-apoptotic functions of bcl-2 and bcl-xL through BH3 binding [89]. Overexpression of the BH3-only molecule BAD renders the cell unable to arrest in G0 and persistently activates cdk2 [92]. Previous study showed that GA in combination with nanoparticle Fe3O4 activates BAD and induces apoptosis in LOVO cells [93].

15.3.20 GA Inhibits Cytochrome c

Cytochrome *c*, an intermediate in apoptosis, is released by the mitochondria in response to proapoptotic stimuli. The studies have shown that GA, induces the expression of cytochrome *c* in colorectal cancer HT-29, bladder cancer T24 and UMUC3, breast cancer MDA-MB-231, and human hepatocellular carcinoma cells [94–96].

15.3.21 GA Induces the Activation of Caspase-3 and Caspase-9

Caspases play a central role in mediating various apoptotic responses. In vitro and in vivo research of GA has shown that it induces the activation of caspase-3 and caspase-9 in various cancer cells including glioma, osteosarcoma, non-small lung cancer, leukemia, lymphoma, breast cancer, pancreatic cancer, melanoma and multiple myeloma and, induces apoptosis [7, 11, 17, 22, 24, 31, 66, 75–77].

15.4 Role of GA in Chronic Diseases

Extensive studies from past one decade have shed light on GA's potential as anti-inflammatory and anticancer agents. So far the focus of the studies have been to identify the molecular targets by which GA exerts its effects, primarily on cancer cells. However, a very recent study showed that GA could be used as an anti-psoriatic agent [97]. Importantly, the molecular mechanism by which GA mediates its effect strongly suggest that it could be used for the prevention and treatment of many organ and tissue disorders, which are associated with inflammation and oxidative stress. GA alleviates oxidative stress, inflammation in chronic diseases and regulates inflammatory and pro-inflammatory pathways related with most chronic diseases.

15.4.1 Cardiovascular Diseases

Cardiovascular Diseases (CVDs), including heart disease, vascular disease and atherosclerosis, are the most critical current global health threat. Epidemiological and clinical trials have shown strong consistent relationships between the inflammation markers and risk of cardiovascular diseases [98]. It is widely appreciated that the key mechanisms in the development of CVDs are inflammation and oxidant stress, activation of pro-inflammatory cytokines, chronic transmural inflammation, and C reactive protein (CRP) [99]. Thus cytokines, other bioactive molecules, and cells that are characteristic of inflammation are believed to be involved in atherogenesis. An elegant recent study by Liu et al. [100] showed that GA inhibits pressure overload or isoproterenol infusion-induced cardiac hypertrophy and fibrosis, through the inhibition of the proteasome and the NF-κB pathway, suggesting that GA treatment may provide a new strategy to treat cardiac hypertrophy and changes in myocardial NF-κB signaling [100].

15.4.2 Rheumatoid Arthritis

Rheumatoid arthritis (RA) could give rise to a systemic chronic inflammatory disorder and may impact many organs and tissues but mainly attack flexible (synovial) joints [101]. It was reported that oxidative stress made an important contribution to joint destruction in RA [102]. ROS is a significant mediator that activates a variety of transcription factors including NF-κB and AP-1, thus regulating the expression of over 500 different genes, such as growth factors, chemokines, cell cycle regulatory molecules, inflammatory cytokines, and anti-inflammatory molecules [103]. Therefore, transcription factors and genes, involved in inflammation and antioxidation, are suspected to play a crucial adjective function in RA. The main treatment of RA is to reduce arthritis reaction, inhibit disease development and irreversible bone destruction, protect the joints and muscle function, and ultimately achieve complete remission or low disease activity. Treatment principles include patient education, early treatment, and combination therapy [104, 105]. Drug therapy includes nonsteroidal anti-inflammatory drugs (NSAIDs), slow-acting antirheumatic drugs, immunosuppressive agents, immune and biological agents, and botanicals. NSAIDs are most common. Our earlier studies strongly suggest that GA is one of the NSAIDs with anti-inflammatory and antioxidant actions both in vivo and in vitro and could be used effectively as anti-RA agent. Recent studies of Cascao et al. [106] support our hypothesis. By using rat RA model, this group showed that GA inhibits RA by inhibiting the levels of cytokines and key inflammatory molecules [106].

15.4.3 Diabetes and Obesity

Type 2 diabetes is a chronic disease where cells have reduced insulin signaling, leading to hyperglycemia, and long-term complications, such as heart, kidney, and liver disease. Recently, more and more studies have shown the critical roles of oxidative stress and inflammatory reactions in the pathogenesis of diabetes. Studies have shown that AMP-activated protein kinase (AMPK) plays a key role in maintaining intracellular and whole-body energy homeostasis. Activation of AMPK has been shown to ameliorate the symptoms of type 2 diabetes and obesity. In vitro studies by Zhao et al. [107] demonstrate that GA, activates AMPK by increasing the phosphorylation of AMPKα and its downstream substrate ACC in various cell lines [107]. This group also showed that GA induced activation of AMPK was associated with increased intracellular ROS level. Collectively, these results suggest that GA may be a novel direct activator of AMPK and could be used as anti-diabetic agent. However, further studies are required to fully evaluate this function of GA.

15.4.4 Psoriasis

Psoriasis is a chronic inflammatory skin disease characterized by thick, red, and scaly lesions on any part of the body, which affects approximately 2 % of the population worldwide [108]. Many cytokines, including interleukin-23(IL-23), IL-17A, TNF-α, IL-6, IL-1β, and IL-22, are also involved in the pathogenesis of psoriasis [109]. Along these lines a recent study showed that GA could be used as an anti-psoriatic agent [97].

15.4.5 Cancer

Inflammation plays key roles in all the ways of tumorigenesis and therapy response [110]. Activation and interaction between STAT3 and NF-κB are very vital in the control of cancer cells and inflammatory cells [111]. TNF-α, VEGF, IL-10, MMP-2 and MMP-9, MCP, CD4+ T, AP-1, Akt, PPAR-γ, MAP kinases, and mTORC1 are also important linking factors between inflammation and cancer [111]. It has been shown that GA suppresses the growth of various cancer cells such as non-small cell lung cancer [112], human hepatocellular carcinoma [113], oral squamous cell carcinoma [114], human breast cancer [86], human malignant melanoma [115], human gastric carcinoma [116], and human leukemia cancer [7] and multiple myeloma [31, 117]. A variety of mechanisms have been proposed by which GA inhibits the proliferation of cancer cells and induces apoptosis. These include inhibition of antiapoptotic proteins Bcl-2 [86, 88] and survivin [118]; induction of apoptosis-associated proteins p53 [119], bax, and procaspase-3 [115]; activation of c-*jun*-NH2-kinase, p38 [20], and GSK-3β [15]; inhibition of topoisomerase II by binding to its ATPase domain [120], downregulation of the MDM2 oncogene and subsequent induction of p21 [119]; suppression of LPS induced COX-2 [10]; and downregulation of human telomerase reverse transcriptase [121]. It has also been shown that GA directly binds to c-myc [122], transferrin receptors [123], and CXCR4 [124]. Recently, a proteomic approach revealed that GA suppresses expression of 14-3-3 protein sigma and stathmin [116]. We have shown earlier that GA inhibits NF-κB and its regulated gene products in human myeloid leukemia [7]; STAT3 and its regulated gene products in MM [31]. Most recently, we showed that GA interacts with CXCR4 and inhibits chemotaxis and osteoclastogenesis in MM [124]. Recently, it is shown that GA is a novel tissue specific proteasome inhibitor, with potency comparable to bortezomib [25]. In addition, recent studies have shown that GA is bioavailable, less toxic, effective, and inhibits development of tumors in animal models, and most importantly it has been approved for phase 2 clinical trial in solid tumors [4, 121, 125, 126]. Since, GA modulates the expression of proteins plays important role in survival, migration, invasion and chemoresistance of multiple myeloma cells (Fig. 15.2), we have been working on the development of GA as anti-myeloma agent.

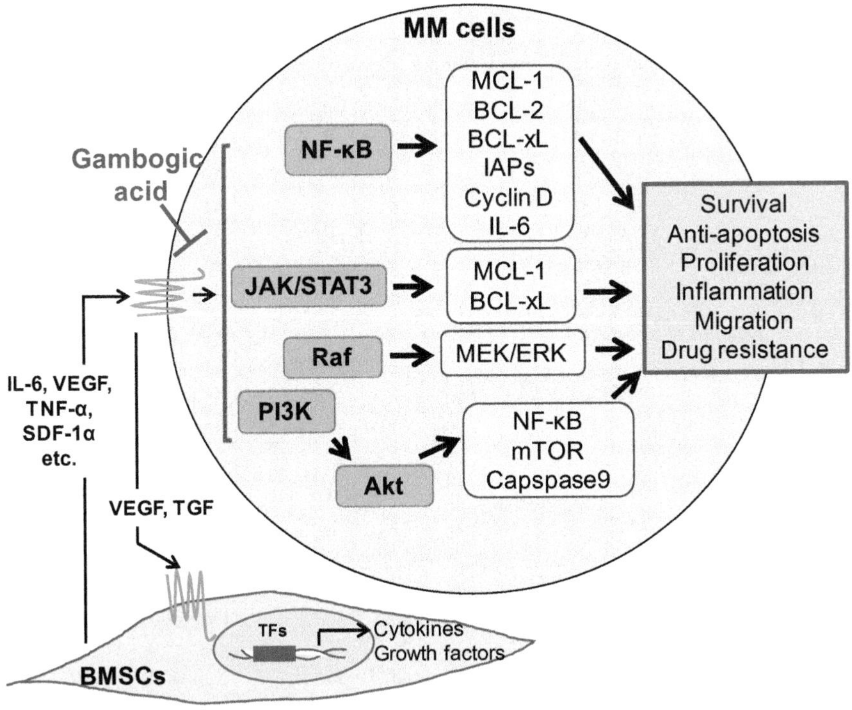

Fig. 15.2 Intimate relationship between multiple myeloma and bone marrow microenvironment. Bone marrow stromal cells secrete cytokine a growth factors, these growth factors activates several pathways in multiple myeloma. Gambogic acid targets these pathways

15.5 Biological Activities of GA in Animal Models

Besides the extensive in vitro demonstrations of GA's anti-proliferative effects, numerous other studies have evaluated its efficacy in various animal models in vivo (Table 15.2). The in vivo studies have investigated the effects of GA on tumor angiogenesis and the biomarkers COX-2 and VEGF in prostate carcinoma [16]. One group demonstrated that systemic administration of GA for 3 weeks to athymic mice bearing non-small lung NCI-H1993 xenografts significantly inhibited tumor growth [127]. Meanwhile, others have shown that GA can suppress the growth of cervical carcinoma [128], modulate the growth of colorectal cancer [129], modulate the growth of prostate cancer in rodents [16], inhibit the growth of human B-cell lymphoma by inducing proteasome inhibition [130] in nude mice, and inhibits hepatocellular carcinoma, multiple myeloma, bladder cancer tumor growth, in part by suppressing angiogenesis, and inducing apoptosis [7, 11, 17, 22, 24, 31, 66, 75–77]. More recent studies have evaluated GA's chemosensitizing effects [118]. Our group evaluated the chemosensitizing effect of GA in combination with paclitaxel, TNF-α, 5-FU on multiple myeloma [7]. Together, these in vivo animal studies clearly suggest GA's anticancer potential when administered either alone or in combination with currently employed chemotherapeutic agents.

Table 15.2 A list of studies describing antitumor effects of gambogic acid in animals

Tumor	Cell line	Route	Dose (mg/kg)	Model	References
Lung	SPC-A1	i.v.	4, 8	Xenograft	[121]
	NCI-H1993	i.p.	10, 20 or 30	Xenograft	[127]
	NCI-H1975	i.v.	8	Xenograft	[137]
	A549	i.p.	8, 16 and 32	Xenograft	[134]
Gastric cancer	BGC-823	i.v.	8	Xenograft	[85]
Cervical carcinoma	HeLa cells	i.p.	2	Xenograft	[128]
Chronic myeloid · leukemia	KBM5	i.p.	3	Xenograft	[24]
Liver	HepG2	i.v.	1.5	Xenograft	[132]
Ovarian	SKOV3		1.0	Xenograft	[133]
Breast	MDA-MB-231	i.v.	4 and 8	Orthotopic	[94]
Hepatoma	H22	i.v.	2, 4 and 8	Xenograft	[125]
	H22	p.o.	12.5, 25, 30 and 50	Xenograft	[125]
	SMMC-7721	i.v.	2, 4, and 8	Xenograft	[131, 136]
Melanoma	B16-F10	i.v.	0.375, 0.75, and 1.5	Orthotopic	[135]
Colon	HT-29	i.v.	5, 10 and 20	Xenograft	[129]

15.6 Biological Activities of GA in Humans

There are no clinical studies so far in USA, however in China GA is in Phase II clinical trial [4, 121, 125, 126]. The plethora of studies clearly suggest GA's potential as anticancer agent. It the opportune time to seriously consider this xanthone in clinical trial especially in USA.

15.7 Conclusions

The spice derived from kokum, the fruit of *Garcinia indica*, is used in Indian cuisines and Ayurvedic medicine. The main component isolated from kokum is GA, which demonstrates thrust quencher, antioxidant, antimicrobial, antiulceration, and anticancer properties. Although GA is a potent, biologically active compound, only a number of studies are carried out in animals and none have been done in humans. Because of its diverse range of biological activity in vitro, more in vivo and clinical studies are warranted to establish its true usefulness as a clinical therapeutic agent in a variety of human diseases.

References

1. Guo Q et al (2006) Toxicological studies of gambogic acid and its potential targets in experimental animals. Basic Clin Pharmacol Toxicol 99(2):178–184
2. Noguer O, Villena J, Lorita J, Vilaro S, Reina M (2009) Syndecan-2 downregulation impairs angiogenesis in human microvascular endothelial cells. Exp Cell Res 315(5):795–808
3. Jang SW et al (2007) Gambogic amide, a selective agonist for TrkA receptor that possesses robust neurotrophic activity, prevents neuronal cell death. Proc Natl Acad Sci USA 104 (41):16329–16334
4. Qi Q et al (2008) Studies on the toxicity of gambogic acid in rats. J Ethnopharmacol 117 (3):433–438
5. Udvadia AJ, Linney E (2003) Windows into development: historic, current, and future perspectives on transgenic zebrafish. Dev Biol 256(1):1–17
6. Zhang HZ et al (2004) Discovery, characterization and SAR of gambogic acid as a potent apoptosis inducer by a HTS assay. Bioorg Med Chem 12(2):309–317
7. Pandey MK et al (2007) Gambogic acid, a novel ligand for transferrin receptor, potentiates TNF-induced apoptosis through modulation of the nuclear factor-kappaB signaling pathway. Blood 110(10):3517–3525
8. Li X et al (2013) Gambogic acid is a tissue-specific proteasome inhibitor in vitro and in vivo. Cell Rep 3(1):211–222
9. Wang Y et al (2014) Methyl jasmonate sensitizes human bladder cancer cells to gambogic acid-induced apoptosis through down-regulation of EZH2 expression by miR-101. Br J Pharmacol 171(3):618–635
10. Palempalli UD et al (2009) Gambogic acid covalently modifies IkappaB kinase-beta subunit to mediate suppression of lipopolysaccharide-induced activation of NF-kappaB in macrophages. Biochem J 419(2):401–409

11. Yang LJ, Chen Y (2013) New targets for the antitumor activity of gambogic acid in hematologic malignancies. Acta Pharmacol Sin 34(2):191–198
12. Franke TF (2008) PI3K/Akt: getting it right matters. Oncogene 27(50):6473–6488
13. Franke TF, Hornik CP, Segev L, Shostak GA, Sugimoto C (2003) PI3K/Akt and apoptosis: size matters. Oncogene 22(56):8983–8998
14. Fruman DA, Rommel C (2014) PI3K and cancer: lessons, challenges and opportunities. Nat Rev Drug Discov 13(2):140–156
15. Li R et al (2009) Gambogic acid induces G0/G1 arrest and apoptosis involving inhibition of SRC-3 and inactivation of Akt pathway in K562 leukemia cells. Toxicology 262(2):98–105
16. Yi T et al (2008) Gambogic acid inhibits angiogenesis and prostate tumor growth by suppressing vascular endothelial growth factor receptor 2 signaling. Cancer Res 68(6):1843–1850
17. Pandey MK et al (2014) Gambogic acid inhibits multiple myeloma mediated osteoclastogenesis through suppression of chemokine receptor CXCR4 signaling pathways. Exp Hematol 42(10):883–896
18. Yang Y, Sun X, Yang Y, Yang X, Zhu H, Dai S, Chen X, Zhang H, Guo Q, Song Y, Wang F, Cheng H, Sun X (2016) Gambogic acid enhances the radiosensitivity of human esophageal cancer cells by inducing reactive oxygen species via targeting Akt/mTOR pathway. Tumour Biol 37(2):1853–1862
19. Ma J et al (2015) Gambogic acid inhibits osteoclast formation and ovariectomy-induced osteoporosis by suppressing the JNK, p38 and Akt signalling pathways. Biochem J 469 (3):399–408
20. Chen J et al (2008) Microtubule depolymerization and phosphorylation of c-Jun N-terminal kinase-1 and p38 were involved in gambogic acid induced cell cycle arrest and apoptosis in human breast carcinoma MCF-7 cells. Life Sci 83(3–4):103–109
21. Lu N et al (2007) Gambogic acid inhibits angiogenesis through suppressing vascular endothelial growth factor-induced tyrosine phosphorylation of KDR/Flk-1. Cancer Lett 258 (1):80–89
22. Wang LH et al (2014) Gambogic acid synergistically potentiates cisplatin-induced apoptosis in non-small-cell lung cancer through suppressing NF-kappaB and MAPK/HO-1 signalling. Br J Cancer 110(2):341–352
23. Yan F et al (2012) Gambogenic acid induced mitochondrial-dependent apoptosis and referred to phospho-Erk1/2 and phospho-p38 MAPK in human hepatoma HepG2 cells. Environ Toxicol Pharmacol 33(2):181–190
24. Shi X et al (2014) Gambogic acid induces apoptosis in imatinib-resistant chronic myeloid leukemia cells via inducing proteasome inhibition and caspase-dependent Bcr-Abl downregulation. Clin Cancer Res 20(1):151–163
25. Parsons SJ, Parsons JT (2004) Src family kinases, key regulators of signal transduction. Oncogene 23(48):7906–7909
26. Benati D, Baldari CT (2008) SRC family kinases as potential therapeutic targets for malignancies and immunological disorders. Curr Med Chem 15(12):1154–1165
27. Aleshin A, Finn RS (2010) SRC: a century of science brought to the clinic. Neoplasia 12 (8):599–607
28. Yu H, Jove R (2004) The STATs of cancer—new molecular targets come of age. Nat Rev Cancer 4(2):97–105
29. Turkson J, Jove R (2000) STAT proteins: novel molecular targets for cancer drug discovery. Oncogene 19(56):6613–6626
30. Clevenger CV (2004) Roles and regulation of stat family transcription factors in human breast cancer. Am J Pathol 165(5):1449–1460
31. Prasad S, Pandey MK, Yadav VR, Aggarwal BB (2011) Gambogic acid inhibits STAT3 phosphorylation through activation of protein tyrosine phosphatase SHP-1: potential role in proliferation and apoptosis. Cancer Prev Res 4(7):1084–1094
32. Pandey MK, Rastogi S, Kale VP, Gowda T, Amin SG (2014) Targeting CXCL12/CXCR4 axis in multiple myeloma. J Hematol Thrombo Dis 2:159

33. Bachelerie F et al (2014) International Union of Basic and Clinical Pharmacology. [corrected]. LXXXIX. Update on the extended family of chemokine receptors and introducing a new nomenclature for atypical chemokine receptors. Pharmacol Rev 66 (1):1–79
34. Murphy PM et al (2000) International union of pharmacology. XXII. Nomenclature for chemokine receptors. Pharmacol Rev 52(1):145–176
35. Hansell CA, Hurson CE, Nibbs RJ (2011) DARC and D6: silent partners in chemokine regulation? Immunol Cell Biol 89(2):197–206
36. Nakayama T et al (2003) Cutting edge: profile of chemokine receptor expression on human plasma cells accounts for their efficient recruitment to target tissues. J Immunol 170(3):1136–1140
37. Balkwill F (2004) Cancer and the chemokine network. Nat Rev Cancer 4(7):540–550
38. Teicher BA, Fricker SP (2010) CXCL12 (SDF-1)/CXCR4 pathway in cancer. Clin Cancer Res 16(11):2927–2931
39. Yang XJ, Seto E (2007) HATs and HDACs: from structure, function and regulation to novel strategies for therapy and prevention. Oncogene 26(37):5310–5318
40. Legube G, Trouche D (2003) Regulating histone acetyltransferases and deacetylases. EMBO Rep 4(10):944–947
41. Qi Q et al (2015) Involvement of RECK in gambogic acid induced anti-invasive effect in A549 human lung carcinoma cells. Mol Carcinog 54(Suppl 1):E13–E25
42. Abbi S, Guan JL (2002) Focal adhesion kinase: protein interactions and cellular functions. Histol Histopathol 17(4):1163–1171
43. Guan JL (2010) Integrin signaling through FAK in the regulation of mammary stem cells and breast cancer. IUBMB Life 62(4):268–276
44. Mitra SK, Schlaepfer DD (2006) Integrin-regulated FAK-Src signaling in normal and cancer cells. Curr Opin Cell Biol 18(5):516–523
45. Guan JL (1997) Role of focal adhesion kinase in integrin signaling. Int J Biochem Cell Biol 29(8–9):1085–1096
46. Sulzmaier FJ, Jean C, Schlaepfer DD (2014) FAK in cancer: mechanistic findings and clinical applications. Nat Rev Cancer 14(9):598–610
47. Tai YL, Chen LC, Shen TL (2015) Emerging roles of focal adhesion kinase in cancer. BioMed Res Int 2015:690690
48. You D et al (2015) FAK mediates a compensatory survival signal parallel to PI3K-AKT in PTEN-null T-ALL cells. Cell Rep 10(12):2055–2068
49. Hu YL et al (2014) FAK and paxillin dynamics at focal adhesions in the protrusions of migrating cells. Sci Rep 4:6024
50. Schlaepfer DD, Jones KC, Hunter T (1998) Multiple Grb2-mediated integrin-stimulated signaling pathways to ERK2/mitogen-activated protein kinase: summation of both c-Src- and focal adhesion kinase-initiated tyrosine phosphorylation events. Mol Cell Biol 18(5):2571–2585
51. Janakiram NB, Rao CV (2012) iNOS-selective inhibitors for cancer prevention: promise and progress. Future Med Chem 4(17):2193–2204
52. Kostourou V et al (2011) The role of tumour-derived iNOS in tumour progression and angiogenesis. Br J Cancer 104(1):83–90
53. Lechner M, Lirk P, Rieder J (2005) Inducible nitric oxide synthase (iNOS) in tumor biology: the two sides of the same coin. Semin Cancer Biol 15(4):277–289
54. Finkel T (2011) Signal transduction by reactive oxygen species. J Cell Biol 194(1):7–15
55. Schieber M, Chandel NS (2014) ROS function in redox signaling and oxidative stress. CB 24 (10):R453–R462
56. Geng J, Xiao S, Zheng Z, Song S, Zhang L (2013) Gambogic acid protects from endotoxin shock by suppressing pro-inflammatory factors in vivo and in vitro. Inflammation research: official journal of the European Histamine Research Society… [et al.] 62(2):165–172
57. Stasinopoulos I, Shah T, Penet MF, Krishnamachary B, Bhujwalla ZM (2013) COX-2 in cancer: Gordian knot or Achilles heel? Front Pharmacol 4:34

58. Greenhough A et al (2009) The COX-2/PGE2 pathway: key roles in the hallmarks of cancer and adaptation to the tumour microenvironment. Carcinogenesis 30(3):377–386
59. Tindall E (1999) Celecoxib for the treatment of pain and inflammation: the preclinical and clinical results. J Am Osteopath Assoc 99(11 Suppl):S13–S17
60. Page-McCaw A, Ewald AJ, Werb Z (2007) Matrix metalloproteinases and the regulation of tissue remodelling. Nat Rev Mol Cell Biol 8(3):221–233
61. Parks WC, Wilson CL, Lopez-Boado YS (2004) Matrix metalloproteinases as modulators of inflammation and innate immunity. Nat Rev Immunol 4(8):617–629
62. Egeblad M, Werb Z (2002) New functions for the matrix metalloproteinases in cancer progression. Nat Rev Cancer 2(3):161–174
63. Gialeli C, Theocharis AD, Karamanos NK (2011) Roles of matrix metalloproteinases in cancer progression and their pharmacological targeting. FEBS J 278(1):16–27
64. Shay G, Lynch CC, Fingleton B (2015) Moving targets: emerging roles for MMPs in cancer progression and metastasis. Matrix Biol 44–46:200–206
65. Qi Q et al (2008) Involvement of matrix metalloproteinase 2 and 9 in gambogic acid induced suppression of MDA-MB-435 human breast carcinoma cell lung metastasis. J Mol Med 86 (12):1367–1377
66. Qi Q et al (2008) Anti-invasive effect of gambogic acid in MDA-MB-231 human breast carcinoma cells. Biochem Cell Biol 86(5):386–395
67. Etienne-Manneville S (2010) From signaling pathways to microtubule dynamics: the key players. Curr Opin Cell Biol 22(1):104–111
68. Dumontet C, Jordan MA (2010) Microtubule-binding agents: a dynamic field of cancer therapeutics. Nat Rev Drug Discov 9(10):790–803
69. Jordan MA, Wilson L (2004) Microtubules as a target for anticancer drugs. Nat Rev Cancer 4 (4):253–265
70. Hochegger H, Takeda S, Hunt T (2008) Cyclin-dependent kinases and cell-cycle transitions: does one fit all? Nat Rev Mol Cell Biol 9(11):910–916
71. Musgrove EA, Caldon CE, Barraclough J, Stone A, Sutherland RL (2011) Cyclin D as a therapeutic target in cancer. Nat Rev Cancer 11(8):558–572
72. Hosokawa Y, Arnold A (1998) Mechanism of cyclin D1 (CCND1, PRAD1) overexpression in human cancer cells: analysis of allele-specific expression. Genes Chromosom Cancer 22 (1):66–71
73. Rouleau M, Patel A, Hendzel MJ, Kaufmann SH, Poirier GG (2010) PARP inhibition: PARP1 and beyond. Nat Rev Cancer 10(4):293–301
74. Helleday T, Petermann E, Lundin C, Hodgson B, Sharma RA (2008) DNA repair pathways as targets for cancer therapy. Nat Rev Cancer 8(3):193–204
75. Krajarng A et al (2015) Apoptosis induction associated with the ER stress response through up-regulation of JNK in HeLa cells by gambogic acid. BMC Complement Altern Med 15:26
76. Thida M, Kim DW, Tran TT, Pham MQ, Lee H, Kim I, Lee JW (2016) Gambogic acid induces apoptotic cell death in T98G glioma cells. Bioorg Med Chem Lett 26(3):1097–1101
77. Yang LJ et al (2012) Effects of gambogic acid on the activation of caspase-3 and downregulation of SIRT1 in RPMI-8226 multiple myeloma cells via the accumulation of ROS. Oncol Lett 3(5):1159–1165
78. Wang X, Lin Y (2008) Tumor necrosis factor and cancer, buddies or foes? Acta Pharmacol Sin 29(11):1275–1288
79. Lee JY, Lee BH, Lee JY (2015) Gambogic acid disrupts toll-like receptor4 activation by blocking lipopolysaccharides binding to myeloid differentiation factor 2. Toxicol Res 31 (1):11–16
80. Liao CH, Sang S, Liang YC, Ho CT, Lin JK (2004) Suppression of inducible nitric oxide synthase and cyclooxygenase-2 in downregulating nuclear factor-kappa B pathway by Garcinol. Mol Carcinog 41(3):140–149
81. Youle RJ, Strasser A (2008) The BCL-2 protein family: opposing activities that mediate cell death. Nat Rev Mol Cell Biol 9(1):47–59

82. Juin P, Geneste O, Gautier F, Depil S, Campone M (2013) Decoding and unlocking the BCL-2 dependency of cancer cells. Nat Rev Cancer 13(7):455–465
83. Gleave ME, Monia BP (2005) Antisense therapy for cancer. Nat Rev Cancer 5(6):468–479
84. Xu J et al (2013) Gambogic acid induces mitochondria-dependent apoptosis by modulation of Bcl-2 and Bax in mantle cell lymphoma JeKo-1 cells. Chin J Cancer Res 25(2):183–191
85. Liu W et al (2005) Anticancer effect and apoptosis induction of gambogic acid in human gastric cancer line BGC-823. World J Gastroenterol 11(24):3655–3659
86. Gu H et al (2009) Gambogic acid reduced bcl-2 expression via p53 in human breast MCF-7 cancer cells. J Cancer Res Clin Oncol 135(12):1777–1782
87. Zhai D et al (2008) Gambogic acid is an antagonist of antiapoptotic Bcl-2 family proteins. Mol Cancer Ther 7(6):1639–1646
88. Zhao L, Guo QL, You QD, Wu ZQ, Gu HY (2004) Gambogic acid induces apoptosis and regulates expressions of Bax and Bcl-2 protein in human gastric carcinoma MGC-803 cells. Biol Pharm Bull 27(7):998–1003
89. Czabotar PE, Lessene G, Strasser A, Adams JM (2014) Control of apoptosis by the BCL-2 protein family: implications for physiology and therapy. Nat Rev Mol Cell Biol 15(1):49–63
90. Ma SB et al (2014) Bax targets mitochondria by distinct mechanisms before or during apoptotic cell death: a requirement for VDAC2 or Bak for efficient Bax apoptotic function. Cell Death Differ 21(12):1925–1935
91. Xie H et al (2009) GA3, a new gambogic acid derivative, exhibits potent antitumor activities in vitro via apoptosis-involved mechanisms. Acta Pharmacol Sin 30(3):346–354
92. Zinkel S, Gross A, Yang E (2006) BCL2 family in DNA damage and cell cycle control. Cell Death Differ 13(8):1351–1359
93. Fang L et al (2012) Synergistic effect of a combination of nanoparticulate Fe3O4 and gambogic acid on phosphatidylinositol 3-kinase/Akt/Bad pathway of LOVO cells. Int J Nanomed 7:4109–4118
94. Li C et al (2012) Gambogic acid promotes apoptosis and resistance to metastatic potential in MDA-MB-231 human breast carcinoma cells. Biochem Cell Biol 90(6):718–730
95. Ishaq M et al (2014) Gambogic acid induced oxidative stress dependent caspase activation regulates both apoptosis and autophagy by targeting various key molecules (NF-kappaB, Beclin-1, p62 and NBR1) in human bladder cancer cells. Biochim Biophys Acta 1840 (12):3374–3384
96. Tang C et al (2009) Downregulation of survivin and activation of caspase-3 through the PI3K/Akt pathway in ursolic acid-induced HepG2 cell apoptosis. Anticancer Drugs 20 (4):249–258
97. Wen J et al (2014) Gambogic acid exhibits anti-psoriatic efficacy through inhibition of angiogenesis and inflammation. J Dermatol Sci 74(3):242–250
98. Costa S, Reina-Couto M, Albino-Teixeira A, Sousa T (2016) Statins and oxidative stress in chronic heart failure. Rev Port J Cardiol 35(1):41–57
99. Urbieta Caceres VH et al (2011) Early experimental hypertension preserves the myocardial microvasculature but aggravates cardiac injury distal to chronic coronary artery obstruction. Am J Physiol Heart Circ Physiol 300(2):H693–H701
100. Liu S et al (2013) Gambogic acid suppresses pressure overload cardiac hypertrophy in rats. Am J Cardiovasc Dis 3(4):227–238
101. McInnes IB, Schett G (2011) The pathogenesis of rheumatoid arthritis. N Engl J Med 365 (23):2205–2219
102. Wruck CJ et al (2011) Role of oxidative stress in rheumatoid arthritis: insights from the Nrf2-knockout mice. Ann Rheum Dis 70(5):844–850
103. Ray PD, Huang BW, Tsuji Y (2012) Reactive oxygen species (ROS) homeostasis and redox regulation in cellular signaling. Cell Signal 24(5):981–990
104. Kahlenberg JM, Fox DA (2011) Advances in the medical treatment of rheumatoid arthritis. Hand Clin 27(1):11–20
105. Forestier R et al (2009) Non-drug treatment (excluding surgery) in rheumatoid arthritis: clinical practice guidelines. Joint Bone Spine 76(6):691–698

106. Cascao R et al (2014) Potent anti-inflammatory and antiproliferative effects of gambogic acid in a rat model of antigen-induced arthritis. Mediat Inflamm 2014:195327
107. Zhao B, Shen H, Zhang L, Shen Y (2012) Gambogic acid activates AMP-activated protein kinase in mammalian cells. Biochem Biophys Res Commun 424(1):100–104
108. Gupta MA, Simpson FC, Gupta AK (2015) Psoriasis and sleep disorders: a systematic review. Sleep Med Rev 29:63–75
109. Coimbra S, Figueiredo A, Castro E, Rocha-Pereira P, Santos-Silva A (2012) The roles of cells and cytokines in the pathogenesis of psoriasis. Int J Dermatol 51(4):389–395; quiz 395–388
110. Aggarwal BB, Shishodia S, Sandur SK, Pandey MK, Sethi G (2006) Inflammation and cancer: how hot is the link? Biochem Pharmacol 72(11):1605–1621
111. Grivennikov SI, Karin M (2010) Dangerous liaisons: STAT3 and NF-kappaB collaboration and crosstalk in cancer. Cytokine Growth Factor Rev 21(1):11–19
112. Zhu X et al (2009) Mechanisms of gambogic acid-induced apoptosis in non-small cell lung cancer cells in relation to transferrin receptors. J Chemother 21(6):666–672
113. Mu R et al (2010) An oxidative analogue of gambogic acid-induced apoptosis of human hepatocellular carcinoma cell line HepG2 is involved in its anticancer activity in vitro. Eur J Cancer Prev 19(1):61–67
114. He D et al (2009) The NF-kappa B inhibitor, celastrol, could enhance the anti-cancer effect of gambogic acid on oral squamous cell carcinoma. BMC Cancer 9:343
115. Xu X et al (2009) Gambogic acid induces apoptosis by regulating the expression of Bax and Bcl-2 and enhancing caspase-3 activity in human malignant melanoma A375 cells. Int J Dermatol 48(2):186–192
116. Wang X et al (2009) Proteomic identification of molecular targets of gambogic acid: role of stathmin in hepatocellular carcinoma. Proteomics 9(2):242–253
117. Wang F et al (2014) Gambogic acid suppresses hypoxia-induced hypoxia-inducible factor-1alpha/vascular endothelial growth factor expression via inhibiting phosphatidylinositol 3-kinase/Akt/mammalian target protein of rapamycin pathway in multiple myeloma cells. Cancer Sci 105(8):1063–1070
118. Wang T et al (2008) Gambogic acid, a potent inhibitor of survivin, reverses docetaxel resistance in gastric cancer cells. Cancer Lett 262(2):214–222
119. Rong JJ et al (2010) Gambogic acid triggers DNA damage signaling that induces p53/p21 (Waf1/CIP1) activation through the ATR-Chk1 pathway. Cancer Lett 296(1):55–64
120. Qin Y et al (2007) Gambogic acid inhibits the catalytic activity of human topoisomerase IIalpha by binding to its ATPase domain. Mol Cancer Ther 6(9):2429–2440
121. Wu ZQ, Guo QL, You QD, Zhao L, Gu HY (2004) Gambogic acid inhibits proliferation of human lung carcinoma SPC-A1 cells in vivo and in vitro and represses telomerase activity and telomerase reverse transcriptase mRNA expression in the cells. Biol Pharm Bull 27 (11):1769–1774
122. Yu J et al (2006) Repression of telomerase reverse transcriptase mRNA and hTERT promoter by gambogic acid in human gastric carcinoma cells. Cancer Chemother Pharmacol 58 (4):434–443
123. Kasibhatla S et al (2005) A role for transferrin receptor in triggering apoptosis when targeted with gambogic acid. Proc Natl Acad Sci USA 102(34):12095–12100
124. Pandey MK, Kale VP, Song C, Sung SS, Sharma AK, Talamo G, Dovat S, Amin SG (2014) Gambogic acid inhibits multiple myeloma mediated osteoclastogenesis through suppression of chemokine receptor CXCR4 signaling pathways. Exp Hematol 42(10):883–896
125. Gu H et al (2008) Gambogic acid induced tumor cell apoptosis by T lymphocyte activation in H22 transplanted mice. Int Immunopharmacol 8(11):1493–1502
126. Chi Y et al (2013) An open-labeled, randomized, multicenter phase IIa study of gambogic acid injection for advanced malignant tumors. Chin Med J 126(9):1642–1646
127. Li D et al (2015) Antitumor activity of gambogic acid on NCI-H1993 xenografts via MET signaling pathway downregulation. Oncol Lett 10(5):2802–2806

128. Yue Q et al (2016) proteomic analysis revealed the important role of vimentin in human cervical carcinoma HeLa cells treated with gambogic acid. MCP 15(1):26–44
129. Huang GM, Sun Y, Ge X, Wan X, Li CB (2015) Gambogic acid induces apoptosis and inhibits colorectal tumor growth via mitochondrial pathways. WJG 21(20):6194–6205
130. Shi X et al (2015) Gambogic acid induces apoptosis in diffuse large B-cell lymphoma cells via inducing proteasome inhibition. Sci Rep 5:9694
131. Yang Y et al (2007) Differential apoptotic induction of gambogic acid, a novel anticancer natural product, on hepatoma cells and normal hepatocytes. Cancer Lett 256(2):259–266
132. Lu N et al (2013) Gambogic acid inhibits angiogenesis through inhibiting PHD2-VHL-HIF-1alpha pathway. Eur J Pharm Sci 49(2):220–226
133. Wang J, Yuan Z (2013) Gambogic acid sensitizes ovarian cancer cells to doxorubicin through ROS-mediated apoptosis. Cell Biochem Biophys 67(1):199–206
134. Li Q et al (2010) Gambogenic acid inhibits proliferation of A549 cells through apoptosis-inducing and cell cycle arresting. Biol Pharm Bull 33(3):415–420
135. Zhao J et al (2008) Inhibition of alpha(4) integrin mediated adhesion was involved in the reduction of B16-F10 melanoma cells lung colonization in C57BL/6 mice treated with gambogic acid. Eur J Pharmacol 589(1–3):127–131
136. Guo QL, You QD, Wu ZQ, Yuan ST, Zhao L (2004) General gambogic acids inhibited growth of human hepatoma SMMC-7721 cells in vitro and in nude mice. Acta Pharmacol Sin 25(6):769–774
137. Wang C, Wang W, Wang C, Tang Y, Tian H (2015) Combined therapy with EGFR TKI and gambogic acid for overcoming resistance in -T790M mutant lung cancer. Oncol Lett 10 (4):2063–2066

Chapter 16
Embelin and Its Role in Chronic Diseases

Hong Lu, Jun Wang, Youxue Wang, Liang Qiao and Yongning Zhou

Abstract *Embelia ribes Burm* of *Myrsinaceae* family has been widely used as an herb in the traditional medicine of India. Embelin is an active component extracted from the fruits of *Embelia ribes*. It has a wide spectrum of biological activities and is not toxic at low dose. This review focuses on the physical–chemical properties and bioactivities of Embelin, as well as its effects on chronic diseases such as tumors, autoimmune inflammatory diseases, parasitic infections, microbial infections, diabetes, obesity, and cardio-cerebral vascular diseases. The underlying mechanisms of the effects are also discussed. As a multiple-targeted therapeutic agent, Embelin has the potential to be used widely for the treatment of a variety of chronic diseases, including malignant tumors.

Keywords Embelin · Anticancer activity · Autoimmune inflammatory diseases · Anthelmintic activity · Antimicrobial activity · Diabetes · Cardio-cerebral vascular diseases

---

H. Lu · J. Wang · L. Qiao · Y. Zhou
Division of Gastroenterology and Hepatology, The First Hospital of Lanzhou University, Lanzhou 730000, Gansu Province, China
e-mail: light199839@163.com

J. Wang
e-mail: whiskey.1210@163.com

Y. Zhou
e-mail: yongningzhou@sina.com

Y. Wang
Department of Physiology, The University of Texas Southwestern Medical Center, Dallas, TX 75390, USA
e-mail: youxuewang@yahoo.com

L. Qiao (✉)
Storr Liver Centre, The Westmead Institute for Medical Research, The University of Sydney at Westmead Hospital, Westmead, NSW 2145, Australia
e-mail: liang.qiao@sydney.edu.au

S.C. Gupta et al. (eds.), *Anti-inflammatory Nutraceuticals and Chronic Diseases*, Advances in Experimental Medicine and Biology 928,
DOI 10.1007/978-3-319-41334-1_16

16.1 Introduction

Embelin (2,5-dihydroxy-3-undecyl-1,4-benzoquinone) also known as embelic acid or emberine, is a major active constituent of the fruits of *Embelia ribes Burm*, which belongs to the *Myrsinaceae* family. It is also found in other plants, such as *Lysimachia punctata* (*Primulaceae*) [104, 105], and *erythrorhiza* (*Oxalidaceae*) [34].

Embelia ribes Burm, also known as false black pepper in English, Vidanda in Sanskrit, and Babrang in Hindi, is widely distributed in India, Sri Lanka, Malaysia, Singapore, and China [45, 124]. It contains benzoquinone derivatives of Embelin and its dimeric form is named Vilangin [90]. It also contains cyclitol quercitol, alkaloid christembine, tannins, as well as fatty ingredients including resinoid, fixed oil, and minute quantities of volatile oils [64, 106, 107]. Embelin is a major component from all the parts of *Embelia Ribes*, including fruits, pericarp, root bark, stem bark, seeds, and leaves [35, 115] with varied quantity ranging from 1.01 to 4.31 % of the weight [105]. The content of Embelin in pericarp, seeds, entirely crushed fruits, and decorticated seeds along with pericarp was found to be 0.39, 4.18, 3.30, and 3.34 % w/w respectively [35].

Embelia ribes has been widely used as an herb in traditional medicine in India since time immemorial. The whole plant is used as an anti-inflammatory and antinociceptive preparation to treat rheumatism, fever, and some skin diseases [89]. The fruits have digestive, carminative, anthelmintic, contraceptive and laxative effects, and are used to treat tumors, ascites, bronchitis, mental diseases, dyspnoea, heart diseases, urinary discharges, jaundice, hemicrania, and worms in wounds. The leaves are astringent, demulcent, and depurative, and are used to treat in pruritus, sore throat, aphthae ulcers of mouth, indolent ulcers, skin diseases, and leprosy. Decoction of the roots is used in the treatment of influenza [45, 139].

The active component from *Embelia ribes* was first isolated more than 4 decades ago (see structure in Fig. 16.1). It was named Embelin, and was later chemically synthesized. Embelin has a wide range of medicinal property, including ant fertile [67], antitumoral [26, 29], anti-inflammatory [60, 137, 138, 144], analgesic [20], antioxidant [129, 149], hepatoprotective [132], wound healing, antibacterial [32], and anticonvulsant activities [77, 78].

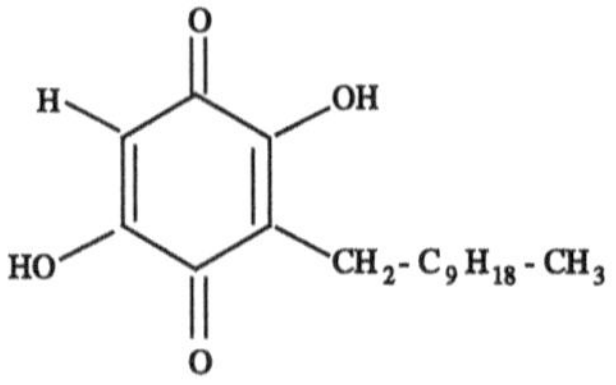

Fig. 16.1 Constitutional formula of Embelin (Molecular formula $C_{17}H_{26}O_4$; Molecular weight 294.39; Melting point 142–143 °C; Appearance Orange solid, Log p (octanol-water) 4.34; Solubility Insoluble in water, but soluble in organic solvents such as DMSO and Ether) [89]

16.2 Physical–Chemical Properties of Embelin

Embelin is a hydroxyl benzoquinone with alkyl substitution and a derivative of para-benzoquinone. Therefore, it has the basic physical–chemical characteristic of para-benzoquinone. It shows orange color, and can be used to dye silk and wool [120]. As a nonpolar molecule, Embelin suffers from erratic bioavailability due to poor aqueous solubility [96, 98, 128], which limits its clinical application. Meanwhile, its long alkyl chain (undecyl) provides it with strong lipophilic ability [69] and high cell membrane permeability [57], which make it more stable and allow it enter the cells easily.

Sublimation and volatility are other major characteristics of Embelin. It does not decompose under normal pressure after being heated, and can be distilled with water vapor, which makes it easy to be extracted and purified.

Embelin is also a phenolic lipid, and is photosensitive. In methanol, it shows a peak absorbance (λ max) at 450 nm [59]. When irradiated with light of the appropriate wavelength, Embelin can be activated and produces anticancer and anti-inflammatory effects through antioxidant activity [58, 59].

16.3 Biological Activities of Embelin

Embelin is a phenolic lipid that can be found as a secondary metabolite not only in plants, but also in fungi, bacteria, and animals both during normal development and in response to stress conditions such as infection, wounding, and UV radiation [115]. It is structurally similar to natural coenzyme Q10 (ubiquinones), and it has antioxidant activity similar to that of coenzyme Q10.

Embelin is also a weak mitochondrial uncoupler that dissociates the electron transport system from ADP phosphorylation and inhibits ATP synthesis [79]. The uncoupling effect also leads to increased oxygen consumption. It may explain why Embelin caused swelling of the mitochondria in rat liver and respiratory inhibition in germinated cowpea. It can also explain why Embelin prevented angiogenesis during tumor growth and wound healing by exhausting the low respiratory reserve of proliferating endothelial cells through uncoupling action [22].

Although Embelin possesses several promising biological activities, preclinical efforts have been hampered because of water insolubility which leads to poor bioavailability by oral route. In order to resolve the solubility issue and improve biological activity, new techniques, such as utilization of the liquisolid compact systems [95], formulation of Embelin–phospholipid complex (EPC) [98], construction of Embelin-loaded thermosensitive injectable hydrogel system [99, 100], and synthesis of Embelin analogues [18, 28, 69, 128] have been tried. Polymeric micelle technique has also been introduced to enhancing the water solubility and bioavailability [27].

Some progresses have been made to improve the solubility and delivery of Embelin. A micelle system was developed through the conjugation of Embelin and polyethylene glycol (PEG) through an aspartic acid bridge. The resulting PEG-Embelin micelles is dual functional and can efficiently deliver both Embelin itself and other hydrophobic antitumor drugs, such as Paclitaxel, which are encapsulated in the micelles. This system has been tested with success in cancer cell line in vitro and animal cancer models in vivo [51, 76]. Diammonium salt of Embelin exists in some plants and can easily be made from purified Embelin. It was found to be highly soluble in water and its biological activities were found to be similar to those of Embelin [28]. It could be an ideal therapeutic agent which can be administered easily.

Toxicity studies revealed that Embelin is safe to use. It did not show toxic effect on human fibroblasts at 20 μg/ml for 72 h in vitro [104]. In the acute toxicity study, no prominent signs of toxicity or death were observed in mice administered orally with crude hydroalcoholic extract of *Embelia ribes* at the dose up to 5000 mg/kg for 24 h [28]. In chronic toxicity study, the administration of Embelin at the dose of 50 mg/kg/day for 14 weeks to Wistar rats did not cause any drastic drop in the blood counts [132]. In another study, administration of Embelin at 10 mg/kg/day for 10 weeks in rats did not show toxic side effects on bone marrow, liver, kidney, and heart [111]. Embelin at doses of 50 mg and 100 mg/kg of body weight/day for 14 days did not cause significant body weight changes, mortality, or apparent signs of toxic effects in mice [115]. Previous studies had also reported the nontoxic nature of Embelin on hematopoietic cells when administered for 6 months in mice, rats, and monkeys [55].

The specifics and details of some biomedicinal activities of Embelin will also be discussed in the following sections.

16.4 Role of Embelin in Chronic Diseases

16.4.1 Anticancer Activity of Embelin

Anticancer effect of Embelin has been studied in various kinds of cancer, including breast cancer [29, 133], prostate cancer [94, 106, 107], hepatic cancer [131, 132], pancreatic cancer [86, 99, 100], colon cancer [24, 25], gastric cancer [141], leukemia [49, 50], and multiple myeloma [47], through in vivo and in vitro experiments. It can effectively inhibit tumor cell proliferation and migration, induce tumor cell apoptosis, and inhibit tumor invasion, metastasis and angiogenesis.

The molecular mechanisms of the anticancer effect of Embelin have also been studied extensively. Multiple signaling pathways have been found to be involved. Embelin was predicted to be a strong inhibitor of XIAP through structure-based computational screening of a traditional herbal medicine three-dimensional structure database [92]. It also downregulates the expression of XIAP [27, 50, 86, 141].

XIAP belongs to inhibitor of apoptosis (IAP) family [119]. It binds to and inhibits the initiator caspase-9 and effector caspase-3, caspase-7, and consequently prevents intrinsic apoptotic pathways [114, 126]. XIAP is overexpressed in various types of cancer cells [136]. Embelin could induce apoptosis of tumor cell through down-regulating expression of XIAP and activating caspase cascades [27, 50, 141]. It could also transform TRAIL-resistant pancreatic cancer cells into TRAIL-sensitive cells by suppressing the expression of XIAP in vitro [86].

Nuclear factor-κB (NF-κB) plays an important role in tumor cell survival and proliferation, as well as tumor angiogenesis, invasion, and inflammation [3, 8, 101]. Embelin blocks NF-κB signaling pathway resulting in the suppression of NF-κB regulated antiapoptotic and metastatic gene products. Embelin inhibits the expression of ICAM-1, MMP-9, COX-2, cyclin D1, c-Myc, and VEGF [25, 122, 141], all of which are regulated by NF-κB and closely related to proliferation, invasion, and angiogenesis of tumors. It also inhibits NF-κB-dependent apoptosis gene products including survivin, XIAP, IAP-1/2, TRAF1, cFLIP and Bcl-2, and downregulates Bcl-xL [65, 94].

Researches showed Embelin suppressed activation of NF-κB not through modifying NF-κB proteins itself but through inhibiting IKK (IκB kinase) activation, IκBα (the inhibitor of NF-κB)-phosphorylation and degradation, and p65 phosphorylation and acetylation, which then inhibited nuclear translocation of NF-κB and expression of the NF-κB-dependent reporter genes [3, 112, 145]. IKK could phosphorylate and degrade IκBα [38]. When IκBα was degraded, NF-κB translocated to the nucleus and activated the transcription of specific genes [41]. These results suggested that Embelin induces apoptosis not only by inhibiting and downregulating XIAP, but also through suppressing NF-κB signaling. XIAP, as a downstream target gene, could be activated by NF-κB [63].

Embelin also regulates activity of the PI3 K/AKT pathway by reducing AKT expression levels, and increases PTEN levels in cancer cell lines in vitro. The PI3 K/Akt pathway contributes to tumor formation through the anti-apoptotic activity of Akt. Akt inhibits apoptosis through phosphorylation of GSK3β, which leads to inactivation of itself [56] and maintains the stabilization of β-catenin [71]. Embelin could suppress β-catenin expression through inhibition of activation of AKT and GSK-3β, and thus promote apoptosis [94]. Suppression of Akt activation could also lead to P53 activation and turn on pro-apoptotic signaling pathways for induction of apoptosis [42]. At the same time, AKT could induce activation of transcriptional factors, such as NF-κB [72]. Further research indicated that AKT could activate IKK, and then cause NF-κB activation and cell survival [61]. The upregulated PTEN can suppress activity of AKT [17].

Embelin upregulates the expression of P53 both in vivo and in vitro [99, 100, 133, 141]. P53 protein, as a key regulator of apoptosis, controls cell cycle progression and DNA repair, and induces apoptosis by regulating the expression of proteins like Bcl-2 and Bax, which concomitantly induce Cytochrome C release and activate Caspase cascades (primarily Caspase 9 and Caspase 3) leading to apoptosis [130].

Embelin inhibits JAK/STAT3 signaling pathways in mouse pancreatic cancer cells through the downregulation of non-receptor protein tyrosine kinases janus-like kinase 2(JAK2) and c-Src kinase [47], which then decrease the phosphorylation of STAT3 in tumor cells [24, 99, 100]. The phosphorylation of STAT3 is mainly dependent on the activation of JAK although the role of c-Src kinase in STAT3 phosphorylation has been demonstrated too [123]. STAT3 has been shown to regulate the expression of tumor-associated genes, such as apoptosis inhibitors (Bcl-xl, Bcl-2, and survivin), cell cycle regulators (cyclin D1), and angiogenesis inducers (VEGF) [2, 47].

PPARγ is a transcriptional factor that belongs to a superfamily of nuclear hormone receptors. It is richly expressed in the normal gastrointestinal epithelium, and plays a vital role in the regulation of differentiation of gastrointestinal epithelial cells [150]. It is also abundantly expressed in colon cancer cells, and activation of PPARγ inhibits proliferation and induces apoptosis in some colon cancer cell lines [25, 73, 127, 148]. Heterozygous loss of PPARγ increased the susceptibility to carcinogen-induced colon cancer and gastric cancer [40]. Embelin effectively suppressed 1,2-Dimethylhydrazine dihydrochloride (DMH)-induced colon carcinogenesis in vivo when PPARγ was present, and this effect could be due to inhibition for NF-κB activity, which is dependent on PPARγ [25].

Akt/mTOR/S6K1 signal pathway is closely related to tumorigenesis, metastasis, and angiogenesis in vitro [9, 82]. Once Akt is stimulated, it can be propagated to mammalian target of rapamycin (mTOR), a key modulator of protein translation [75]. S6K1 is a downstream component of mTOR signaling pathway and a key mTOR effector for tumor cell growth and proliferation [31]. The upregulated expression of S6K1 gene indicates a poor prognosis in patients with cancer [84]. Embelin was found to inhibit the tumor growth and induce tumor cell apoptosis through the suppression of Akt/mTOR/S6K1 signaling cascades in human prostate cancer cells [65].

In rat model of N-nitrosodimethylamine (DENA)-initiated and phenobarbital (PB)-promoted hepatocarcinogenesis, Embelin (50 mg/kg/day) blocked the induction of hepatic hyperplastic nodules, prevented body weight loss, and improved the markers of hepatic function (ALT, AST, ALP, TBIL) and hypoproteinemia [131], suggesting its preventive effect on tumor formation. In this model of hepatocarcinogenesis, a significant decrease in the hepatic glutathione antioxidant defense, an increase in lipid peroxidation and histological alterations such as dysplasia and atypical cells with abnormal chromatin pattern were observed. Embelin was able to improve or even reverse these biochemical and pathological changes possibly through free radical scavenging and antioxidant activity [132]. Embelin's radical scavenging activity has been found to be better than that of α-tocopherol, a well-known scavenger of peroxyl radical [57].

The immune system plays a crucial role in tumor microenvironment, and numerous cytokines and growth factors produced by inflammatory cells or immune cells can affect the regulation of genes that mediate proliferation, prevent apoptosis, and thereby promote carcinogenesis [81]. NF-kB plays a central role in mediating the link between inflammation and cancer development, and exerts a procarcinogenic effect principally on immune (myeloid) cells and epithelial cells [62]. Activated NF-κB regulates the expression of IL-6, TNF-α, IFN-γ, IL-1β, IL-8, and some other cytokines [54, 113].

The level of IL-6 in tumors is directly correlated with increased necrosis, proliferation, and vascular invasion, and the level of circulating IL-6 is highly correlated with poor survival. Moreover, exogenous and endogenous IL-6 can effectively activate JAK/STAT pathway [24, 74]. IL-6 associates with inflammatory cells and immune suppressive cells including Th1, Th2, Th17, regulatory T cell (Treg), and myeloid-derived suppressor cells (MDSCs) [93, 99, 100]. Embelin suppresses immune suppressive IL-17A$^+$ cells, GM-CSF$^+$ cells, MDSCs and Treg by inhibiting IL-6 secretion [99, 100]. It decreases the levels of IL-1β, IL-17a, and IL-23a, and inhibits the infiltration of CD4$^+$ T cells and macrophages in colonic tissues [24]. IL-17-producing effector T helper (Th17) cells are crucial for inflammation and may have a potential role in carcinogenesis [142, 147]. The roles of IL-6 and IL-23 in the maturation of Th17 cells have been identified [10].

TNF-α can stimulate accumulation of inflammatory cells via induction of expression of adhesion molecules such as ICAM-1 in neighboring endothelial cells, and give rise to production of secondary cytokines [60], resulting in expansion of inflammatory reactions. TNF-α can also activate NF-κB by degrading IκBα [3]. So, the relationship between TNF-α and tumor is beyond doubt. TNF-α is synthetized as a membrane anchored protein (pro-TNF-α), and the soluble component of pro-TNF-α is then released into the extracellular space by the action of a protease called converting enzyme (TACE) [91]. Embelin could decrease the level of TNF-α through blocking the expression of TACE in human breast cancer cells [29].

Embelin could inhibit osteoclastogenesis, which is related to bone loss induced by RANKL and tumor cells, such as multiple myeloma and breast cancer cells in vitro, through the suppression of NF-κB activation [112]. Thereby, Embelin could be used for patients with secondary bone lesions associated with various cancers.

In summary, Embelin has antitumor effect on a variety of cancers, and it executes its antitumor effect through multiple pathways (Fig. 16.2). The use of multi-target drugs has been increasingly accepted because of clearer realization that cancer is caused by dysregulation of multiple pathways [83]. Sorafenib and Sunitinib are examples of multi-target drugs that modulate several tyrosine kinases/signal transduction pathways. Embelin has a great potential for the treatment and prevention of cancer.

16.4.2 Embelin and Autoimmune Inflammatory Diseases

Rheumatoid arthritis, inflammatory bowel disease (IBD), psoriasis, multiple sclerosis (MS), and autoimmune encephalomyelitis (AE) are all included in the category of autoimmune inflammatory diseases, and possess common clinical characteristics, namely unknown etiology, immune correlation, and the lack of

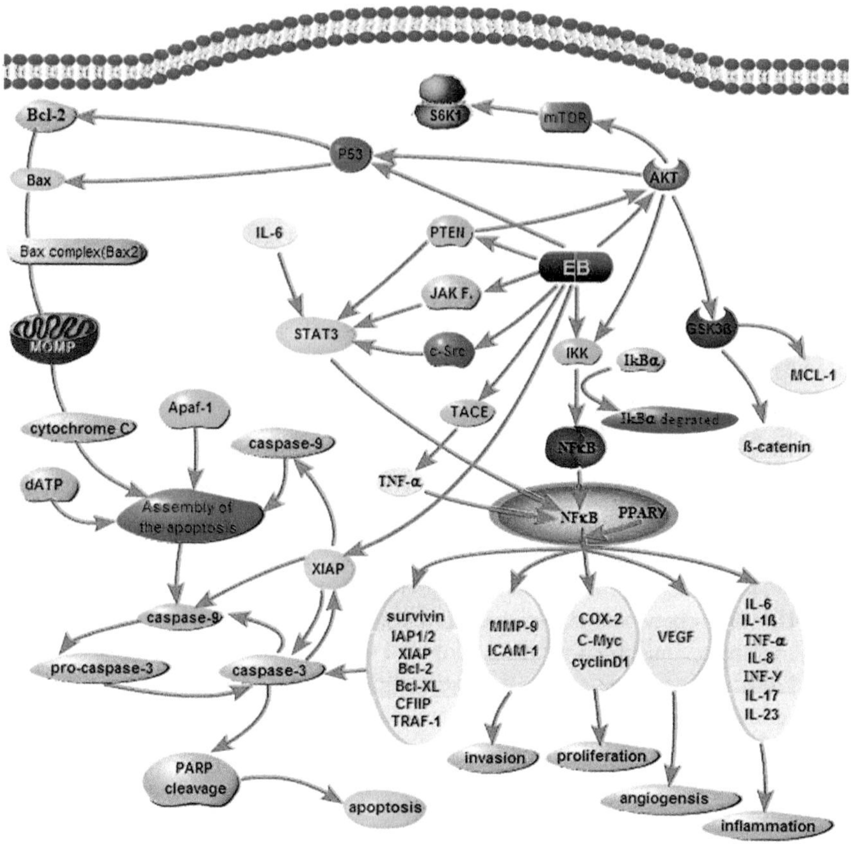

Fig. 16.2 Schematic diagrams showing antitumor mechanism of Embelin. *EB* Embelin, *XIAP* X-chromosome linked inhibitor of apoptosis protein, *NF-κB* Nuclear factor-κB, *IκBα* the inhibitor of NF-κB, *IKK* IκB kinase, *AKT* protein kinase B, *GSK3β* glycogen synthase kinase-3β, *JAK* janus-like kinase, *PPARγ* peroxisome proliferator-activated receptor gamma, *mTOR* mammalian target of rapamycin, *S6K1* ribosomal S6 kinase 1, *STAT3* signal transducer and activator of transcription 3

effective therapeutic agents with few side effects. *Embelia ribes* have been shown to relieve the symptoms of fever and skin diseases for many years. The effects of Embelin on ulcerative colitis, psoriasis, autoimmune encephalomyelitis, rheumatoid arthritis and the underlying mechanisms have also been studied.

Embelin was found to be effective in treating acetic acid-induced ulcerative colitis in rats. It relieved symptoms such as body weight loss, diarrhea, and gross intestinal bleeding. It decreased wet weight of the colon tissue [7] and alleviated colonic shortening and splenomegaly [68], indicating the improvement of the inflammation of colon. It decreased the colonic myeloperoxidase (MPO) activity and lipid peroxides (LPO), as well as serum lactate dehydrogenase (LDH). It also increased the reduced glutathione (GSH) in this rat ulcerative colitis model [7, 137, 138]. Wet weight of the colon tissue is considered as a reliable indicator of the extent of the inflammation in colitis. MPO exists abundantly in the neutrophils, and the levels of colonic MPO reflect the infiltration of activated neutrophils in colon which in turn reflect the severity of the colitis [21]. LPO is the product of membrane lipid peroxidation, and it can cause further lipid peroxidation and generate more reactive metabolites through self propagation chain reaction. LPO exhausts cellular antioxidants and accelerates the development of inflammation and ulceration. GSH can block free radical damage, enhance the antioxidant activity, facilitate the transport of amino acids, and play a critical role in detoxification [44]. The elevation of LDH in serum indicates enhanced production of lactic acid [80] and increased release of LDH by damaged cells.

Pro-inflammatory cytokines (TNF-α, IFN-γ, IL-1β, IL-6 and IL-12), and anti-inflammatory cytokines (IL-4, IL-10, IL-11) play a central role during the occurrence and development of IBD [46, 121]. TNF-α can disrupt the epithelial barrier, induce the apoptosis of epithelial cells, and stimulate the secretions of chemokines from intestinal epithelial cells. It can also activate immune system of the bowel through recruiting and activating neutrophils and macrophages [15]. IL-1β can increase the infiltration of inflammatory cells into the intestine. Embelin was found to ameliorated colitis by suppressing the level of TNF-α, IL-1β, and IL-6 in the colonic tissues of mice with dextran sulfate sodium (DSS)-induced colitis [68].

Epidermal keratinocytes are known to participate in immune and inflammatory reactions by producing a variety of cytokines including TNF-α, which plays a crucial role in autoimmune diseases of skin, such as psoriasis. TNF-α released from keratinocytes promotes the accumulation of inflammatory cells. Embelin could inhibit topical edema, and decrease skin thickness, tissue weight, and MPO activity in phorbol ester (TPA)-induced inflammation in mouse ear, which serves as a model of psoriasis. The possible mechanism might be the blockage of the production of pro-inflammatory cytokines (TNF-α, IL-1β) by keratinocytes [60].

Experimental Autoimmune Encephalomyelitis (EAE) is an autoimmune disorder of the CNS that serves as an animal model for human MS [66]. Dendritic cells (DCs) play a definitive role in the induction and maintenance of self-tolerance, and the absence of these cells can lead to autoimmune inflammatory diseases, such as MS. Transforming growth factor-beta (TGF-β) signaling in DCs was found to be a prerequisite for the control of autoimmune encephalomyelitis [146], and it could program DCs into a tolerogenic state [16], and thereby limit the inflammatory response and promote the recovery from EAE [52]. Embelin was shown to significantly increase TGF-β/β-catenin signaling, decrease STAT3 phosphorylation in DCs, maintain DCs in their tolerogenic state, and block the expression of pro-inflammatory factors (IFN-γ, IL-12, IL-6, and IL-23), which lead to the improvement of the EAE clinical score and alleviation of CNS inflammation and demyelination [144].

The effect of Embelin on rheumatoid arthritis was also affirmed. Embelin was found to reduce inflammation and bone erosion in a mouse model of inflammatory arthritis possibly through the induction of apoptosis [30] and suppression of osteoclastogenesis [112].

To summarize, Embelin has anti-inflammatory and immunomodulatory effects, and can be potential treatment for autoimmune inflammatory diseases.

16.4.3 Anthelmintic Activity of Embelin

Embelia ribes Burm has been used as an anthelminthic remedy in India for a long time. The fruits of *Embelia ribes* are widely used to expel the adult stage *beef tapeworm* and other intestinal parasites [23, 39]. The ethanolic extract from the seeds of *Embelia ribes* (10–200 μg/mL) exhibited potent anthelmintic activity against roundworm *Rhabditis pseudoelongata* in vitro [43]. Crude hydroalcoholic extract from the fruits showed significant anthelmintic activities against *the dwarf tapeworm* (*Hymenolepis nana*) in vivo and against *hookworm larva* and *Necator americanus* in vitro [28]. Diammonium salt of Embelin showed anthelmintic activity against intestinal cestodes (*Hymenolepis diminuta* and *Hymenolepis microstoma*), trematode (*Echinostoma caproni*), nematode (*Heligmosomoides polygyrus*), and *hookworm larva* in vitro. The in vivo anthelmintic activity of diammonium salt of Embelin against *Hymenolepis diminuta* and *Hymenolepis nana* was also confirmed. However, the anthelmintic activity against *Hymenolepis microstoma, Echinostoma caproni,* or *Heligmosomoides polygyrus* was not confirmed [6, 28]. In addition, Embelin was moderately active against *Leishmania amazonensis* and *Leishmania braziliensis* lysing 70 % of the parasites at 100 μg/ml, and potently active against *Trypanosoma cruzi trypomastigotes* with 100 % lysis at 100 μg/ml in vitro [34].

16.4.4 Antimicrobial Activity of Embelin

The crude extracts from *Embelia ribes* have displayed moderate antibacterial activity against *Salmonella typhi*, *Staphylococcus aureus*, *Enterobacter aerogenes*, and *Klebsiella pneumoniae* [5, 109, 135].

Embelin was found to suppress *Escherichia coli* and methicillin-sensitive and methicillin-resistant strains of *Staphylococcus aureus* with minimal inhibitory concentration(MIC) values of 50, 250, and 62 μg/ml respectively [34]. At high concentration (100 μg/disk), it significantly inhibited the growth of *Staphylococcus aureus*, *Streptococcus pyogenes*, *Shigella flexneri*, *Shigella sonnei,* and *Pseudomonas aeruginosa*; and was moderately effective against *Salmonella typhi*, *Shigella boydii,* and *Proteus mirabilis* [19]. Further study indicated Embelin showed bactericidal activity against Gram positive organisms, and bacteriostatic activity against Gram negative organisms [108].

In combination, Embelin and oxacillin showed synergistic antimicrobial effects against 4 (ATCC 29213, ATCC 43300, EMRSA15, and TRSA2) out of 9 *Staphylococcus aureus* strains (fractional inhibitory concentration sum (ΣFIC) indices 0.203–0.477). Embelin and tetracycline combination were bactericidal against 3 (ATCC 43300, MRSA4, and TRSA2) out of 9 strains (ΣFIC 0.400–0.496). Both combinations showed an additive effect in most of the strains with no occurrence of antagonism. Addition of Embelin completely reversed the resistances to Oxacillin and tetracycline in ATCC 43300, MRSA1, MdRSA2, and MdRSA3, which are multi-drug-resistant strains [115].

Streptococcus mutans plays a significant role in dental infection by effectively utilizing sugars and synthesizing large amounts of exopolysaccharides, which are indispensable in adhesion of bacteria and accumulation of biofilm. The organized structure and mechanisms of biofilm are responsible for the emergence of drug resistant bacteria [70]. Embelin could block the biofilm formation of *Streptococcus mutans,* and is expected to become novel drug candidates for treating oral infections caused by *S. mutans* [32].

The crude extracts from *Embelia ribes* have displayed moderate antifungal activity against *Candida albican, Candida tropicalis, Candida parapsilosis,* and *Aspergillus fumigatus* [110, 134]. Embelin exhibited good inhibitory activity against *Candida tropicalis* [110, 134], and *Candida albican* [87] with MIC50 values of 700 and 120 mg/L, respectively, by means of EUCAST (European Committee for Antifungal Susceptibility Tests). The MIC_{50} values were below 700 mg/L for *Candida albican, Candida tropicalis, Candida parapsilosis, Candida albidus,* and *Aspergillus Flavus* by NCCLS (The National Committee for Clinical Laboratory Standards, USA) method [134]. Embelin also showed antifungal activity against dermatophytic fungi *Epidermophyton floccosum, Microsporum canis, Microsporum gypseum, Trichophyton mentagrophytes,* and *Trichophyton rubrum* with MICs ranging from 50 to 100 μg/ml using agar dilution method [34].

The methanol extract of *Embelia ribes* was proven to be active on hepatitis C virus (HCV) protease (PR) with ≥ 90 % inhibition at 100 μg/ml, and the active component Embelin was found to be a potent HCV-PR inhibitors with an IC_{50} value of 21 μM [37, 102].

In summary, *Embelia ribes* and Embelin have antibacterial, antifungal, and antiviral activities in vitro. Animal researches are needed to study the in vivo effect of Embelin before clinical application can be considered.

16.4.5 Embelin and Its Antidiabetic Properties

Ethanolic extract of *Embelia ribes* improved hyperglycaemia, and decreased serum insulin, lactate dehydrogenase, creatinine in Wistar rats with streptozotocin (40 mg/kg, intravenously)-induced diabetes. It also decreased systolic blood pressure and heart rate, as well as total cholesterol and triglycerides in these diabetic rats [14].

In rats with alloxan-induced diabetic, oral administration of Embelin (25 and 50 mg/kg) for 21 days significantly decreased fasting blood glucose, improved body weights, and restored biochemical parameters such as TGL, TC, TB, CR, LDH, ALP, VLDL, TP, and albumin. It also significantly improved and almost normalized the histological changes of liver, kidney, and pancreas in these diabetic rats. However, the antidiabetic activity of Embelin (50 mg/kg) was found to be inferior to that of glibenclamide (10 mg/kg) [77, 78, 88].

The underlying mechanism of the antidiabetic effect of *Embelia ribes* and Embelin might be the protection of β-cells against reactive oxygen species-mediated damage by enhancing cellular antioxidant defense. It is indicated the antioxidant defense system is weakened in STZ-induced diabetic rats [14, 88], and the islet β-cells are susceptible to damage caused by oxygen free radicals. Increases of lipid peroxides (LPO), superoxide dismutase (SOD) and catalase (CAT) indicate an oxidative stress condition, and glutathione (GSH) is one of the primary defenses that counteract the oxidative stress. Extract of *Embelia ribes* at the dose of 100 mg/kg and 200 mg/kg increased SOD, CAT and GSH levels in pancreatic tissue of diabetic rats [11, 13, 14]. Embelin was found to decrease the malondialdehyde (MDA), restore depleted GSH as well as antioxidant enzymes SOD and CAT in liver and pancreatic tissues of STZ-induced diabetic rats [14, 36, 88], suggesting that antidiabetic activity of Embelin is at least partially due to the improvement of the oxidation defense mechanism, which protects islet β-cell against oxidative damage.

It is documented that cytokines TNF-α and IL-6 are associated with insulin resistance [85]. TNF-α could induce serine phosphorylation of insulin receptor substrate-1 (IRS-1), interfere with normal tyrosine phosphorylation and insulin signaling, which causes insulin resistance [48]. The high level of IL-6 is also related with decreased insulin sensitivity in skeletal muscles and liver, and IL-6 could block IRS phosphorylation, which ultimately lead to decreased gluconeogenesis and increased glycogenolysis [33]. Embelin decreased the levels of cytokines TNF-α and IL-6 in STZ-induced diabetic rats [88], and therefore improved insulin resistance and normalized the metabolism of glucose and lipid.

PPARγ is the molecular target to treat T2DM, and its expression is downregulated in multiple tissues in insulin resistance and diabetes [103]. Embelin induced PPARγ expression in the epididymal adipose tissue of rats with HFD+STZ-induced diabetes. It also caused plasma membrane translocation and activation of glucose transporter protein 4 (GLUT4), and relative increases in the expressions of PI3K and p-Akt, implying that Embelin increased insulin-mediated PI3K/p-Akt signaling dependent glucose uptake in adipose tissue through the translocation and subsequent activation of GLUT4 [36]. GLUT4, along with GLUT1, plays an important role in tissue glucose uptake and body glucose homeostasis regulation [143].

Embelin has also been used to treat obesity, which is a risk factor of T2DM. It prevents body weight gain, visceral fat accumulation, and blood pressure increase. It also decreased serum levels of leptin in the murine model of high fat diet (HFD)-induced obesity [12].

Embelin also exhibited nephroprotective and anti-polyuric effects in rats with lithium-induced nephrogenic diabetes insipidus (NDI). It increased body weight, and decreased plasma and urine creatinine, blood urea nitrogen levels, and urine protein levels. Embelin, as a potent antioxidant, seemed to protect kidneys through promoting antioxidant status as evidenced by the increased level of GSH in kidneys [117].

16.4.6 Embelin and Cardio-Cerebral Vascular Diseases

Aqueous extract of *Embelin Ribes* exhibited cardioprotective effect, and it ameliorated myocardial injury through enhancing the antioxidant defense in isoproterenol (ISO)-induced myocardial infarction in rats [11, 13]. Recently, Embelin was also found to have cardioprotective effect [118, 149]. It significantly decreased the serum levels of cardiac enzymes such as CK-MB, LDH, and AST in rats with ISO-induced myocardial infarction. It also decreased serum levels of lipids and lipoproteins, and improved histopathological changes such as myocardial degeneration and necrosis. The underlying mechanism of this cardioprotective activity of Embelin might be the recovery of myocardial mitochondrial respiratory enzyme activities, the enhancement of antioxidant defense status, and the inhibition of mitochondria dependent apoptotic damage [118].

It is known that inflammation is one of the most vital factors which results in ventricular dysfunction following myocardial ischemia–reperfusion injury [53, 116]. Increased expression of inflammatory cytokines is highly correlated with the deterioration of myocardial function [140]. It could trigger the systematic inflammatory response syndrome (SIRS), and lead to myocardial dysfunction and multiple organ failure (MOF). In a rabbit model of myocardial ischemia–reperfusion injury following cardiac arrest (CA), Embelin downregulated the expression of pro-inflammatory cytokines TNF-α, IL-1β, and IL-6 through inhibition of NF-κB in myocardial tissues. It blocked apoptosis and necrosis of myocardium, and improved cardiac function and hemodynamics following resuscitation [149]. This observation indicates that Embelin may protect the heart against myocardial ischemia–reperfusion injury via its anti-inflammatory abilities.

The fruits of *Embelia ribes* are traditionally used as a brain tonic to treat mental disorders in India. The ethanolic extract of Embelia ribes fruits was also proven to have potent neuroprotective effects [4]. The protective effect of Embelin on global ischemia/reperfusion-induced brain injury was validated using an experimental rat model. Pretreatment with Embelin (25 and 50 mg/kg) normalized locomotor activity and hanging latency time and decreased beam walking latency. The treatment also reduced lipid peroxidation, increased the total thiol content and glutathione-S-transferase activity in brain, and decreased the area of infraction. The antioxidant activity of Embelin might be the foundation of its neuroprotective effect [137, 138].

It has been proved that Embelin was effective in the treatment of seizure, epilepsy, and anxiety in animals. It has anticonvulsant activity against both grand mal and petit mal epilepsy. In animal experiment, Embelin inhibited seizures induced by maximal electroshock and pentylenetetrazole in a dose-dependent manner. The anticonvulsant activity of Embelin was comparable to that of phenytoin and diazepam [77, 78]. Embelin also showed a dose-dependent anxiolytic effect in animal experiment [1].

16.5 Conclusion

Embelin, as a bioactive ingredient of *Embelia ribes Burm*, possesses higher medicinal value. It can suppress the growth, invasion, and metastasis of malignant tumors; inhibit inflammatory; and ameliorate infections of bacteria, viruses, and parasites. It is also antidiabetic, neuroprotective and cardioprotective. It has the potential in the treatment of malignant tumor, autoimmune diseases, infections, diabetes, and obesity, as well as cardio-cerebral vascular diseases. Further in vivo animal studies and well-designed clinical trials are needed to validate the clinical application.

Acknowledgments This work was supported by the grant "The Model for Prevention and Control of Malignant Tumor in Area with High Incidence from Wuwei Gansu Province" (National Science and Technology Program, Grant Code: 2012GS620101 to YN Zhou).

Conflict of interest The authors declare no conflict of interest.

References

1. Afzal M, Gupta G, Kazmi I, Rahman M, Upadhyay G, Ahmad K, Imam F, Pravez M, Anwar F (2012) Evaluation of anxiolytic activity of embelin isolated from Embelia ribes. Biomed Aging Pathol 2:45–47
2. Aggarwal BB, Sethi G, Ahn KS, Sandur SK, Pandey MK, Kunnumakkara AB, Sung B, Ichikawa H (2006) Targeting Signal-Transducer-and-Activator-of-Transcription-3 for Prevention and Therapy of Cancer. Ann N Y Acad Sci 1091:151–169
3. Ahn KS, Sethi G, Aggarwal BB (2007) Embelin, an inhibitor of X chromosome-linked inhibitor-of-apoptosis protein, blocks nuclear factor-kappaB (NF-kappaB) signaling pathway leading to suppression of NF-kappaB-regulated antiapoptotic and metastatic gene products. Mol Pharmacol 71:209–219
4. Ansari MN, Bhandari U (2008) Protective effect of Embelia ribes Burm on methionine-induced hyperhomocysteinemia and oxidative stress in rat brain. Indian J Exp Biol 46:521–527
5. Awino O, Kiprono P, Keronei K, Kaberia F, Obala A (2014) Antimicrobial Activity of 2,5-Dihydroxy-3-methyl-1,4-benzoquinone from Embelia schimperi. Zeitschrift Für Naturforschung C 63:47–50

6. BØgh HO, Andreassen JR, Lemmich J (1996) Anthelmintic usage of extracts of Embelia schimperi from Tanzania. J Ethnopharmacol 50:35–42
7. Badamaranahalli SS, Kopparam M, Bhagawati ST, Durg S (2015) Embelin lipid nanospheres for enhanced treatment of ulcerative colitis–Preparation, characterization and in vivo evaluation. Eur J Pharm Sci 76:73–82
8. Baker RG, Hayden MS, Ghosh S (2011) NF-κB, inflammation, and metabolic disease. Cell Metab 13:11–22
9. Bartlett JMS (2010) Biomarkers and Patient Selection for PI3K/Akt/mTOR targeted therapies: current status and future directions. Clin Breast Cancer 10:S86–S95
10. Bettelli E, Carrier Y, Gao W, Korn T, Strom TB, Oukka M, Weiner HL, Kuchroo VK (2006) Reciprocal developmental pathways for the generation of pathogenic effector TH17 and regulatory T cells. Nature 441:235–238
11. Bhandari U, Ansari MN, Islam F (2008) Cardioprotective effect of aqueous extract of Embelia ribes Burm fruits against isoproterenol-induced myocardial infarction in albino rats. Indian J Exp Biol 9:35–40
12. Bhandari U, Chaudhari HS, Bisnoi AN, Kumar V, Khanna G, Javed K (2013) Anti-obesity effect of standardized ethanol extract of Embelia ribes in murine model of high fat diet-induced obesity. PharmaNutrition 1:50–57
13. Bhandari U, Jain N, Ansari MN, Pillai KK (2008) Beneficial effect of Embelia ribes ethanolic extract on blood pressure and glycosylated hemoglobin in streptozotocin-induced diabetes in rats. Fitoterapia 79:351–355
14. Bhandari U, Jain N, Pillai KK (2007) Further studies on antioxidant potential and protection of pancreatic beta-cells by Embelia ribes in experimental diabetes. Exp Diabetes Res 2007 (ID: 15803)
15. Bischoff SC, Lorentz A, Schwengberg S, Weier G, Raab R, Manns MP (1999) Mast cells are an important cellular source of tumour necrosis factor alpha in human intestinal tissue. Gut 44:643–652
16. Bryan VL, Zachary TB, Robert CF, Nir H, James JC, Marianne B (2011) TGF-β suppresses β-catenin-dependent tolerogenic activation program in dendritic cells. PLoS ONE 6:e20099
17. Cantley LC, Neel BG (1999) New insights into tumor suppression: PTEN suppresses tumor formation by restraining the phosphoinositide 3-kinase/AKT pathway. Proc Natl Acad Sci 96:4240–4245
18. Chen J, Nikolovska-Coleska Z, Wang G, Qiu S, Wang S (2006) Design, synthesis, and characterization of new embelin derivatives as potent inhibitors of X-linked inhibitor of apoptosis protein. Bioorg Med Chem Lett 16:5805–5808
19. Chitra M, Shyamala Devi CS, Sukumar E (2003) Antibacterial activity of embelin. Fitoterapia 74(4):401–403
20. Chitra M, Sukumar E, Suja V, Devi CSS (1994) Antitumor, anti-Inflammatory and analgesic property of embelin, a plant product. Chemotherapy 40:109–113
21. Choudhary S, Keshavarzian A, Yong S, Wade M, Bocckino S, Day BJ, Banan A (2001) Novel antioxidants zolimid and AEOL11201 ameliorate colitis in rats. Dig Dis Sci 46:2222–2230
22. Coutelle O, Hornig-Do HT, Witt A, Andree M, Schiffmann LM, Piekarek M, Brinkmann K, Seeger JM, Liwschitz M, Miwa S, Hallek M, Kronke M, Trifunovic A, Eming SA, Wiesner RJ, Hacker UT, Kashkar H (2014) Embelin inhibits endothelial mitochondrial respiration and impairs neoangiogenesis during tumor growth and wound healing. EMBO Mol Med 6:624–639
23. D'Avigdor E, Wohlmuth H, Asfaw Z, Awas T (2014) The current status of knowledge of herbal medicine and medicinal plants in Fiche, Ethiopia. J Ethnobiol Ethnomed 10:1–33
24. Dai Y, Jiao H, Teng G, Wang W, Zhang R, Wang Y, Hebbard L, George J, Qiao L (2014) Embelin reduces colitis-associated tumorigenesis through limiting IL-6/STAT3 signaling. Mol Cancer Ther 13:1206–1216

25. Dai Y, Qiao L, Chan KW, Yang M, Ye J, Ma J, Zou B, Gu Q, Wang J, Pang R, Lan HY, Wong BC (2009) Peroxisome proliferator-activated receptor-gamma contributes to the inhibitory effects of Embelin on colon carcinogenesis. Cancer Res 69:4776–4783
26. Danquah M, Duke CB 3rd, Patil R, Miller DD, Mahato RI (2012) Combination therapy of antiandrogen and XIAP inhibitor for treating advanced prostate cancer. Pharm Res 29:2079–2091
27. Danquah M, Li F, Duke CB 3rd, Miller DD, Mahato RI (2009) Micellar delivery of bicalutamide and embelin for treating prostate cancer. Pharm Res 26:2081–2092
28. Debebe Y, Tefera M, Mekonnen W, Abebe D, Woldekidan S, Abebe A, Belete Y, Menberu T, Belayneh B, Tesfaye B, Nasir I, Yirsaw K, Basha H, Dawit A, Debella A (2015) Evaluation of anthelmintic potential of the Ethiopian medicinal plant Embelia schimperi Vatke in vivo and in vitro against some intestinal parasites. BMC Complement Altern Med 15:187
29. Dhanjal JK, Nigam N, Sharma S, Chaudhary A, Kaul SC, Grover A, Wadhwa R (2014) Embelin inhibits TNF-α converting enzyme and cancer cell metastasis: molecular dynamics and experimental evidence. BMC Cancer 14:775
30. Dharmapatni AA, Cantley MD, Marino V, Perilli E, Crotti TN, Smith MD, Haynes DR (2015) The X-linked inhibitor of apoptosis protein inhibitor embelin suppresses inflammation and bone erosion in collagen antibody induced arthritis mice. Mediators Inflamm 2015(2): 1–10 (ID: 564042)
31. Dowling RJ, Sonenberg N (2010) Downstream of mTOR: translational control of cancer. In: mTOR pathway and mTOR inhibitors in cancer therapy. Humana Press, pp. 201–216.
32. Dwivedi D, Singh V (2015) Effects of the natural compounds embelin and piperine on the biofilm-producing property of Streptococcus mutans. J Tradit Complement Med. http://www.elsevier.com/locate/jtcme
33. Emanuelli B, Peraldi P, Filloux C, Sawka-Verhelle D, Hilton D, Van Obberghen E (2000) SOCS-3 is an insulin-induced negative regulator of insulin signaling. J Biol Chem 275:15985–15991
34. Feresin GE, Tapia A, Sortino M, Zacchino S, Arias ARd, Inchausti A, Yaluff G, Rodriguez J, Theoduloz C, Schmeda-Hirschmann G (2003) Bioactive alkyl phenols and embelin from *Oxalis erythrorhiza*. J Ethnopharmacol 88:241–247
35. Ferreria GM, Laddha KS (2013) Histochemical localization of embelin in fruits of *Embellia Ribes Brum* and its quantification. Int J Pharma Biosci Technol 1:16–19
36. Gandhi GR, Stalin A, Balakrishna K, Ignacimuthu S, Paulraj MG, Vishal R (2013) Insulin sensitization via partial agonism of PPARgamma and glucose uptake through translocation and activation of GLUT4 in PI3K/p-Akt signaling pathway by embelin in type 2 diabetic rats. Biochim Biophys Acta 1830:2243–2255
37. Ghazi H, Hirotsugu M, Norio N, Masao H, Nobuko K, Kunitada S (2000) Inhibitory effects of sudanese medicinal plant extracts on hepatitis C virus (HCV) protease. Phytother Res 14:510–516
38. Ghosh S, Karin M (2002) Missing pieces in the NF-κB puzzle. Cell 109:S81–S96
39. Giday M, Asfaw Z, Woldu Z (2009) Medicinal plants of the Meinit ethnic group of Ethiopia: an ethnobotanical study. J Ethnopharmacol 124:513–521
40. Girnun GD, Smith WM, Drori S, Sarraf P, Mueller E, Eng C, Nambiar P, Rosenberg DW, Bronson RT, Edelmann W (2002) APC-dependent suppression of colon carcinogenesis by PPARγ. Proc Natl Acad Sci 99:13771–13776
41. Golan-Goldhirsh A, Gopas J (2013) Plant derived inhibitors of NF-κB. Phytochem Rev 13:107–121
42. Gottlieb TM, Leal JF, Seger R, Taya Y, Oren M (2002) Cross-talk between Akt, p53 and Mdm2: possible implications for the regulation of apoptosis. Oncogene 21:1299–1303
43. Gp C (2012) Anthelmintic activity of fruits of Embelia ribes Burm. Int J Pharm Chem Sci 1:1680–1681

44. Gustafson DL, Swanson JD, Pritsos CA (1993) Modulation of glutathione and glutathione dependent antioxidant enzymes in mouse heart following doxorubicin therapy. Free Radic Res Commun 19:111–120
45. Harish GU, Danapur V, Jain R, Patell VM (2012) Endangered medicinal plant *Embelia ribes Burm*.f.—a review. Pharmacognosy Journal 4:6–19
46. Hendrickson BA, Ranjana G, Cho JH (2002) Clinical aspects and pathophysiology of inflammatory bowel disease. Clin Microbiol Rev 15:79–94
47. Heo JY, Kim HJ, Kim SM, Park KR, Park SY, Kim SW, Nam D, Jang HJ, Lee SG, Ahn KS, Kim SH, Shim BS, Choi SH, Ahn KS (2011) Embelin suppresses STAT3 signaling, proliferation, and survival of multiple myeloma via the protein tyrosine phosphatase PTEN. Cancer Lett 308:71–80
48. Hotamisligil GS, Peraldi P, Budavari A, Ellis R, White MF, Spiegelman BM (1996) IRS-1-mediated inhibition of insulin receptor tyrosine kinase activity in TNF-α-and obesity-induced insulin resistance. Science 271:665–670
49. Hu R, Yang Y, Liu Z, Jiang H, Zhu K, Li J, Xu W (2015) The XIAP inhibitor Embelin enhances TRAIL-induced apoptosis in human leukemia cells by DR4 and DR5 upregulation. Tumour Biol 36:769–777
50. Hu R, Zhu K, Li Y, Yao K, Zhang R, Wang H, Yang W, Liu Z (2011) Embelin induces apoptosis through down-regulation of XIAP in human leukemia cells. Med Oncol 28:1584–1588
51. Huang Y, Lu J, Gao X, Li J, Zhao W, Sun M, Stolz DB, Venkataramanan R, Rohan LC, Li S (2012) PEG-derivatized embelin as a dual functional carrier for the delivery of paclitaxel. Bioconjug Chem 23:1443–1451
52. Issazadeh S, Mustafa M, Ljungdahl Å, Höjeberg B, Dagerlind Å, Elde R, Olsson T (1995) Interferon γ, interleukin 4 and transforming growth factor β in experimental autoimmune encephalomyelitis in Lewis rats: dynamics of cellular mRNA expression in the central nervous system and lymphoid cells. J Neurosci Res 40:579–590
53. Ivan L, Mehran M, Jean-Daniel C, Luc-Marie J, Christian S, Bénédicte B, Alain C, Alain R, Pierre C, Simon W (2002) Reversible myocardial dysfunction in survivors of out-of-hospital cardiac arrest. J Am Coll Cardiol 40:2110–2116
54. Jeon Y-J, Kim B-H, Kim S, Oh I, Lee S, Shin J, Kim T-Y (2013) Rhododendrin ameliorates skin inflammation through inhibition of NF-κB, MAPK, and PI3K/Akt signaling. Eur J Pharmacol 714:7–14
55. Johri R, Dhar S, Pahwa G, Sharma S, Kaul J, Zutshi U (1990) Toxicity studies with potassium embelate, a new analgesic compound. Indian J Exp Biol 28:213–217
56. Jope RS, Johnson GVW (2004) The glamour and gloom of glycogen synthase kinase-3. Trends Biochem Sci 29:95–102
57. Joshi R, Kamat JP, Mukherjee T (2007) Free radical scavenging reactions and antioxidant activity of embelin: biochemical and pulse radiolytic studies. Chem Biol Interact 167:125–134
58. Joy B, Kumar SN, Radhika AR, Abraham A (2015) Embelin (2,5-Dihydroxy-3-undecyl-p-benzoquinone) for photodynamic therapy: study of their cytotoxicity in cancer cells. Appl Biochem Biotechnol 175:1069–1079
59. Joy B, Nishanth Kumar S, Soumya MS, Radhika AR, Vibin M, Abraham A (2014) Embelin (2,5-dihydroxy-3-undecyl-p-benzoquinone): a bioactive molecule isolated from Embelia ribes as an effective photodynamic therapeutic candidate against tumor in vivo. Phytomedicine 21:1292–1297
60. Kalyan Kumar G, Dhamotharan R, Kulkarni NM, Mahat MY, Gunasekaran J, Ashfaque M (2011) Embelin reduces cutaneous TNF-alpha level and ameliorates skin edema in acute and chronic model of skin inflammation in mice. Eur J Pharmacol 662:63–69
61. Kane LP, Smith SV, Stokoe D, Weiss A (1999) Induction of NF-kappaB by the Akt/PKB kinase. Curr Biol 9:601–604
62. Karin M, Greten FR (2005) NF-κB: linking inflammation and immunity to cancer development and progression. Nat Rev Immunol 5:749–759

63. Karin M, Lin A (2002) NF-κB at the crossroads of life and death. Nat Immunol 3:221–227
64. Khan MI, Ahmed A, Akram M, Mohiuddin E, Khan U, Ayaz S, Shah S, Asif M, Ghazala S, Ahmed K (2010) Monograph of *Embelia ribes Burm.* F. Afr J Plant Sci 4:503–505
65. Kim SW, Kim SM, Bae H, Nam D, Lee JH, Lee SG, Shim BS, Kim SH, Ahn KS, Choi SH, Sethi G, Ahn KS (2013) Embelin inhibits growth and induces apoptosis through the suppression of Akt/mTOR/S6K1 signaling cascades. Prostate 73:296–305
66. Krishnamoorthy G, Wekerle H (2009) EAE: an immunologist's magic eye. Eur J Immunol 39(8):2031–2035
67. Kumar D, Kumar A, Prakash O (2012) Potential antifertility agents from plants: a comprehensive review. J Ethnopharmacol 140:1–32
68. Kumar GK, Dhamotharan R, Kulkarni NM, Honnegowda S, Murugesan S (2011) Embelin ameliorates dextran sodium sulfate-induced colitis in mice. Int Immunopharmacol 11:724–731
69. Lamblin M, Sallustrau A, Commandeur C, Cresteil T, Felpin F-X, Dessolin J (2012) Synthesis and biological evaluation of hydrophilic embelin derivatives. Tetrahedron 68:4655–4663
70. Lewis K (2001) Riddle of biofilm resistance. Antimicrob Agents Chemother 45:999–1007
71. Li M, Wang X, Meintzer MK, Laessig T, Birnbaum MJ, Heidenreich KA (2000) Cyclic AMP promotes neuronal survival by phosphorylation of glycogen synthase kinase 3β. Mol Cell Biol 20:9356–9363
72. Li Y, Sarkar FH (2002) Inhibition of nuclear factor κB activation in PC3 cells by genistein is mediated via Akt signaling pathway. Clin Cancer Res 8:2369–2377
73. Liang Q, Yun D, Gu Q, Chan KW, Bing Z, Ma J, Wang J, Lan HY, Wong BCY (2008) Down-regulation of X-linked inhibitor of apoptosis synergistically enhanced peroxisome proliferator-activated receptor γ ligand-induced growth inhibition in colon cancer. Mol Cancer Ther 7:2203–2211
74. Liu A, Liu Y, Li PK, Li C, Lin J (2011) LLL12 inhibits endogenous and exogenous interleukin-6-induced STAT3 phosphorylation in human pancreatic cancer cells. Anticancer Res 31:2029–2035
75. Lopiccolo J, Blumenthal GM, Bernstein WB, Dennis PA (2008) Targeting the PI3K/Akt/mTOR pathway: effective combinations and clinical considerations. Drug Resist Updates 11:32–50
76. Lu J, Huang Y, Zhao W, Marquez RT, Meng X, Li J, Gao X, Venkataramanan R, Wang Z, Li S (2013) PEG-derivatized embelin as a nanomicellar carrier for delivery of paclitaxel to breast and prostate cancers. Biomaterials 34:1591–1600
77. Mahendran S, Badami S, Maithili V (2011) Evaluation of antidiabetic effect of embelin from Embelia ribes in alloxan induced diabetes in rats. Biomed Prev Nutr 1:25–31
78. Mahendran S, Thippeswamy BS, Veerapur VP, Badami S (2011) Anticonvulsant activity of embelin isolated from *Embelia ribes*. Phytomedicine 18:186–188
79. Makawiti DW, Konji VN, Olowookere JO (1990) Interaction of benzoquinones with mitochondria interferes with oxidative phosphorylation characteristics. FEBS Lett 266:26–28
80. Manna S, Bhattacharyya D, Basak D, Mandal T (2004) Single oral dose toxicity study of a-cypermethrin in rats. Indian J Pharmacol 36:25
81. Mantovani A, Allavena P, Sica A, Balkwill F (2008) Cancer-related inflammation. Nature 454:436–444
82. Mcauliffe PF, Meric-Bernstam F, Mills GB, Gonzalez-Angulo AM (2010) Deciphering the role of PI3K/Akt/mTOR pathway in breast cancer biology and pathogenesis. Clin Breast Cancer 10:S59–S65
83. Mencher SK, Wang LG (2005) Promiscuous drugs compared to selective drugs (promiscuity can be a virtue). BMC Clin Pharmacol 5:3
84. Mj VDV (2004) Overexpression of P70 S6 kinase protein is associated with increased risk of locoregional recurrence in node-negative premenopausal early breast cancer patients. Br J Cancer 90:1543–1550

85. Moller DE (2000) Potential role of TNF-alpha in the pathogenesis of insulin resistance and type 2 diabetes. Trends Endocrinol Metab TEM 11:212–217
86. Mori T, Doi R, Kida A, Nagai K, Kami K, Ito D, Toyoda E, Kawaguchi Y, Uemoto S (2007) Effect of the XIAP inhibitor embelin on TRAIL-induced apoptosis of pancreatic cancer cells. J Surg Res 142:281–286
87. Muris JJF, Cillessen SAGM, Wim V, Houdt IS, Kummer JA, Van Krieken JHJM, Jiwa NM, Jansen PM, Kluin-Nelemans HC, Van Ossenkoppele GJ (2005) Immunohistochemical profiling of caspase signaling pathways predicts clinical response to chemotherapy in primary nodal diffuse large B-cell lymphomas. Blood 105:2916–2923
88. Naik SR, Niture NT, Ansari AA, Shah PD (2013) Anti-diabetic activity of embelin: involvement of cellular inflammatory mediators, oxidative stress and other biomarkers. Phytomedicine 20:797–804
89. Narayanaswamy R, Gnanamani A (2014) 2, 5-dihydroxy-3-undecyl-1, 4-benzoquinone (Embelin)-a second solid gold of India- A review. Int J Pharm Pharm Sci 6:23–30
90. Narayanaswamy R, Shymatak M, Chatterjee S, Wai LK, Arumugam G (2014) Inhibition of angiogenesis and nitric oxide synthase (NOS), by Embelin & Vilangin using in vitro, in vivo and in silico STUDIES. Adv Pharm Bull 4:543
91. Newton R, Solomon K, Covington M, Decicco C, Haley P, Friedman S, Vaddi K (2001) Biology of TACE inhibition. Ann Rheum Dis 60:iii25–iii32
92. Nikolovska-Coleska Z, Xu L, Hu Z, Tomita Y, Li P, Roller PP, Wang R, Fang X, Guo R, Zhang M, Lippman ME, Yang D, Wang S (2004) Discovery of embelin as a cell-permeable, small-molecular weight inhibitor of XIAP through structure-based computational screening of a traditional herbal medicine three-dimensional structure database. J Med Chem 47:2430–2440
93. Oh K, Lee O-Y, Shon SY, Nam O, Ryu PM, Seo MW, Lee D-S (2013) A mutual activation loop between breast cancer cells and myeloid-derived suppressor cells facilitates spontaneous metastasis through IL-6 trans-signaling in a murine model. Breast Cancer Res 15:R79
94. Park N, Baek HS, Chun Y-J (2015) Embelin-induced apoptosis of human prostate cancer cells is mediated through modulation of Akt and β-catenin signaling. PLoS ONE 10: e0134760
95. Parmar K, Patel J, Sheth N (2014) Fabrication and characterization of liquisolid compacts of Embelin for dissolution enhancement. J Pharm Invest 44:391–398
96. Parmar K, Patel J, Sheth N (2015) Self nano-emulsifying drug delivery system for Embelin: design, characterization and in-vitro studies. Asian J Pharm Sci. http://www.elsevier.com/locate/AJPS
97. Patel RK, Patel VR, Patel MG (2012) Development and validation of a RP-HPLC method for the simultaneous determination of embelin, rottlerin and ellagic acid in Vidangadi churna. J Pharm Anal 2:366–371
98. Pathan RA, Bhandari U (2010) Preparation & characterization of embelin–phospholipid complex as effective drug delivery tool. J Incl Phenom Macrocycl Chem 69:139–147
99. Peng M, Huang B, Zhang Q, Fu S, Wang D, Cheng X, Wu X, Xue Z, Zhang L, Zhang D, Da Y, Dai Y, Yang Q, Yao Z, Qiao L, Zhang R (2014) Embelin inhibits pancreatic cancer progression by directly inducing cancer cell apoptosis and indirectly restricting IL-6 associated inflammatory and immune suppressive cells. Cancer Lett 354:407–416
100. Peng M, Xu S, Zhang Y, Zhang L, Huang B, Fu S, Xue Z, Da Y, Dai Y, Qiao L, Dong A, Zhang R, Meng W (2014) Thermosensitive injectable hydrogel enhances the antitumor effect of embelin in mouse hepatocellular carcinoma. J Pharm Sci 103:965–973
101. Perkins ND (2012) The diverse and complex roles of NF-κB subunits in cancer. Nat Rev Cancer 12:121–132
102. Phuong do T, Ma CM, Hattori M, Jin JS (2009) Inhibitory effects of antrodins A-E from Antrodia cinnamomea and their metabolites on hepatitis C virus protease. Phytother Res 23:582–584
103. Plutzky J (2003) PPARs as therapeutic targets: Reverse cardiology? Science 302:406–407

104. Podolak I, Galanty A, Janeczko Z (2005) Cytotoxic activity of embelin from *Lysimachia punctata*. Fitoterapia 76:333–335
105. Podolak I, Strzałka M (2008) Qualitative and quantitative LC profile of embelin and rapanone in selected *Lysimachia* species. Chromatographia 67:471–475
106. Poojari R (2014) Embelin—a drug of antiquity: shifting the paradigm towards modern medicine. Expert Opin Investig Drugs 23:427–444
107. Poojari RJ (2014) Embelin, a small molecule quinone with a co-clinical power for castrate-resistant prostate cancer. Front Pharmacol 5:184
108. Radhakrishnan N (2011) A potential antibacterial agent Embelin, a natural benzoquinone extracted from Embelia ribes. Biol Med 3(2):1–7
109. Rani P, Khullar N (2004) Antimicrobial evaluation of some medicinal plants for their anti-enteric potential against multi-drug resistant Salmonella typhi. Phytother Res 18:670–673
110. Rathi SG, Bhaskar VH, Patel PG (2010) Antifungal activity of *Embelia ribes* plant extracts. Int J Pharm Biol Res 1:6–10
111. Rathinam KKS, Ramiah N (1976) Studies on the antifertility activity of embelin. J Res Ind Med Yoga Homeop 11:84–90
112. Reuter S, Prasad S, Phromnoi K, Kannappan R, Yadav VR, Aggarwal BB (2010) Embelin suppresses osteoclastogenesis induced by receptor activator of NF-κB ligand and tumor cells in vitro through inhibition of the NF-κB cell signaling pathway. Mol Cancer Res 8:1425–1436
113. Rhodus NLCB, Myers S, Miller L, Ho V, Ondrey F (2005) The feasibility of monitoring NF-κB associated cytokines: TNF-alpha, IL-1alpha, IL-6, and IL-8 in whole saliva for the malignant transformation of oral lichen planus. Mol Carcinog 44:77–82
114. Riedl S, Renatus M, Schwarzenbacher R, Zhou Q, Sun C, Fesik S, Liddington R, Salvesen G (2001) Structural basis for the inhibition of caspase-3 by XIAP. Cell 104:791–800
115. Rondevaldova J, Leuner O, Teka A, Lulekal E, Havlik J, Van Damme P, Kokoska L (2015) In vitro antistaphylococcal effects of *Embelia schimperi* extracts and their component embelin with oxacillin and tetracycline. Evid Based Complement Alternat Med 2015:1–7 (ID: 175983)
116. Ruiz-Bailén M, Hoyos EAD, Ruiz-Navarro S, Díaz-Castellanos MÁ, Rucabado-Aguilar L, Gómez-Jiménez FJ, Martínez-Escobar S, Moreno RM, Fierro-Rosón J (2005) Reversible myocardial dysfunction after cardiopulmonary resuscitation. Resuscitation 66:175–181
117. Sahu AK, Gautam MK, Deshmukh PT, Kushwah LS, Silawat N, Akbar Z, Muthu MS (2012) Effect of embelin on lithium-induced nephrogenic diabetes insipidus in albino rats. Asian Pac J Trop Dis 2:S729–S733
118. Sahu BD, Anubolu H, Koneru M, Kumar JM, Kuncha M, Rachamalla SS, Sistla R (2014) Cardioprotective effect of embelin on isoproterenol-induced myocardial injury in rats: possible involvement of mitochondrial dysfunction and apoptosis. Life Sci 107:59–67
119. Salvesen GS, Duckett CS (2002) IAP proteins: blocking the road to death's door. Nat Rev Mol Cell Biol 3:401–410
120. Samatha S, Vasudevan TN (1996) *Embelia ribes Burm.* as a source of red colorant. J Sci Ind Res 55:888–889
121. Sandro A, Gabriele BP (2005) Biologic therapy for inflammatory bowel disease. Drugs 65:2253–2286
122. Schaible AM, Traber H, Temml V, Noha SM, Filosa R, Peduto A, Weinigel C, Barz D, Schuster D, Werz O (2013) Potent inhibition of human 5-lipoxygenase and microsomal prostaglandin E2 synthase-1 by the anti-carcinogenic and anti-inflammatory agent embelin. Biochem Pharmacol 86:476–486
123. Schreiner SJ, Schiavone AP, Smithgall TE (2002) Activation of STAT3 by the Src family kinase Hck requires a functional SH3 domain. J Biol Chem 277:45680–45687
124. Shankarmurthy K, Krishna V, Maruthi K, Rahiman B (2004) Rapid adventitious organogenesis from leaf segments of *Embelia ribes Burm.*-a threatened medicinal plant. TAIWANIA-TAIPEI- 49:194–200

125. Shelar RMC, Tekale P, Katkar K, Naik V, Suthar A, Chauhan VS (2009) Embelin: an HPLC method for quantitative estimation in *Embelia ribes Burm.* F. Int J Pharm Clin Res 1:146–149
126. Shi Y (2009) Structural biology of programmed cell death. In: Essentials of apoptosis. Springer, pp. 95–118
127. Shimada T, Kojima K, Yoshiura K, Hiraishi H, Terano A (2002) Characteristics of the peroxisome proliferator activated receptor γ (PPARγ) ligand induced apoptosis in colon cancer cells. Gut 50:658–664
128. Singh B, Guru SK, Sharma R, Bharate SS, Khan IA, Bhushan S, Bharate SB, Vishwakarma RA (2014) Synthesis and anti-proliferative activities of new derivatives of embelin. Bioorg Med Chem Lett 24:4865–4870
129. Singh D, Singh R, Singh P, Gupta RS (2009) Effects of embelin on lipid peroxidation and free radical scavenging activity against liver damage in rats. Basic Clin Pharmacol Toxicol 105:243–248
130. Slee EA, Harte MT, Kluck RM, Wolf BB, Casiano CA, Newmeyer DD, Wang H-G, Reed JC, Nicholson DW, Alnemri ES (1999) Ordering the cytochrome c–initiated caspase cascade: hierarchical activation of caspases-2,-3,-6,-7,-8, and-10 in a caspase-9–dependent manner. J Cell Biol 144:281–292
131. Sreepriya M, Bali G (2005) Chemopreventive effects of embelin and curcumin against N-nitrosodiethylamine/phenobarbital-induced hepatocarcinogenesis in Wistar rats. Fitoterapia 76:549–555
132. Sreepriya M, Bali G (2006) Effects of administration of Embelin and Curcumin on lipid peroxidation, hepatic glutathione antioxidant defense and hematopoietic system during N-nitrosodiethylamine/Phenobarbital-induced hepatocarcinogenesis in Wistar rats. Mol Cell Biochem 284:49–55
133. Sumalatha KR, Abiramasundari G, Chetan GK, Divya T, Sudhandiran G, Sreepriya M (2014) XIAP inhibitor and antiestrogen embelin abrogates metastasis and augments apoptosis in estrogen receptor positive human breast adenocarcinoma cell line MCF-7. Mol Biol Rep 41:935–946
134. Suthar M, Patel R, Hapani K, Patel A (2009) Screening of *Embelia ribes* for antifungal activity. Int J Pharm Sci Drug Res 1:203–206
135. Tambekar DH, Khante BS, Chandak BR, Titare AS, Boralkar SS, Aghadte SN (2009) Screening of antibacterial potentials of some medicinal plants from Melghat forest in India. Afr J Tradit Complement Altern Med 6:228–232
136. Tamm I, Kornblau SM, Segall H, Krajewski S, Welsh K, Kitada S, Scudiero DA, Tudor G, Qui YH, Monks A, Andreeff M, Reed JC (2000) Expression and prognostic significance of IAP-family genes in human cancers and myeloid leukemias. Clin Cancer Res 6:1796–1803
137. Thippeswamy BS, Mahendran S, Biradar MI, Raj P, Srivastava K, Badami S, Veerapur VP (2011) Protective effect of embelin against acetic acid induced ulcerative colitis in rats. Eur J Pharmacol 654:100–105
138. Thippeswamy BS, Nagakannan P, Shivasharan BD, Mahendran S, Veerapur VP, Badami S (2011) Protective effect of embelin from *Embelia ribes Burm.* against transient global ischemia-induced brain damage in rats. Neurotox Res 20:379–386
139. Varier PS (2006) Indian medicinal plants a compendium of 500 species, vol 2. Orient Longman (Pvt) Ltd., Chennai, pp 368–371
140. Vinten-Johansen J, Jiang R, Reeves JG, Mykytenko J, Deneve J, Jobe LJ (2007) Inflammation, proinflammatory mediators and myocardial ischemia-reperfusion Injury. Hematol Oncol Clin North Am 21:123–145
141. Wang DG, Sun YB, Ye F, Li W, Kharbuja P, Gao L, Zhang DY, Suo J (2014) Anti-tumor activity of the X-linked inhibitor of apoptosis (XIAP) inhibitor embelin in gastric cancer cells. Mol Cell Biochem 386:143–152
142. Wang L, Yi TM (2009) IL-17 can promote tumor growth through an IL-6-Stat3 signaling pathway. J Exp Med 206:1431–1438

143. Watson RT, Makoto K, Pessin JE (2004) Regulated membrane trafficking of the insulin-responsive glucose transporter 4 in adipocytes. Endocr Rev 25:177–204
144. Xue Z, Ge Z, Zhang K, Sun R, Yang J, Han R, Peng M, Li Y, Li W, Zhang D, Hao J, Da Y, Yao Z, Zhang R (2014) Embelin suppresses dendritic cell functions and limits autoimmune encephalomyelitis through the TGF-beta/beta-catenin and STAT3 signaling pathways. Mol Neurobiol 49:1087–1101
145. Yang T, Lan J, Huang Q, Chen X, Sun X, Liu X, Yang P, Jin T, Wang S, Mou X (2015) Embelin sensitizes acute myeloid leukemia cells to TRAIL through XIAP inhibition and NF-kappaB inactivation. Cell Biochem Biophys 71:291–297
146. Yasmina L, Terrence T, David J, Elise T, Yisong W, Kuchroo VK, Flavell RA (2008) TGF-β signaling in dendritic cells is a prerequisite for the control of autoimmune encephalomyelitis. Proc Natl Acad Sci USA 105:10865–10870
147. Yen D, Cheung J, Scheerens H, Poulet F, McClanahan T, McKenzie B, Kleinschek MA, Owyang A, Mattson J, Blumenschein W, Murphy E, Sathe M, Cua DJ, Kastelein RA, Rennick D (2006) IL-23 is essential for T cell-mediated colitis and promotes inflammation via IL-17 and IL-6. J Clin Invest 116:1310–1316
148. Yoshizumi T, Ohta TI, Terada I, Fushida S, Fujimura T, Nishimura G, Shimizu K, Yi S, Miwa K (2004) Thiazolidinedione, a peroxisome proliferator-activated receptor-gamma ligand, inhibits growth and metastasis of HT-29 human colon cancer cells through differentiation-promoting effects. Int J Oncol 25:631–639
149. Zhao ZG, Tang ZZ, Zhang WK, Li JG (2015) Protective effects of embelin on myocardial ischemia-reperfusion injury following cardiac arrest in a rabbit model. Inflammation 38:527–533
150. Zou B, Qiao L, Wong BC (2009) Current understanding of the role of PPARgamma in gastrointestinal cancers. PPAR Res 2009(1):121-132. (ID: 816957)

Chapter 17
Butein and Its Role in Chronic Diseases

Ziwei Song, Muthu K. Shanmugam, Hanry Yu and Gautam Sethi

Abstract Natural compounds isolated from various plant sources have been used for therapeutic purpose for centuries. These compounds have been routinely used for the management of various chronic ailments and have gained considerable attention because of their significant efficacy and comparatively low side effects. Butein, a chacolnoid compound that has been isolated from various medicinal plants has exhibited a wide range of beneficial pharmacological effects, such as anti-inflammatory, anticancer, antioxidant, and anti-angiogenic in diverse disease models. This article briefly summarizes the past published literature related to the therapeutic and protective effects of butein, as demonstrated in various models of human chronic diseases. Further analysis of its important cellular targets, toxicity, and pharmacokinetic profile may further significantly expand its therapeutic application.

Keywords Butein · Anticancer · Inflammation · Angiogenesis · Antioxidant

---

Z. Song · H. Yu
Department of Physiology, Yong Loo Lin School of Medicine, MD9-04-11,
2 Medical Drive, Singapore 117597, Singapore

M.K. Shanmugam · G. Sethi (✉)
Department of Pharmacology, Yong Loo Lin School of Medicine,
National University of Singapore, Singapore 117600, Singapore
e-mail: phcgs@nus.edu.sg

H. Yu
Institute of Biotechnology and Nanotechnology, A*STAR, The Nanos,
#04-01, 31 Biopolis Way, Singapore 138669, Singapore

H. Yu
Singapore-MIT Alliance for Research and Technology, 1 CREATE Way,
#10-01 CREATE Tower, Singapore 138602, Singapore

H. Yu
Mechanobiology Institute, National University of Singapore, T-Lab, #05-01,
5A Engineering Drive 1, Singapore 117411, Singapore

S.C. Gupta et al. (eds.), *Anti-inflammatory Nutraceuticals and Chronic Diseases*,
Advances in Experimental Medicine and Biology 928,
DOI 10.1007/978-3-319-41334-1_17

17.1 Introduction

Plant-derived natural compounds and their derivatives have been used as therapeutic agents over the centuries. However, their exact chemical structures, functions as well as molecular targets are not completely known as of yet. Their high therapeutic efficiency and low side effects have made themselves ideal alternatives of synthetic drugs [4, 56]. Thus extensive qualitative and quantitative tests have been done to evaluate and to extend their therapeutic potential as drug candidates. Butein, a plant polyphenol (2′,3,4,4′-2′,4′,3,4- or 3,4,2′,4′-tetrahydroxychalcone), with the chemical structure shown in Fig. 17.1, has been reported to exhibit several important pharmacological effects, such as anti-inflammatory, anti-cancer, anti-oxidant, and anti-angiogenic [5, 33, 37, 50, 58]. It was first found in *Toxicodendronverniciﬂuum* (formerly called *RhusVerniciflua Stokes*, RVS), a tree widely used as a local food additive and therapeutic supplement in South East Asia [62]. It can also be isolated from the heartwood of *Dalbergiaodorifera*, the seed of *Cyclopiasubternata* and the stems of *Semecarpusanacardium*, as well as many other plants [41]. The various plant sources of butein are shown in Table 17.1 [60].

The first dietary butein supplement Inh-AR, launched by Megabol, is a sport pro-hormone supplement to control estrogen production by inhibiting aromatase [1]. Its activities in aromatase inhibition and estrogen regulation have also made butein a promising candidate for breast cancer treatment. Besides cancer [2, 30, 73], it also has exhibited promising effects in the treatment of many other chronic diseases, including inflammation [63], glaucoma [14], cardiovascular diseases [9], and metabolic complications [48]. Although molecular mechanisms underlying its various reported pharmacological effects remain to be elucidated, butein has been found to modulate several important cellular signaling pathways involved in etiology of chronic diseases. Meanwhile, it exhibits low toxicity against normal cells, thereby indicating its potential both as a chemopreventive and chemotherapeutic agent [28, 71]. In this chapter, we have briefly summarized various published reports related to the pharmacological properties and biological activities of butein, and emphasized on its therapeutic effects against various chronic diseases.

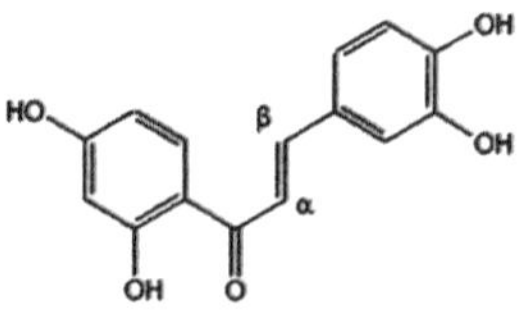

Fig. 17.1 The chemical structure of butein

Table 17.1 Plant sources of butein [60]

Family	Plant	Part
Adoxaceae	Viburnum propinquum Hemsl.	Leaves
Anacardiaceae	Cotinuscoggygria Scop.	Heartwood
	Searsiaverniciflua Stokes Syn.	Stem bark
	Toxicodendronvernicifluum (Stokes) FA Barkley	Stem bark
	Semecarpusanacardium L.	Stem bark
Asparagaceae	Sansevierialiberica Ger. and Labr.	Rhizomes
Asteraceae	Bidensbipinnata L.	Flowers
	Bidenspilosa L.	Whole plant
	Bidenstripartita L.	Whole plant
	Coreopsis douglasii (DC.) HM Hall	Flowers
	Coreopsis gigantean (Kellogg) HM Hall	Flowers
	Coreopsis maritime (Nutt.) Hook. f.	Flowers
	Coreopsis petrophiloides BL Rob. & Greenm.	Flowers
	Coreopsis lanceolata L.	Flowers
	Cosmos sulfurous Cav.	Flowers
	Dahlia variabilisDesf.	Flowers
	Dahlia coccinea Cav.	Petals
	VernoniaanthelminticaWilld	Seeds
Fabaceae	Acacia pycnathaBenth.	Heartwood
	Adenantherapavonina L.	Wood
	Bauhinia purpurea L.	Seeds
	Butea frondosaRoxb.	Flowers
	Butea monosperma (Lam.) Taub.	Flowers
	Caragana intermedia Kuang & HC Fu Syn.	Whole plant
	CaraganakorshinskiiKom.	
	Cyclopiasubternata Vogel Syn.	Seeds
	Cyclopiafalcata (Harv.) Kies	
	Dalbergiaodorifera TC Chen	Heartwood
	DipteryxlacuniferaDucke	Fruits
	Millettianitida var. hirsutissima Z. Wei	Stems
	Millettiaspeciosa Champ.	Roots
	Sophoraalopecuroides L.	Whole plant
	Viciafaba L.	Fruits
Pinaceae	AbiespindrowRoyle ex D. Don	Stems
Rubiaceae	Hydnophytumformicarum Jack.	Tubers
Schisandraceae	Schisandrapropinqua (Wall.) Baill	Whole plant
Solanaceae	Solanum lycopersicum Lam.	Fruits

17.2 Physiochemical Properties of Butein

As a flavonoid compound, butein exhibits the various common structure features and biological activities shared by the flavonoid family. Flavonoids are known to provide health benefits, such as disease prevention, antioxidant activities, and chemoprevention [63, 66]. These compounds can be classified into different groups based upon their specific structural features, and each group has different biological activities and efficiency. Butein belongs to the chaloconoid subgroup of flavonoid family, with two aromatic carbon rings linked together by the α,β-unsaturated carbonyl group and a double bond [7]. Chemical and physical properties of butein are summarized below in Table 17.2.

There are several studies on the structural-activity relationship of butein, providing new insights into the specific chemical structural features that exhibit diverse biological activities. Studies show that the position of hydroxyl groups on aromatic carbon rings is crucial for the bioactivities of chalcone compounds [53], and that the double bond at C2–C3 as well as the 4-oxo functional group contributes to the inflammatory activities of flavonoids [22]. In addition, a study to compare butein and luteolin (two flavonoid compounds without and with C ring structures, respectively) proves that, butein is more effective in the induction of heme oxygencase-1 (HO-1) and the suppression of NF-κB activation, thus suppressing LPS-induced inflammatory responses in the macrophage RAW264.7 cells. This report clearly indicates that although both flavonoids exhibit anti-inflammatory activities, but the C ring structure of butein contributes to its significantly higher efficacy [63].

Table 17.2 Chemical and physical properties of butein

Molecular formula	$C_{15}H_{12}O_5$
Molecular weight	272.25278 g/mol
Exact mass	272.068473 g/mol
Monoisotopic mass	272.068473 g/mol
XLogP3	2.8
Hydrogen bond donor count	4
Hydrogen bond acceptor count	5
Rotatable bond count	3
Topological polar surface area	98 A^2
Heavy atom count	20
Formal charge	0
Complexity	367
Isotope atom count	0
Defined atom stereocenter count	0
Undefined atom stereocenter count	0
Defined bond stereocenter count	1
Undefined bond stereocenter count	0
Covalently bonded unit count	1

Source: [51]

17.3 Role of Butein Against Chronic Diseases

As a multi-targeted compound with diverse biological effects, butein has been reported to target several important cell signaling pathways. Although the underlying mechanisms and molecular targets remain to be elucidated, published results indicate that butein exhibit therapeutic effects on several chronic diseases including inflammation, cancer, cardiovascular diseases, and metabolic complications. This section briefly summarizes its reported therapeutic effects against various chronic ailments.

17.3.1 Inflammatory Diseases

Inflammation is body's primary protective response against harmful foreign stimuli. The primary purpose of inflammation is beneficial: to clear out damaged tissues and to initiate the healing process. However, aberrant inflammatory response can lead to some severe complications such as cancers [41], cardiovascular diseases and rheumatoid arthritis [10, 40]. It is known that the activation of nuclear factor-κB (NF-κB) regulates the production of many pro-inflammatory mediators. NF-κB can be activated by extracellular stimuli and later translocate from cytoplasm to nucleus [63]. As stated in the previous section, butein suppresses lipopolysaccharide (LPS)-induced inflammatory responses in the macrophage RAW264.7 cells by dose-dependently inhibiting various enzymes and pro-inflammatory mediators, including nitrite [26], tumor necrosis factor-α (TNF-α) [26, 37], COX-1 [59], COX-2 [37], inducible nitric oxide synthase (iNOS) [63], PGE-2 [26], and nitric oxide (NO) [26, 43] production. It is hypothesized that these anti-inflammatory effects are mediated by suppression of deregulated activation of NF-κB and JNK1/2 signaling pathways [26]. It also induces the expression of HO-1, an enzyme that inhibits NF-κB activation in macrophages [63].

Besides suppressing NF-κB in macrophage RAW264.7 cells, butein also inhibits the activation of NF-κB in human mast cells leading to the decreased production of TNF-α, IL-6, and IL-8 [58], and in adipocytes by blocking IKKβ, a NF-κB upstream kinase [68]. And it also abrogates ß-glucuronidase and lysozyme in rat neutrophils [5]. Moreover, it also exhibits anti-inflammatory effects on lung epithelial A549 cells by inhibiting TNF-α-induced ROS generation, NF-κB activation, MAPK phosphorylation and Akt phosphorylation, and by decreasing TNF-α-induced monocyte cell adhesion to lung epithelial cells [58]. In addition, it also reduces IL-8 secretion and MMP-7 expression in intestinal epithelial HT-29 cells, and suppresses the E-selectin expression in human umbilical vein endothelial cells [38]. It also exhibits significant activity against bowel inflammatory diseases by decreasing the expression of IL-6, IL-1β, interferon (IFN)-γ, and MMP-9 in IL-10 deficient mice [41].

17.3.2 Cancer

As stated above, butein can interfere with tumor progression by suppressing inflammatory reactions [52]. It is also well recognized as a promising anticancer agent and functions by inhibiting cellular growth, migration as well as by promoting apoptosis. Its anticancer effects have been reported against various tumor cells, including breast cancer [67], colon cancer [74], leukemia [31], melanoma [15], osteosarcoma cells [24], prostate cancer [30], hepatocellular carcinoma [57], lung cancer [42], and neuroblastoma cells [8]. Its anticancer effects are achieved by modulating various critical cellular signaling pathways and enzymes involved in tumorigenesis and apoptosis. It is well established that PI3K/Akt/mTOR is one of the major signaling pathways regulating cell survival and motility [17]. And its activation plays a key role in tumor cell growth and invasion [6, 17]. Butein can significantly suppress PI3K/Akt phosphorylation in human prostate cancer cells [30] and cervical cancer cells [2]. It is also found to downregulate MMP-9 and uPA expression by inhibiting Akt/mTOR/p70S6K, thus acting as antimetastatic agent [46].

Various studies also show that butein induces reactive oxygen species (ROS) production, which is also critical for cell apoptosis, cell senescence and cell division [65]. It has been reported that it induces G2/M phase cell cycle arrest in hepatoma cells by regulating ROS level, JNK expression, ATM, and Chk activity [50]. It also induces ROS generation, ERK1/2, and p38MAPK suppression in triple-negative breast cancer MDA-MB-231 cells [72]. Similarly, it causes apoptosis of neutroblastoma cells by increasing ROS level and modulating various enzymes [8]. And it also shows antiproliferative and apoptotic activities in HeLa human cervical cancer cells, by inhibiting the expression of PI3K, Akt and mTOR phosphorylation, and by inducing the ROS generation [2]. These effects were further confirmed in vivo in a nude mouse model, where it significantly suppressed cervical tumor growth with limited side effects by inhibiting PI3K/Akt/mTOR activation and increasing ROS generation [2]. It also increases caspase-3, -8, -9 activities in neutroblastoma cells and caspase-3 activity in HeLa cells, the expression of which is critical for apoptosis [31]. Moreover, Bcl-2 downregulation is also observed in butein-induced apoptosis of neutroblastoma cells [8]. It is also shown that butein increases Bax while suppressing Bcl-2 expression in Hela cells. Bax and Bcl-2 are both critical enzymes for apoptosis, and the Bax/Bcl-2 ratio contributes to the butein-induced apoptosis [2].

Another critical molecule involved in the anticancer activity of butein is the signal transducer and activator of transcription 3 (STAT3), a transcription factor. STAT3 can regulate the NF-κB signaling pathway, and thus plays a major role in the inflammation-related tumorigenesis [21, 76]. It is activated by IL6/JAK signaling pathway [29]. The IL6/JAK/STAT3 mechanism has been found to participate in the progression of various malignant tumors, such as prostate cancer, breast cancer, and myeloma [41]. Butein inhibits the IL6/JAK/STAT3 pathway by suppressing c-Src and JAK1/JAK2 activation, and by inhibiting Bcl-xL, Bcl-2, and cyclin D1 expression [57]. Moreover, it blocks the ERK1/2 and NF-κB signaling pathways in human bladder cancer cells, which inhibits the cell proliferation and tumor invasion [78]. It also negatively regulates NK-κB activation by modulating critical molecules such as TNFα1, TRADD, TRAF2, NIK, TAK1/TAB17.1, and IKK-β [55]. Besides STAT3, matrix metalloproteinase (MMP) is also critical in tumor cell apoptosis, tumor progression, and invasion. It has been found that butein suppresses the activation of MMP-9 in prostate cancer cells [18, 35], and the activation of MMP-2 and MMP-9 in Hela cells [2]. Butein is also noted to inhibit both MMP-9 activity and STAT3 activation in Colo 205 cells [41], which indicates its possible therapeutic potential for treating bowel inflammation-induced colon cancer.

There are several critical enzymes and molecules regulated by butein in various tumor cell lines. For example, glutathione-s -transferase (GST), an enzyme that reduces H_2O_2-induced oxidative stress, is significantly increased after butein treatment in human caucasian neuroblastoma IMR-32 cells [77]. And it also suppresses some other enzymes critical for tumorigenesis, such as histone deacetylase enzymes [54], aromatase [67] and recombinant human aldo-keto reductase family [61]. And butein can inhibit DNA, RNA, and protein synthesis by reducing the cellular uptake of thymidine, uridine, and leucine of cancer cells [74]. Moreover, butein treatment suppresses colony formation in UACC-812 human breast cancer cells co-cultured with fibroblasts [34]. And it induces apoptosis in U937 human leukemia cells by modulating caspase 3-dependent pathways [23].

17.3.3 Cardiovascular Diseases

Cardiovascular diseases are one of the leading causes of mortality worldwide [49]. They are also closely associated with various other complications, such as obesity and diabetes [20]. Butein has been found to exhibit cardiovascular protection effects by improving blood circulation, in which platelets aggregation and thrombosis play a key role. It has been reported that butein also exhibits anti-thrombin effects by inhibiting the blood coagulation drawn from New Zealand white rabbits [43]. It also inhibits ADP-induced platelet aggregation [43] and adrenalin-induced secondary aggregation in human plasma [45]. Besides its anti-platelet effects, butein can also suppress the viability and motility of vascular smooth muscle cells, both of which can lead to atherosclerosis by thickening the blood vessels [9]. This activity is further confirmed in vivo in animal models of phenylephrine-induced contracted rat aorta [75] and balloon-injured rat carotid arteries [8].

17.3.4 Diabetes and Metabolic Complications

Diabetes is a group of metabolic diseases caused by either insufficient supply of insulin (Type I diabetes mellitus) or aberrant cellular response to insulin (Type II diabetes mellitus). Butein can significantly suppress diabetes induced by streptozotocin [44]. It also has been found to have protective effects on functional pancreatic beta-cells and rat islets. Type I diabetes is mainly caused by beta-cell destruction, in which various inflammatory cytokines are involved, including IL-1β, TNF-α, IFN-γ, etc. [25]. Moreover, it protects the cellular activity of beta cells by inhibiting cytokine-mediated cell death, NO production, iNOS expression, and NF-κB translocation [25], thus indicating its potential for Type I diabetes mellitus prevention.

17.3.5 Liver Diseases

It has been reported that butein is also active in liver fibrosis prevention, by increasing albumin production [16] and inhibiting hepatic stellate cell proliferation [69]. In vivo data shows that butein can reduce hydroxyproline and malondialdehyde levels in liver fibrosis mouse model induced by CCl_4 [36]. It can also decrease the toxicity caused by ethanol in hepatic stellate cells and hepatoma HepG2 cells [64], indicating its potential to prevent alcohol-related liver complications, such as cirrhosis, fatty liver, and alcoholic hepatitis. The effects to decrease alcohol-induced toxicity are achieved by suppressing ROS production, MMP-1 and -2 inhibitors in HSCs. It has been also found that butein inhibits the JNK/p38 MAPK signaling pathway and upregulates NF-κB [64]. Moreover, butein inhibits rat hepatocyte apoptosis by decreasing PARP cleavage, DNA fragmentation, and caspase activation [60].

17.3.6 Other Protective and Therapeutic Effects

Butein has been found to have therapeutic effects against the initiation and progression of several other major human diseases. For example, it has anti-HIV effects by causing around 58 % inhibition of HIV-1 protease [70]. It can also suppress ICAM-1 expression and increase leukocyte function-associated antigen-1 positive cells in nephritic glomeruli [19]. And it can decreases the protein level in urine and cholesterol level in plasma, thus indicating its therapeutic potential for nephropathy, a kidney disease which can be caused by either IgA deposition in glomerulus or chemotherapy agents [60]. Moreover, it is potential drug candidate for tuberculosis, as it can inhibit myocolic acids production and HadB activity, by blocking the activity of *Mycobacteriumbovis* BCG, a myobacteria that causes tuberculosis [3]. It also shows protective effects in several neuronal cell lines. It largely reduces the toxicity induced by glutamate in mouse HT22 neuronal cells [11, 12]. And it can be a potential pain killer by inhibiting SNARE-complex, a critical enzyme involved in the synaptic vesicle transmission [27].

17.4 Preclinical Studies

Although the therapeutic effects of butein have been demonstrated in various in vitro models of different cell lines as mentioned above, yet it still need to be further confirmed in vivo in order to have practical application. And several studies have reassured its bioactivities in animals. It is revealed that the tumorigenesis of xenograft cervical tumors can be inhibited in nude mice with minor side effects, by intraperitoneal injection of butein [2]. Similarly, extracts from *RhusVerniciflua Stokes* (RVS) containing butein has been shown to decrease lung cancer tumor size in a xenograft mouse model. It inhibits angiogenesis and suppresses tumor growth, by inhibiting VEGF activity which indicates its potential for treating angiogenesis dependent cancers [13]. Moreover, injection of butein significantly reduces the colonic inflammation in IL-10-/- mice with drug-induced colitis [41]. Also, butein has shown to prevent drug-induced acute renal failure in rats, indicating its potential for nephropathy treatment [60]. Additionally, it also has exhibited protective effects in rat models with spinal cord injury [47] and CCl_4-induced liver fibrosis [36], which is, again, consistent with respective in vitro results. There are few preclinical trials to analyze the possible therapeutic potential of butein in humans. Extracts from RVS with butein significantly reduced the tumor size in an 82 years old patient after 5 months of treatment [39]. Gastric cancer has always been one of the leading diseases, and the effect of conventional therapies such as surgical resection is limited for elderly patients. So RVS extracts containing butein can be an ideal alternative treatment. Also, this finding indicates that the therapeutic effects of butein can also be elevated and optimized in a combination with other useful flavonoid compounds. Extracts from RVS with butein significantly reduced the tumor size in a 82-years-old patient after 5 months of treatment [39]. Gastric cancer has always been one of the leading diseases, and the effect of conventional therapies such as surgical resection is limited for elderly patients. So RVS extracts containing butein can be an ideal alternative treatment. Also, this finding also indicates that the therapeutic effects of butein can also be elevated and optimized in a combination with other useful flavonoid compounds.

17.5 Conclusions

Herbal medicine can be traced back to hundreds of years ago, and our ancestors use different plants with different bioactivities in different combinations. However, the ancient application of herbal medicine is solely based on experience, without qualitative or quantitative tests. With the development of drug testing techniques, the chemical structures and activities of these therapeutic compounds have been extensively studied, by using high throughput screening and various in vitro as well as in vivo models. Butein is a multi-target compound that can exhibit a wide array of beneficial effects by modulating a wide variety of cellular signal transduction

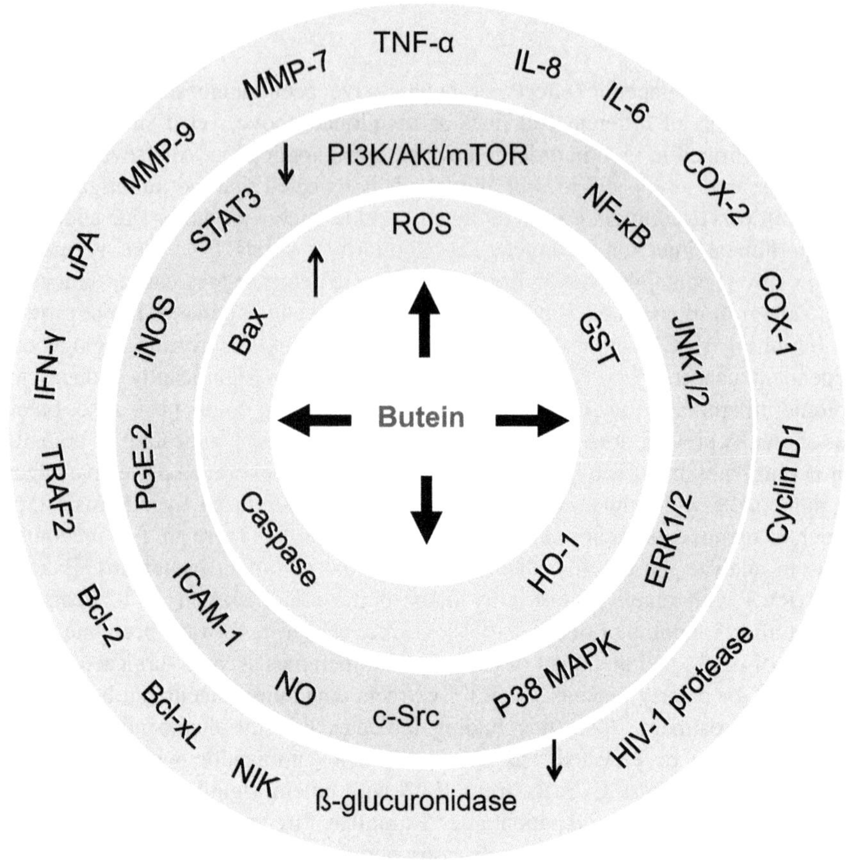

Fig. 17.2 Major signaling pathways and enzymes regulated by butein, ↓ indicates inhibition or downregulation; ↑ indicates activation or upregulation. The molecules and pathways in the *inner circle* are all upregulated or activated, while those in the *outer two circles* are downregulated or inhibited by butein

cascades (Fig. 17.2). Its therapeutic effects have been validated in various cell lines as well as mice models. However, neither Food and Drug Administration (FDA) in US nor European Food Safety Authority (EFSA) has approved it as a therapeutic drug. The only formulation containing butein available at present is Inh-AR, a dietary supplement. There are many structure-activity studies on butein to reveal the relationship between its chemical structural features and reported pharmacological effects [22, 53, 63]. These studies provides in-depth understanding of its observed biological effects and may also aid to synthesize similar compounds in future that can achieve the same, or even better, therapeutic effects with better pharmacokinetic profile. Although butein has many beneficial effects and low side effects, its toxicity still needs to be elucidated. It is shown that the *RhusVerniciflua Stokes*, one of the original sources of butein, can cause severe skin complications [32], thereby indicating that butein may also have potential adverse effects. However, there is currently lack of relevant toxicity studies with this therapeutic agent. Overall, butein appears to be a promising drug candidate because of its various beneficial effects and therapeutic actions against major human chronic diseases. However, additional clinical trials are needed to validate its safety and efficacy so that it can be rapidly applied for human use in near future.

Acknowledgments This work was supported by National University Health System Bench to Bedside grant to GS.

References

1. Ambozik S (2012) Aromatase in the dock. http://www.megabol.com/aromatase.html
2. Bai X, Ma Y, Zhang G (2015) Butein suppresses cervical cancer growth through the PI3K/AKT/mTOR pathway. Oncol Rep 33(6):3085–3092
3. Brown AK, Papaemmanouil A, Bhowruth V, Bhatt A, Dover LG, Besra GS (2007) Flavonoid inhibitors as novel antimycobacterial agents targeting Rv0636, a putative dehydratase enzyme involved in Mycobacterium tuberculosis fatty acid synthase II. Microbiology 153(Pt 10):3314–3322
4. Butler MS (2004) The role of natural product chemistry in drug discovery. J Nat Prod 67 (12):2141–2153
5. Chan SC, Chang YS, Wang JP, Chen SC, Kuo SC (1997) Three new flavonoids and antiallergic, anti-inflammatory constituents from the heartwood of *Dalbergia odorifera*. Planta Med 64:153–158
6. Chen YL, Law PY, Loh HH (2005) Inhibition of PI3K/Akt signaling: an emerging paradigm for targeted cancer therapy. Curr Med Chem Anti Cancer Agents 5:575–589
7. Chen W, Song J, Guo P, Wen Z (2006) Butein, a more effective antioxidant than α-tocopherol. J Mol Struct (Thoechem) 763(1–3):161–164
8. Chen YH, Yeh CW, Lo HC, Su SL, Hseu YC, Hsu LS (2012) Generation of reactive oxygen species mediates butein-induced apoptosis in neuroblastoma cells. Oncol Rep 27(4):1233–1237
9. Chen YN, Huang TF, Chang CH, Hsu CC, Lin KT, Wang SW, Peng HC, Chung CH (2012) Antirestenosis effect of butein in the neointima formation progression. J Agric Food Chem 60 (27):6832–6838
10. Chen TY, Sun HL, Yao HT, Lii CK, Chen HW, Chen PY, Li CC, Liu KL (2013) Suppressive effects of *Indigofera suffruticosa* Mill extracts on lipopolysaccharide-induced inflammatory responses in murine RAW 264.7 macrophages. Food Chem Toxicol 55:257–264
11. Cho N, Choi JH, Yang H, Jeong EJ, Lee KY, Kim YC, Sung SH (2012) Neuroprotective and anti-inflammatory effects of flavonoids isolated from *Rhus verniciflua* in neuronal HT22 and microglial BV2 cell lines. Food Chem Toxicol 50(6):1940–1945
12. Cho N, Lee KY, Huh J, Choi JH, Yang H, Jeong EJ, Kim HP, Sung SH (2013) Cognitive-enhancing effects of *Rhus verniciflua* bark extract and its active flavonoids with neuroprotective and anti-inflammatory activities. Food Chem Toxicol 58:355–361
13. Choi WC, Lee JH, Lee EO, Lee HJ, Yoon SW, Ahn KS, Kim SH (2006) Study on antiangiogenic and antitunor activities of processed *Rhus verniciflua* Stokes extract. Korean J Oriental Physiol Pathol 20(4):825–829

14. Choi SJ, Lee MY, Jo H, Lim SS, Jung SH (2012) Preparative isolation and purification of neuroprotective compounds from *Rhus verniciflua* by high speed counter-current chromatography. Biol Pharm Bull 35(4):559–567
15. Cui Z, Song E, Hu DN, Chen M, Rosen R, McCormick SA (2012) Butein induces apoptosis in human uveal melanoma cells through mitochondrial apoptosis pathway. Curr Eye Res 37 (8):730–739
16. Dong MS, Jung NC, Na CS (2004) Composition comprising phenolic compound for preventing and treating liver cirrhosis. Patent no.: WO2004002471 A1
17. Fresno Vara JA, Casado E, de Castro J, Cejas P, Belda-Iniesta C, Gonzalez-Baron M (2004) PI3K/Akt signalling pathway and cancer. Cancer Treat Rev 30(2):193–204
18. Garg P, Vijay-Kumar M, Wang L, Gewirtz AT, Merlin D, Sitaraman SV (2009) Matrix metalloproteinase-9-mediated tissue injury overrides the protective effect of matrix metalloproteinase-2 during colitis. Am J Physiol Gastrointest Liver Physiol 296(2):G175–G184
19. Hayashi K, Nagamatsu T, Honda S, Suzuki Y (1996) Butein (3,4,2',4'-tetrahydroxychalcone) ameliorates experimental anti-glomerular basement membrane antibody-associated glomerulonephritis (3). Eur J Pharmacol 316:297–306
20. Highlander P, Shaw GP (2010) Current pharmacotherapeutic concepts for the treatment of cardiovascular disease in diabetics. Ther Adv Cardiovasc Dis 4(1):43–54
21. Hodge DR, Hurt EM, Farrar WL (2005) The role of IL-6 and STAT3 in inflammation and cancer. Eur J Cancer 41(16):2502–2512
22. Ishikawa YT, Goto M, Yamaki K (2003) Inhibitory effects of several flavonoids on E-selectin expression on human umbilical vein endothelial cells stimulated by tumor necrosis factor-α. Phytother Res 17:1224–1227
23. Iwashita KK, Kobori M, Yamaki K, Tsushida T (2000) Flavonoids inhibit cell growth and in B16 melanoma 4A5 Cells induce apoptosis. Biosci Biotechnol Biochem 64(9):1813–1820
24. Jang HS, Kook SH, Son YO, Kim JG, Jeon YM, Jang YS, Choi KC, Kim J, Han SK, Lee KY, Park BK, Cho NP, Lee JC (2005) Flavonoids purified from *Rhus verniciflua* Stokes actively inhibit cell growth and induce apoptosis in human osteosarcoma cells. Biochim Biophys Acta 1726(3):309–316
25. Jeong GS, Lee DS, Song MY, Park BH, Kang DG, Lee HS, Kwon KB, Kim YS (2011) Butein from *Rhus verniciflua* protects pancreatic b cells against cytokine-induced toxicity mediated by inhibition of nitric oxide formation. Biol Pharm Bull 34(1):97–102
26. Jung CH, Kim JH, Hong MH, Seog HM, Oh SH, Lee PJ, Kim GJ, Kim HM, Um JY, Ko SG (2007) Phenolic-rich fraction from *Rhus verniciflua* Stokes (RVS) suppress inflammatory response via NF-kappaB and JNK pathway in lipopolysaccharide-induced RAW 264.7 macrophages. J Ethnopharmacol 110(3):490–497
27. Jung CH, Kweon DH, Shin YK, Yang YS (2011) Polyphenol compounds with modulating neurotransmitter release. Patent no.: US8263643 B2
28. Kang DG, Lee AS, Mun YJ, Woo WH, Kim YC, Sohn EJ, Moon MK, Lee HS (2004) Butein ameliorates renal concentrating ability in cisplatin-induced acute renal failure in rats. Biol Pharm Bull 27(3):366–370
29. Kato T (2011) Stat3-driven cancer-related inflammation as a key therapeutic target for cancer immunotherapy. Immunotherapy 3(5):587–591
30. Khan N, Adhami VM, Afaq F, Mukhtar H (2012) Butein induces apoptosis and inhibits prostate tumor growth in vitro and in vivo. Antioxid Redox Signal 16(11):1195–1204
31. Kim NY, Pae HO, Oh GS, Kang TH, Kim YC, Rhew HY, Chung HT (2001) Butein, a plant polyphenol, induces apoptosis concomitant with increased caspase-3 activity, decreased Bcl-2 expression and increased Bax expression in HL-60 cells. Pharmacol Toxicol 88:261–266
32. Kim KH, Moon E, Choi SU, Pang C, Kim SY, Lee KR (2015) Identification of cytotoxic and anti-inflammatory constituents from the bark of *Toxicodendron vernicifluum* (Stokes) F.A. Barkley. J Ethnopharmacol 162:231–237

33. Kojima R, Kawachi M, Ito M (2015) Butein suppresses ICAM-1 expression through the inhibition of IkappaBalpha and c-Jun phosphorylation in TNF-alpha- and PMA-treated HUVECs. Int Immunopharmacol 24(2):267–275
34. Kook SH, Son YO, Chung SW, Lee SA, Kim JG, Jeon YM, Lee JC (2007) Caspase-independent death of human osteosarcoma cells by flavonoids is driven by p53-mediated mitochondrial stress and nuclear translocation of AIF and endonuclease G. Apoptosis 12(7):1289–1298
35. Lakatos G, Sipos F, Miheller P, Hritz I, Varga MZ, Juhasz M, Molnar B, Tulassay Z, Herszenyi L (2012) The behavior of matrix metalloproteinase-9 in lymphocytic colitis, collagenous colitis and ulcerative colitis. Pathol Oncol Res 18(1):85–91
36. Lee SH, Nan JX, Zhao YZ, Woo SW, Park EJ, Kang TH, Seo GS, Kim YC, Sohn DH (2003) The chalcone butein from *Rhus verniciflua* shows antifibrogenic activity. Planta Med 69:990–994
37. Lee SH, Seo GS, Sohn DH (2004) Inhibition of lipopolysaccharide-induced expression of inducible nitric oxide synthase by butein in RAW 264.7 cells. Biochem Biophys Res Commun 323(1):125–132
38. Lee SH, Seo GS, Jin XY, Ko G, Sohn DH (2007) Butein blocks tumor necrosis factor alpha-induced interleukin 8 and matrix metalloproteinase 7 production by inhibiting p38 kinase and osteopontin mediated signaling events in HT-29 cells. Life Sci 81(21–22):1535–1543
39. Lee SH, Choi SC, Kim KS, Park JW, Lee SH, Yoon SW (2010) Shrinkage of gastric cancer in an elderly patient who received *Rhus verniciflua* Stokes extract. J Altern Complement Med 16 (4):497–500
40. Lee DS, Li B, Im NK, Kim YC, Jeong GS (2013) 4,2',5'-trihydroxy-4'-methoxychalcone from *Dalbergia odorifera* exhibits anti-inflammatory properties by inducing heme oxygenase-1 in murine macrophages. Int Immunopharmacol 16(1):114–121
41. Lee SD, Choe JW, Lee BJ, Kang MH, Joo MK, Kim JH, Yeon JE, Park JJ, Kim JS, Bak YT (2015) Butein effects in colitis and interleukin-6/signal transducer and activator of transcription 3 expression. World J Gastroenterol 21(2):465–474
42. Li Y, Ma C, Qian M, Wen Z, Jing H, Qian D (2014) Butein induces cell apoptosis and inhibition of cyclooxygenase2 expression in A549 lung cancer cells. Mol Med Rep 9(2):763–767
43. Liao XL, Luo JG, Kong LY (2013) Flavonoids from *Millettia nitida* var. hirsutissima with their anticoagulative activities and inhibitory effects on NO production. J Nat Med 67(4):856–861
44. Lim SS, Jung SH, Ji J, Shin KH, Keum SR (2001) Synthesis of avonoids and their effects on aldose reductase and sorbitol accumulation in streptozotocin-induced diabetic rat tissues. J Pharm Pharmacol 53:653–668
45. Lin CN, Lin TH, Hsu MF, Wang JP, Ko FN, Teng CM (1997) 2',5'-Dihydroxychalcone as a potent chemical cyclooxygenase inhibitor mediator and cyclooxygenase inhibitor. J Pharm Pharmacol 49:530–536
46. Liu SC, Chen C, Chung CH, Wang PC, Wu NL, Cheng JK, Lai YW, Sun HL, Peng CY, Tang CH, Wang SW (2014) Inhibitory effects of butein on cancer metastasis and bioenergetic modulation. J Agric Food Chem 62(37):9109–9117
47. Lu M, Wang S, Han X, Lv D (2013) Butein inhibits NF-kappaB activation and reduces infiltration of inflammatory cells and apoptosis after spinal cord injury in rats. Neurosci Lett 542:87–91
48. Martineau LC (2012) Large enhancement of skeletal muscle cell glucose uptake and suppression of hepatocyte glucose-6-phosphatase activity by weak uncouplers of oxidative phosphorylation. Biochim Biophys Acta 1820(2):133–150
49. Mendis S, Puska P, Norrving B (2011) Global Atlas on cardiovascular disease prevention and control. World Health Organization, 3–18

50. Moon DO, Choi YH, Moon SK, Kim WJ, Kim GY (2010) Butein suppresses the expression of nuclear factor-kappa B-mediated matrix metalloproteinase-9 and vascular endothelial growth factor in prostate cancer cells. Toxicol In Vitro 24(7):1927–1934
51. National Center for Biotechnology Information (2005) CID=5281222.PubChem compound database. https://pubchem.ncbi.nlm.nih.gov/compound/5281222
52. Neergheen VS, Bahorun T, Taylor EW, Jen LS, Aruoma OI (2010) Targeting specific cell signaling transduction pathways by dietary and medicinal phytochemicals in cancer chemoprevention. Toxicology 278(2):229–241
53. Nerya O, Musa R, Khatib S, Tamir S, Vaya J (2004) Chalcones as potent tyrosinase inhibitors: the effect of hydroxyl positions and numbers. Phytochemistry 65(10):1389–1395
54. Orlikova B, Schnekenburger M, Zloh M, Golais F, Diederich M, Tasdemir D (2012) Natural chalcones as dual inhibitors of HDACs and NF-kappaB. Oncol Rep 28(3):797–805
55. Pandey MK, Sandur SK, Sung B, Sethi G, Kunnumakkara AB, Aggarwal BB (2007) Butein, a tetrahydroxychalcone, inhibits nuclear factor (NF)-kappaB and NF-kappaB-regulated gene expression through direct inhibition of IkappaBalpha kinase beta on cysteine 179 residue. J Biol Chem 282(24):17340–17350
56. Paterson I, Anderson E (2005) The renaissance of natural products as drug candidates. Science 310:451–453
57. Rajendran P, Ong TH, Chen L, Li F, Shanmugam MK, Vali S, Abbasi T, Kapoor S, Sharma A, Kumar AP, Hui KM, Sethi G (2011) Suppression of signal transducer and activator of transcription 3 activation by butein inhibits growth of human hepatocellular carcinoma in vivo. Clin Cancer Res 17(6):1425–1439
58. Rasheed Z, Akhtar N, Khan A, Khan KA, Haqqi TM (2010) Butrin, isobutrin, and butein from medicinal plant *Butea monosperma* selectively inhibit nuclear factor-kappaB in activated human mast cells: suppression of tumor necrosis factor-alpha, interleukin (IL)-6, and IL-8. J Pharmacol Exp Ther 333(2):354–363
59. Selvam C, Jachak SM, Bhutani KK (2004) Cyclooxygenase inhibitory flavonoids from the stem bark of *Semecarpus anacardium* Linn. Phytother Res 18:582–584
60. Semwal RB, Semwal DK, Combrinck S, Viljoen A (2015) Butein: from ancient traditional remedy to modern nutraceutical. Phytochem Lett 11:188–201
61. Song DG, Lee JY, Lee EH, Jung SH, Nho CW, Cha KH, Koo SY, Pan CH (2010) Inhibitory effects of polyphenols isolated from *Rhus verniciflua* on Aldo-keto reductase family 1 B10. BMB Rep 43:268–272
62. Song NJ, Yoon HJ, Kim KH, Jung SR, Jang WS, Seo CR, Lee YM, Kweon DH, Hong JW, Lee JS, Park KM, Lee KR, Park KW (2013) Butein is a novel anti-adipogenic compound. J Lipid Res 54(5):1385–1396
63. Sung J, Lee J (2015) Anti-inflammatory activity of butein and luteolin through suppression of NFkappaB activation and induction of heme oxygenase-1. J Med Food 18(5):557–564
64. Szuster-Ciesielska A, Mizerska-Dudka M, Daniluk J, Kandefer-Szerszen M (2013) Butein inhibits ethanol-induced activation of liver stellate cells through TGF-beta, NFkappaB, p38, and JNK signaling pathways and inhibition of oxidative stress. J Gastroenterol 48(2):222–237
65. Valko M, Leibfritz D, Moncol J, Cronin MT, Mazur M, Telser J (2007) Free radicals and antioxidants in normal physiological functions and human disease. Int J Biochem Cell Biol 39 (1):44–84
66. Vitaglione P, Morisco F, Caporaso N, Fogliano V (2005) Dietary antioxidant compounds and liver health. Crit Rev Food Sci Nutr 44(7–8):575–586
67. Wang Y, Chan FL, Chen S, Leung LK (2005) The plant polyphenol butein inhibits testosterone-induced proliferation in breast cancer cells expressing aromatase. Life Sci 77 (1):39–51
68. Wang Z, Lee Y, Eun JS, Bae EJ (2014) Inhibition of adipocyte inflammation and macrophage chemotaxis by butein. Eur J Pharmacol 738:40–48
69. Woo SW, Lee SH, Kang HC, Park EJ, Zhao YZ, Kim YC, Sohn DH (2003) Butein suppresses myofibroblastic differentiation of rat hepatic stellate cells in primary culture. J Pharm Pharmacol 55(3):347–352

70. Xu HX, Wan M, Dong H, But PP, Foo LY (2000) Inhibitory activity of flavonoids and tannins against HIV-1 protease I. Biol Pharm Bull 23(9):1072–1076
71. Yadav VR, Prasad S, Sung B, Aggarwal BB (2011) The role of chalcones in suppression of NF-kappaB-mediated inflammation and cancer. Int Immunopharmacol 11(3):295–309
72. Yang LH, Ho YJ, Lin JF, Yeh CW, Kao SH, Hsu LS (2012) Butein inhibits the proliferation of breast cancer cells through generation of reactive oxygen species and modulation of ERK and p38 activities. Mol Med Rep 6(5):1126–1132
73. Yang PY, Hu DN, Lin IC, Liu FS (2015) Butein shows cytotoxic effects and induces apoptosis in human ovarian cancer cells. Am J Chin Med 43(4):769–782
74. Yit CC, Das NP (1994) Cytotoxic effect of butein on human colon adenocarcinoma cell proliferation. Cancer Lett 82:65–72
75. Yu SM, Cheng ZJ, Kuo SC (1995) Endothelium-dependent relaxation of rat aorta by butein, a novel cyclic AMP-specific phosphodiesterase inhibitor. Eur J Pharmacol 280:69–77
76. Yu H, Pardoll D, Jove R (2009) STATs in cancer inflammation and immunity: a leading role for STAT3. Nat Rev Cancer 9(11):798–809
77. Zhang K, Wong KP (1997) Glutathione conjugation of chlorambucil: measurement and modulation by plant polyphenols. Biochem J 325:417–422
78. Zhang L, Chen W, Li X (2008) A novel anticancer effect of butein: inhibition of invasion through the ERK1/2 and NF-kappa B signaling pathways in bladder cancer cells. FEBS Lett 582(13):1821–1828

Chapter 18
Garcinol and Its Role in Chronic Diseases

Amit K. Behera, Mahadeva M. Swamy, Nagashayana Natesh and Tapas K. Kundu

Abstract The various bioactive compounds isolated from leaves and fruits of Garcinia sps plants, have beencharacterized and experimentally demonstrated to be anti-oxidant, anti-inflammatory and anti-cancer in nature.Garcinol, a polyisoprenylated benzophenone, obtained from plant Garcinia indica has been found to be aneffective inhibitor of several key regulatory pathways (e.g., NF-kB, STAT3 etc.) in cancer cells, thereby being ableto control malignant growth of solid tumours in vivo. Despite its high potential as an anti-neoplastic modulator ofseveral cancer types such as head and neck cancer, breast cancer, hepatocellular carcinoma, prostate cancer,colon cancer etc., it is still in preclinical stage due to lack of systematic and conclusive evaluation ofpharmacological parameters. While it is promising anti-cancer effects are being positively ascertained fortherapeutic development, studies on its effectiveness in ameliorating other chronic diseases such ascardiovascular diseases, diabetes, allergy, neurodegenerative diseases etc., though seem favourable, are veryrecent and require in depth scientific investigation.

Keywords STAT3 · Epigenetic enzymes · Inflammation · Tumorigenesis

18.1 Introduction

Garcinol (camboginol) is a natural compound originally extracted from dried fruit rind of *Garcinia indica* (Clusiaceae) (Fig. 18.1). The plant *Garcinia indica* (also known as kokum) has been utilized in culinary field, cosmetics, and confectionary industries and most importantly in Ayurvedic medicine. The plant has been immensely valued for its medicinal utility. In traditional Indian Ayurvedic

A.K. Behera · M.M. Swamy · T.K. Kundu (✉)
Transcription and Disease Laboratory, Molecular Biology and Genetics Unit,
Jawaharlal Nehru Centre for Advanced Scientific Research, Jakkur P.O.,
Bangalore 560064, India
e-mail: tapas@jncasr.ac.in

N. Natesh
Central Government Health Scheme Dispensary, No. 3, Basavanagudi, Bangalore, India

S.C. Gupta et al. (eds.), *Anti-inflammatory Nutraceuticals and Chronic Diseases*,
Advances in Experimental Medicine and Biology 928,
DOI 10.1007/978-3-319-41334-1_18

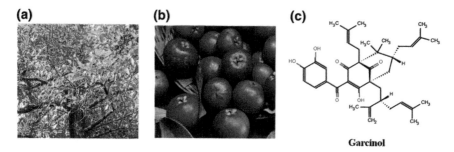

Garcinol

Fig. 18.1 **a** Image of *Garcinia indica* tree. **b** Ripe fruits of *Garcinia indica*. **c** Chemical structure of garcinol

practices, leaves and fruits of this plant have been used for treatment of inflammatory ailments and digestive disorders [1]. As per Ayurvedic classical texts, it has been mentioned as cardiac tonic, anti-helminthic and used in intestinal disorders, hemorrhoids, tumors, etc. [2]. Many groups have put efforts to identify and characterize the biological function and medicinal value of different phytochemicals obtained from this plant. Different studies have independently demonstrated that garcinol possesses antibacterial, antioxidant, gastroprotective, and most importantly, antineoplastic properties. Recent investigations have revealed that garcinol treatment significantly affects multiple biological pathways, suggesting its potent therapeutic role in multitude of human disorders.

The diseases which are persistent and long lasting, such as cancer, cardiovascular diseases, diabetes, arthritis, neurodegenerative diseases, allergies, etc., are included in the group of chronic diseases. With current advancement in medical science, complete cure is not possible for the pathological conditions seen in chronic diseases. However, with medical intervention controlling measures could be taken so as to alleviate the pathological severity or retard the progression of the disease. As a result the inevitable outcome of mortality in case of such diseases could be delayed. Several of the chronic diseases could be prevented on the grounds of healthy lifestyle. Thus, self-awareness and personal management of illness also could help to avoid complications and increase survival. Nevertheless, researchers have been putting constant efforts to find cures for such diseases. In the field of drug development for human diseases, naturally available compounds and small molecules derived from medicinal plant sources have been under investigation in last few decades. On a similar basis, there have been several preclinical studies carried out with garcinol testifying and underscoring its value with therapeutic promises in manifold human disorders including chronic diseases, which will be discussed in subsequent sections.

18.2 Physicochemical Properties of Garcinol

Biochemical Properties: According to one investigation, the role of functional groups namely 13,14-dihydroxy, present on garcinol, seems to be important in regulating its anticancer activity in context of oral cancer. In this study it has been revealed that 13,14-dimethoxy derivative of garcinol has very little effect in regulating cell cycle and apoptosis of SCC15 cell line compared to unmethylated garcinol. The mechanism behind this difference has been attributed to the ability of garcinol to bind and inhibit 5-lipoxygenase (5-Lox), where hydroxyl groups at C13 and C14 seem to be critical in interaction with the catalytic domain of 5-Lox [3]. Importance of C-13 and C-14 has been further shown by another study, where substitution of C-13 and C-14 of isogarcinol (an intramolecular cyclization product of garcinol) could enhance the specificity of the molecule in context of inhibition of histone acetyltransferase (HAT) activity [4]. It has been further discussed in Sect. 18.7.

Pharmacokinetic Properties: According to the calculation by Guide to Pharmacology (IUPHAR/BPS) online tool, Garcinol has four hydrogen bond acceptors and three hydrogen bond donors. It has 10 rotatable bonds. Its 2-D structure would have topological polar surface area of 111.9 $Å^2$. It displays an octanol–water partition coefficient: log P of 10.07. The number of Lipinski's rules broken is 2, making it pharmacologically less amenable to be an orally active drug, which is a theoretical prediction.

There have been very few studies toward understanding of bioavailability of garcinol. According to one investigation, effect of garcinol seems to be more effective in the absence of serum in in vitro cell culture system. The addition of 10 % FBS (fetal bovine serum) to medium leads to approximately 10-fold decrease in IC_{50} value of garcinol for HCT116 cell growth. Addition of BSA (bovine serum albumin) protein to media showed similar effect, indicating interaction of garcinol with serum proteins. However, no such effect was observed with cambogin (found in *Garcinia cambogia,* having similar but not identical structure with that of garcinol). Cellular uptake assessment studies showed that intracellular garcinol level in HT-29 and HCT116 cells was 2–5-fold more than that of cambogin after incubation in serum-free Hank's balanced salt solution for 1 h. However, in the presence of FBS the intracellular level of garcinol was dramatically reduced under similar experimental conditions [5].

Pharmacokinetic properties of garcinol with respect to its absorption, metabolism, tissue distribution, excretion and physiological toxicity, etc. are needed to be investigated in animal model before considering for clinical trial toward therapeutic advancement, despite its promising anticancer properties.

18.3 Modulation of Cell Signaling Pathways by Garcinol

Garcinol has been demonstrated to inhibit HATs such as p300 and PCAF both in vitro and in vivo; as a result it could suppress HAT-dependent transcription from chromatin. It was further shown by microarray analysis that inhibition of HAT with treatment of garcinol could suppress expression of majority of genes tested at global level in HeLa cells. Several of downregulated genes were revealed to be proto-oncogenes, justifying anticancer property of garcinol [6]. Garcinol treatment has been shown to cause upregulation of several tumor suppressor miRNAs, of which miR-200c was found to target and downregulate Notch1 in pancreatic CSCs [7]. The administration of garcinol has been shown to cause significant reduction in expression level of cyclooxygenase-2 (COX-2), cyclin D1, and vascular endothelial growth factor, which is proposed to occur via inhibition of the extracellular signal-regulated protein kinase 1/2, PI3K/Akt and Wnt/β-catenin signaling pathways [8, 9] (Fig. 18.2).

Garcinol has been shown by several groups to target and inhibit STAT3 signaling pathway. The first report on this aspect has shown that garcinol treatment could reduce STAT3 expression as well as the levels of phosphorylated STAT3 in breast, prostate, and pancreatic cancer cell lines [10]. This finding has been confirmed by other groups and it has been further demonstrated that garcinol could inhibit acetylation and dimerization of STAT3, thereby negatively affecting its nuclear localization and DNA-binding ability thus transcriptional property of STAT3 in cell [11] (Fig. 18.3). In breast cancer, it inhibited Wnt-beta-catenin pathway which acts as a pro-survival signaling pathway in aggressive cancers. Beta-catenin level was

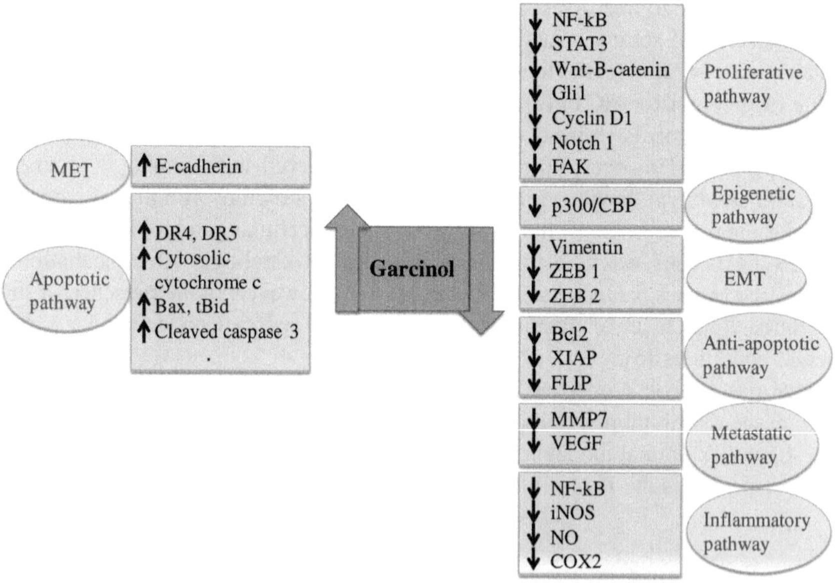

Fig. 18.2 Different cellular pathways positively and negatively regulated by garcinol in cell. *DR4* death receptor 4, *Bax* Bcl2-associated X Protein, *tBid* truncated BH3 interacting-domain death agonist, *NF-kB* nuclear factor kappa light chain enhancer of activated B cells, *STAT3* signal transducer and activator of transcription 3, *FAK* focal adhesion kinase, *CBP* CREB-binding protein, *ZEB1* zinc finger E-box-binding homeobox 1, *Bcl2* B-cell lymphoma 2, *XIAP* X-linked inhibitor of apoptosis protein, *FLIP* FLICE-like inhibitory protein, *MMP7* matrix metalloproteinase-7, *VEGF* vascular endothelial growth factor, *iNOS* inducible nitric oxide synthase, *NO* nitric oxide, *COX-2* cyclooxygenase-2

decreased at both cytoplasmic and nuclear level with increase in phosphorylated form of beta-catenin (which is targeted for degradation) upon treatment with garcinol in MDA-MB-231 and BT-549 cells. There was concomitant reduction in expression of cyclin D1 which is a downstream target of beta-catenin [12].

Pro-apoptotic role of garcinol has been demonstrated by several groups in various cancer cell lines. Multiple reports demonstrate that garcinol treatment could lead to downregulation of NF-kB pathway, which appears to be the underlying mechanism in the induction of apoptosis [13, 14]. However, there are other reports which show modulation of a different pathway to activate apoptosis. According to one such study, it can lead to loss of membrane potential of mitochondria and release of cytochrome c to cytoplasm, which in turn triggers intrinsic apoptotic pathway with activation of caspase 9 and 3 in human leukemia HL60 cells [15]. Yet another study finds that it could upregulate the expression of death receptors: DR4 and DR5 could sensitize the colon cancer cells, e.g., HCT116 and HT29 cells toward TNF-related apoptosis-inducing ligand (TRAIL)-induced apoptosis. According to this report, garcinol could induce activation of caspase 8, which

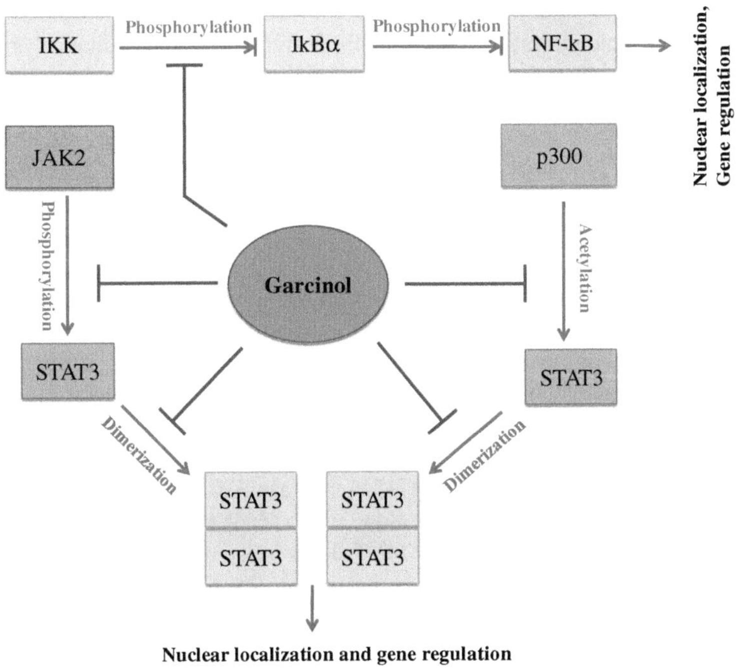

Fig. 18.3 Scheme to show the mechanism through which garcinol suppresses NF-kB and STAT3 pathways. Garcinol inhibits IKK activity, resulting in reduced degradation and increased accumulation of IkBα, which in turn phosphorylates NF-kB and leads to degradation of NF-kB. Garcinol inhibits both phosphorylation and acetylation of STAT3 by JAK2 and p300, respectively, which reduces the nuclear localization of STAT3. Garcinol also directly binds to STAT3 and impairs the dimerization and thus DNA-binding and transcriptional regulation ability of STAT3

subsequently helps in activation of intrinsic apoptotic pathway [16]. This study highlights significance of combinatorial therapy where garcinol could play an important role to potentiate TRAIL-induced apoptosis in TRAIL-resistant cancer cells. Garcinol has been found to inhibit double-strand break (DSB) repair including nonhomologous end joining (NHEJ) in HeLa cervical cancer cells as well as A549 lung cancer cells and enhance the incidence of senescence induced by ionizing radiation (IR), exhibiting radiosensitization properties [17].

18.4 Role of Garcinol in Chronic Diseases

Cancer: Garcinol has been revealed by many groups to be anticarcinogenic and pro-apoptotic in several cancers, such as prostate cancer, colorectal cancer, breast cancer, pancreatic cancer, head and neck cancer, liver cancer, etc. In a hamster chick pouch model of oral cancer induced by 7,12-dimethylbenz[a]anthracene (DMBA), treatment with garcinol suppressed 5-Lox pathway, thereby leukotriene B4 (LTB4) biosynthesis led to reduction in cell proliferation, cancer lesions, and the growth of visible tumor [18]. Parallel studies in head and neck cancer have led to the understanding that it could inhibit STAT3 and NF-kB signaling pathway in head and neck cancer [19]. Researchers have been able to demonstrate that it could also suppress activation of the kinases involved in subsequent activation of STAT3, e.g., c-Src, JAK1, and JAK2. Moreover, it could inhibit activation of positive regulators of NF-kB such as transforming growth factor-β-activated kinase 1 (TAK1) and IKK (IkB kinase) and prevent phosphorylation and degradation of negative regulator of NF-kB such as IkBα (nuclear factor of kappa light polypeptide gene enhancer in B-cell inhibitor, alpha). By blocking activation of pro-survival and anti-apoptotic pathways (such as STAT3 and NF-kB pathways), garcinol was demonstrated to be able to inhibit growth of HNSCC in nude mice. Apart from inhibiting growth of tumor cells in xenograft of MDA-MB-231 cells in SCID mice, it also inhibits epithelial to mesenchymal transition (EMT) process which is necessary for metastasis of cancer cells. Garcinol treatment has been found to decrease the expression of the mesenchymal markers such as vimentin, ZEB1, and ZEB2 in aggressive breast cancer cell lines MDA-MB-231 and BT-549, and can lead to increased expression of miR-200 and let-7 family of miRNAs along with E-cadherin favoring the process of mesenchymal to epithelial transition (MET) [12].

A study involving pancreatic cancer stem-like cells shows that garcinol could significantly suppress stem-like properties of PANC-1 side population (exhibiting cancer stem-like cell properties) as well as metastatic potential by downregulating the expressions of Notch1, ABCG2, Mcl-1, Gli-1, and EZH2. Moreover, it could upregulate tumor suppressor miR-200c which was revealed to target and downregulate Notch 1 [7]. It exhibited enhanced bioactivity with high level of synergism with curcumin in reducing proliferation and inducing apoptosis in pancreatic cancer (PaCa) cells in vitro [20]. Garcinol induces apoptosis in hepatocellular carcinoma

Hep3B cells (deficient for p53), where it has been demonstrated to activate death receptor and mitochondrial apoptotic pathway with significant activation of caspase 9 and 3. It could lead to accumulation of reactive oxygen species (ROS), endoplasmic reticulum (ER) stress modulator GADD153 (growth arrest and DNA damage inducible gene 153), increased Bax2/Bcl-2 ratio, elevated tBid (truncated Bid), and caspase 8 in cancer cell. This study highlights the therapeutic application of garcinol in the context of p53-independent apoptosis [21]. Garcinol also suppressed the growth of prostate cancer cell lines such as LNCaP, C4-2B, and PC3 in vitro and could induce apoptotic cell death. This chemopreventive nature of garcinol was demonstrated to occur via inhibition of NF-kB pathway [13]. Study with colorectal cancer cell line HT-29 shows that garcinol can lead to inhibition of tyrosine phosphorylation of focal adhesion kinase (FAK), which is a mediator of integrin-regulated intracellular signaling in adherent cells, thus impairing cellular proliferation and migration. It also inhibited expression of MMP7 (matrix metalloproteinase 7) in HT-29 cells, thereby leading to inhibition of invasiveness of the cancerous cells. Researchers were also able to demonstrate that it could lead to inhibition of growth promoting c-Src, MAPK/ERK, and PI3K/Akt signaling pathways and can cause release of cytochrome c from mitochondria to cytosol and induction of apoptosis in HT-29 colorectal cells [22].

Diabetes: Diabetes is a pathological condition characterized by prolonged and high levels of sugar in blood of the patient. Either inadequate production of insulin or inability of cells of body to respond to insulin for proper metabolism of sugar or both could lead to diabetes. Diabetic condition is known to cause damage in small blood vessels to the eye, kidney, and nerves causing diabetic retinopathy, diabetic nephropathy, and diabetic neuropathy, respectively, with damage to respective organs. Investigations have revealed marked hyperacetylation of histones in several organs of diabetic rats such as retina. One study has successfully targeted histone acetylation in retinal Müller glia cells grown in a diabetes-like concentration of glucose, which would mimic pathogenesis of diabetic retinopathy. In this report the researchers show that garcinol treatment could lead to reduction in histone acetylation, consequently suppressing expression of the pro-inflammatory factors implicated in diabetic retinopathy [23]. With a similar perspective, curcumin analog C66 has been found to prevent diabetic nephropathy in mice via inhibition of HAT activity of p300/CBP, which seems to be one of important mechanisms modulated by curcumin and its analogs to exert antidiabetic effects [24–26], further emphasizing the significance of garcinol in the prospects of treatment of diabetic complications as a modulator of HATs. Another line of research indicates that garcinol could also target the process of adipogenesis and reduce accumulation of lipids in 3T3-L1 cells [27]. With further research anti-adipogenic effect of garcinol could be exploited to manage obesity, which is known to increase the risk of type 2 diabetes.

Cardiovascular Diseases: Many cardiovascular diseases result in cardiac fibrosis which in turn leads to thickening and stiffening of cardiac muscle in the progression to heart failure. It has been found that excessive expression of collagen-1 (which normally provides structural support to heart) in cardiac fibroblasts in fibrotic condition could be inhibited by treatment with garcinol which would target acetyltransferase p300/CBP, required for basal expression of Collagen1 [28]. Thus garcinol might be useful as a part of chemoprevention therapy in retarding cardiac fibrosis in cardiovascular diseases. Similar line of research with other HAT inhibitors further corroborates and favors the idea of suppression of HAT in the context of cardiovascular diseases. For instance, anacardic acid, a reported inhibitor of p300/PCAF [29], was found to reverse cardiac hypertrophy induced by ethanol in fetal mice [30]. Investigation on the mechanism revealed that anacardic acid could suppress the over-expression of NKX2.5, Cx43, and β-MHC genes (involved in fetal heart development) induced by alcohol via inhibition of HATs. Yet another study demonstrates that phenylephrine (PE)-induced cardiac hypertrophy is mediated by HAT activity of p300/CBP, inhibition of which by anacardic acid could prevent hypertrophic stimulation in primary neonatal cardiomyocytes [31]. Thus utilization of HAT inhibitors such as garcinol with proper and validated combination with other chemical modulators such as anacardic acid could be considered for further research to develop therapeutics to ameliorate cardiovascular diseases.

Neurodegenerative Diseases: Garcinol could enhance neuronal survival by modulating ERK pathway and promote neurite growth in epidermal growth factor (EGF)-responsive neural precursor cell [32]. Antioxidant nature of garcinol has been experimentally demonstrated by many groups. Garcinol can scavenge hydroxyl-free radicals and can relieve oxidative stress in the cell; a concept which has been tested to verify whether it can confer neuroprotection against damaging effects of free radicals. Indeed garcinol was found to reduce inducible nitric oxide synthase (iNOS) level (induced by lipopolysaccharide) in primary astrocytes and could enhance survival of neurons in neuron–astrocyte co-culture system [33]. This finding raises the possibility of garcinol being considered in development of therapeutics for neurodegenerative diseases such as Alzheimers's, Parkinson's to attenuate oxidative stress-induced neurotoxicity.

Allergy: Beneficiary role of garcinol has been investigated in certain allergic conditions such as asthma. Asthma is a chronic inflammatory disease of respiratory tract which can be induced by alcohol, aspirin, and exercise or triggered by the presence of allergens in workplace such as wood dust, spray paint, latex, isocyanates, smoke, and air pollutants. Symptoms of asthma include shortness of breath, coughing, wheezing associated with reversible airflow obstruction, and bronchospasm. Environmental factors play a very important role in determining nature of allergy. Thus, alteration in epigenetic mechanisms from genetic interaction with environment could determine severity of pathophysiological outcome. It has been observed that acetylation marks on H3 and H4, site specifically H3K9, H3K14, H3K27, H3K18, and H4K16, were significantly increased on Notch1 promoter in case of asthmatic lung $CD4^+$ T cells compared to control group, concomitant to increased activity of p300 and PCAF and decreased activity of HDAC1 and HDAC2. In an attempt to reverse this condition researchers have used garcinol as an inhibitor of HAT and successfully reduced the acetylation marks on Notch1 promoter, thereby achieving reduction in expression level of Notch1 in asthmatic T cells. Further investigation on asthmatic parameters with garcinol intervention showed that it could significantly suppress the levels of inflammatory cytokines such as IL4, IL5, and IL13 in asthmatic lung T cells [34]. This study indicates that with further investigation garcinol might prove to have applications in treatment of asthma.

18.5 Biological Activities of Garcinol in Animal Models

In situ studies of colon carcinogenesis induced by azoxymethane (AOM) in male F344 rats showed that dietary garcinol administration at doses of 0.01 and 0.05 % could suppress expression of iNOS and COX-2 as well as reduce O(2)(-) and NO generation and ultimately could achieve 26 and 40 % reduction in frequency of aberrant crypt foci (ACF) development, respectively. Significant reduction in proliferating cell nuclear antigen (PCNA) index in ACF was also observed with garcinol treatment. Garcinol administration in such cases was also seen to enhance activities of liver glutathione *S*-transferase (GST) and quinone reductase (QR), which play an important role in detoxification process of body [35]. In a similar vein, another study demonstrates chemopreventive properties of garcinol in colitis-associated colon cancer, where garcinol treatment could successfully reverse dextran sulfate sodium (DSS)-induced colitis/inflammation-related colon tumorigenesis in male ICR mice [8]. In context of hepatocellular carcinoma (HCC), researchers have shown that treatment with garcinol could successfully inhibit growth of HCC in athymic nude mice through suppression of STAT3 signaling [11]. Garcinol was found to inhibit autophagy (0–6 h duration of treatment) via activation of PI3K/Akt and mTOR pathway and induce apoptosis in PC-3 human prostate cancer cells. Additionally, garcinol exhibited antitumor activity in xenograft mouse model of prostate cancer, where it could achieve 80 % tumor reduction [36]. Studies performed with animal models of cancer with garcinol have been summarized in Table 18.1.

18.6 Biological Activities of Garcinol in Humans

Garcinol is still in preclinical stage. There have been numerous in vitro studies with cell lines of human origin as well as in animal models for different human diseases, to assess efficacy of garcinol toward development of chemoprevention modalities. However, there has not been any systematic study on human as a whole organism. A commercially available medicinal product called GarCitrin® (an extract obtained from *Garcinia cambogia*) contains 5 % of garcinol as constituent along with minimum of 50 % of hydroxycitric acid (HCA). The major purpose of using GarCitrin® relies on activity of HCA to block biosynthesis of fatty acids and lipogenesis thus aiding in weight management in an individual [37]. Although it is

Table 18.1 Physico-chemical properties of garcinol

Molecular weight: 602.36
Chemical formula: $C_{38}H_{50}O_6$
Composition: C (75.71 %), H (8.36 %), and O (15.93 %)
IUPAC name: (1S,5R,7R)-3-[(3,4-dihydroxyphenyl)(hydroxy)methylidene]-6,6-dimethyl-1-[(2S)-5-methyl-2-(prop-1-en-2-yl)hex-4-en-1-yl]-5,7-bis(3-methylbut-2-en-1-l)bicycle [3.3.1] nonane-2,4,9-trione
Structure: isoprenylated benzophenone
Density: 1.1 ± 0.1 g/cm^3
Melting point: 122 °C
Optical rotation: [α] 22 D—143°
Solubility: Up to 100 mM in DMSO and up to 100 mM in ethanol
ACD/Labs Percepta platform based predication
Boiling point: 710.8 ± 60.0 °C at 760 mmHg
Vapor pressure: 0.0 ± 2.4 mmHg at 25 °C
Enthalpy of vaporization: 109.1 ± 3.0 kJ/mol
Molar refractivity: 175.6 ± 0.3 cm^3
Polarizability: 69.6 ± 0.5 10–24 cm^3
Surface tension: 43.8 ± 3.0 dyne/cm
Molar volume: 541.1 ± 3.0 cm^3

hypothesized that combination of garcinol with HCA would enhance bioavailability of HCA, however, there have not been any scientific investigation to determine exact effect of garcinol in this context.

18.7 Derivatives and Analogs of Garcinol

High cytotoxicity of garcinol has prompted several groups to explore the availability of bioactive compounds with analogous chemical structures as well as synthesizing derivatives on garcinol scaffold with better biological utility. According to one such study, mono-substituted isogarcinol (IG: an intramolecular cyclization product of garcinol) derivatives, LTK-13 (14-isopropoxy IG), LTK-14 (14-methoxy IG), and LTK-19 (13,14 disulfoxy IG) were specific inhibitors of p300-HAT compared to parental compound, which inhibits both p300 and PCAF HAT activity. Further investigation with the derivative LTK14, which is specific inhibitor of p300 and non-toxic to cells, showed that it could suppress HIV multiplication in T lymphocytes via HAT inhibition [4]. Another study, in context of cancer, showed that two oxidative derivatives of garcinol namely, garcim-1 and garcim-2, possessed greater inhibitory potential on growth of colon cancer cells [5].

Compounds from different species of *Garcinia* genus having similar structures also have been isolated and found to be exhibiting similar biological activities,

Table 18.2 Summary of *in vivo* cancer chemopreventive studies with garcinol

Types of cancer	Cell considered for xenograft	Animal	Pathway/genes targeted by garcinol	References
HNSCC	CAL27	Mouse	Inhibition of NF-kB pathway	Li et al. [39]
Prostate	PC-3	Mouse	Activation of Apoptosis, inhibition of autophagy, Activation of p-mTOR and p-PI3 Kinase/Akt pathway	Wang et al. [36]
Hepato-cellular	PLC/PRF5	Mouse	Inhibition of STAT3 signaling	Sethi et al. [11]
Colon	In situ (induction by DSS)	Mouse	Inhibition of PI3K/Akt and Wnt/beta-catenin pathway, inhibition of inflammation	Tsai et al. [8]
HNSCC	CAL27	Mouse	Inhibition of NF-kB and STAT3 signaling pathway	Li et al. [19]
Oral	In situ (induced by DMBA)	Hamster	Inhibition of 5-lipoxygenase pathway	Chen et al. [18]
Breast	MDA-MB-231	Mouse	Suppression of NF-kB and Wnt-beta-catenin pathway	Ahmad et al. [12]
Breast	MDA-MB-231	Mouse	Inhibition of STAT3 signaling	Ahmad et al. [10]
Tongue	In situ (induced by 4-NQO)	Rat	Suppression of cyclooxygenase (COX) expression	Yoshida et al. [9]
Colon	In situ (induced by azoxymethane)	Rat	Inhibition of iNOS and COX expression and suppression of free radical [O(2)(-) and NO] generation.	Tanaka et al. [35]

In situ: chemicals used to induce carcinogenesis at the relevant sites or organs in the animal
4NQO 4-nitroquinoline 1-oxide, *DMBA* 7,12-dimethylbenz[a]anthracene, *DSS* dextran sulfate sodium

underscoring the pharmaceutical importance of the molecular scaffold of garcinol (Fig. 18.1) . Few of such compounds showing therapeutic values have been listed in Table 18.2. Among polyphenol analogs of garcinol, chalcones have been emphasized for their structural similarity and biological activity. Structurally, chalcones possess aromatic rings and α,β-unsaturated ketone system, but not isoprenyl group present in garcinol. Biologically, similar to garcinol, chalcones are potent antioxidants, and anti-inflammatory in nature. Chalcones have been shown to target NF-kB and Akt pathway in cells and exhibit antitumor activity in several human cancer cell lines [38].

Table 18.3 Structural bioactive analogs and polyphenol precursors of garcinol isolated from *Garcinia* sps

Name of Garcinia sp.	Name of the compound isolated	Chemical structure	Biological activity	References
Garcinia indica, *Garcinia ovalifolia*, *Garcinia mangostana*	Isogarcinol	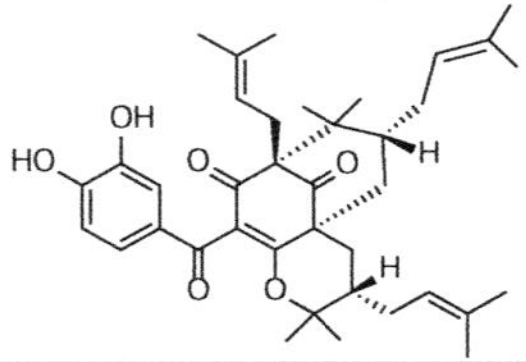	(a) Anticancer, pro-apoptotic (b) Immuno-suppressant	(a) Pieme et al. [40] (b) Fu et al. [41]
Garcinia assigu	Gracinol 13-*O*-methyl ether	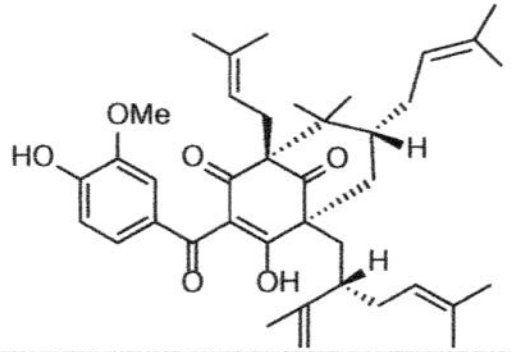	Cancer chemopreventive	Ito et al. [42]
Garcinia achachairu Rusby	Guttiferone A	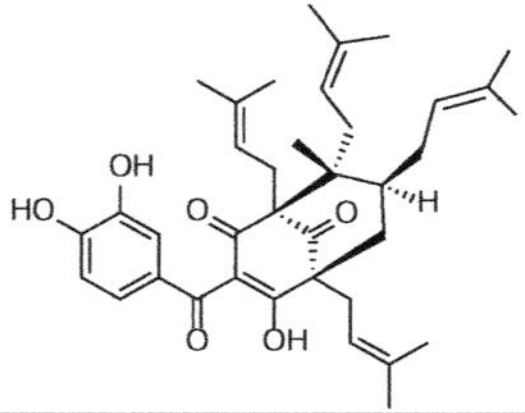	(a) Neuroprotective (b) Anticancer (c) Gastroprotective	(a) Nuñez-Figueredo et al. [43] (b) Pardo-Andreu et al. [44] (c) Niero et al. [45]
Garcinia yunnanensis	Oblongifolin	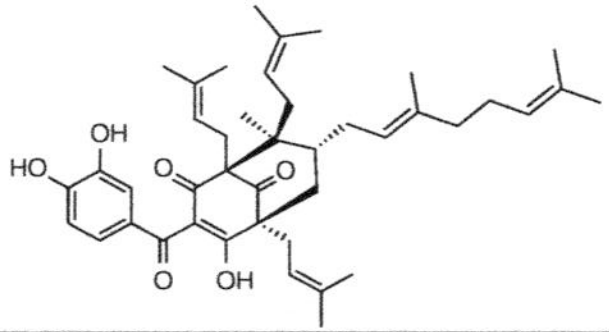	(a) Anticancer, pro-apoptotic (b) Anti-metastatic (c) Antiallergic	(a) Feng et al. [46] (b) Wang et al. [47] (c) Lu et al. [48]

(continued)

Table 18.3 (continued)

Name of Garcinia sp.	Name of the compound isolated	Chemical structure	Biological activity	References
Garcinia xanthochymus	Xanthochymol	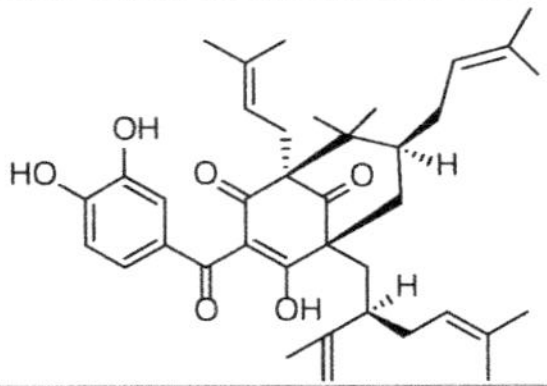	Anticancer Pro-apoptotic	Matsumoto et al. [49], Einbond et al. [50]
Garcinia brasiliensis	7-Epiclusianone	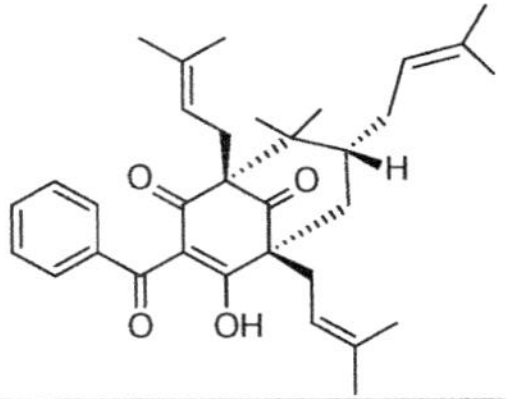	Anticancer effect on glioblastoma	Sales et al. [51]
Garcinia multiflora	Garcimultiflorone D	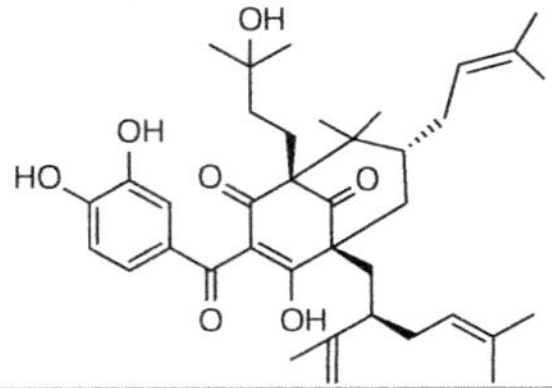	Pro-apoptotic	Liu et al. [52]
Garcinia hanburyi	Gambogic acid[a]	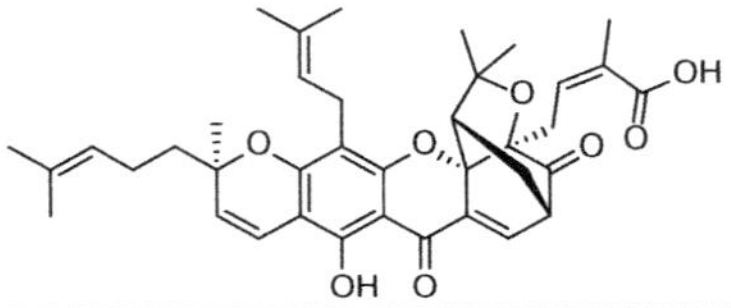	Anticancer and pro-apoptotic effect on (a) Lung cancer (b) Chronic myelogenous leukemia (c) Colorectal cancer	(a) Wang et al. [53] (b) Shi et al. [54] (c) Wen et al. [55]

(continued)

Table 18.3 (continued)

Name of Garcinia sp.	Name of the compound isolated	Chemical structure	Biological activity	References
Garcinia kola	Kolaviron	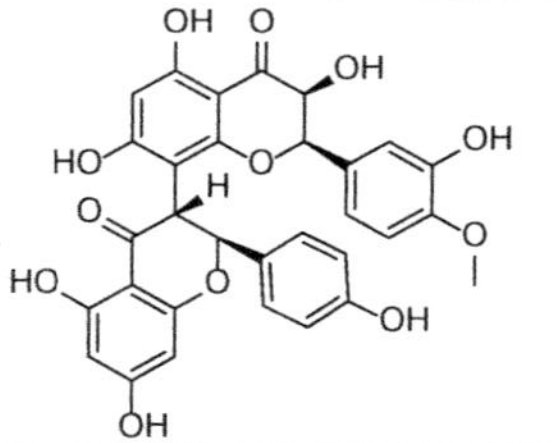	Antidiabetic and hypoglycemic	Iwu et al. [56], Oyenihi et al. [57]
Garcinia mangostana	Alpha-Mangostin	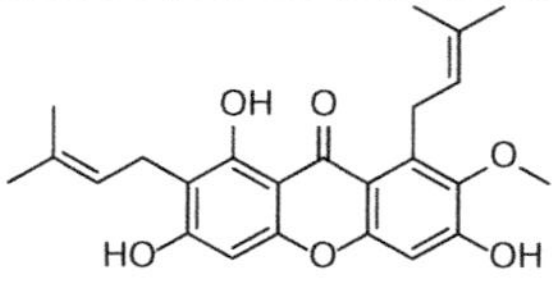	(a) Anti-inflammatory, cytoprotective and anti-apoptotic in SH-SY5Y cells (b) Anticancer (c) Anti-invasive	(a) Janhom and Dharmasaroja [58] (b) Hafeez et al. [59] (c) Wang et al. [60]
Garcinia nujiangensis	Nujiangexanthone A	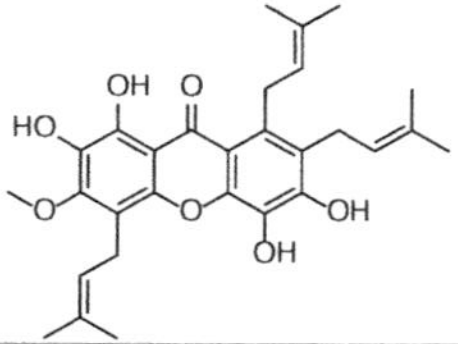	Antiasthmatic effect	Lu et al. [61]

[a]Approved by the Chinese Food and Drug Administration for the treatment of lung cancer and is in Phase II clinical trials [62]

18.8 Conclusions

Among several natural compounds isolated from fruit rind of *Garcinia indica*, garcinol has been found to be the major component responsible for medicinal utility of the plant. Initial studies showed potent antioxidant and anti-inflammatory properties of garcinol. Further, in vitro and in vivo studies in animal models have demonstrated its role as an effective anticancer agent in multitude of cancers, such as prostate, colon, head and neck, pancreatic, and breast cancers. Therapeutic potential of garcinol has been found not to be limited to cancers alone. Several scientific researches indicate that it could exhibit benefits in many other chronic diseases such as cardiovascular disorders, diabetes, neurodegenerative diseases, and certain allergies such as asthma. However, majority of investigations carried out with garcinol have explored and emphasized on its promising antineoplastic properties. Researchers have identified and elucidated the molecular targets of garcinol in different cancer cells and explained the basis of antitumor activity of garcinol. It could suppress the growth in cancer cells via inhibition of several of pro-survival pathways such as NF-kB, STAT3, and Akt/PI3K pathways and simultaneously can induce apoptotic cell death. Additionally, it inhibits epithelial to mesenchymal transition and metastasis of cancer cells and favors mesenchymal to epithelial transition. Despite several animal studies justifying therapeutic role of garcinol in last decade, it is still in preclinical stage of drug development due to lack of proper pharmacokinetic studies. Further investigations are required to determine toxicological aspects of garcinol and assess the parameters encompassing its bio-metabolism such as absorption, systemic and/or localized distribution, and excretion at the level of whole organism. It is important to understand the biologically effective dosage or concentrations of garcinol for a specific disease, route of administration, and temporal scheme of administration for better bioavailability in whole organism, for ultimate development toward clinical applications. Proper pharmacological assessment of garcinol could shed light into its relative propensity of being effective as a future drug and encourage researchers to look for structural analogs and synthesize derivatives of garcinol to improve on the limitations and make it more effective and amenable for clinical therapy.

Acknowledgments TKK was supported by grants from Department of Biotechnology, Govt. of India (Chromatin and Disease: Programme support (grant number: Grant BT/01/CEIB/10/III/01). TKK is a recipient of the Sir J.C. Bose National Fellowship, Department of Science and Technology, Government of India. AKB is a Senior Research Fellow of the Council of Scientific and Industrial Research, Government of India. We acknowledge contribution of Prof. Gautam Sethi, from NUS, Singapore for in vivo experiments on hepatocellular carcinoma with garcinol as part of collaborative research with us. GS was supported by grants from National Medical Research Council of Singapore [Grant R-184-000-211-213].

References

1. Baliga MS, Bhat HP, Pai RJ et al (2011) The chemistry and medicinal uses of the underutilized Indian fruit tree *Garcinia indica* Choisy (kokum): a review. Food Res Intern 44(7):1790–1799
2. Charaka samhita text, suthrasthaana, chapter 4th and 27th, Bhava prakasha text
3. Han CM, Zhou XY, Cao J et al (2015) 13,14-Dihydroxy groups are critical for the anti-cancer effects of garcinol. Bioorg Chem 60:123–129
4. Mantelingu K, Reddy BA, Swaminathan V et al Specific inhibition of p300-HAT alters global gene expression and represses HIV replication. Chem Biol 14(6):645–57
5. Hong J, Kwon SJ, Sang S et al (2007) Effects of garcinol and its derivatives on intestinal cell growth: inhibitory effects and autoxidation-dependent growth-stimulatory effects. Free Radic Biol Med 42(8):1211–1221
6. Balasubramanyam K, Altaf M, Varier RA et al (2004) Polyisoprenylated benzophenone, garcinol, a natural histone acetyltransferase inhibitor, represses chromatin transcription and alters global gene expression. J Biol Chem 279(32):33716–33726
7. Huang CC, Lin CM, Huang YJ et al (2015) Garcinol downregulates Notch1 signaling via modulating miR-200c and suppresses oncogenic properties of PANC-1 cancer stem-like cells. Biotechnol Appl Biochem. doi:10.1002/bab.1446
8. Tsai ML, Chiou YS, Chiou LY et al (2014) Garcinol suppresses inflammation-associated colon carcinogenesis in mice. Mol Nutr Food Res 58(9):1820–1829
9. Yoshida K, Tanaka T, Hirose Y et al (2005) Dietary garcinol inhibits 4-nitroquinoline 1-oxide-induced tonguecarcinogenesis in rats. Cancer Lett 221(1):29–39
10. Ahmad A, Sarkar SH, Aboukameel A et al (2012) Anti-cancer action of garcinol in vitro and in vivo is in part mediated through inhibition of STAT-3 signaling. Carcinogenesis 33 (12):2450–2456
11. Sethi G, Chatterjee S, Rajendran P et al (2014) Inhibition of STAT3 dimerization and acetylation by garcinol suppresses the growth of human hepatocellular carcinoma in vitro and in vivo. Mol Cancer 13:66
12. Ahmad A, Sarkar SH, Bitar B et al (2012) Garcinol regulates EMT and Wnt signaling pathways in vitro and in vivo, leading to anticancer activity against breast cancer cells. Mol Cancer Ther 11(10):2193–2201
13. Ahmad A, Wang Z, Wojewoda C et al (2011) Garcinol-induced apoptosis in prostate and pancreatic cancer cells is mediated by NF- kappaB signaling. Front Biosci (Elite Ed) 3:1483–1492
14. Ahmad A, Wang Z, Ali R et al (2010) Apoptosis-inducing effect of garcinol is mediated by NF-kappaB signaling in breast cancer cells. J Cell Biochem 109(6):1134–1141
15. Pan MH, Chang WL, Lin-Shiau SY et al (2001) Induction of apoptosis by garcinol and curcumin through cytochrome c release and activation of caspases in human leukemia HL-60 cells. J Agric Food Chem 49(3):1464–1474
16. Prasad S, Ravindran J, Sung B et al (2010) Garcinol potentiates TRAIL-induced apoptosis through modulation of death receptors and antiapoptotic proteins. Mol Cancer Ther 9(4):856–868
17. Oike T, Ogiwara H, Torikai K et al (2012) Garcinol, a histone acetyltransferase inhibitor, radiosensitizes cancer cells by inhibiting non-homologous end joining. Int J Radiat Oncol Biol Phys 84(3):815–821
18. Chen X, Zhang X, Lu Y et al (2012) Chemoprevention of 7,12-dimethylbenz[a]anthracene (DMBA)-induced hamster cheek pouch carcinogenesis by a 5-lipoxygenase inhibitor, garcinol. Nutr Cancer 64(8):1211–1218
19. Li F, Shanmugam MK, Chen L (2013) Garcinol, a polyisoprenylated benzophenone modulates multiple proinflammatory signaling cascades leading to the suppression of growth and survival of head and neck carcinoma. Cancer Prev Res (Phila) 6(8):843–54
20. Parasramka MA, Gupta SV (2012) Synergistic effect of garcinol and curcumin on antiproliferative and apoptotic activity in pancreatic cancer cells. J Oncol 2012:709739

21. Cheng AC, Tsai ML, Liu CM et al (2010) Garcinol inhibits cell growth in hepatocellular carcinoma Hep3B cells through induction of ROS-dependent apoptosis. Food Funct 1(3):301–307
22. Liao CH, Sang S, Ho CT et al (2005) Garcinol modulates tyrosine phosphorylation of FAK and subsequently induces apoptosis through down-regulation of Src, ERK, and Akt survival signaling in human colon cancer cells. Cell Biochem 96(1):155–169
23. Kadiyala CS, Zheng L, Du Y et al (2012) Acetylation of retinal histones in diabetes increases inflammatory proteins: effects of minocycline and manipulation of histone acetyltransferase (HAT) and histone deacetylase (HDAC). J Biol Chem 287(31):25869–25880
24. Wang Y, Wang Y, Luo M et al (2015) Novel curcumin analog C66 prevents diabetic nephropathy via JNK pathway with the involvement of p300/CBP-mediated histone acetylation. Biochim Biophys Acta 1852(1):34–46
25. Yun JM, Jialal I, Devaraj S (2011) Epigenetic regulation of high glucose-induced proinflammatory cytokine production in monocytes by curcumin. J Nutr Biochem 22(5):450–458
26. Pham TX, Lee J (2012) Dietary regulation of histone acetylases and deacetylases for the prevention of metabolic diseases. Nutrients 4(12):1868–1886
27. Hsu CL, Lin YJ, Ho CT et al (2012) Inhibitory effects of garcinol and pterostilbene on cell proliferation and adipogenesis in 3T3-L1 cells. Food Funct 3(1):49–57
28. Chan EC, Dusting GJ, Guo N et al (2010) Prostacyclin receptor suppresses cardiac fibrosis: role of CREB phosphorylation. J Mol Cell Cardiol 49(2):176–185
29. Balasubramanyam K, Swaminathan V, Ranganathan A et al (2003) Small molecule modulators of histone acetyltransferase p300. J Biol Chem 278(21):19134–19140
30. Peng C, Zhang W, Zhao W, Zhu J, Huang X, Tian J (2015) Alcohol-induced histone H3K9 hyperacetylation and cardiac hypertrophy are reversed by a histone acetylases inhibitor anacardic acid in developing murine hearts. Biochimie 113:1–9
31. Davidson SM, Townsend PA, Carroll C et al (2005) The transcriptional coactivator p300 plays a critical role in the hypertrophic and protective pathways induced by phenylephrine in cardiac cells but is specific to the hypertrophic effect of urocortin. ChemBioChem 6(1):162–170
32. Weng MS, Liao CH, Yu SY et al (2011) Garcinol promotes neurogenesis in rat cortical progenitor cells through the duration of extracellular signal-regulated kinase signaling. J Agric Food Chem 59(3):1031–1040
33. Liao CH, Ho CT, Lin JK (2005) Effects of garcinol on free radical generation and NO production in embryonic rat cortical neurons and astrocytes. Biochem Biophys Res Commun 329(4):1306–1314
34. Cui ZL, Gu W, Ding T et al (2013) Histone modifications of Notch1 promoter affect lung $CD4^+$ T cell differentiation in asthmatic rats. Int J Immunopathol Pharmacol 26(2):371–381
35. Tanaka T, Kohno H, Shimada R et al (2000) Prevention of colonic aberrant crypt foci by dietary feeding of garcinol in male F344 rats. Carcinogenesis 21(6):1183–1189
36. Wang Y, Tsai ML, Chiou LY et al (2015) Antitumor activity of garcinol in human prostate cancer cells and xenograft mice. J Agric Food Chem 63(41):9047–9052
37. Heymsfield SB, Allison DB, Vasselli JR et al (1998) Garcinia cambogia (hydroxycitric acid) as a potential antiobesity agent: a randomized controlled trial. JAMA 280(18):1596–1600
38. Padhye S, Ahmad A, Oswal N et al (2009) Emerging role of Garcinol, the antioxidant chalcone from *Garcinia indica* Choisy and its synthetic analogs. J Hematol Oncol 2:38
39. Li F, Shanmugam MK, Siveen KS et al (2015) Garcinol sensitizes human head and neck carcinoma to cisplatin in a xenograft mouse model despite downregulation of proliferative biomarkers. Oncotarget 6(7):5147–5163
40. Pieme CA, Ambassa P, Yankep E et al (2015) Epigarcinol and isogarcinol isolated from the root of *Garcinia ovalifolia* induce apoptosis of human promyelocytic leukemia (HL-60 cells). BMC Res Notes 8(1):700
41. Fu Y, Zhou H, Wang M et al (2014) Immune regulation and anti-inflammatory effects of isogarcinol extracted from *Garcinia mangostana* L. against collagen-induced arthritis. J Agric Food Chem 62(18):4127–4134

42. Ito C, Itoigawa M, Miyamoto Y et al (2003) Polyprenylated benzophenones from *Garcinia assigu* and their potential cancer chemopreventive activities. J Nat Prod 66(2):206–209
43. Nuñez-Figueredo Y, García-Pupo L, Ramírez-Sánchez J et al (2012) Neuroprotective action and free radical scavenging activity of guttiferone-A, a naturally occurring prenylatedbenzophenone. Arzneimittelforschung 62(12):583–589
44. Pardo-Andreu GL, Nuñez-Figueredo Y, Tudella VG et al (2011) The anti-cancer agent guttiferone-A permeabilizes mitochondrial membrane: ensuing energetic and oxidative stress implications. Toxicol Appl Pharmacol 253(3):282–289
45. Niero R, Dal Molin MM, Silva S et al (2012) Gastroprotective effects of extracts and guttiferone A isolated from *Garcinia achachairu* Rusby (Clusiaceae) against experimentally induced gastric lesions in mice. Naunyn Schmiedebergs Arch Pharmacol 385(11):1103–1109
46. Feng C, Zhou LY, Yu T et al (2012) A new anticancer compound, oblongifolin C, inhibits tumor growth and promotes apoptosis in HeLa cells through Bax activation. Int J Cancer 131(6):1445–1454
47. Wang X, Lao Y, Xu N et al (2015) Oblongifolin C inhibits metastasis by up-regulating keratin 18 and tubulins. Sci Rep 5:10293
48. Lu Y, Cai S, Tan H et al (2015) Inhibitory effect of oblongifolin C on allergic inflammation through the suppression of mast cell activation. Mol Cell Biochem 406(1–2):263–271
49. Matsumoto K, Akao Y, Kobayashi E et al (2003) Cytotoxic benzophenone derivatives from Garcinia species display a strong apoptosis-inducing effect against human leukemia cell lines. Biol Pharm Bull 26(4):569–571
50. Einbond LS, Mighty J, Kashiwazaki R et al (2013) Garcinia benzophenones inhibit the growth of human colon cancer cells and synergize with sulindac sulfide and turmeric. Anticancer Agents Med Chem 13(10):1540–1550
51. Sales L, Pezuk JA, Borges KS et al (2015) Anticancer activity of 7-epiclusianone, a benzophenone from *Garcinia brasiliensis*, in glioblastoma. BMC Complement Altern Med 15(1):393
52. Liu X, Yu T, Gao XM et al (2010) Apoptotic effects of polyprenylated benzoylphloroglucinol derivatives from the twigs of Garcinia multiflora. J Nat Prod 73(8):1355–1359
53. Wang LH, Yang JY, Yang SN et al (2014) Suppression of NF-κB signaling and P-glycoprotein function by gambogic acid synergistically potentiates adriamycin-induced apoptosis in lung cancer. Curr Cancer Drug Targets 14(1):91–103
54. Shi X, Chen X, Li X et al (2014) Gambogic acid induces apoptosis in imatinib-resistant chronic myeloid leukemia cells via inducing proteasome inhibition and caspase-dependent Bcr-Abl downregulation. Clin Cancer Res 20(1):151–163
55. Wen C, Huang L, Chen J et al (2015) Gambogic acid inhibits growth, induces apoptosis, and overcomes drug resistance in human colorectal cancer cells. Int J Oncol 47(5):1663–1671
56. Iwu MM, Igboko OA, Okunji CO et al (1990) Antidiabetic and aldose reductase activities of biflavanones of Garcinia kola. J Pharm Pharmacol 42(4):290–292
57. Oyenihi OR, Brooks NL, Oguntibeju OO (2015) Effects of kolaviron on hepatic oxidative stress in streptozotocin induced diabetes. BMC Complement Altern Med 15:236
58. Janhom P, Dharmasaroja P (2015) Neuroprotective effects of Alpha-Mangostin on MPP(+)-induced apoptotic cell death in neuroblastoma SH-SY5Y cells. J Toxicol 2015:919058
59. Hafeez BB, Mustafa A, Fischer JW et al (2014) α-Mangostin: a dietary antioxidant derived from the pericarp of *Garcinia mangostana* L. inhibits pancreatic tumor growth in xenograft mouse model. Antioxid Redox Signal 21(5):682–699
60. Wang JJ, Sanderson BJ, Zhang W (2012) Significant anti-invasive activities of α-mangostin from the mangosteen pericarp on two human skin cancer cell lines. Anticancer Res 32(9):3805–3816
61. Lu Y, Cai S, Nie J et al (2015) The natural compound nujiangexanthone A suppresses mast cell activation and allergic asthma. Biochem Pharmacol 100:61–72
62. Chi Y, Zhan XK, Yu H et al (2013) An open-labeled, randomized, multicenter phase IIa study of gambogic acid injection for advanced malignant tumors. Chin Med J (Engl) 126(9):1642–1646

Chapter 19
Morin and Its Role in Chronic Diseases

Krishnendu Sinha, Jyotirmoy Ghosh and Parames C. Sil

Abstract Chronic diseases can be referred to the long-term medical conditions which are mostly progressive in nature, i.e., it deteriorates over time. Diabetes, arthritis, heart disease, stroke, cancer, and chronic respiratory problems (e.g., COPD) are not a few examples of chronic diseases and chronic diseases are the leading causes of death and disability all over the world. Chronic diseases and conditions are among the most common, costly, and preventable of all health problems. Affordable cost, presence mostly in the consumables, and minimal side effects make the naturally occurring compounds interesting and attractive for pharmacological study in recent years. Plants produce diverse types of low molecular weight products mainly for the defense purpose. Among them, the group of secondary metabolites related to a polyphenolic group has been named flavonoids and are of great interest due to their incredible pharmacological properties. In these regard, due to its potent anti-inflammatory, anti-apoptotic and many important pharmacological properties (relevant to chronic diseases, e.g., urate transporter inhibitor related to gout, modulator of immunosystem related to chronic hypersensitivity, etc.), morin [morin hydrate:2-(2,4-dihydroxyphenyl)-3,5,7-trihydroxy-4H-1-benzopy ran-4-one; 3,5,7, 20,40 pentahydroxyflavone], widely found among the Moraceae family, considered as one of the most important key bioflavonols. However, little is known about the molecular mechanisms of its action on such conditions. In this chapter, we have summarized most of the findings, if not all, available till date.

K. Sinha · P.C. Sil (✉)
Division of Molecular Medicine, Bose Institute, P-1/12, CIT Scheme VII M, Kolkata 700054, West Bengal, India
e-mail: parames@jcbose.ac.in; parames_95@yahoo.co.in

K. Sinha
Department of Zoology, Jhargram Raj College, Government of West Bengal, Jhargram 721507, West Bengal, India

J. Ghosh
Chemistry Department, Banwarilal Bhalotia College Asansol, Ushagram, Asansol 713303, West Bengal, India

S.C. Gupta et al. (eds.), *Anti-inflammatory Nutraceuticals and Chronic Diseases*, Advances in Experimental Medicine and Biology 928,
DOI 10.1007/978-3-319-41334-1_19

Keywords Morin · Chronic diseases · Anti-inflammatory · Antioxidant · Cellular signaling

19.1 Introduction

Affordable cost, presence mostly in the consumables, and minimal side effects make the naturally occurring compounds interesting and attractive for pharmacological study in recent years. Plants produce diverse types of low molecular weight products mainly for the defense purpose. Among them, the group of secondary metabolites related to a polyphenolic group has been named flavonoids and are of great interest due to their incredible pharmacological properties [14, 24]. These compounds are consumed regularly as a part of the diet, present in flowers, tea, red wine, fruits, nuts, herbs, vegetables, seeds, spices, stems, etc. and are known to possess a number of biological and pharmacological activities like anti-hepatotoxic, anti-inflammatory, antiulcer, antioxidant, etc., and also have the ability to inhibit various enzyme activities [12, 27]. Among these, morin [morin hydrate:2-(2,4-dihydroxyphenyl)-3,5,7-trihydroxy-4H-1-benzopy ran-4-one; 3,5,7,20,40 pentahydroxyflavone] (Fig. 19.1) is belonging to the group of flavonols (a class of flavonoids having 3-hydroxyflavon backbone) found in the branches of white mulberry (*Morus alba* L), osage orange (*Maclura pomifera*), almond (*Psidium guajava*), fig (*Chlorophora tinctoria*), mill (*Prunus dulcis*), old fustic (*Maclura tinctoria*), and other family members of Moraceae along with sweet chestnut (*Castanea sativa, family Fagaceae*) [4, 35]. This compound exhibits different types of pharmacological activities, like free radical scavenging, anti-inflammatory, xanthine oxidase inhibitor property, protective effect on DNA from damage caused by free radicals, prevention of low-density lipoprotein oxidation, anticancer activity, etc. [14, 35]. Further studies both in in vitro and in vivo indicate that it possesses numerous add on health benefits. However, no article has yet been published that comprises and explains its botanical origin and pharmacological activities in spite of the current research progress made on

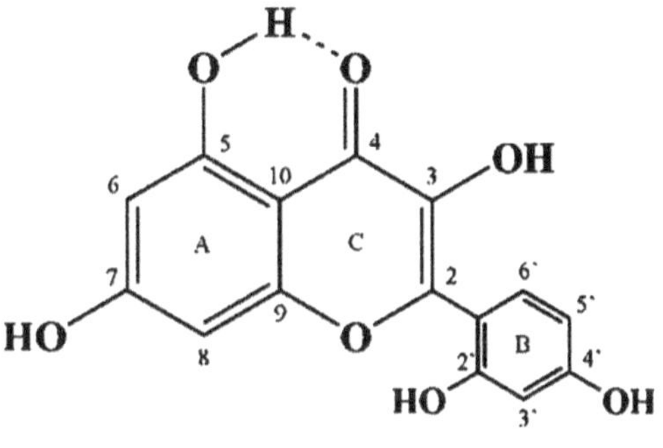

Fig. 19.1 Molecular structure of morin [Reprinted from Biochim. Biophys. Acta [General Subjects] 1850:769–783; with the permission from Elsevier; License Number: 3764180672838]

pharmacological/biological activities of morin. So, in this chapter, we would like to compile the known pharmacological activities of morin on different chronic diseases. Morin is thought to be a major bioactive molecule which could be used for the prevention of hepatotoxicity. Also, the protective effects of this molecule against oxidative stress and inflammation were investigated in some earlier studies [14]. In addition, a number of other beneficial pharmacological effects including the prevention of low-density lipoprotein oxidation, immunomodulation (the downregulation of immune responses), inhibition of xanthine oxidase, and anticancer activity were also reported [11, 14, 25, 34, 35, 46]. All these properties justify its validity as an agent in the pharmacological treatment of several chronic diseases. Chronic diseases are long-term medical conditions that are generally progressive [27]. Diseases like inflammatory bowel disease, COPD, diabetes, myocardial infraction (MI), several neurological diseases, chronic environmental pollutant-mediated toxicity, cancer, etc. can be considered as chronic diseases [27]. Reports from Centers for Disease Control and Prevention showed up to 2012, about 117 million people in US had one or more chronic health conditions and every one of four adults had two or more chronic health conditions (http://www.cdc.gov/chronicdisease/overview/). They also reported 7 of the top 10 causes of death in 2010 were chronic diseases, whereas 2 of these chronic diseases—heart disease and cancer—together accounted for nearly 48 % of all deaths. Obesity is another serious health concern. During 2009–2010, more than one-third of adults, or about 78 million people, were obese. Other very crucial chronic disease conditions are arthritis, diabetes-related kidney failure, etc. where among 53 million adults with a clinical diagnosis of arthritis, more than 22 million have trouble with their daily activities due to arthritis (http://www.cdc.gov/chronicdisease/overview/). However, the possibility of preventing or controlling cancer using flavonoids from fruits has created a considerable amount of interest as high intake of vegetables and fruits and is reported to be associated with low incidence of cancer [30, 38]. Results from a number of studies suggest that phytochemicals can safely modulate the biology of the cancer cells and induce cancer cell death. Some properties of this molecule have also been reported that may regulate the inflammatory responses and halt carcinogenesis and cancer progression [20]. However, little is known about the molecular mechanisms of the anticancer effects of this unique molecule [30].

19.2 Physciochemical Properties of Morin

Morin has a molecular weight of 302.2357 g/mol, exact mass of 302.042653 g/mol, monoisotopic mass of 302.042653 g/mol, molecular formula of $C_{15}H_{10}O_7$, XLogP3 of 1.5, hydrogen bond donor count of 5, hydrogen bond acceptor count of 7, rotatable bond count of 1, topological polar surface area of 127 A^2, heavy atom count of 22, formal charge of 0, complexity of 488, isotope atom count of 0, defined atom stereocenter count of 0, undefined atom stereocenter count of 0, defined bond stereo center count of 0, undefined bond stereo center count of 0, a covalently bonded unit count of 1, and experimental melting point 303.5 °C [5]. Morin is a naturally occurring molecule (can also be synthesized) and it inhibits or retard the oxidation of a substance to which it is added. It counteracts the harmful and damaging effects of oxidation in animal tissues. The structure [Fig. 19.1] of morin hydrate shows that it is an isomeric form of quercetin. Quercetin and morin both have OH in position 3, a carbonyl group in position 4, and a resorcinol moiety. However, there is a difference in the hydroxylation pattern on B-ring. In morin, the hydroxylation is at the meta-position (in Morin), whereas it is in the ortho position in quercetin. For all its groups and an ortho hydroxylation pattern on B-ring, quercetin is regarded to have the highest antioxidant potential of the flavonoids but morin hydrate has also been demonstrated to have higher effectiveness of certain oxidative processes. Morin is soluble in methanol (50 mg ml^{-1}) and generously soluble in alcohol whereas faintly soluble in ether and acetic acid. It is also soluble in aqueous alkaline solutions and gives intense yellow color. This color changes to brown upon water exposure. It is also soluble in water (0.25 mg/ml, 20 °C; 0.94 mg/ml, 100 °C). In respect to pharmacokinetic study, Hou et al. investigated and compared the pharmacokinetics of morin and its isomer quercetin in rats. Parent forms and their glucuronides and sulfates in serum were studied. They found that after oral dosing of both the parent forms, morin, and its glucuronides, and sulfates were present in the blood stream and a nonlinear pharmacokinetics was observed for morin. On the other hand, negligible bioavailability of quercetin is presented as its glucuronides and sulfates were only detected in the blood and the metabolites showed linear pharmacokinetics at the two doses studied. The total AUC of parent form with conjugated metabolites showed that the extent of absorption of morin was threefold compared to that of quercetin. Hou et al. [18] proved that the fates of the flavonols were markedly affected by difference in hydroxylation pattern on B-ring. Xie et al. showed how morin interacted with human serum albumin (HSA). The interaction has been investigated using fluorescence, Fourier transform, infrared spectroscopic approaches, and UV absorption [45]. Under the physiological condition, there is a specific binding site on HSA for morin, and the binding affinity was found to be $1.13 \pm 0.11 \times 10^{-5}$ L Mol^{-1}. The intrinsic fluorescence of morin was noticeably boosted in the presence of HSA due to excited-state proton transfer. The level of protonation of the hydroxyl groups played a significant role during the morin–HSA binding process and it was evident from the fact that with the increase of the buffer pH from 6.4 to 8.4, binding ability of morin to protein decreased. The interaction between morin and HSA induced an apparent decline of the protein α-helix and β-sheet structures [45].

19.3 Role of Morin in Chronic Diseases: Modulation of Cell Signaling Pathways in Animal and Human Model

Morin proves itself effective against many chronic diseases. An increasing number of studies showed that morin significantly modulate different cell signaling pathways related to chronic pathophysiological conditions, including gastrointestinal complications, diabetes, cardiovascular disease, cancer, arthritis, neurodegenerative disease, and several inflammatory diseases. As various oxidative stress-related disorders are led by inflammation, antioxidant and anti-inflammatory activities of morin play a critical role in the therapeutic process of these disorders. Different studies prove that morin is effective against several chronic diseases like chronic neurodegenerative disease, chronic cardiovascular pathophysiology, chronic gastrointestinal pathophysiology, chronic hypersensitivity and immunological disorders, cancer and several oxidative stress-related chronic pathophysiological disorders, arthritis, diabetes, and related pathophysiology. Morin alters the levels of phosphorylated Akt kinase, Erk1/2, AIF release, cytosolic Bax, and regulated the NF-κB's nuclear translocation, and acts against the imbalances in the levels/activities of different enzymes (e.g., elastase), inflammatory mediators, proinflammatory cytokines, inflammatory enzymes, glycoproteins, reactive oxygen species, lysosomal acid hydrolases, and transcription factors (e.g., NF-κB, p65, and AP1) to produce the desirable effects. Also, different others pathways are involved in morin's protective actions and these are described extensively in the following sections.

19.3.1 Morin Against Chronic Neurodegenerative Disease

Excessive glutamate receptors activation (i.e., excitotoxicity) leads to acute and chronic neurological disorders including stroke. The neuroprotective role of two natural polyphenol antioxidants, mangiferin and morin, has been previously reported in a model of ischemic brain damage using an in vitro model of excitotoxic neuronal death involving N-Methyl-D-aspartate (NMDA) receptor over activation [15]. Campos-Esperza et al. [7] showed the intricate molecular details of the neuroprotection exert by morin. They found that morin significantly reduced the reactive oxygen species formation while activate the antioxidant enzyme system, and reinstate the altered mitochondrial membrane potential to its basal state. They also observed that morin could inhibit glutamate-induced calpains activation, normalized the levels of phosphorylated Akt kinase and Erk1/2. It also inhibited AIF release from mitochondria, restored the normalized level of cytosolic Bax, and regulated the NF-κB's nuclear translocation. These changes ultimately lead to reduction of apoptotic neuronal death induced by glutamate. These results, based on excellent antioxidant and anti-apoptotic properties of morin, support the clinical application of morin as a trial neuroprotector in the pathology involving excitotoxic neuronal death [7]. Zhang et al. investigated the neuroprotective effects of morin on 1-methyl-4-phenylpyridinium ion (MPP+)-induced apoptosis in neuronal differentiated PC12 cells as well as in a 1-methyl-4-phenyl-1, 2, 3, 6-tetrahydropyridine (MPTP) mouse model of Parkinson disease (PD) where they found that MPP+, in PC12 cells, induced ROS formation and apoptosis, whereas morin significantly attenuated the MPP+-induced loss of cell viability, apoptosis, and inhibit ROS formation. In mice model, morin significantly attenuated the MPTP-induced nigrostriatal lesions, dopaminergic neuronal death, striatal dopamine depletion, and permanent behavioral deficits. The results clearly suggest the neuroprotective actions of this unique molecule both in vitro and in vivo and indicate the possibility of being a novel therapeutic agent for the treatment of PD and other neurodegenerative diseases [49].

Ammonia is considered as a potent neurotoxin. It has been intensely associated in the pathogenesis of hepatic encephalopathy. Subash and Subramaniam evaluated the chronotherapeutic effect of morin, on ammonium chloride (AC)-induced hyperammonemia in a rat model. Morin significantly ameliorate AC-induced pathophysiological changes in respect to the circulating levels of urea, ammonia, hydroperoxides (HP), thiobarbituric acid reactive substances (TBARS), liver markers [aspartate transaminase (AST), alanine transaminase (ALT), and alkalinephosphatase (ALP)], superoxide dismutase (SOD), glutathione peroxidase (GPx), catalase (CAT), reduced glutathione (GSH), and vitamins A, C, and E. The authors speculated that the chronotherapeutic effect of morin in hyperammonemic rats might be due to temporal variations of lipid peroxidation and of antioxidants, urea cycle enzymes, etc., temporal variations of metabolic enzymes involved in the degradation of morin and the temporal variation in its bioavailability [36].

19.3.2 Morin Against Arthritis

In Ghanaian traditional medicine, leaf extracts of *Ficus exasperata* P. Beauv. (Moraceae) have been and are being commonly used for the treatment of various pathological states including inflammatory disorders. The main active ingredient in all the extracts is morin. A recent study was conducted to evaluate the antiarthritic effect of an ethanolic extract of *F. exasperata* (FEE) in an arthritis model (using rats) in which the disease was induced by the Freund's adjuvant [3]. For this study, dexamethasone and methotrexate were used as positive controls. Like these positive controls, FEE also showed significant dose-dependent antiarthritic properties in adjuvant-induced arthritis. In addition, like antirheumatic drug methotrexate and the steroidal anti-inflammatory agent dexamethasone, FEE was found to significantly reduce the arthritic edema in the lateral paw of the animals and prevented the spread of the edema from the lateral to the contralateral paws, suggesting the protective role of the extract in inhibiting systemic spread. In rat brain homogenates, the extract has been reported to exhibit reducing activity, scavenge DPPH radical, and prevent lipid peroxidation. Detection of phenol in the extract suggests that the ethanolic extract of these leaves probably exerts antiarthritic activity after oral administration and it also has antioxidant properties; combination of the both may contribute to its beneficial activity [3]. Zeng et al. [48] investigated the effect of morin on type II collagen-induced arthritis (CIA) in rats and also explored the underlying molecular mechanisms of synovial angiogenesis. Morin significantly attenuated arthritic development which is specified by reduction of paw swelling and arthritis scores. Morin also noticeably reduced the serum levels of proinflammatory cytokines, e.g., interleukin (IL)-6 (IL6), tumor necrosis factor-α (TNFα), etc. Along with that, it increased the level of anti-inflammatory cytokine interleukin-10 and improved pathological changes of joints as evident from histology. Morin also distinctly inhibited expression of vascular endothelial growth factor (VEGF), basic fibroblast growth factor, and CD31 in synovial membrane tissues. It also reduced the serum levels of VEGF in CIA rats. In in vitro study, morin also significantly inhibited VEGF-induced human umbilical vein endothelial cells migration and tube formation. These results nicely showed that morin had antirheumatoid potential which it exerts probably by inhibiting synovial [48]. Sultana and Rasool proved that the combination therapy of morin along with a NSAID was very effective in suppressing the pathogenesis of rheumatoid arthritis (RA), against adjuvant-induced arthritis (an experimental model for RA) in rats. They found that imbalances in the levels/activities of elastase, inflammatory mediators (TNFα, IL1β, MCP1, VEGF, and PGE2), paw edema, glycoproteins (hexose and hexosamine), urinary constituents (hydroxyproline and glycosaminoglycans), reactive oxygen species (LPO and NO), lysosomal acid hydrolases (acid phosphatase, N-acetylglucosaminidase, β-galactosidase, and cathepsin D), proinflammatory cytokines (TNFα, IL1β, IL17, IL6, and MCP1), inflammatory enzymes (iNOS and COX2), RANKL, and transcription factors (NF-κB, p65, and AP1) were regulated back effectively to near control level by morin and indomethacin, which were elevated in case of RA. Their findings were supported by histopathological and radiological analysis, whereas body weight, bone collagen, and the antioxidant status [superoxide dismutase (SOD), catalase (CAT), glutathione peroxidase (GPx), glutathione, and ceruloplasmin)] were found to be decreased in RA and that was restored back by the combinatorial therapy [37]. Gout is a general systemic joint disorder where hyperuricemias is a hallmark of gout [3]. A serum uric acid level above 9 mg dL^{-1} is considered as gouty arthritis [6]. Pathological manifestation of gout follows over production or decreased excretion of uric acid (purine metabolic end product) [26]. Urate–anion transporter (URAT1) in the brush border membrane of the proximal tubule in kidney is the main transporter involved in the maintenance of serum uric acid level by reabsorbing the urate from the lumen to the cytosol in kidney tubules [9, 14]. Different drugs including xanthine oxidase inhibitors (e.g., allopurinol), inhibitors of urate reabsorption at proximal renal tubule-like probenecid, benzbromarone, etc. are being used in the treatment of gout. However, some undesirable side effects like hepatotoxicity are associated with the benzbromarone and other agents having hypouricemic activity [14]. Certain natural herbs were reported to have the xanthine oxidase inhibitor activity along with other types of mechanisms and those are helpful in the treatment of gouty arthritis and hyperuricemia-related disorders. Morin hydrate is one of them having the xanthine oxidase inhibitor activity and the other type of mechanism which can reduce the rheumatic disorders [14]. The urate reabsorption inhibitory effect of morin at the brush border of proximal renal tubule membrane vesicles explains the above-said action of morin on the kidney [46]. Wijeratne et al. [43] using oxonate-induced hyperuricemic rat model showed the uricosuric activity of morin hydrate. Above-mentioned information suggest that morin has been used in the treatment of rheumatic disorders.

19.3.3 Morin Against Chronic Cardiovascular Pathophysiologies

Cardiovascular diseases (CVD) are the major cause of chief mortality worldwide due to its complicated nature. Among CVD disorder, MI is a major one. If there is imbalance between the coronary supply and its myocardial demand, then myocardial infarction takes place and it causes necrosis of the myocardial tissue. Morin shows cardiovascular protection in isoproterenol (ISO)-induced myocardial infarction in rats and this protection is attributed to its free radical scavenging activity by the polyphenolic group [2]. It also shows significant beneficial effect on lipid profiles, blood pressure, and serum glucose levels from the high-fat diet-induced hypertensive rats. ISO, which is a synthetic catecholamine, has been documented to produce severe stress in the myocardium, resulting in myocardial infarction, if it is administered in supramaximal doses. Cardiac necrosis due to the administration of ISO includes increased oxygen consumption, calcium overload and accumulation, increased myocardial cAMP levels, alterations of membrane permeability, and increase in lipid peroxides level [2]. Al-Numair et al. reported that morin pretreatment (20, 40, and 80 mg/kg, respectively) daily for a period of 30 days decreases significantly the activities of cardiac marker enzymes such as lactate dehydrogenase, creatine kinase, aspartate transaminase and creatine kinase-MB, membrane bound enzymes (such as calcium-dependent adenosine triphosphatase), sodium potassium-dependent adenosine triphosphatase, and magnesium-dependent adenosine triphosphatase, in serum. Calcium-dependent adenosine triphosphatase and magnesium-dependent adenosine triphosphatase were increased, whereas the activity of sodium potassium-dependent adenosine triphosphatase was found to decrease in the heart. At the same time it also showed a significant decrease in glycoprotein (hexosamine, fucose, hexose, and sialic acid) levels in serum and heart. ISO administration disrupts the redox balance and produces myocardial infarction via free radical-mediated β-adreno-receptor mechanism. However, positive alterations of these biochemical parameters were successfully achieved with morin pretreatment daily for a period of 30 days. From their studies, the authors concluded that morin has a protective role in ISO-induced MI in rats and the observed effects might be due to the free radical scavenging, antioxidant, and membrane-stabilizing properties of morin [2]. These beneficial effects of morin are due to its multitude of biological function such as antioxidant, anti-inflammatory, and free radical scavenging activity. Another group of investigators also conducted a study to prove the cardio-protective benefits of this flavonoid in ISO-induced myocardial infarcted rats. A significant increase in the levels of cardiac markers was detected in ISO-induced myocardial infarcted rats although morin pretreated animals could regulate the abnormalities in electrocardiograph and biomarkers. Results also showed an increased lipid peroxidation product in ISO-induced myocardial infarcted rats. The animals, pretreated with morin, however, showed reduction of lipid peroxidation. Histopathological studies supported all these observations as pretreatment with morin-inhibited myocardial damage. Combining, the results of the above-mentioned studies proved that the pretreatment of morin exhibits protective effect and are rational to understand its beneficial effects on cardio-protection against myocardial injury. The results also indicate the cardio-protective ability of morin [31]. However, till now, the molecular mechanism of its protective actions is not crystal clear, and it requires more studies to prove its inherent molecular mechanisms.

The protective effect of morin against deoxycorticosterone acetate (DOCA)-induced hypertension was recently investigated in male Wistar rats. DOAC salt hypertensive rats showed considerably increased systolic and diastolic blood pressure in association with considerably increased systolic and diastolic blood, AST, ALP, ALT, GGT, urea, uric acid, and creatinine levels in the plasma. However, morin effectively lowered all the enzymes' level up to that of the control. The study indicates antihypertensive effect of morin [32]. In vitro studies have established that oxidized low-density lipoprotein (ox-LDL) has increased atherogenicity compared to native LDL. Upon oxidative modification of LDL, alteration in its structure allows LDL to be taken up by scavenger receptors on smooth muscle, macrophage, and endothelial cells. This lead to the formation of lipid-laden foam cells which is the hallmark of primary atherosclerotic lesions. Naderi et al. found that morin significantly inhibits in vitro LDL oxidation. Thus, they proved that morin would probably be helpful to prevent atherosclerosis [28]. In a study, Wu et al. demonstrated that morin hydrate significantly reduced the tissue necrosis in post-ischemic and reperfused rabbit hearts by >50 %. They showed that, besides scavenging oxyradicals, morin hydrate discreetly inhibits a free radical generating enzyme xanthine oxidase, from the ischemic endothelium. However, they also speculate that morin hydrate may chelate some metal ions which help in further oxyradical formation and thus inhibiting the process of oxidative stress generation [44].

19.3.4 Morin Against Chronic Gastrointestinal Pathophysiology

Galvez et al. reported that morin possesses intestinal anti-inflammatory activity in the chronic stages of trinitrobenzenesulphonic acid model of rat colitis. They showed that the morin administration enabled tissue recovery following a colonic insult with trinitrobenzenesulphonic acid. It also reduced myeloperoxidase activity, colonic leukotriene B4, and interleukin-1b levels, improved colonic oxidative stress, and inhibited colonic nitric oxide synthase activity [11]. In another study it has been shown that morin significantly ameliorate nonsteroidal anti-inflammatory drug (NSAID)-induced gastropathy in a rat model [35] (Fig. 19.2a, b). The gastroprotective action of morin is primarily attributed to its potent antioxidant nature. Morin also significantly inhibits indomethacin (IND)-induced inflammatory responses and gastric damage. IND induces ROS production which indirectly leads to NF-κB activation. A simultaneous proinflammatory response gets initiated leading to neutrophil infiltration. Activated NF-κB increases the redox burden by inhibiting catalase production and inducing iNOS production. On the other hand, increased TNF-α and IL-1β activate NF-κB. This produces ROS and creates a positive feedback loop. However, morin effectively inhibits ROS production, scavenges free radicals, and chelates noxious Fe^{2+}. Besides, morin pretreatment effectively inhibits IND-mediated NF-κB activation by inhibiting IKK activation. Thus, it reduces proinflammatory cytokine production, related to apoptosis and gastric damage. Morin also prevents downregulation of catalase and thus helps to restore the cellular redox homeostasis (Fig. 19.3). In conclusion, this study provides evidence that morin has significant potential as a therapeutic intervention for IND-induced gastric mucosal injury. From the study it can be said that future detailed pharmacokinetic and pharmacodynamic studies are expected to establish morin as a gastroprotective agent [35]. The main inflammatory parameters in the intestinal inflammation are free radicals, nitric oxide, leuckotrienes, etc. and are responsible for the production of inflammatory mediators in the intestinal inflammatory conditions [11]. Morin hydrate has been shown to inhibit nitric oxide synthase activity and the leukotriene-b4 synthesis [17]. Moreover, because of its inhibitory effect on the myeloperoxidase activity, the intestinal inflammation marker of neutrophil infiltration activity was evidently increased [16]. Inhibition of IL-1β, one of the proinflammatory cytokines responsible for the induction of inducible nitric oxide synthase (iNOS) activity in enterocytes, is another important anti-inflammatory activity attributed to the morin hydrate [33]. Inflammatory bowel disease (IBD) is a chronic phase of inflammatory disorder and is known to be associated with two closely related conditions (Crohn's disease and Ulcerative colitis) in the intestine. Synthesis and upregulation of proinflammatory mediators (such as reactive oxygen species, cytokines and platelet-activating factors, etc.) are the main aetiological events that occurred in the development of IBD. 5-amino salicylic acid and local or systemic gluco-corticosteroids are the drugs which are nowadays used for the management of IBD to exert their benefit through various mechanisms [40]. Experimentally, rats were imparted colitis by single injection of colonic instillation of the hapten trinitrobenzene sulphonic acid dissolved in ethanol and the colitic animals were treated with morin hydrate which showed the beneficial effect on 4th week following colitis insult [11]. Myeloperoxidase, IL-β4, interleukin-1β (IL-1β) synthesis, glutathione (GSH) and malondialdehyde (MDA) levels, and nitric oxide synthase (NOS) activity are different biochemical mediators reported to be involved in the colonic inflammation [14]. Inhibition of the

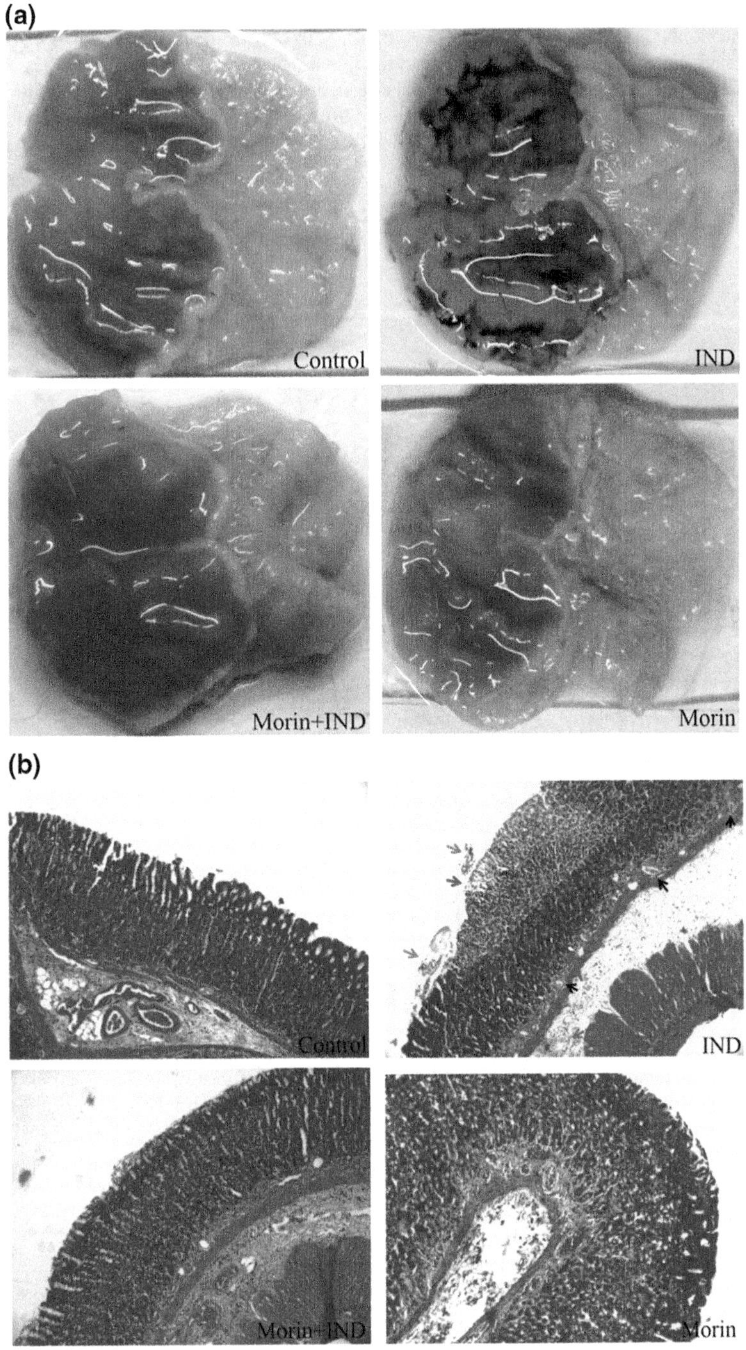
(a)
Control
IND
Morin+IND
Morin
(b)
Control
IND
Morin+IND
Morin

◀ **Fig. 19.2** Effect of morin on gastric mucosa in IND-induced gastric injury. Control: vehicle treatment alone; IND: IND treatment alone; morin + IND: treatment with morin IND; Morin: morin treatment alone. **a** Open stomach showing injured mucosa. Note that the injury (in the form of reddish black ulcers of different sizes) is highest in the IND (red arrows) and morin almost completely prevented the ulceration. **b** Sections of gastric mucosa were stained with hematoxylin–eosin. The IND group showed marked changes with outward mucosal damage (*red arrow*), presence of inflammatory exudates (*green arrows*), extensive vasocongestion (*black arrows*), and damaged submucosa (*blue arrow*) [Reprinted from Biochim. Biophys. Acta [General Subjects] 1850:769–783; with the permission from Elsevier; License Number: 3764180672838]

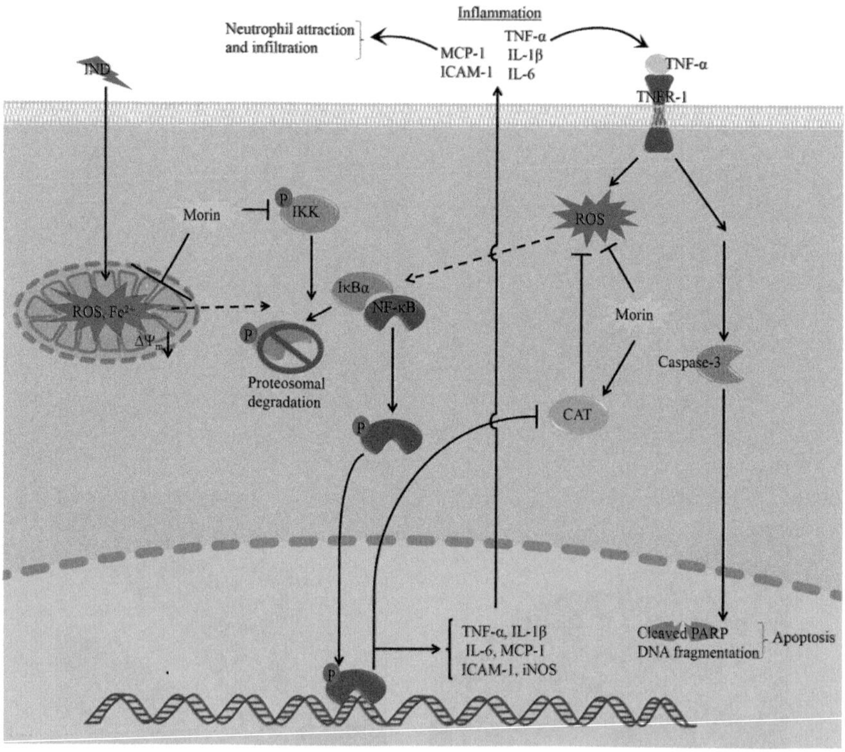

Fig. 19.3 Graphical representation of molecular mechanisms of gastroprotective action of morin against IND-induced gastropathy in rats ('Solid arrows' indicating stimulatory interaction; 'blunt arrow' indicates inhibitory interaction; 'broken arrows' indicate plausible mechanisms) [Reprinted from Biochim. Biophys. Acta [General Subjects] 1850:769–783; with the permission from Elsevier; License Number: 3764180672838]

synthesis of most important cytokine, IL-1β, decreased in the NOS and free radicals involved in the inflammatory cascade are believed to be the factors involved in the anti-inflammatory activity of morin.

19.3.5 Morin Against Diabetes and Related Pathophysiology

Noor et al. [29] showed that morin hydrate inhibits amyloid formation by human islet amyloid polypeptide (IAPP, amylin) and disaggregates preformed IAPP amyloid fibers that were evident from transmission electron microscopy (TEM) and right-angle light scattering. IAPP is responsible for type-2 diabetes-related islet amyloid formation and is also evident in islet cell transplants leading to graft failure. Human IAPP have fewer inhibitors and it is extremely amyloidogenic. However, due to the specific substitution pattern on the B-ring, morin hydrate signifies a novel type of IAPP amyloid inhibitor [29]. Vanitha et al. [41] found that morin significantly reduced the blood glucose and enhanced the serum insulin levels in experimentally induced type I diabetic rats. Morin dose dependently reduced glucose-6-phosphatase, fructose-1,6-bisphosphatase, hexokinase, and glucose-6-phosphate dehydrogenase activities in liver. It significantly protected pancreatic islets' overall morphology as well as preserve insulin-positive cells in diabetic rats. From the study it is evident that morin might be advantageous in the treatment of diabetes and regulation of carbohydrate metabolic enzyme activities. It is of prime importance in the pathophysiological conditions [41]. Abuohashish et al. [1] found the putative advantageous effect of morin on diabetic osteopenia in rats which they suggested might be due to both the anti-inflammatory and antioxidant properties. They found that morin is particularly effective in bone metabolic disorder which is a major chronic problem in age-related disease. In case of diabetic rats significant bone loss was observed at the level of bone turnover parameters including osteocalcin (OC), bone alkaline phosphatase (bALP), and collagen type 1 cross-linked C-telopeptide (CTX). However, the study showed that morin treatment obviously attenuated these elevations in those parameters [1]. A significant impairment in trabecular bone microarchitecture, density, and other morphometric parameters have been detected by performing bone micro-CT scan of diabetic rats, and those were efficiently ameliorated by morin treatment. Besides, in diabetic rats, serum levels of glucose, TBARS, IL-1β, IL-6, and TNF-α were significantly elevated, while that of insulin and GSH was decreased. These changes were bring back to normal after 5 weeks morin treatment, suggesting the protective effect of morin against diabetic-induced osteopenia [1].

19.3.6 Morin Against Chronic Hypersensitivity and Immunological Disorders

Kim et al. showed that morin suppressed IgE-mediated allergic responses in a mouse model. It inhibited production of TNF-α, IL-4, and degranulation of antigen (Ag)-stimulated mast cells. They also found that morin inhibited the phosphorylation of Syk which plays a very important role in the Syk activation. Morin also inhibits activation of linker for activation of T cells (LAT) in rat basophilic leukemia (RBL)-2H3 cells and bone marrow-derived mast cells (BMMCs) along with the inhibition of p38, Akt and the MAP kinases, ERK1/2, JNK, and Fyn kinase. With further investigations, their results suggest that the morin suppresses the IgE-mediated allergic response by principally inhibiting Fyn kinase in mast cells [23]. Findings of Fang et al. [10] indicated that morin might have the ability to regulate immune response through modulating the cytokine profiles exhibited in chronic immunotoxic pathophysiology. They have shown that morin and its derivatives (sulfates/glucuronides) were effective on LPS-activated RAW 264.7 cells (macrophages) in reducing NO, TNF-α, and IL-12 production. Moreover, phagocytic activities of the peripheral blood cells were significantly lowered in the morin-treated cells in respect to control. These lowering in the NO production and reduced macrophage phagocytic activities corresponded to LPS-resistant state is very important to treat various chronic autoimmune diseases [10].

19.3.7 Morin Against Cancer and Several Oxidative Stress-Related Chronic Pathophysiological Disorders

Recently, attention has been given on the anti-cancer activity of morin in various kinds of cancers. For example, it exerted protective effect on chemically produced rat tongue carcinogenesis [20] and inhibited phorbol ester-induced transformation of rat hepatocytes.[19]. Besides, by inhibiting the lipoxygenase pathway, this molecule could inhibit the peroxisome-proliferated activator receptor-induced keratinocyte differentiation [39]. The inhibitory activity of this molecule was reported during the release of inflammatory cytokines (such as IL-8, IL-6, and TNF) from mast cells [21]. In an in vivo study, morin hydrate showed anticancer activity in cancer models (like inhibit the growth of COLO205 cells in nude mice) [8]. The transcription factor NF-κB is known to be involved in various kinds of cell proliferation, cell survival, tumorigenesis, and inflammation. Induction of NF-κB activation pathway induced by TNF, ceramide, lipopolysaccharide, IL-1, phorbol 12-myristate 13-acetate, and H_2O_2 was reported to be suppressed by morin. The process involved the inhibition of IκB (inhibitory subunit of NF-κB) kinase that leads to suppression of phosphorylation and degradation of IκBα and consequently nuclear translocation of p65 occurs. NF-κB-dependent reporter gene expression [activated by TNF receptor (TNFR), TNF, TNFR-associated factor 2, TNFR1-associated death domain, NF-κB-inducing kinase, IκB kinase, and the p65 subunit of NF-κB] was also reported to be inhibited by morin hydrate. Besides, it could also downregulate the NF-κB-related products that are involved in the cell survival (i.e., inhibitor of apoptosis proteins 1 & 2, survivin, X-chromosome-linked IAP, and BcL-xL), invasion (matrix metalloproteinase-9), and proliferation (cyclin D1 and cyclooxygenase-2) [14].

Zeng et al. in their study demonstrated that morin hydrate acts as a broad-spectrum antioxidant as it scavenges both xanthine oxidase/hypoxanthine-generated oxyradicals and also nonenzymatic, nitrogen-derived radicals. They showed the effectiveness of morin hydrate on rabbit corneal endothelial cells against oxyradicals and nitric oxide-induced damage. This way morin hydrate might be helpful in preventing free radical-induced damage in chronic corneal problems and also in its effective preservation [47]. In a study, Hsiang et al. [19] found that morin, in a dose-dependent manner, reticent (terephthalic acid) TPA-induced cellular transformation in Chang liver cells. TPA-induced AP-1 activity, while through the inhibition of p38 kinase, morin inhibited the AP-1. Moreover, morin induced the S-phase which suggests that a cell cycle checkpoint was activated by morin to block DNA synthesis as a protective measure against TPA-induced genotoxicity. Their study established this molecule as a potent anti-hepatocellular transformation agent that inhibited cellular transformation [19]. Kim et al. proved that morin has excellent antioxidant and anti-inflammatory nature for which it can be considered as an excellent agent against the chronic diseases. They proved that morin extensively modulate reactive species (RS)-induced NF-κB activation through its RS scavenging activity. Their findings indicate that morin neutralizes RS in vitro, inhibits *t*-BHP-induced RS generation, and represses redox-sensitive transcription factor NF-κB activation through reduced DNA binding activity, nuclear translocation of p65/p50, and IκBα phosphorylation. More precisely, it can be said from their study that, in endothelial cells, suppression of the NF-κB cascade by morin was modulated through the ERK and p38 MAPKs pathways and morin's antioxidant effect, as a consequence, extended the expression level of NF-κB-dependent proinflammatory genes, thereby reducing COX-2, iNOS, and 5-LOX [22]. During the metabolic process, a limited range of various metals for the enzymatic and nonenzymatic process in organic and inorganic forms are required. However, various heavy metals, like mercury, (known as a wide-spread environmental pollutant) can cause severe alterations in humans and animals [13, 14]. Morin hydrate has been shown to protect various organs from mercuric chloride-induced toxicity. Moreover, it exerts protective effects on the alterations of serum markers like LDH, AST, and ACP levels which are increased in renal nephritis and renal infarction [42]. Kidney is a multipurpose organ in the body. It is in control for excretion of metabolic wastes from the body and for the regulation of homeostasis (e.g., acid base balance, electrolyte balance, water balance, calcium level, blood pressure) in the body. However, when the metabolites are more toxic than its precursor, they can lead to severe toxication which ultimately remains responsible for kidney damage [14]. Humans are exposed to these heavy metals in many ways in daily life. Mercury is one of them causing kidney damage. Morin, in such cases, could be used as an effective antioxidant. Morin possesses a variety of biological functions against oxidative stress-induced damage, such as cardiovascular cells, glomerular mesangial cells, hepatocytes, oligo dendrocytes, and in neurons [42, 44].

19.4 Conclusions

From the diverse studies reviewed in this article, morin emerged as a useful natural flavone in the management of different chronic pathophysiological conditions. Despite these direct pharmacological activities, morin could help to detect parameters related to severe chronic diseases. It could also be used as an excellent and novel pathological detection tool. Recently, fluorescence-based, time saving, stain with morin hydrate has been developed and it stains phospho-proteins in one-dimensional SDS-PAGE where Al^{3+} was used as a "fixed bridge.'. With the help of this novel quantification method based on kinetic measurement of the fluorescence decrease of Al^{3+}–morin complex it can be used to determine the bisphosphonate content in plasma samples. This method would upkeep research on the development of drug delivery systems for the related bisphosphonates. However, despite the in vivo and in vitro studies, trying to elucidate the mechanisms of action morin, in future, more studies are required to clearly understand the precise molecular mechanism with great depth. Detailed preclinical studies and its clinical experimentations are also extremely needed to provide a basis for potential expediency of this gift of nature, morin, in the treatment and mitigation of chronic diseases.

References

1. Abuohashish HM, Al-Rejaie SS, Al-Hosaini KA, Parmar MY, Ahmed MM (2013) Alleviating effects of morin against experimentally-induced diabetic osteopenia. Diabetol Metab Syndr 5:1
2. Al-Numair KS, Chandramohan G, Alsaif MA (2012) Pretreatment with morin, a flavonoid, ameliorates adenosine triphosphatases and glycoproteins in isoproterenol-induced myocardial infarction in rats. J Nat Med 66:95–101
3. Amo-Barimah A, Woode E, Boakye-Gyasi E, Ainooson G, Abotsi W (2010) Antiarthritic and antioxidant effects of the leaf extract of *Ficus exasperata* P. Beauv. (Moraceae). Pharmacognosy Res 2:89–97.
4. Basile A, Sorbo S, Giordano S, Ricciardi L, Ferrara S, Montesano D, Cobianchi RC, Vuotto M, Ferrara L (2000) Antibacterial and allelopathic activity of extract from Castanea sativa leaves. Fitoterapia 71:S110–S116
5. Bradley J-C, Lang AS, Williams AJ, Curtin E (2011) ONS open melting point collection. Available from Nature Precedings. http://dx.doi.org/10.1038/npre.2011.6229.1
6. Campion EW, Glynn RJ, Delabry LO (1987) Asymptomatic hyperuricemia. Risks and consequences in the Normative Aging Study. Am J Med 82:421–426
7. Campos-Esparza MR, Sanchez-Gomez MV, Matute C (2009) Molecular mechanisms of neuroprotection by two natural antioxidant polyphenols. Cell Calcium 45:358–368
8. Chen Y-C, Shen S-C, Chow J-M, Ko CH, Tseng S-W (2004) Flavone inhibition of tumor growth via apoptosis in vitro and in vivo. Int J Oncol 25:661–670
9. Enomoto A, Kimura H, Chairoungdua A, Shigeta Y, Jutabha P, Cha SH, Hosoyamada M, Takeda M, Sekine T, Igarashi T (2002) Molecular identification of a renal urate–anion exchanger that regulates blood urate levels. Nature 417:447–452

10. Fang S-H, Hou Y-C, Chang W-C, Hsiu S-L, Chao P-DL, Chiang B-L (2003) Morin sulfates/glucuronides exert anti-inflammatory activity on activated macrophages and decreased the incidence of septic shock. Life Sci 74:743–756
11. Galvez J, Coelho G, Crespo M, Cruz T, Rodríguez-Cabezas M, Concha A, Gonzalez M, Zarzuelo A (2001) Intestinal anti-inflammatory activity of morin on chronic experimental colitis in the rat. Aliment Pharmacol Ther 15:2027–2039
12. Gladding PA, Webster MW, Farrell HB, Zeng IS, Park R, Ruijne N (2008) The antiplatelet effect of six non-steroidal anti-inflammatory drugs and their pharmacodynamic interaction with aspirin in healthy volunteers. Am J Cardiol 101:1060–1063
13. Goldstein RS, Schnellmann RG (1996) Toxic responses of the kidney. In: Klaassen CD, (ed.), Casarett and Doull's toxicology: the basic science of poisons, 5th edn. Mc Graw Hill, Kansas, pp 417–442
14. Gopal JV (2013) Morin hydrate: botanical origin, pharmacological activity and its applications: a mini-review. Pharmacogn J 5:123–126
15. Gottlieb M, Leal-Campanario R, Campos-Esparza MR, Sánchez-Gómez MV, Alberdi E, Arranz A, Delgado-García JM, Gruart A, Matute C (2006) Neuroprotection by two polyphenols following excitotoxicity and experimental ischemia. Neurobiol Dis 23:374–386
16. Grisham MB (1992) A comparative analysis of two models of colitis in rats. Gastroenterology 102:1524–1534
17. Hogaboam C, Jacobson K, Collins S, Blennerhassett M (1995) The selective beneficial effects of nitric oxide inhibition in experimental colitis. Am J Physiol Gastrointest Liver Physiol 268: G673–G684
18. Hou Y, Chao P, Ho H, Wen C, Hsiu S (2003) Profound difference in pharmacokinetics between morin and its isomer quercetin in rats. J Pharm Pharmacol 55:199–203
19. Hsiang C-Y, Wu S-L, Ho T-Y (2005) Morin inhibits 12-O-tetradecanoylphorbol-13-acetate-induced hepatocellular transformation via activator protein 1 signaling pathway and cell cycle progression. Biochem Pharmacol 69:1603–1611
20. Kawabata K, Tanaka T, Honjo S, Kakumoto M, Hara A, Makita H, Tatematsu N, Ushida J, Tsuda H, Mori H (1999) Chemopreventive effect of dietary flavonoid morin on chemically induced rat tongue carcinogenesis. Int J Cancer 83:381–386
21. Kempuraj D, Madhappan B, Christodoulou S, Boucher W, Cao J, Papadopoulou N, Cetrulo CL, Theoharides TC (2005) Flavonols inhibit proinflammatory mediator release, intracellular calcium ion levels and protein kinase C theta phosphorylation in human mast cells. Br J Pharmacol 145:934–944
22. Kim JM, Lee EK, Park G, Kim MK, Yokozawa T, Yu BP, Chung HY (2010) Morin modulates the oxidative stress-induced NF-κB pathway through its anti-oxidant activity. Free Radical Res 44:454–461
23. Kim JW, Lee JH, Hwang BY, Mun SH, Ko NY, Kim DK, Kim B, Kim HS, Kim YM, Choi WS (2009) Morin inhibits Fyn kinase in mast cells and IgE-mediated type I hypersensitivity response in vivo. Biochem Pharmacol 77:1506–1512
24. Kuhnau J (1976) Flavonoids. A class of semi-essential food components: Their role in human nutrition. In: World review of nutrition and dietetics. World Rev Nutr Diet 24:117–191
25. Lian T-W, Wang L, Lo Y-H, Huang I-J, Wu M-J (2008) Fisetin, morin and myricetin attenuate CD36 expression and oxLDL uptake in U937-derived macrophages. Biochim Biophys Acta Mol Cell Biol Lipids 1781:601–609
26. Lioté F (2003) Hyperuricemia and gout. Curr Rheumatol Rep 5:227–234
27. Middleton E, Kandaswami C, Theoharides TC (2000) The effects of plant flavonoids on mammalian cells: implications for inflammation, heart disease, and cancer. Pharmacol Rev 52:673–751

28. Naderi GA, Asgary S, Sarraf-Zadegan N, Shirvany H (2003) Anti-oxidant effect of flavonoids on the susceptibility of LDL oxidation. Mol Cell Biochem 246:193–196
29. Noor H, Cao P, Raleigh DP (2012) Morin hydrate inhibits amyloid formation by islet amyloid polypeptide and disaggregates amyloid fibers. Protein Sci 21:373–382
30. Park C, Lee WS, Go S-I, Nagappan A, Han MH, Hong SH, Kim GS, Kim GY, Kwon TK, Ryu CH (2014) Morin, a flavonoid from Moraceae, induces apoptosis by induction of BAD protein in human leukemic cells. Int J Mol Sci 16:645–659
31. Pogula BK, Maharajan MK, Oddepalli DR, Boini L, Arella M, Sabarimuthu DQ (2012) Morin protects heart from beta-adrenergic-stimulated myocardial infarction: an electrocardiographic, biochemical, and histological study in rats. J Physiol Biochem 68:433–446
32. Prahalathan P, Kumar S, Raja B (2012) Effect of morin, a flavonoid against DOCA-salt hypertensive rats: a dose dependent study. Asian Pac J Trop Biomed 2:443–448
33. Salzman A, Denenberg AG, Ueta I, O'Connor M, Linn SC, Szabó C (1996) Induction and activity of nitric oxide synthase in cultured human intestinal epithelial monolayers. Am J Physiol Gastrointest Liver Physiol 270:G565–G573
34. Singh MP, Jakhar R, Kang SC (2015) Morin hydrate attenuates the acrylamide-induced imbalance in antioxidant enzymes in a murine model. Int J Mol Med 36:992–1000
35. Sinha K, Sadhukhan P, Saha S, Pal PB, Sil PC (2015) Morin protects gastric mucosa from nonsteroidal anti-inflammatory drug, indomethacin induced inflammatory damage and apoptosis by modulating NF-κB pathway. Biochim Biophys Acta Gen Subj 1850:769–783
36. Subash S, Subramanian P (2012) Chronotherapeutic effect of morin in experimental chronic hyperammonemic rats. Int J Nutr Pharmacol Neurol Dis 2:266
37. Sultana F, Rasool M (2015) A novel therapeutic approach targeting rheumatoid arthritis by combined administration of morin, a dietary flavanol and non-steroidal anti-inflammatory drug indomethacin with reference to pro-inflammatory cytokines, inflammatory enzymes, RANKL and transcription factors. Chem Biol Interact 230:58–70
38. Surh Y-J (2004) Transcription factors in the cellular signaling network as prime targets of chemopreventive phytochemicals. Cancer Res Treat 36:275
39. Thuillier P, Brash A, Kehrer J, Stimmel J, Leesnitzer L, Yang P, Newman R, Fischer S (2002) Inhibition of peroxisome proliferator-activated receptor (PPAR)-mediated keratinocyte differentiation by lipoxygenase inhibitors. Biochem J 366:901–910
40. Travis S, Jewell D (1994) Salicylates for ulcerative colitis—their mode of action. Pharmacol Ther 63:135–161
41. Vanitha P, Uma C, Suganya N, Bhakkiyalakshmi E, Suriyanarayanan S, Gunasekaran P, Sivasubramanian S, Ramkumar K (2014) Modulatory effects of morin on hyperglycemia by attenuating the hepatic key enzymes of carbohydrate metabolism and β-cell function in streptozotocin-induced diabetic rats. Environ Toxicol Pharmacol 37:326–335
42. Venkatesan R, Sadiq AM, Kumar JS, Lakshmi GR, Vidhya R (2010) Effect of Morin on mercury chloride induced nephrotoxicity. Ecoscan 4:193–196
43. Wijeratne SS, Abou-Zaid MM, Shahidi F (2006) Antioxidant polyphenols in almond and its coproducts. J Agric Food Chem 54:312–318
44. Wu T-W, Fung K-P, Zeng L-H, Wu J, Hempel A, Grey AA, Camerman N (1995) Molecular properties and myocardial salvage effects of morin hydrate. Biochem Pharmacol 49:537–543
45. Xie M-X, Long M, Liu Y, Qin C, Wang Y-D (2006) Characterization of the interaction between human serum albumin and morin. Biochim Biophys Acta Gen Subj 1760:1184–1191
46. Yu Z, Fong WP, Cheng CH (2007) Morin (3,5,7,2′,4′-pentahydroxyflavone) exhibits potent inhibitory actions on urate transport by the human urate anion transporter (hURAT1) expressed in human embryonic kidney cells. Drug Metab Dispos 35:981–986
47. Zeng L, Rootman D, Burnstein A, Wu J, Wu T (1998) Morin hydrate: a better protector than purpurogallin of corneal endothelial cell damage induced by xanthine oxidase and SIN-1. Curr Eye Res 17:149–152

48. Zeng N, Tong B, Zhang X, Dou Y, Wu X, Xia Y, Dai Y, Wei Z (2015) Antiarthritis effect of morin is associated with inhibition of synovial angiogensis. Drug Dev Res 76:463–73
49. Zhang Z-T, Cao X-B, Xiong N, Wang H-C, Huang J-S, Sun S-G, Wang T (2010) Morin exerts neuroprotective actions in Parkinson disease models in vitro and in vivo. Acta Pharmacol Sin 31:900–906

Chapter 20
Ellagic Acid and Its Role in Chronic Diseases

Giuseppe Derosa, Pamela Maffioli and Amirhossein Sahebkar

Abstract Ellagic acid is a natural anti-oxidant phenol found in numerous fruits and vegetables, in particular pomegranate, persimmon, raspberry, black raspberry, strawberry, peach, plumes, nuts (walnuts, almonds), and wine. The anti-proliferative and anti-oxidant properties of ellagic acid have prompted research into its potential health benefits. The aim of this chapter will be to summarize potential benefits of ellagic acid supplementation in chronic diseases.

Keywords Ellagic acid · Cancer · Chronic inflammation · Diabetes

G. Derosa (✉) · P. Maffioli
Department of Internal Medicine and Therapeutics, University of Pavia,
Fondazione IRCCS Policlinico S. Matteo, P.Le C. Golgi, 2, 27100 Pavia, Italy
e-mail: giuseppe.derosa@unipv.it

G. Derosa
Center for Prevention, Surveillance, Diagnosis and Treatment of Rare Diseases,
Fondazione IRCCS Policlinico San Matteo, Pavia, Italy

G. Derosa
Center for the Study of Endocrine-Metabolic Pathophysiology and Clinical Research,
University of Pavia, Pavia, Italy

G. Derosa
Laboratory of Molecular Medicine, University of Pavia, Pavia, Italy

P. Maffioli
PhD School in Experimental Medicine, University of Pavia, Pavia, Italy

A. Sahebkar
Biotechnology Research Center, Mashhad University of Medical Sciences,
Mashhad, Iran

A. Sahebkar (✉)
Department of Medical Biotechnology, School of Medicine,
Mashhad University of Medical Sciences, P.O. Box: 91779-48564, Mashhad, Iran
e-mail: sahebkara@mums.ac.ir; amir_saheb2000@yahoo.com

S.C. Gupta et al. (eds.), *Anti-inflammatory Nutraceuticals and Chronic Diseases*,
Advances in Experimental Medicine and Biology 928,
DOI 10.1007/978-3-319-41334-1_20

20.1 Introduction

A diet rich in polyphenols, which are found in fruits and vegetables, is strongly associated with a reduced risk for developing chronic diseases such as cancer and cardiovascular disease [1]. Ellagic acid is a natural phenol anti-oxidant found in numerous fruits and vegetables. Ellagic acid is a dimeric derivative of gallic acid and rarely occurs free in diet crops, but usually occurs in food products conjugated with glycoside moiety (glucose, xylose) or forms part of ellagitannins (polymeric molecules) [2, 3]. These compounds usually occur in fruits (pomegranates, persimmon, raspberries, black raspberries, strawberries, peach, plumes), nuts (walnuts, almonds), vegetables, and wine. Ellagitannins are the bioactive polyphenols present in pomegranate; however, they are not absorbed intact by the human gut, but they can be hydrolyzed to ellagic acid by colonic gastrointestinal flora [3, 4]. The anti-proliferative and anti-oxidant properties of ellagic acid have prompted research into its potential health benefits. The aim of this chapter will be to summarize potential benefits of ellagic acid supplementation.

20.2 Physiochemical Properties of Ellagic Acid

Ellagic acid (2,3,7,8-tetrahydroxy-chromeno[5,4,3-cde]chromene-5,10-dione, $C_{14}H_6O_8$) (Fig. 20.1) was first discovered in 1831. It is a highly thermostable molecule, with a melting point of 350 °C, with a molecular weight of 302.197 g/mol, slightly soluble in water, alcohol, and ether, but soluble in caustic potash [5]. Ellagic acid is a weak acid, which is ionized at physiological pH [5]. It structurally presents four rings representing the lipophilic domain, four phenolic groups, and two lactones, which form hydrogen-bond sides and act as electron acceptors, respectively, and that represent the hydrophilic domain.

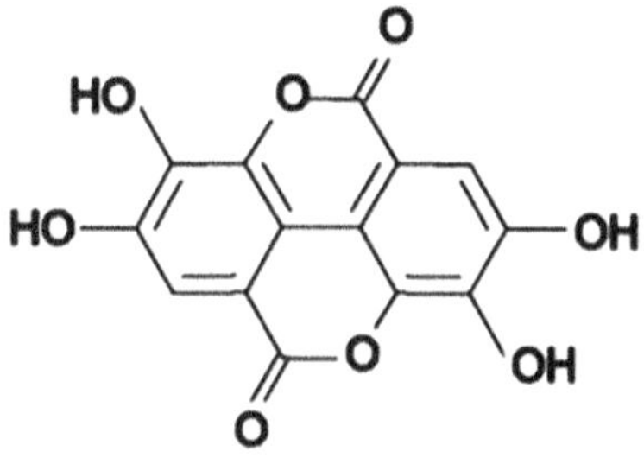

Fig. 20.1 Ellagic acid structure

20.3 Role of Ellagic Acid in Chronic Diseases

20.3.1 Ellagic Acid and Inflammation

Ellagic acid proved to have anti-inflammatory effects in acute or chronic model of ulcerative colitis [6]. In the study by Marin et al., the acute model of ulcerative colitis was represented by female Balb/C mice treated with dextran sulfate sodium (DSS) (5 %) for 7 days, while concomitantly receiving a dietary supplement of ellagic acid (2 %). In the chronic ulcerative colitis model, instead, female C57BL/6 mice received 4-week-long cycles of DSS (1 and 2 %) interspersed with week-long recovery periods along with a diet supplemented with ellagic acid (0.5 %). In acute model, ellagic acid slightly ameliorated disease severity as observed both macroscopically and through the reduction of inflammatory mediators including interleukin-6, tumor necrosis factor-α (TNF-α), and interferon-γ. In the chronic model, ellagic acid significantly inhibited the progression of the disease, reducing intestinal inflammation and decreasing histological scores. Daily treatment with dietary ellagic acid significantly reduced cyclooxygenase-2 (COX-2) and inducible nitric oxide synthase (iNOS) expression in colon tissue in a chronic model of DSS-induced colitis. This action of ellagic acid is noteworthy, because COX-2 and iNOS activation produce excessive inflammatory mediators which may be detrimental to the integrity of the colon and contribute to the development of intestinal damage. These data are consistent with those of other studies conducted by Rosillo et al. [7]. Similarly, these authors showed that ellagic acid administration reduced the expression of both COX-2 and iNOS in a model of Cronh's disease induced by administration of trinitrobenzenesulfonic acid (TNBS) in rats. Myeloperoxidase activity and pro-inflammatory cytokines, such as TNF-α production, were correlated with the development of colonic inflammation and dietary ellagic acid, as well as pomegranate enriched with or without ellagic acid, was able to diminish both parameters. Ellagic acid probably acts on NF-κB family. NF-κB activation actively contributes to the development and maintenance of intestinal inflammation, promoting the expression of various pro-inflammatory cytokines including interleukins-1, -2, -6, -8, -12, and TNF-α. NF-κB activation also mediates the transcription of pro-inflammatory genes such as COX-2 and iNOS. In the study by Rosillo et al. [7], the nuclear protein expression of NF-κB p65, involved in ulcerative colitis and Crohn's disease, was drastically decreased upon dietary treatment with ellagic acid and ellagic acid-enriched pomegranate extract.

20.3.2 Role of Ellagic Acid in Cancer

The anti-cancer effect of ellagic acid has been studied in many human cancer cell lines including those of skin, esophageal, and colon cancer where it exhibited anti-proliferative activity, with the ability to cause cell cycle arrest and induce apoptosis [8]. Ellagic acid takes part in various DNA maintenance reactions preventing genomic instability which otherwise leads to cancer [9]. Ellagic acid has an anti-proliferative effect and induces apoptosis via a mitochondrial pathway in Caco-2 cells, an in vitro model for colon cancer, without interfering with the normal colon cells [3]. In particular, a study exploring the activity of ellagic acid demonstrated that it could induce apoptosis in 1,2-dimethyl hydrazine (DMH)-induced colon carcinoma and participate in a wide range of DNA maintenance reactions that prevent genomic instability [8]. Ellagic acid prevents PI3K/Akt activation that, in turn, results in the modulation of its downstream Bcl-2 family proteins [8] involved in the activation of the intrinsic apoptotic pathway [3]. Bax expression and caspase-3 activation were noted after ellagic acid supplementation leading to elevation of cytochrome c levels and finally cell death [3].

20.3.3 Ellagic Acid and Liver Protection

Ellagic acid possesses anti-oxidant, anti-hepatotoxic, anti-steatosic, anti-cholestatic, anti-fibrogenic, anti-hepatocarcinogenic, and anti-viral properties that improve the hepatic architectural and functions against toxic and pathological conditions. Hepatotoxicity refers to liver dysfunction or liver damage associated with exposure to drugs or xenobiotics. Ellagic acid increases anti-oxidant response through the transcriptional activation of nuclear erythroid 2-related factor 2 (Nrf2), and indirectly having a scavenging activity against a variety of reactive oxygen species. Moreover, ellagic acid inhibits alcohol-induced liver cell damage increasing the anti-oxidant levels, scavenging free radicals, and stabilizing cell membranes as reported by Devipriya et al. [10]. They showed that in female albino Wistar rats, weighing treated with ellagic acid against alcohol-induced damage, there was an inhibition of alcohol-induced toxicity by improving body weight, restoring anti-oxidant status, modulating micronutrients, and attenuating the lipid levels in the circulation. Administration of ellagic acid effectively reduced the level of lipids in the circulation, preventing lipid peroxidation [11]. This was confirmed by Yu et al. [12] which reported that ellagic acid supplementation reduced the elevations of plasma cholesterol in hyperlipidemic rabbits. It can be speculated that ellagic acid might have decreased the activity of 3-hydroxy-3-methylglutaryl coenzyme A (HMG CoA) reductase, or enhanced the rate of lipid degradative process and increased the hepatic bile acids and fecal neutral sterol and thus decreased the level of other lipids.

Ellagic acid has revealed potential activities against HBV infection as reported by Pathak et al. [13] which identified that ellagic acid inhibits the HBx-induced transcriptional activation for replication of the virus. Recently, the anti-viral activity of ellagic acid against HCV was described by Reddy et al. [14], and Ajala et al. [15]; these authors demonstrated that ellagic acid inhibits NS3/4A protease activity in vitro, suggesting an interaction between ellagic acid with the unconventional Zn-binding site present in the core region of the enzyme, blocking its activity.

20.3.4 Ellagic Acid and Advanced Glycation End Products

It has been reported that the gradual build-up of advanced glycation end products (AGEs) in body tissues is a major contributor to many progressive diseases including diabetic complications [16] and Alzheimer's disease [17, 18]. AGE-modified plasma proteins could bind to AGE receptors (RAGE) on the surface of the cell, activate cell signaling, and lead to the production of reactive oxygen species and inflammatory factors. Moreover, proteins on the extracellular matrix crosslink with other matrix components, leading to a loss in their function.

As mentioned above, pomegranate fruit, which is a rich source of phenolics, in particular ellagitannins, showed anti-oxidant and anti-inflammatory effects. Taking into account the effects on AGE, pomegranate fruit juice and extracts have been shown to exert neuro-protective effects by ameliorating symptoms of Alzheimer's disease potentially caused by the abnormal accumulation of AGEs in the brain [19]. This finding was further supported by Rojanathammanee et al. [20], who determined whether a dietary intervention with ellagic acid could attenuate microgliosis in a rat model of Alzheimer's disease. Three months of pomegranate feeding lowered TNF-α concentrations in brain, and lowered nuclear factor of activated T-cell (NFAT) transcriptional activity compared with controls. Immunocytochemistry showed that pomegranate, but not control-fed mice, had attenuated microgliosis and amyloid β plaque deposition, involved in Alzheimer's disease.

20.3.5 Ellagic Acid and Diabetes

Ellagic acid seems to play an anti-diabetic activity through the action on β-cells of pancreas, stimulating insulin secretion and decreasing glucose intolerance. This effect of ellagic acid was reported by Fatima et al. [21]. Treatment with *Emblica officinalis* extract, rich in ellagic acid, has been reported to result in a significant decrease in the fasting blood glucose in a dose- and time-dependent manner in diabetic rats. Ellagic acid significantly increased serum insulin in diabetic rats in a dose-dependent manner. Insulin-to-glucose ratio was also increased by *Emblica officinalis* treatment. Immunostaining of pancreas showed that *Emblica officinalis* extract (250 mg/kg) increased β-cell size, but a higher dose of 500 mg/kg increased β-cells number in diabetic rats. Moreover, *Emblica officinalis* extract significantly increased plasma total anti-oxidants and liver GSH and TBARS. Elevation in glucose tolerance by ellagic acid suggested that ellagic acid probably works by stimulating insulin secretion from pancreatic β-cells. These results infer that ellagic acid may exert anti-diabetic activity through the action on β-cells of pancreas resulting in an increase in β-cell size and number, increasing anti-oxidant status, decreasing blood glucose, increasing serum insulin, and β-cell morphology, and morphometry [21].

20.4 Conclusions

Ellagic acid seems to be a very promising agent for the treatment of chronic diseases, especially ulcerative colitis, Cronh's disease, Alzheimer's disease, and diabetes. Ellagic acid also seems to have hepatoprotective and anti-cancer properties. The anti-diabetic potential of ellagic acid makes it a potentially interesting alternative to traditional glucose-lowering medications and a strong candidate for diabetic drug research. However, detailed toxicity evaluations need to be performed before any therapeutic application in humans could be suggested. Proof-of-concept safety and efficacy trials are also warranted to verify the interesting preclinical findings. Further studies are needed to see if the very good results observed in animal will be confirmed in humans.

References

1. Zamora-Ros R, Knaze V, Luján-Barroso L, Slimani N, Romieu I, Fedirko V, de Magistris MS, Ericson U, Amiano P, Trichopoulou A, Dilis V, Naska A, Engeset D, Skeie G, Cassidy A, Overvad K, Peeters PH, Huerta JM, Sánchez MJ, Quirós JR, Sacerdote C, Grioni S, Tumino R, Johansson G, Johansson I, Drake I, Crowe FL, Barricarte A, Kaaks R, Teucher B, Bueno-de-Mesquita HB, van Rossum CT, Norat T, Romaguera D, Vergnaud AC, Tjønneland A, Halkjær J, Clavel-Chapelon F, Boutron-Ruault MC, Touillaud M, Salvini S, Khaw KT, Wareham N, Boeing H, Förster J, Riboli E, González CA (2011) Estimated dietary intakes of flavonols, flavanones and flavones in the European Prospective Investigation into Cancer and Nutrition (EPIC) 24 hour dietary recall cohort. Br J Nutr 106(12):1915–1925
2. Seeram NP, Zhang Y, McKeever R, Henning SM, Lee RP, Suchard MA, Li Z, Chen S, Thames G, Zerlin A, Nguyen M, Wang D, Dreher M, Heber D (2008) Pomegranate juice and extracts provide similar levels of plasma and urinary ellagitannin metabolites in human subjects. J Med Food 11(2):390–394
3. Larrosa M, Tomás-Barberán FA, Espín JC (2006) The dietary hydrolysable tannin punicalagin releases ellagic acid that induces apoptosis in human colon adenocarcinoma Caco-2 cells by using the mitochondrial pathway. J Nutr Biochem 17(9):611–625
4. Gil MI, Tomás-Barberán FA, Hess-Pierce B, Holcroft DM, Kader AA (2000) Antioxidant activity of pomegranate juice and its relationship with phenolic composition and processing. J Agric Food Chem 48(10):4581–4589
5. Bala I, Bhardwaj V, Hariharan S, Kumar MN (2006) Analytical methods for assay of ellagic acid and its solubility studies. J Pharm Biomed Anal 40(1):206–210
6. Marín M, Giner RM, Ríos JL, Recio MC (2013) Intestinal anti-inflammatory activity of ellagic acid in the acute and chronic dextrane sulfate sodium models of mice colitis. J Ethnopharmacol 150(3):925–934
7. Rosillo MA, Sánchez-Hidalgo M, Cárdeno A, Aparicio-Soto M, Sánchez-Fidalgo S, Villegas I, de la Lastra CA (2012) Dietary supplementation of an ellagic acid-enriched pomegranate extract attenuates chronic colonic inflammation in rats. Pharmacol Res 66 (3):235–242
8. Umesalma S, Sudhandiran G (2011) Ellagic acid prevents rat colon carcinogenesis induced by 1, 2 dimethyl hydrazine through inhibition of AKT-phosphoinositide-3 kinase pathway. Eur J Pharmacol 660(2–3):249–258
9. Xu YM, Deng JZ, Ma J, Chen SN, Marshall R, Jones SH, Johnson RK, Hecht SM (2003) DNA damaging activity of ellagic acid derivatives. Bioorg Med Chem 11:1593–1596

10. Devipriya N, Sudheer AR, Menon VP (2007) Dose-response effect of ellagic acid oncirculatory antioxidants and lipids during alcohol-induced toxicity in experimental rats. Fundam Clin Pharmacol 21:621–630
11. Singh K, Khanna AK, Chander R (1999) Hepatoprotective activity of ellagic acid carbon tetrachloride induced hepatotoxicity in rats. Indian J Exp Biol 37:1025–1026
12. Yu YM, Chang WC, Wu CS, Chiang SY (2005) Reduction of oxidative stress and apoptosis in hyperlipidemic rabbits by ellagic acid. J Nutr Biochem 16:675–681
13. Pathak RK, Baunthiyal M, Taj G, Kumar A (2014) Virtual screening of natural inhibitors to the predicted HBx protein structure of Hepatitis B Virus using molecular docking for identification of potential lead molecules for liver cancer. Bioinformation 10:428–435
14. Reddy BU, Mullick R, Kumar A, Sudha G, Srinivasan N, Das S (2014) Small molecule inhibitors of HCV replication from Pomegranate. Sci Rep 4:1–10
15. Ajala OS, Jukov A, Ma CM (2014) Hepatitis C virus inhibitory hydrolysable tanninsfrom the fruits of Terminalia chebula. Fitoterapia 99:117–123
16. Ulrich P, Cerami A (2001) Protein glycation, diabetes, and aging. Recent Prog Horm Res 56:1–21
17. Yan SD, Chen X, Fu J, Chen M, Zhu H, Roher A, Slattery T, Zhao L, Nagashima M, Morser J, Migheli A, Nawroth P, Stern D, Schmidt AM (1996) RAGE and amyloid-beta peptide neurotoxicity in Alzheimer's disease. Nature 382(6593):685–691
18. Srikanth V, Maczurek A, Phan T, Steele M, Westcott B, Juskiw D, Münch G (2011) Advanced glycation endproducts and their receptor RAGE in Alzheimer's disease. Neurobiol Aging 32 (5):763–777
19. Liu W, Ma H, Frost L, Yuan T, Dain JA, Seeram NP (2014) Pomegranate phenolics inhibit formation of advanced glycation endproducts by scavenging reactive carbonyl species. Food Funct 5(11):2996–3004
20. Rojanathammanee L, Puig KL, Combs CK (2013) Pomegranate polyphenols and extract inhibit nuclear factor of activated T-cell activity and microglial activation in vitro and in a transgenic mouse model of Alzheimer disease. J Nutr 143(5):597–605
21. Fatima N, Hafizur RM, Hameed A, Ahmed S, Nisar M, Kabir N (2015) Ellagic acid in Emblica officinalis exerts anti-diabetic activity through the action on β-cells of pancreas. Eur J Nutr. doi:10.1007/s00394-015-1103-y

Author Index

S.C. Gupta et al. (eds.), *Anti-inflammatory Nutraceuticals and Chronic Diseases*,
Advances in Experimental Medicine and Biology 928,
DOI 10.1007/978-3-319-41334-1